Lessons from the ICU
Under the Auspices of the European Society
of Intensive Care Medicine

Maurizio Cecconi, Head Dept Anesthesia and ICU,
Humanitas Research Hospital,
Rozzano, Milano, Italy *Series Editor*

Daniel De Backer, Dept Intensive Care Erasme University,
Université Libre de Bruxelles, Bruxelles,
Brussels Hoofdst.ge., Belgium *Series Editor*

Lessons from the ICU is a Book Series published by Springer under the auspices of the *European Society of Intensive Care Medicine* (ESICM). The aim of the Series is to provide focused and state-of-the-art reviews of central topics in Intensive Care. Ultimately, its mission is to transfer the latest knowledge to the bedside in order to improve patient outcomes. Accordingly, the ESICM has also developed *Lessons from the ICU* with the vision or providing the best resources for everyone working in Intensive Care.

Each volume presents a comprehensive review of topical issues in Intensive Care. The volumes are intended to cover the majority of aspects that intensive care professionals are likely to encounter in the course of their career. Books offer an excellent guide for residents who are new to the ICU, and for allied professionals, senior consultants as well as nurses and allied healthcare professionals.

The chapters are organized in a way that allows the reader to quickly familiarize or reacquaint themselves with the pathophysiological background before moving on to diagnosis and treatment. Each chapter includes a list of Take Home Messages, as well as practical examples that apply theoretical knowledge in real clinical scenarios. Each volume in the Series is edited by international Key Opinion Leaders in Intensive Care, and each chapter is written by experts in the field.

In summary, this Series represents a valuable contribution to fill the gap in the current Intensive Care literature by providing top-quality literature reviews that can be easily digested and used at the bedside to improve patient outcomes.

More information about this series at http://www.springer.com/series/15582

Michael R. Pinsky
Jean-Louis Teboul
Jean-Louis Vincent
Editors

Hemodynamic Monitoring

ESICM
EUROPEAN SOCIETY OF INTENSIVE CARE MEDICINE

Springer

Editors
Michael R. Pinsky
Critical Care Medicine Dept.
University of Pittsburgh
Pittsburgh, PA
USA

Jean-Louis Teboul
Bicetre University Hospital
Paris South University
Le Kremlin-Bicêtre
France

Jean-Louis Vincent
Department of Intensive Care
Erasme University Hospital
Brussels
Belgium

ISSN 2522-5928 ISSN 2522-5936 (electronic)
Lessons from the ICU
ISBN 978-3-319-69268-5 ISBN 978-3-319-69269-2 (eBook)
https://doi.org/10.1007/978-3-319-69269-2

Library of Congress Control Number: 2019930093

This Springer imprint is published by the registered company Springer Nature Switzerland AG
The registered company address is: Gewerbestrasse 11, 6330 Cham, Switzerland

The editors wish to dedicate this volume to all our teachers who through hard work and dedication mentored us through our careers, our colleagues who have been with us always on this journey of shared patient care, and to our patients, for whose optimal care and comfort is our never-ending goal.

Foreword

Critical illness often presents problems of such complexity that the bedside clinician is forced to integrate information from many data streams into the management decision. As the 'evidence-based' investigational paradigm gained traction and eventual dominance in medicine, initial hope was entertained by many intensivists that solid evidence from trials, together with advanced imaging and the laboratory data, would generate effective 'rules' to guide practice. In fact, well-designed and conducted clinical trials (RCTs) do characterize general behaviors and may provide defensible starting points for making some choices, especially if positive. To this point however, we have been disappointed by RCT output; fundamentally, such problems are too imprecisely defined, complicated, interactive, and labile to allow RCTs, 'snapshot' imaging, and biomarkers – even considered together – to reliably direct the next best step for the individual patient.

Effective life support needs a more 'personalized' approach that adheres to established principles aimed at supporting the patient's own efforts to recover homeostasis and viability. Our decisions must remain flexible; within the physical boundaries of the ICU, the principles of therapeutic challenge, frequent reassessment, continual re-evaluation, and timely mid-course correction remain fundamental elements of the intensivist's art. Moment-by-moment access to key information relevant to the patient's status is central to well-timed interventions. Successful management still depends upon having a firm grasp of the physiology of critical illness, coupled with the ability to expertly integrate and act upon monitored information from key indicators that reflect cardiopulmonary functioning. A few foundational elements of critical care physiology share precedence over the others, but none is more important than the circulation.

This important volume, written by the foremost experts of our field and directed toward bedside management, is a wide-ranging compendium of in-depth chapters that address essential cardiovascular physiology as well as the pragmatics of diagnosing, monitoring, and supporting the circulatory system. The mechanistic basis for clinical decision making is emphasized throughout. Cardio-respiratory management of the critically ill has advanced rather impressively in recent decades, and such progress is clearly evident in the attention given to such up-to-date topics as bedside ultrasound, assessment of the microcirculation and perfusion adequacy, advanced monitoring options, and extracorporeal circulatory assistance and gas exchange. The chapters of this book are not meant to be read sequentially from cover to cover (even though such an exercise might prove highly rewarding), but rather to be accessed in a focused manner as specific clinical issues arise in patient care or when knowledge gaps need to be filled.

In this current exciting age of rapidly expanding knowledge of genetic and molecular sciences, exhaustive statistical analyses, empirical evidence gathering, RCTs and meta-analysis, it sometimes seems that our attention as practitioners has been diverted from understanding the 'why?' to the 'what and how'?. I congratulate the editors and authors for addressing both in admirable fashion. It is refreshing and most welcome to see a definitive work based upon the often neglected but invaluable middle ground of applied pathophysiology. Mastery of physiology will always be needed to unravel our most difficult clinical challenges and remains the foundation of intelligent critical care.

John J. Marini
Minneapolis/St. Paul, MN, USA

Preface

An essential aspect of the care of the critically ill patient is to identify cardiovascular insufficiency, treat it, and know when to stop over resuscitation while also attending to the various other aspects of pathology that each patient brings to the clinical environment. No two patents are alike in their presentation of acute illness, response to therapy, or potential for a good outcome from the treatment of disease and a minimal amount of treatment-associated morbidities. Furthermore, most people, if they live long enough, will experience some acute potentially life-taking process that if not treated correctly and rapidly will result in death or morbidity before their time. These realities make the practice of critical care medicine one of the most demanding of all medical specialties, and also one of its greatest attractions in the recruitment of dedicated and passionate bedside clinicians.

Within this context, this volume has been crafted to systematically address all aspects of hemodynamic monitoring-related cardiovascular diagnosis and management. Part I of this volume addresses the essential aspects of the physiology and pathophysiology of cardiovascular insufficiency. The authors of these eleven chapters are some of the leading clinical investigators in the field with many years of bedside clinical experience and an impressive publication record of clinical trials and basic science companion studies. Although these chapters are arranged in a progressive sequence to supplement each other, the reader can pick and choose specific chapters of interest based on their perceived knowledge gaps or focused areas of interest.

Part II of this volume assumes the reader is cognizant of the underlying physiology and pathophysiology and goes directly into their use in clinical assessment. Because once a basic understanding of physiology is present, real-time knowledge of the patient allows diagnosis to become personalized by addressing the unique aspects of each patient as they face life-threatening disease processes. These five integrated chapters require an understanding of the underlying physiology but then take that plane and elevate it to clinical decision making and prognosis. This section in the volume represents a unique series of chapters relative to other critical care medicine textbooks, and we hope its utility to direct patient care will be innately obvious to the reader.

Part III addresses the specific measures made by various monitoring devices because at the end of the day hemodynamic monitoring is monitoring with specific devices that report specific information over time. Thus the focus on specific monitoring modality and physiologic parameter discussed in these twelve chapters bring the physiology of Part I and the pathophysiologic assessments in Part II into reality at the bedside.

Part IV addresses the very real question of what to do and why. Targeting specific therapeutic end points assumes that their achievement will reduce morbidity and mortality. But what therapies to give and why? These questions are addressed in these three very focused chapters.

Finally, in Part V, patients usually fit into broad groupings of acute illness based on the fundamental pathophysiologic processes that initiated their instability. Acute heart failure, septic shock, ARDS, neurologic emergencies, postoperative problems, and recently the need for extracorporeal support. They reflect the present-day disease state/processes commonly seen in the intensive care unit. These chapters serve to solidify the prior chapters into a complete set, leaving the bedside clinician with insight and hopeful perspective as to what to expect, to monitor, and how to apply that monitoring.

The editors are profoundly grateful to the authors of this book for their excellent contributions and knowledge base that made these chapters what they are; the senior editors of the European Society of Intensive Care Medicine, who oversaw the creation of this book within their series; and the publisher, Springer, for their support and dedication to this very important and clinically relevant opus.

Michael R. Pinsky
Pittsburgh, PA, USA

Jean-Louis Teboul
Le Kremlin-Bicêtre, France

Jean-Louis Vincent
Brussels, Belgium

Contents

IV Basic Goals in Clinical Practice

V Choosing the Right Hemodynamic Therapy

Contributors

Darryl Abrams
Division of Pulmonary, Allergy, and Critical Care
Columbia University College of Physicians
and Surgeons/New York-Presbyterian Hospital
New York, NY, USA
da2256@cumc.columbia.edu

Gareth L. Ackland
Translational Medicine and Therapeutics,
William Harvey Research Institute, Barts and
The London School of Medicine and Dentistry
Queen Mary University of London
John Vane Science Centre
London, UK
g.ackland@qmul.ac.uk

David Antcliffe
Imperial College London
London, UK
d.antcliffe@imperial.ac.uk

Massimo Antonelli, MD
Department of Anesthesiology
and Intensive Care Medicine
Fondazione Policlinico Universitario
A.Gemelli- Università Cattolica
del Sacro Cuore – Roma
Rome, ItalyMassimo.Antonelli@Unicatt.it

Pierre Asfar
Medical Intensive Care Department
University Hospital of Angers
Angers, France
piasfar@chu-angers.fr

Hollmann D. Aya
Critical Care Department
St Bartholomew's Hospital – Heart Center
Barts Health NHS Trust
London, UK
hollmann.aya@nhs.net

Daniel De Backer
Department of Intensive Care
CHIREC Hospitals, Université Libre de Bruxelles
Brussels, Belgium
ddebacke@ulb.ac.be

Jan Bakker, MD, PhD, FCCP, FCCM
Department of Pulmonary and Critical Care
New York University
New York, NY, USA

Division of Pulmonary, Allergy,
and Critical Care Medicine
Columbia University Medical Center
New York, NY, USA

Department of Intensive Care Adults
Erasmus MC University Medical Center
Rotterdam, The Netherlands

Department of Intensive Care
Pontificia Universidad Católica de Chile
Santiago, Chile
jan.bakker@erasmusmc.nl

Nicolas Bréchot, MD, PhD
Medical–Surgical ICU, Hôpital Pitié–Salpêtrière,
Assistance Publique–Hôpitaux de Paris
Paris Cedex, France

INSERM U1050, Centre for Interdisciplinary
Research in Biology (CIRB), College de France
CNRS, INSERM, PSL Research University
Paris, France
icolas.brechot@aphp.fr

David Carpio, MD
Departamento de Medicina Intensiva
Facultad de Medicina, Pontificia Universidad
Católica de Chile
Santiago, Chile
dcarpio14@hotmail.com

Ricardo Castro, MD, MPH
Departamento de Medicina Intensiva
Facultad de Medicina, Pontificia Universidad
Católica de Chile
Santiago, Chile
rcastro.med@gmail.com

Maurizio Cecconi
IRCCS Istituto Clinico Humanitas
Rozzano, MI, Italy
Humanitas University
Pieve Emanuele, MI, Italy
maurizio.cecconi@hunimed.eu

Francesco Cipulli
Department of Anesthesiology,
Emergency and Intensive Care Medicine
University of Göttingen
Göttingen, Germany
francescocipulli@libero.it

Alain Combes, MD, PhD
Medical–Surgical ICU, Hôpital Pitié–Salpêtrière
Assistance Publique–Hôpitaux de Paris
Paris Cedex, France
Sorbonne University, UPMC Univ Paris 06,
INSERM, UMRS_1166-iCAN,
Institute of Cardiometabolism and Nutrition
Paris Cedex, France
alain.combes@psl.aphp.fr

Nadia Corcione
Fondazione IRCCS Ca' Granda Ospedale
Maggiore Policlinico
Milan, Italy
nadia.corcione@gmail.com

Maxime Coutrot, MD
Medical–Surgical ICU, Hôpital Pitié–Salpêtrière
Assistance Publique–Hôpitaux de Paris
Paris Cedex, France
maxime.coutrot@aphp.fr

Ilaria Alice Crippa, MD
Department of Intensive Care
Hopital Erasme, Université Libre de
Bruxelles (ULB)
Brussels, Belgium
ilaria.alice.crippa@gmail.com

Antonio M. Dell'Anna, MD
Department of Anesthesiology
and Intensive Care Medicine
Fondazione Policlinico Universitario
A.Gemelli- Università Cattolica del Sacro
Cuore – Roma
Rome, Italy
anthosdel@yahoo.it

Julien Demiselle
Medical Intensive Care Department
University Hospital of Angers
Angers, France
jdemiselle@gmail.com

Gary Duclos
Aix-Marseille Université
Marseille, France
gary.duclos@ap-hm.fr

Eleonora Duscio
Department of Anesthesiology,
Emergency and Intensive Care Medicine
University of Göttingen
Göttingen, Germany
eleonora.duscio@gmail.com

Mark R. Edwards
University Hospital Southampton NHS
Foundation Trust and University of Southampton
Southampton, UK
mark.edwards2@uhs.nhs.uk

Ina Filipović-Grčić, MD
Department of Anesthesiology and Intensive Care
European Medical Center-General
Hospital Dubrovnik
Dubrovnik, Croatia
inafg@yahoo.com

Francesco Fiorini
Imperial College London
London, UK
francesco.fiorini16@imperial.ac.uk

Manuel Ignacio Monge García
Unidad de Cuidados Intensivos,
Hospital SAS de Jerez de la Frontera
Jerez de la Frontera, Spain
ignaciomonge@gmail.com

Luciano Gattinoni
Department of Anesthesiology, Emergency and Intensive Care Medicine
University of Göttingen
Göttingen, Germany
gattinoniluciano@gmail.com

Guillaume Geri
Medico-Surgical ICU,
Ambroise Paré Hospital, APHP
Boulogne-Billancourt, France

Versailles Saint Quentin University
INSERM U1018, Team 5
Paris, France
guillaume.geri@aphp.fr

Anthony C. Gordon
Imperial College London
London, UK
anthony.gordon@imperial.ac.uk

Giacomo Grasselli
University of Milan
Milan, Italy
giacomo.grasselli@unimi.it

Sebastian A. Haas
Department of Anesthesiology and Intensive Care Medicine
Rostock University Medical Center
Rostock, Germany
Sebastian.haas@med.uni-rostock.de

Glenn Hernández, MD, PhD
Departamento de Medicina Intensiva
Facultad de Medicina
Pontificia Universidad Católica de Chile
Santiago, Chile
glennguru@gmail.com

Peter Buhl Hjortrup
Department of Intensive Care
Copenhagen University Hospital Rigshospitalet
Copenhagen, Denmark
peter.buhl.hjortrup@regionh.dk

Alexa Hollinger
The University Hospital of Basel
Basel, Switzerland
alexa.hollinger@usb.ch

Alexander Kobzik, MD
Department of Critical Care Medicine
University of Pittsburgh
Pittsburgh, PA, USA
kobzikaj@upmc.edu

Jonathan Lacey
University College London
London, UK
jonathan.lacey.16@ucl.ac.uk

Marc Leone
Aix-Marseille Université
Marseille, France
marc.leone@ap-hm.fr

Becky X Lou, MD
Zucker School of Medicine at Hofstra/Northwell Health
New Hyde Park, NY, USA
becky.x.lou@gmail.com

Sheldon Magder
Department of Critical Care
McGill University Health Centre
Montreal, QC, Canada
sheldon.magder@muhc.mcgill.ca

Marco Maggiorini
University Hospital Zürich
Zürich, Switzerland
klinmax@usz.uzh.ch

Manu L. N. G. Malbrain
Vrije Universiteit Brussel (VUB)
Ixelles, Belgium
manu.malbrain@telenet.be

Paul E. Marik, MD, FCCM, FCCP
Division of Pulmonary and Critical Care Medicine
Eastern Virginia Medical School
Norfolk, VA, USA
marikpe@evms.edu

Claude Martin
Aix-Marseille Université
Marseille, France
claude.martin@ap-hm.fr

Paul H. Mayo, MD
Zucker School of Medicine at Hofstra/Northwell Health
New Hyde Park, NY, USA
mayosono@gmail.com

Katherine McAndrew
Department of Intensive Care Medicine
St George's University Hospitals NHS Foundation Trust
London, UK
katherinemcandrew@hotmail.co.uk

Alexandre Mebazaa
Hôpitaux Lariboisière Saint Louis University Hospitals
Paris, France
alexandre.mebazaa@lrb.aphp.fr

Zsolt Molnar, MD, PhD
Department of Anesthesiology and Intensive Therapy
University of Szeged
Szeged, Hungary
zsoltmolna@gmail.com

Xavier Monnet
Medical Intensive Care Unit, Bicêtre Hospital
Paris-Sud University Hospitals
Inserm UMR_S999, Paris-Sud University
Le Kremlin-Bicêtre, France

Service de réanimation médicale
Hôpital de Bicêtre
Le Kremlin-Bicêtre, France
xavier.monnet@aphp.fr

Monty Mythen
University College London
London, UK
m.mythen@ucl.ac.uk

Marton Nemeth, MD, PhD
Department of Anesthesiology and Intensive Therapy
University of Szeged
Szeged, Hungary
nemethmarton85@gmail.com

Lee S. Nguyen
Critical Care Medicine Department
CMC Ambroise Paré
Neuilly-sur-Seine, France
nguyen.lee@icloud.com

Gustavo A. Ospina-Tascón
Department of Intensive Care Medicine
Fundación Valle del Lili - Universidad ICESI
Cali, Colombia
gusospin@gmail.com

Didier Payen, MD, PhD
University Paris 7 Denis Diderot, Sorbonne Cité
UMR INSERM 1109, Hôpital Lariboisière, AP-HP
Paris, France
dpayen1234@orange.fr

Rupert M. Pearse
Queen Mary's University of London Barts & The London School of Medicine and Dentistry
London, UK

Adult Critical Care Unit, Royal London Hospital
London, UK
r.pearse@qmul.ac.uk

Anders Perner
Department of Intensive Care
Copenhagen University Hospital Rigshospitalet
Copenhagen, Denmark
Anders.Perner@regionh.dk

Antonio Pesenti
University of Milan
Milan, Italy
antonio.pesenti@unimib.it

Michael R. Pinsky, MD
Department of Critical Care Medicine
University of Pittsburgh
Pittsburgh, PA, USA
pinsky@pitt.edu

Peter Radermacher
Institut für Anästhesiologische Pathophysiologie und Verfahrensentwicklung
Universitätsklinikum
Ulm, Germany
peter.radermacher@uni-ulm.de

Daniel A. Reuter
Department of Anesthesiology and Intensive Care Medicine
Rostock University Medical Center
Rostock, Germany
Daniel.reuter@med.uni-rostock.de

Andrew Rhodes
Department of Intensive Care Medicine
St George's University Hospitals NHS Foundation Trust
London, UK
andrewrhodes@nhs.net

Federica Romitti
Department of Anesthesiology, Emergency and Intensive Care Medicine
University of Göttingen
Göttingen, Germany
fromitti@icloud.com

Arnoldo Santos
CIBER de enfermedades respiratorias (CIBERES)
Madrid, Spain

Surgical Sciences Department, Hedenstierna Laboratory, Uppsala University
Uppsala, Sweden
asantosoviedo@yahoo.es

Bernd Saugel
Department of Anesthesiology
Center of Anesthesiology and Intensive Care Medicine, University Medical Center Hamburg-Eppendorf
Hamburg, Germany
bcs.muc@gmx.de

Thomas W. L. Scheeren
Department of Anaesthesiology
University of Groningen
University Medical Center Groningen
Groningen, The Netherlands
t.w.l.scheeren@umcg.nl

Matthieu Schmidt
Medical-Surgical Intensive Care Unit
Hôpital Pitié-Salpêtrière, Assistance Publique-Hôpitaux de Paris
Paris, France

Sorbonne University Paris, INSERM
Institute of Cardiometabolism and Nutrition
UMRS_1166-ICAN
Paris, France
matthieu.schmidt@aphp.fr

Mervyn Singer
Bloomsbury Institute of Intensive Care Medicine, University College London
London, UK
m.singer@ucl.ac.uk

Pierre Squara
Critical Care Medicine Department
CMC Ambroise Paré
Neuilly-sur-Seine, France
pierre.squara@orange.fr

Fabio Silvio Taccone, MD, PhD
Department of Intensive Care
Hopital Erasme
Université Libre de Bruxelles (ULB)
Brussels, Belgium
ftaccone@ulb.ac.be

Jukka Takala, MD, PhD
Department of Intensive Care Medicine
Inselspital, Bern University Hospital
University of Bern
Bern, Switzerland
jukka.takala@insel.ch

Jean-Louis Teboul
Medical Intensive Care Unit, Bicêtre Hospital,
Paris-Sud University Hospitals
Inserm UMR_S999, Paris-Sud University
Le Kremlin-Bicêtre, France
jean-louis.teboul@aphp.fr

Flavia Torrini, MD
Department of Anesthesiology
and Intensive Care Medicine
Fondazione Policlinico Universitario
A.Gemelli- Università Cattolica del Sacro
Cuore – Roma
Rome, Italy
torrini.flavia@gmail.com

Francesco Vasques
Department of Anesthesiology,
Emergency and Intensive Care Medicine
University of Göttingen
Göttingen, Germany
francesco.vasques@hotmail.it

Antoine Vieillard-Baron
Medico-Surgical ICU
Ambroise Paré Hospital, APHP
Boulogne-Billancourt, France
Versailles Saint Quentin University
INSERM U1018, Team 5
Paris, France
antoine.vieillard-baron@aphp.fr

Jean-Louis Vincent
Department of Intensive Care
Erasme University Hospital
Université Libre de Bruxelles
Brussels, Belgium
jlvincent@intensive.org

Physiology and Pathophysiology

Contents

Introduction to "Hemodynamic Monitoring"

Jukka Takala

M. R. Pinsky et al. (eds.), *Hemodynamic Monitoring*, Lessons from the ICU,
https://doi.org/10.1007/978-3-319-69269-2_1

1

The primary goal of intensive care medicine is the prevention, reduction, and removal of temporary risk of death in acutely ill patients, including patients exposed to risk of death due to surgery and other therapeutic interventions. Cardiovascular organ dysfunction or failure is, after respiratory failure, the most common organ function problem in intensive care unit (ICU) patients [1]. The central role of hemodynamic monitoring in the ICU armamentarium is therefore self-evident. In this context monitoring implies observing continuously or continually changes in physiologic variables over time to reveal changes in organ function, to prompt therapeutic interventions, and to evaluate response to therapeutic interventions. Monitoring per se cannot be expected to improve patient outcomes – only timely applied right interventions can do so [2].

Hemodynamic monitoring and diagnostics are different entities, sharing common features and overlapping, if diagnostics are frequently repeated. Monitoring tools, such as cardiac output monitors or pulmonary artery catheter, may help to establish diagnosis, and diagnostic tools, such as echocardiography, can be used repeatedly to monitor cardiovascular function and response to treatment at least over short periods of time. Measurements and diagnostic evaluations that were intermittently done in the past (e.g., cardiac output, venous oximetry) can now be performed continually or continuously. Echocardiography, traditionally a diagnostic tool, has an established role in perioperative monitoring of cardiac surgery patients. Barriers for its use for monitoring ICU patients are disappearing with increased availability of equipment and trained operators, although operator dependence and the need for frequent repetitions remain limitations. The introduction of miniature transesophageal echocardiography probes is likely to facilitate echocardiography-based continual monitoring also in the ICU [3].

The use of dynamic assessment of circulation is a fundamental component of hemodynamic monitoring. The principle of observing the physiology, inducing a perturbation, and observing the response was emphasized by Max Harry Weil in 1965, when he described the use of fluid challenge in shock: "The effect of fluid replacement on the clinical status of the patient in shock is gauged by objective changes in circulation, such as blood pressure, mental alertness, urine flow, peripheral venous filling, and appearance and texture of the skin" [4]. In this elegant paper, the today well-known limitations of static values of hemodynamic variables are discussed with great insight. In the last decades, the physiology underlying dynamic hemodynamic assessments and their limitations in monitoring the circulation have been established. Instead of using the fluid challenge to perturb the circulation, many of the current approaches try to predict the response to a fluid challenge in order to avoid unnecessary fluid loading. All these dynamic approaches are based on the principle of assessing "preload dependence." This can be done by observing respiratory cycle-dependent variations in intravascular pressures, vascular diameters, and stroke volume or its surrogates or by directly observing the effect of a volume shift induced by passive leg raising on these variables. The practical aspects of these of methods as well as their limitations are discussed elsewhere in this book. Two major issues deserve to be mentioned already here: first, to be preload or volume responsive is normal and does not indicate the need for volume; second, hypovolemia and right heart failure may both manifest as left heart preload dependence.

The quest for less invasive hemodynamic monitoring has been driven by the goal to reduce the risks of invasive techniques, to reduce the need of special skills and resources, and to make hemodynamic monitoring more widely available. This has been facilitated by major evolution in signal processing, transducer and imaging technology, and in understanding physiology. Wireless transducers and biosensors, and body area networks make remote monitoring technically possible, although their routine clinical application is still confronted with technical and logistic problems [5].

Another trend in hemodynamic monitoring has been the focus on microcirculation. Research tools used for studying pathophysiology of microcirculation and peripheral tissue perfusion have so far failed to break through into clinical monitoring. In order to monitor peripheral tissue perfusion in the clinical setting, traditional clinical variables to monitor circulation have had a renaissance. These include skin temperature, central to peripheral skin temperature difference, capillary refill time, and evaluation of skin mottling [6]. These simple measurements can be used for monitoring hemodynamics without any special equipment, and at same time, they are amenable for new senor technologies.

Integration of hemodynamic monitoring data to provide relevant information for therapeutic decisions becomes a major challenge, when the amount of available data increases. At the moment, such integration can be achieved using clinical information systems to display pathophysiologically relevant combinations of data. The development of intelligent alarms is the next step and can help to apply hemodynamic monitoring outside the ICU [7].

Despite all the exciting new developments in technology, the variety of available monitoring devices, and the improved understanding of pathophysiology, the most important challenge remains: What should be the hemodynamic targets? Hemodynamic monitoring can only reveal changes in cardiovascular function, and the interpretation of such changes may prompt therapeutic interventions. What are the right interventions and what should be their targets remain disappointedly unclear. The application of fixed hemodynamic targets in large-scale randomized controlled trials has given little if any definitive answers [8]. The risks of overzealous hemodynamic support with fluids and vasoactive drugs have also been demonstrated. Given the complexity of hemodynamic pathophysiology, it is very unlikely that any fixed numeric targets for all patients are appropriate. Rather, assessing response to treatment should consider changes in the individual patient's clinical status and signs of tissue perfusion, such as mental alertness, skin temperature and capillary refill, and urine flow, and objective changes in hemodynamic variables provided by hemodynamic monitoring and imaging.

References

1. Moreno R, Vincent JL, Matos R, Mendonça A, Cantraine F, Thijs L, et al. The use of maximum SOFA score to quantify organ dysfunction/failure in intensive care. Results of a prospective, multicentre study. Intensive Care Med. 1999;25:686–96.
2. Takala J. The pulmonary artery catheter: the tool versus treatments based on the tool. Crit Care. 2006;10:162. https://doi.org/10.1186/cc5021.
3. Vignon P, Merz TM, Vieillard-Baron A. Ten reasons for performing hemodynamic monitoring using transesophageal echocardiography. Intensive Care Med. 2017;43:1048–51. https://doi.org/10.1007/s00134-017-4716-1.
4. Weil MH, Shubin H, Rosoff L. Fluid repletion in circulatory shock: central venous pressure and other practical guides. JAMA. 1965;192:668–74.
5. Rathore MM, Ahmad A, Paul A, Wan J, Zhang D. Real-time medical emergency response system: exploiting IoT and big data for public health. J Med Syst. 2016;40:283. https://doi.org/10.1007/s10916-016-0647-6.
6. Lima A, Bakker J. Clinical assessment of peripheral circulation. Curr Opin Crit Care. 2015;21(3):226–31.
7. Kang MA, Churpek MM, Zadravecz FJ, Adhikari R, Twu NM, Edelson DP. Real-time risk prediction on the wards: a feasibility study. Crit Care Med. 2016;44:1468–73.
8. The PRISM Investigators. Early, goal-directed therapy for septic shock — a patient-level meta-analysis. N Engl J Med. 2017;376:2223–34. https://doi.org/10.1056/NEJMoa1701380.

Shock: Definition and Recognition

Antonio M. Dell'Anna, Flavia Torrini, and Massimo Antonelli

M. R. Pinsky et al. (eds.), *Hemodynamic Monitoring*, Lessons from the ICU,
https://doi.org/10.1007/978-3-319-69269-2_2

Learning Ojectives

In this chapter, we will discuss the definition of shock both from the physiological and clinical point of view. We will categorize shock states according to patient cardiac output. Then we will analyze the available tools to diagnose shock and to start appropriate therapies.

2

2.1 Introduction

Circulatory Shock is one of the most common cause of admission to the ICU with a prevalence of 30% for patient already in the ICU [1].

Patients are defined in shock when tissue oxygen demand is not coupled with oxygen supply [2]. From a clinical point of view, shock is often associated with low blood pressure. Hypotension is one of the most common clinical presentations of the shock states, even though its presence does not always represent a "conditio sine qua non." Markers of peripheral hypoperfusion [3] or other signs such as tachycardia not related to pain or anxiety or fever may be other alert signs to identify patients in shock [2].

The main feature of shock condition is the decrease in oxygen utilization at cellular level with impaired cellular metabolism and consequent derangements from normal physiology. If this situation is not promptly corrected, it leads to cellular "energetic failure" [4] which implies arrest of all metabolic functions and multiple organ failure.

In this chapter we will discuss the shock definitions, referring both to the classical definition and exploring cellular and metabolic alterations that characterize the shock states. The different types of shock will be analyzed, trying to highlight their main features and recognition criteria reported into the most recent guidelines.

2.2 Definition

Many diseases may ultimately lead to a condition of shock, with impairment of the organ perfusion and onset of multiple organ failure (MOF). From a pathophysiological point of view, shock is classically defined as a condition in which oxygen supply is inadequate to peripheral oxygen demand [3]. However, shock may be also defined as a condition in which hypotension is associated with a variable degree of organ derangement (i.e., oliguria, mottled skin, confusion, dyspnea, etc.). Regardless of the definition, the relationship between oxygen delivery (DO_2) and oxygen consumption (VO_2) remains essential [5, 6].

DO_2 is the amount of oxygen delivered by the heart to the cells:

$$DO_2 = CO \times CaO_2 \tag{2.1}$$

where CO is the cardiac output and CaO_2 is the arterial oxygen content, calculated as shown in the following Eq. (2.2):

$$CaO_2 = (Hb \times SaO_2 \times 1.34) + (PaO_2 \times 0.003) \tag{2.2}$$

where Hb is the hemoglobin concentration, SaO_2 the arterial O_2 saturation, and PaO_2 arterial partial pressure of oxygen. These equations underline how, besides CO, Hb and SaO_2 play the major role in determining DO_2, more than PaO_2, which contributes to a minor extent. Similarly, VO_2 is calculated as follows:

$$VO_2 = CO \times (CaO_2 - CvO_2) \tag{2.3}$$

where

$$CvO_2 = (Hb \times SvO_2 \times 1.34) + (PvO_2 \times 0.003) \tag{2.4}$$

and SvO_2 is mixed venous oxygen saturation and PvO_2 mixed venous partial pressure of oxygen.

Rearranging Eq. (2.3) excluding the negligible contribution of dissolved oxygen in the formula for CaO_2 and CvO_2 calculation, VO_2 may be also rewritten as follows:

$$VO_2 = CO \times Hb \times (SaO_2 - SvO_2) \times 1.34 \tag{2.5}$$

The difference between arterial and mixed venous saturation (SaO_2 – SvO_2) is also defined as oxygen extraction rate (O_2ER) and identifies the amount of oxygen extracted by peripheral tissues during each cardiac cycle. As shown in ◘ Fig. 2.1a, global VO_2 remains constant, while DO_2 decreases until a critical point, defined as critical O_2ER. Below this point VO_2 decreases linearly with DO_2. This kind of relationship is possible because physiologically DO_2 is fivefold higher than VO_2, so that delivery reduction can be tolerated by

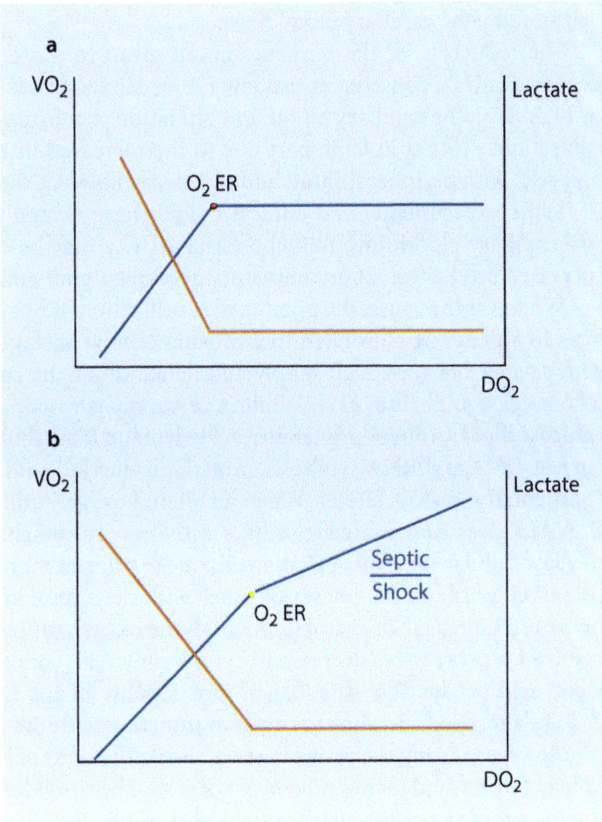

◘ **Fig. 2.1** **a** This figure shows the relationship between oxygen delivery and consumption. After critical O_2 extraction rate (O_2ER) has been reached, oxygen consumption declines along with oxygen delivery. At the same point, anaerobic metabolism becomes more significant, and blood lactate level increases. DO_2 oxygen delivery, VO_2 oxygen consumption, O_2ER oxygen extraction rate. **b** This figure shows the relationship between oxygen delivery and consumption in septic shock patients. Compared to classical relationship seen in ◘ Fig. 2.1a, curves are steeper and shifted higher and rightward. This implies an earlier increase in blood lactate level and a decrease in oxygen consumption that occurs since the first phase of shock. DO_2 oxygen delivery, VO_2 oxygen consumption, O_2ER oxygen extraction rate increasing O_2 extraction. After critical O_2ER has been reached, aerobic metabolism begins to be impaired, and a shift toward anaerobic metabolism occurs with increased lactic acid production (Fig. 2.1a). This kind of behavior of DO_2/VO_2 is preserved in many shock conditions except for septic shock which is the most common distributive shock (see subsequent paragraph – Fig. 2.1b). Indeed, in that case, critical O_2ER is shifted higher and rightward, while the slope of the curves is much more pronounced (Fig. 2.1b).

However, the earliest phases of the shock states may not imply an alteration of global VO_2. Peripheral organs react very differently to reduced blood flow, because of their different physiology. The heart, for instance, has a very high O_2ER so that oxygen consumption is essentially dependent upon coronary blood flow, whose decline will generate a decrease of the aerobic metabolism, with impaired contractility [7]. On the contrary, the kidneys that receive a very high amount of blood flow (approximately 25% of CO) extract a very low amount of oxygen, being able to tolerate a longer period of cold ischemia [8]. Finally, during septic shock, especially after the initial phases, very low O_2ER along with high DO_2 may occur, and this condition has been associated with poor survival [9, 10].

Considered all the limits of the classical definitions, it may be useful reformulating the shock definition moving from general hemodynamics to the cellular level. Regardless the cause and the feature of each type of shock (that we will discuss in the next paragraph), shock states may be all defined as conditions implying an altered oxygen utilization at cellular level. Focusing the attention on the last part of the oxygen distribution chain, we can understand that two main mechanisms are responsible for shock establishment: the reduction of the oxygen amount available to the cells and the inability to use the oxygen delivered by the capillary blood flow.

The reduction of the oxygen amount given to the cells may be primarily due to a decrease of DO_2 consequent to a low CO or Hb decrease. In septic shock, despite normal or high DO_2, the capillary blood flow alterations determine very low cellular oxygen concentrations. This is in large part due to the increased distance between perfused vessels and cells with peripheral shunt and reduced cellular O_2 availability.

Some experimental and clinical models have shown that even in condition of normal capillary blood flow, mitochondrial activity may be consistently reduced, due to an increased production of inflammatory cytokines, eminently common in septic shock [4].

Whatever the cause, the poor oxygen utilization, if not promptly treated, rapidly translates in an energetic problem that impairs cellular metabolism. In this context, the delicate balance between ATP supply and demand may be considered as the central part of a complex equilibrium [11]. While ATP supply is essentially related to O_2 and substrate (glucose, lipid, protein) availability, ATP demand is attributable to many cellular functions such as DNA and RNA synthesis, protein production, and transmembrane pump activity (particularly Na/K ATPase). When an altered oxygen utilization occurs, ATP concentration decreases, and energetic cellular activities are somehow hierarchically "hibernated," to allow cellular survival. ATP demand due to transmembrane pump function is in general preserved until the last phases of shock with the aim of keeping constant the transmembrane physiological electrical gradient. If the oxygen utilization impairment is not rapidly resolved, a progressive decrease in cytoplasmic ATP concentration occurs with increased lactic acid production. The loss of functionality of the transmembrane pumps induces cellular alterations, leading to organ dysfunction with the classical clinical signs of shock.

However, during the early phases of shock, the signs of hemodynamic impairment such as hypotension and tachycardia may not always be so evident. Therefore, oxygen deficit and the increased anaerobic metabolism with a certain degree of organ dysfunction may occur before the classical hemodynamic signs. This has been highlighted in the latest guidelines regarding septic shock definitions, where the recognition of altered mentation, tachypnea, and systolic blood pressure below 100 mmHg (the so-called quick SOFA, qSOFA) [12] may anticipate the occurrence of the classical septic shock symptoms. In other cases, hemodynamic impairment is the cause of cellular oxygen deficit, and hemodynamic alterations slightly precede or go along with signs of anaerobic metabolism and organ failure.

In all cases, early treatment of the cause of shock and prompt correction of its hemodynamic derangements may stop the progression toward MOF and death.

2.3 Shock Classification

Shock states have always been classified according to patient's CO. The rationale behind this approach is that CO is representative of O_2 delivery in the condition of stable hemoglobin and arterial saturation.

SvO_2 is another parameter which may be used to assess the existence of an imbalance between oxygen demand and supply, as well as the adequacy of CO. Normal value is about 65–70% [13]. In low-CO shock, SvO_2 values are typically decreased, while in distributive shock, they are increased.

According to the underlying cause, we can identify four principal types of shock, each one characterized by difference in hemodynamic parameters such as CO, SvO_2, central venous pressure (CVP), systemic vascular resistance (SVR), and echocardiographic signs (▫ Table 2.1):

2.3.1 Low-CO States

In low-CO shock the common problem is the inadequacy of oxygen transport.

2.3.1.1 Hypovolemic Shock

It occurs in about 16% of ICU patients. It is attributable to internal or external fluid loss, and it is the most common cause of shock in trauma patients.

In hypovolemic shock, CO is usually low, because of the decreased preload; SvO_2 is low because O_2 extraction increases in response to the decrease in DO_2, as shown in ▫ Fig. 2.1a; CVP is also low; and SVR are high in the attempt to keep mean arterial pressure (MAP) at normal or quasi-normal value.

Echocardiography signs are the small volumes of the cardiac chambers and normal or high contractility.

2.3.1.2 Cardiogenic Shock

It regards about 16% of ICU patients. It derives from ventricular failure caused by different pathological conditions (i.e., acute myocardial infarction, end-stage cardiomyopathy, arrhythmias, valvular heart disease, myocarditis).

In this kind of shock, CO is low, because contractility is impaired; SvO_2 is low, because O_2ER is increased, like in hypovolemic shock; CVP is high because of the increased end-diastolic volume caused by both the inability of the failing heart to empty cardiac chambers at the end of systole and to a certain degree diastolic impairment related to the loss of ATP production, causing an increase in end-diastolic pressure. SVR are usually high in order to keep MAP at normal values.

Table 2.1 Principal characteristics of different types of shock

	Low cardiac output			High cardiac output
	Hypovolemic	Cardiogenic	Obstructive	Distributive
Filling pressure	Low	High	High	Low/normal
End-diastolic volumes	Low	High	Low (high in pulmonary embolism)	Low/Normal
SVR	High	High	High	Low
MAP	Normal/low (last phases)	High/normal/low	Low	Low
SvO_2	Low	Low	Low	High
Echocardiography	Small cardiac chambers, preserved contractility	Dilated cardiac chambers, impaired contractility	In tamponade: pericardial effusion, small right and left ventricles In tension pneumothorax: small cardiac chambers In pulmonary embolism: small left ventricle, compressed by the dilated right ventricle	Normal cardiac chambers, preserved contractility (unless septic cardiomyopathy occurs)
Clinical signs	Cold and pale skin and extremities, tachycardia, and increased respiratory rate	Cold extremities, dyspnea, peripheral edema, jugular vein distension	Jugular vein distention, dyspnea, increased respiratory rate, tachycardia	Mottled skin, tachycardia, elevated or reduced body temperature

SVR systemic vascular resistance, *MAP* mean arterial pressure, *SvO_2* mixed venous oxygen saturation

Echocardiography signs are represented by dilated ventricles and poor contractility.

2.3.1.3 Obstructive Shock

Less frequent than the other types of shock (about 2% of ICU patients).

It is caused by an obstruction, such as pericardial tamponade, pulmonary embolism, or tension pneumothorax.

CO is typically low because preload is low (pericardial tamponade, tension pneumothorax) or because there is an obstruction to the ventricle efflux (pulmonary embolism). SvO_2 is low as in the other types of low-CO shocks, because of the increase in O_2ER. CVP is typically high, with different underlying mechanisms: the increase in pleural pressure (tension pneumothorax), the rise of end-diastolic volume (pulmonary embolism), and the decreased diastolic compliance (pericardial tamponade). SVR are usually high in order to keep adequate MAP.

Echocardiographic picture of tamponade is characterized by pericardial effusion, small right and left ventricles, and dilated inferior vena cava; in pulmonary embolism, dilated right ventricle and small left ventricle are present; in tension pneumothorax, the hallmark is the compression of the right and left ventricles with small cardiac chambers.

2.4 High-CO States

In high-CO shock, the main problem is in the periphery, as DO_2 is generally preserved but O_2ER is impaired.

2.4.1 Distributive Shock

It represents the most common type of shock in ICU patients, accounting for 64% of admission for shock (62% septic and 2% non-septic). It is characterized by a systemic vasodilation due to either a release of inflammatory factors during sepsis or anaphylaxis or a decrease in sympathetic tone in neurogenic shock.

Clinical signs and parameters are the opposite from other types of shock. CO is typically high, because of the hyperdynamic state caused by the decrease in SVR. SvO_2 is high because of the decrease in O_2ER in the periphery and to the increase in DO_2 related to the high CO. CVP can be low or normal. MAP is typically low, at least in the latest phases. Echocardiography in general shows normal cardiac chambers and preserved or increased contractility (unless septic cardiomyopathy occurs).

Septic shock is the most common shock an intensivist has to deal with. Unfortunately, in some cases the correction of hemodynamic derangements may not be effective.

Underlying mechanisms of septic shock are complex and not entirely clear. The alteration of peripheral O2 metabolism can be either caused by a primary pathological mitochondrial and cellular dysfunction or indirectly caused by microvascular alterations with consequent hypoxic cellular damage.

2.5 Shock Recognition

Early recognition of patient in shock is of a paramount importance in order to reduce morbidity and mortality [12]. Prompt interventions aiming to restore normal hemodynamics and correcting the cause of shock may effectively change the clinical course of the disease [14] (◘ Table 2.2).

The clinical evaluation and physical exam are the first steps to individuate patients at risk or patients already in shock.

Medical history can often suggest the underlying cause, for example, a history of coronary artery disease may suggest a cardiogenic shock, while elevated body temperature and dyspnea may indicate a septic shock. Similarly, after a trauma a patient is likely to suffer from hypovolemic shock because of blood loss or obstructive shock due to tension pneumothorax. Various types of shock can occur in combination, like the distributive (neurogenic) shock after a traumatic spinal injury.

Some alert signs may be useful clinical tools for an early identification of shock. Hypotension is in most of cases the sign that draws the attention of the clinician and is

2

Table 2.2 Diagnostic tools available to diagnose shock state

Diagnostic tool	Advantages	Limits
Clinical signs	Available bedside Easy to detect	Low specificity
Lactate	Good marker of tissue hypoperfusion Available with ABG point of care Reliable prognostic value Trend over time has a prognostic value	Possibility of false positive Relatively slow normalization (hours)
$ScvO_2$-SvO_2	Available with ABG point of care Good marker of O_2 debt in conditions of low DO_2	Normal values do not guarantee adequate perfusion
CO_2 gap	Available with ABG point of care Correlates CO to metabolism	pH and temperature derangements may alter its interpretationABGs must be drawn exactly at the same time
Respiratory quotient	Reliable marker of anaerobic CO_2 production May predict response in terms of O_2 consumption	CO_2 content is complex to calculate bedside
Echocardiography	Available bedside Useful to identify different types of shock	It requires a skilled operator It does not give any functional information

ABG arterial blood gas analysis, *CO* cardiac output, *$ScvO_2$* central venous oxygen saturation, *SvO_2* mixed venous oxygen saturation, *CO_2 gap* difference in central venous-to-arterial carbon dioxide tension, *respiratory quotient* ratio between venous and arterial carbon dioxide content and difference in arterial-to-venous oxygen content [$R = (CvCO_2 - CaCO_2)/(CaO_2 - CvO_2)$]

often considered one of the principal manifestations of shock. However, it can be a relatively late sign in some circumstances and the degree of hypotension does not necessarily correlate with the degree of shock if it is not accompanied by other markers of hypoxia.

Clinical examination should be complete and accurate when shock is suspected. Many clinical alterations are common in shock states, and some of them reflect organ dysfunction due to tissue hypoperfusion, while others are related to whole body response [2].

Some of the typical signs are:

- Mottled and clammy skin (especially in low-CO states)
- Altered mental status (confusion, disorientation, epilepsy, coma)
- Oliguria (urine output <0.5 ml per kilogram of body weight per hour).

Further signs like tachycardia, dyspnea, increased respiratory rate, jugular venous distention, and peripheral edema are often present but are related more to the response of the body to the ongoing shock conditions more than to the shock per se.

The importance of a thorough clinical examination has been recently highlighted in the last published guidelines for sepsis and septic shock management, where the new “quick SOFA” (qSOFA) score has been introduced to individuate those patients who are likely to be septic [12] and at risk of shock mainly outside the ICU. As mentioned, this score includes systolic arterial pressure below 100 mmHg, respiratory rate above 22/min, and altered mental status. If two out of three of such signs are present, sepsis should be suspected.

Arterial hypotension, though very common in shock, deserves a brief comment, because its role in diagnosis and as a target of therapy has been extensively discussed over the last years.

The first question to be addressed is whether all the patients in shock are actually hypotensive. Looking at the most recent guidelines on septic and cardiogenic shock, a positive answer should be given. Indeed, septic shock may be defined as a septic condition in which hypotension persists despite adequate volume resuscitation, with lactate >2 mmol/L [12]. Cardiogenic shock is defined as a state of ineffective cardiac output caused by a primary cardiac disorder with both clinical and biochemical manifestations of inadequate tissue perfusion [15]. In recent trials, pragmatic definition always included a systolic arterial pressure below 90 mmHg. Considering shock with low CO, hypotension may be mostly evident only during the most severe phases, as the homeostatic mechanisms will try to keep mean arterial pressure at a normal level by increasing SVR. In this situation, the increase in SVR is useful to maintain a minimal level of cardiac and cerebral perfusion but may be detrimental for other organ perfusion, decreasing blood flow and increasing oxygen debt [16]. Many patients with acute cardiac failure may develop signs of peripheral anaerobic metabolism without hypotension [17]. On the contrary, elevated MAP may be detrimental because it will impair systolic ejection of the failing heart, worsening oxygen delivery. Along the same way, patients with acute hemorrhage will try to keep MAP within the normal value by increasing adrenergic tone which will recruit unstressed volume from venous reservoir and increase arterial tone. However, if the hemorrhage is not promptly controlled, this compensatory mechanism becomes deleterious, and it will lead to multiple organ failure (MOF) and death. Hypotension can be evident either only in the last phase or if blood loss is more than a half of the circulating blood volume [18].

In conclusion we may say that hypotension is frequently associated with shock conditions, but in many cases, shock may initiate without low blood pressure, and it may be a very late sign of shock.

Another point is if all the hypotensive states may be considered as shock states. On this purpose, though most of acute hypotensions are attributable to shock, not necessarily low blood pressure is related to the impaired organ perfusion. For example, in case of deep sedation, whole body metabolic functions are put at rest and oxygen demand decreases significantly. Hence lower blood pressure might be tolerated without alterations of organ perfusion. However, if very low MAP (i.e., 45–50 mmHg) can be safely accepted for patients without clear signs of organ hypoperfusion is still on debate [19, 20], so it is reasonable to check the causes of low blood pressure for their prompt correction.

The last, and maybe more important, aspect is the clear definition of hypotension. In most guidelines and trials [12, 15, 21], hypotension is defined as systolic blood pressure below 90 mmHg or MAP below 65 mmHg. Such definition comes from the assumption that below a certain MAP, organ blood flow becomes dependent upon pressure, while above that point the blood flow can be considered constant [22]. The thresholds represent a mean among thousands of values and cannot be considered adequate for all patients. While patients with normal or constitutional low blood pressure may easily tolerate MAP below 65 mmHg, those who are hypertensive may not be able to adapt their blood flow regulation even when the MAP is above 65 mmHg [23]. In addition, one threshold can be adequate for some organs, but is not necessarily considered appropriate for the whole body. Rules allowing autoregulation for each organ are different [22], and the most important regulator of organ blood flow – i.e., metabolic control – can vary widely in shock condition, changing completely normal physiology. Even if a general threshold of 65 mmHg may be considered theoretically adequate, only a thorough examination of the patient that includes the evaluation of peripheral hypoperfusion can really define the lower acceptable value of MAP in particular cases. This is even more important considering that the need of a specific blood pressure essentially derives from the need of our cardiovascular system to preferentially direct the blood flow toward the organs, according to their metabolic needs [24]. Accordingly, during sport, a decrease of SVR to increase the peripheral blood flow in certain organs is coupled with a CO increase, to keep MAP stable and guarantee a good organ perfusion. On the contrary, when a decrease of SVR is not due to an increase in metabolic demand but to a dysregulated response (i.e., like in septic shock), the CO increase is not coupled anymore to the real metabolic demands of our peripheral tissue. In summary, hypotension is the most common alert sign during shock; however it can be evident sometimes only in the latest phases of the disease. Similarly, a general threshold of MAP to define shock has been adopted, but it can vary widely from patient to another, and only other signs can tell the clinician if that blood pressure needs to be increased or not.

Other data, coming from blood sample analysis, may lead toward the diagnosis of shock even in the absence of other clear clinical signs or can help to confirm the clinical suspicion.

Among them, arterial lactate level is the most commonly used in clinical practice. Lactic acid is produced also in physiological conditions, but its production is increased in condition of anaerobic metabolism and/or when its hepatic elimination is impaired [25, 26]. Absolute blood lactate values have been associated with a worse outcome in all kinds of shock, and their persistence over time despite treatments has been associated to higher mortality rate [27–29]. Values above 2 mmol/L are considered alert signs associated with increased mortality up to 40%, especially if associated with hypotension [12]. Values above 4 mmol/L have been associated with higher mortality rate in septic shock regardless of other clinical conditions [30].

If the patient has a central venous line or a pulmonary artery catheter, central or mixed venous SO_2 may be measured ($ScvO_2$ and SvO_2, respectively). In clinical practice, measurement of $ScVO_2$ is used as a surrogate of SvO_2. $ScVO_2$ reflects the oxygen extraction only from the upper part of the body (since it is measured in the superior vena cava). Even though their values are not completely interchangeable [31], both represent peripheral O_2ER of the body and may guide therapies. If they are very low (<70% and 65%, respectively), they may indicate that an increase in DO_2 is mandatory [32]. In 2001 a pivotal paper showed that patients with septic shock and very low $ScvO_2$ had lower mortality if a protocol aiming to keep SvO_2 above 70% was applied in the first 6 h after emergency admission [33]. Unfortunately, three more recent trials failed to replicate the same results [21, 34–36] so that $ScvO_2$ optimization has been waived from the last guidelines. However, in such trials, baseline $ScvO_2$ was already >70%, making useless a protocol aiming at ScvO2 optimization [37]. In many shock conditions, particularly in septic shock, $ScvO_2$ appears normal or even high even if an oxygen debt is developing, as shown by an increase in other markers of organ perfusion (i.e., lactate). Some papers have even shown that higher $ScvO_2$ in septic patients are related to higher mortality [10], maybe because it mirrors an impairment of peripheral oxygen extraction [38]. In conclusion, we should keep in mind that low $ScvO_2$ values need to be corrected, while normal or high values do not necessarily correlate a good organ perfusion in shock condition.

The difference between mixed venous and arterial pCO_2 (CO_2 gap) and CO is inversely correlated [39], so that an increase in CO_2 gap is a marker of inadequate CO. More recently some authors have shown that central venous CO_2 may be a valid surrogate of mixed venous CO_2 for CO_2 gap calculation [40]. A value of CO_2 gap >6 mmHg is an alert sign indicating a low cardiac output with peripheral CO_2 stagnation [41]. CO_2 gap varies more rapidly than lactate and ScvO2 could be used as an early marker of peripheral oxygen supply impairment. It has been proposed as a tool for diagnosis and a goal for therapy [42].

The ratio between CO_2 gap and arterial-venous difference in oxygen content ($C_{(a-v)}O_2$) can be considered as a surrogate of the respiratory quotient (R), where the numerator is the difference in CO_2 content instead in CO_2 partial pressure. Many authors [43, 44] have shown that a ratio >1.7 can effectively individuate patients who are developing an oxygen debt and require CO increase. Recent papers [45] have also shown that patients with higher ratio and higher lactate are more likely to die in course of septic shock.

Echocardiography is a very useful diagnostic tool in patients in shock. It can be performed bedside and allows to confirm diagnosis of shock (i.e., myocardial infarction or pericardial tamponade) and to define the type of shock, as discussed previously. It can also show left and right ventricular function, stroke volume, and possible valvular diseases.

Most severe shocks require advanced hemodynamic monitoring. Data coming from such tools may help to classify the shock and adopt the most appropriate therapies. In particular, CO may differentiate between low and high flow shock states, while cardiac filling pressure or intrathoracic volumes may indicate if the cause of low CO is primarily cardiac or hypovolemic.

Take-Home Messages

- Shock is a particular condition in which a problem in oxygen utilization at cellular level induces a variable degree of organ dysfunction.
- Shock states are usually classified according to CO and etiology of the low CO. Particularly three shocks with low CO (hypovolemic, cardiogenic, and obstructive) and one with high CO (distributive) are classically defined.
- Some clinical signs evaluable at the bedside may help clinician to define shock conditions.
- Hypotension is the most common sign of shock but is not always the first sign.
- The lactate increase and the CO_2 gap are important markers of shock states and may guide therapy and reassessment along with echocardiography.

2.6 Self-Evaluation Questions

1. What is the definition of shock?
2. How many types of shock exist and what are the differences among them?
3. How does hypotension correlate to shock states?
4. What are the main clinical signs of shock?
5. How many diagnostic tools do we have and how can we use them?
6. What is the role of lactate in shock diagnosis and treatment?

2

References

1. Vincent JL, Sakr Y, Sprung CL, Ranieri VM, Reinhart K, Gerlach H, Moreno R, Carlet J, Le Gall JR, Payen D, Sepsis Occurrence in Acutely Ill Patients I. Sepsis in European intensive care units: results of the SOAP study. Crit Care Med. 2006;34:344–53.
2. Vincent JL, De Backer D. Circulatory shock. N Engl J Med. 2013;369:1726–34.
3. Vincent JL, Dufaye P, Berre J, Leeman M, Degaute JP, Kahn RJ. Serial lactate determinations during circulatory shock. Crit Care Med. 1983;11:449–51.
4. Brealey D, Brand M, Hargreaves I, Heales S, Land J, Smolenski R, Davies NA, Cooper CE, Singer M. Association between mitochondrial dysfunction and severity and outcome of septic shock. Lancet. 2002;360:219–23.
5. Dantzker D. Oxygen delivery and utilization in sepsis. Crit Care Clin. 1989;5:81–98.
6. Schumacker PT, Cain SM. The concept of a critical oxygen delivery. Intensive Care Med. 1987;13:223–9.
7. Ardehali A, Ports TA. Myocardial oxygen supply and demand. Chest. 1990;98:699–705.
8. O'Connor PM. Renal oxygen delivery: matching delivery to metabolic demand. Clin Exp Pharmacol Physiol. 2006;33:961–7.
9. Vincent JL, Van der Linden P. Septic shock: particular type of acute circulatory failure. Crit Care Med. 1990;18:S70–4.
10. Textoris J, Fouche L, Wiramus S, Antonini F, Tho S, Martin C, Leone M. High central venous oxygen saturation in the latter stages of septic shock is associated with increased mortality. Crit Care. 2011;15:R176.
11. Carre JE, Singer M. Cellular energetic metabolism in sepsis: the need for a systems approach. Biochim Biophys Acta. 2008;1777:763–71.
12. Singer M, Deutschman CS, Seymour CW, Shankar-Hari M, Annane D, Bauer M, Bellomo R, Bernard GR, Chiche JD, Coopersmith CM, Hotchkiss RS, Levy MM, Marshall JC, Martin GS, Opal SM, Rubenfeld GD, van der Poll T, Vincent JL, Angus DC. The third international consensus definitions for sepsis and septic shock (Sepsis-3). JAMA. 2016;315:801–10.
13. Kandel G, Aberman A. Mixed venous oxygen saturation. Its role in the assessment of the critically ill patient. Arch Intern Med. 1983;143:1400–2.
14. Cecconi M, De Backer D, Antonelli M, Beale R, Bakker J, Hofer C, Jaeschke R, Mebazaa A, Pinsky MR, Teboul JL, Vincent JL, Rhodes A. Consensus on circulatory shock and hemodynamic monitoring. Task force of the European Society of Intensive Care Medicine. Intensive Care Med. 2014;40:1795–815.
15. van Diepen S, Katz JN, Albert NM, Henry TD, Jacobs AK, Kapur NK, Kilic A, Menon V, Ohman EM, Sweitzer NK, Thiele H, Washam JB, Cohen MG, American Heart Association Council on Clinical Cardiology; Council on Cardiovascular and Stroke Nursing; Council on Quality of Care and Outcomes Research; and Mission: Lifeline. Contemporary management of cardiogenic shock: a scientific statement from the American Heart Association. Circulation. 2017;136:e232–68.
16. Harjola VP, Mullens W, Banaszewski M, Bauersachs J, Brunner-La Rocca HP, Chioncel O, Collins SP, Doehner W, Filippatos GS, Flammer AJ, Fuhrmann V, Lainscak M, Lassus J, Legrand M, Masip J, Mueller C, Papp Z, Parissis J, Platz E, Rudiger A, Ruschitzka F, Schafer A, Seferovic PM, Skouri H, Yilmaz MB, Mebazaa A. Organ dysfunction, injury and failure in acute heart failure: from pathophysiology to diagnosis and management. A review on behalf of the Acute Heart Failure Committee of the Heart Failure Association (HFA) of the European Society of Cardiology (ESC). Eur J Heart Fail. 2017;19:821–36.
17. Attana P, Lazzeri C, Picariello C, Dini CS, Gensini GF, Valente S. Lactate and lactate clearance in acute cardiac care patients. Eur Heart J Acute Cardiovasc Care. 2012;1:115–21.
18. Kortbeek JB, Al Turki SA, Ali J, Antoine JA, Bouillon B, Brasel K, Brenneman F, Brink PR, Brohi K, Burris D, Burton RA, Chapleau W, Cioffi W, Collet e Silva Fde S, Cooper A, Cortes JA, Eskesen V, Fildes J, Gautam S, Gruen RL, Gross R, Hansen KS, Henny W, Hollands MJ, Hunt RC, Jover Navalon JM, Kaufmann CR, Knudson P, Koestner A, Kosir R, Larsen CF, Livaudais W, Luchette F, Mao P, JH MV, Meredith JW, Mock C, Mori ND, Morrow C, Parks SN, Pereira PM, Pogetti RS, Ravn J, Rhee P, Salomone JP, Schipper IB, Schoettker P, Schreiber MA, Smith RS, Svendsen LB, Taha W, van Wijngaarden-Stephens M, Varga E, Voiglio EJ, Williams D, Winchell RJ, Winter R. Advanced trauma life support, 8th edition, the evidence for change. J Trauma. 2008;64:1638–50.
19. Walsh M, Devereaux PJ, Garg AX, Kurz A, Turan A, Rodseth RN, Cywinski J, Thabane L, Sessler DI. Relationship between intraoperative mean arterial pressure and clinical outcomes after noncardiac surgery: toward an empirical definition of hypotension. Anesthesiology. 2013;119:507–15.

20. van Waes JA, van Klei WA, Wijeysundera DN, van Wolfswinkel L, Lindsay TF, Beattie WS. Association between intraoperative hypotension and myocardial injury after vascular surgery. Anesthesiology. 2016;124:35–44.
21. The Pro CI. A randomized trial of protocol-based care for early septic shock. N Engl J Med. 2014;370(18):1683–93.
22. Carlson BE, Arciero JC, Secomb TW. Theoretical model of blood flow autoregulation: roles of myogenic, shear-dependent, and metabolic responses. Am J Physiol Heart Circ Physiol. 2008;295:H1572–9.
23. Asfar P, Meziani F, Hamel JF, Grelon F, Megarbane B, Anguel N, Mira JP, Dequin PF, Gergaud S, Weiss N, Legay F, Le Tulzo Y, Conrad M, Robert R, Gonzalez F, Guitton C, Tamion F, Tonnelier JM, Guezennec P, Van Der Linden T, Vieillard-Baron A, Mariotte E, Pradel G, Lesieur O, Ricard JD, Herve F, du Cheyron D, Guerin C, Mercat A, Teboul JL, Radermacher P, Investigators S. High versus low blood-pressure target in patients with septic shock. N Engl J Med. 2014;370:1583–93.
24. Magder SA. The highs and lows of blood pressure: toward meaningful clinical targets in patients with shock. Crit Care Med. 2014;42:1241–51.
25. Tapia P, Soto D, Bruhn A, Alegria L, Jarufe N, Luengo C, Kattan E, Regueira T, Meissner A, Menchaca R, Vives MI, Echeverria N, Ospina-Tascon G, Bakker J, Hernandez G. Impairment of exogenous lactate clearance in experimental hyperdynamic septic shock is not related to total liver hypoperfusion. Crit Care. 2015;19:188.
26. Hernandez G, Tapia P, Alegria L, Soto D, Luengo C, Gomez J, Jarufe N, Achurra P, Rebolledo R, Bruhn A, Castro R, Kattan E, Ospina-Tascon G, Bakker J. Effects of dexmedetomidine and esmolol on systemic hemodynamics and exogenous lactate clearance in early experimental septic shock. Crit Care. 2016;20:234.
27. Jones AE, Shapiro NI, Trzeciak S, Arnold RC, Claremont HA, Kline JA, Emergency Medicine Shock Research Network (EMShockNet) Investigators. Lactate clearance vs central venous oxygen saturation as goals of early sepsis therapy: a randomized clinical trial. JAMA. 2010;303:739–46.
28. Jansen TC, van Bommel J, Schoonderbeek FJ, Sleeswijk Visser SJ, van der Klooster JM, Lima AP, Willemsen SP, Bakker J, LACTATE study group. Early lactate-guided therapy in intensive care unit patients: a multicenter, open-label, randomized controlled trial. Am J Respir Crit Care Med. 2010;182:752–61.
29. Rhodes A, Evans LE, Alhazzani W, Levy MM, Antonelli M, Ferrer R, Kumar A, Sevransky JE, Sprung CL, Nunnally ME, Rochwerg B, Rubenfeld GD, Angus DC, Annane D, Beale RJ, Bellinghan GJ, Bernard GR, Chiche JD, Coopersmith C, De Backer DP, French CJ, Fujishima S, Gerlach H, Hidalgo JL, Hollenberg SM, Jones AE, Karnad DR, Kleinpell RM, Koh Y, Lisboa TC, Machado FR, Marini JJ, Marshall JC, Mazuski JE, McIntyre LA, McLean AS, Mehta S, Moreno RP, Myburgh J, Navalesi P, Nishida O, Osborn TM, Perner A, Plunkett CM, Ranieri M, Schorr CA, Seckel MA, Seymour CW, Shieh L, Shukri KA, Simpson SQ, Singer M, Thompson BT, Townsend SR, Van der Poll T, Vincent JL, Wiersinga WJ, Zimmerman JL, Dellinger RP. Surviving sepsis campaign: international guidelines for management of sepsis and septic shock: 2016. Intensive Care Med. 2017;43:304.
30. Casserly B, Phillips GS, Schorr C, Dellinger RP, Townsend SR, Osborn TM, Reinhart K, Selvakumar N, Levy MM. Lactate measurements in sepsis-induced tissue hypoperfusion: results from the surviving sepsis campaign database. Crit Care Med. 2015;43:567–73.
31. van Beest PA, van Ingen J, Boerma EC, Holman ND, Groen H, Koopmans M, Spronk PE, Kuiper MA. No agreement of mixed venous and central venous saturation in sepsis, independent of sepsis origin. Crit Care. 2010;14:R219.
32. Kelly KM. Does increasing oxygen delivery improve outcome? Yes. Crit Care Clin. 1996;12:635–44.
33. Rivers E, Nguyen B, Havstad S, Ressler J, Muzzin A, Knoblich B, Peterson E, Tomlanovich M, Early Goal-Directed Therapy Collaborative Group. Early goal-directed therapy in the treatment of severe sepsis and septic shock. N Engl J Med. 2001;345:1368–77.
34. ARISE Investigators; ANZICS Clinical Trials Group, Peake SL, Delaney A, Bailey M, Bellomo R, Cameron PA, Cooper DJ, Higgins AM, Holdgate A, Howe BD, Webb SA, Williams P. Goal-directed resuscitation for patients with early septic shock. N Engl J Med. 2014;371:1496–506.
35. Mouncey PR, Osborn TM, Power GS, Harrison DA, Sadique MZ, Grieve RD, Jahan R, Harvey SE, Bell D, Bion JF, Coats TJ, Singer M, Young JD, Rowan KM, Pro MTI. Trial of early, goal-directed resuscitation for septic shock. N Engl J Med. 2015;372:1301–11.
36. Investigators P, Rowan KM, Angus DC, Bailey M, Barnato AE, Bellomo R, Canter RR, Coats TJ, Delaney A, Gimbel E, Grieve RD, Harrison DA, Higgins AM, Howe B, Huang DT, Kellum JA, Mouncey PR, Music E, Peake SL, Pike F, Reade MC, Sadique MZ, Singer M, Yealy DM. Early, goal-directed therapy for septic shock – a patient-level meta-analysis. N Engl J Med. 2017;376:2223–34.

37. Dell'Anna AM, Taccone FS. Early-goal directed therapy for septic shock: is it the end? Minerva Anestesiol. 2015;81:1138–43.
38. De Backer D, Donadello K, Sakr Y, Ospina-Tascon G, Salgado D, Scolletta S, Vincent JL. Microcirculatory alterations in patients with severe sepsis: impact of time of assessment and relationship with outcome. Crit Care Med. 2013;41:791–9.
39. Bakker J, Vincent JL, Gris P, Leon M, Coffernils M, Kahn RJ. Veno-arterial carbon dioxide gradient in human septic shock. Chest. 1992;101:509–15.
40. Mallat J, Benzidi Y, Salleron J, Lemyze M, Gasan G, Vangrunderbeeck N, Pepy F, Tronchon L, Vallet B, Thevenin D. Time course of central venous-to-arterial carbon dioxide tension difference in septic shock patients receiving incremental doses of dobutamine. Intensive Care Med. 2014;40:404–11.
41. Dres M, Monnet X, Teboul JL. Hemodynamic management of cardiovascular failure by using PCO(2) venous-arterial difference. J Clin Monit Comput. 2012;26:367–74.
42. Vallet B, Pinsky MR, Cecconi M. Resuscitation of patients with septic shock: please "mind the gap"! Intensive Care Med. 2013;39:1653–5.
43. Monnet X, Julien F, Ait-Hamou N, Lequoy M, Gosset C, Jozwiak M, Persichini R, Anguel N, Richard C, Teboul JL. Lactate and venoarterial carbon dioxide difference/arterial-venous oxygen difference ratio, but not central venous oxygen saturation, predict increase in oxygen consumption in fluid responders. Crit Care Med. 2013;41:1412–20.
44. Mallat J, Lemyze M, Meddour M, Pepy F, Gasan G, Barrailler S, Durville E, Temime J, Vangrunderbeeck N, Tronchon L, Vallet B, Thevenin D. Ratios of central venous-to-arterial carbon dioxide content or tension to arteriovenous oxygen content are better markers of global anaerobic metabolism than lactate in septic shock patients. Ann Intensive Care. 2016;6:10.
45. Ospina-Tascon GA, Umana M, Bermudez W, Bautista-Rincon DF, Hernandez G, Bruhn A, Granados M, Salazar B, Arango-Davila C, De Backer D. Combination of arterial lactate levels and venous-arterial CO2 to arterial-venous O 2 content difference ratio as markers of resuscitation in patients with septic shock. Intensive Care Med. 2015;41:796–805.

Assessing the Adequacy of Cardiac Output

Jean-Louis Vincent

M. R. Pinsky et al. (eds.), *Hemodynamic Monitoring*, Lessons from the ICU,
https://doi.org/10.1007/978-3-319-69269-2_3

3

Learning Objectives

- To appreciate that there is no single value or range of values of cardiac output that is adequate for every individual all the time. Adequacy of cardiac output changes continuously.
- To understand how multiple factors, including tissue perfusion and oxygenation, interact to determine the (in)adequacy of cardiac output in individual patients.
- To be able to explain the four determinants of cardiac output—heart rate, preload, afterload, and myocardial contractility—and how these can be optimized when cardiac output is inadequate.

3.1 Introduction

The cardiac output is a measure of the amount of blood pumped by the heart every minute and is an essential determinant of systemic oxygen delivery (DO_2) and cellular oxygen supply. DO_2 needs to constantly adapt to changing tissue oxygen requirements, so that, if the cardiac output is inadequate, tissue hypoxia may occur leading to organ dysfunction and failure. However, determining the adequacy of cardiac output is not always easy, notably because oxygen requirements vary among patients and in the same patient at different times. Indeed, one cannot talk about a "normal" cardiac output value; rather one should consider cardiac output values as being adequate or inadequate for that individual at that point in time. Interpretation of the cardiac output therefore needs to take into account other factors, including tissue perfusion and oxygenation (◘ Fig. 3.1).

3.2 Cardiac Output as an Essential Component of DO_2

As mentioned, DO_2 is determined by cardiac output and the arterial oxygen content, which is itself determined by the hemoglobin concentration and its oxygen saturation. Hence, a relatively high cardiac output in the presence of hypoxemia and/or anemia does not guarantee a high DO_2 and may indeed be inadequate. By contrast, a low cardiac output is always associated with a low DO_2 because the hemoglobin concentration cannot increase acutely and the oxygen saturation cannot increase to more than 100%.

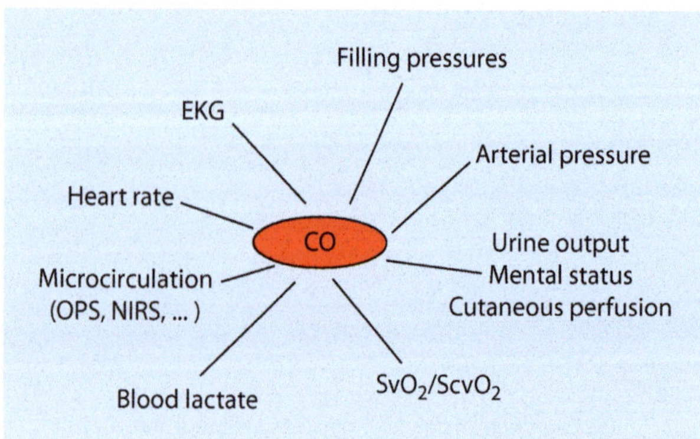

◘ **Fig. 3.1** Some of the factors that can indicate the (in) adequacy of cardiac output. *OPS* orthogonal polarization spectral imaging, *NIRS* near-infrared spectroscopy, SvO_2 mixed venous oxygen saturation, $ScvO_2$ central venous oxygen saturation, *EKG* electrocardiogram

Cardiac output is an adaptive value: it can and must adjust constantly according to the oxygen requirements of the body. Physiologically, it changes continuously in every individual: it is lowest in the middle of the night when asleep and highest during strenuous exercise. If a critically ill patient is sedated and anesthetized, cardiac output may therefore be relatively low but still perfectly adequate. An apparently "low" cardiac output therefore does not necessarily mean that treatment is needed to increase it—it may be sufficient for that patient under those conditions.

Cardiac output will increase in response to anxiety and exercise, as oxygen requirements increase. It must also increase to compensate for a reduction in arterial oxygen content. For example, when climbing a high mountain, the hypoxemia that occurs as a result of the lower atmospheric oxygen will be compensated for by an increase in cardiac output in a healthy, fit individual, so that there is virtually no tissue hypoxia, even at the top of Everest [1]. Likewise, normovolemic anemia can be very well tolerated by compensatory increases in cardiac output, with tissue hypoxia sufficient to cause hyperlactatemia only occurring when hemoglobin levels decrease as low as 4 g/dL [2].

3.3 Essential Questions When Interpreting a Cardiac Output Value

When assessing adequacy of cardiac output, it is not sufficient to look just at the cardiac output value—other factors need to be taken into account, notably related to the presence/absence of adequate tissue blood flow and to the degree of compensation already present. We will consider these two aspects separately, although clearly they may overlap.

3.3.1 Is There a Critical Reduction in Tissue Perfusion?

Many individuals walk around with a low cardiac output. They may not walk fast, but they can complete all their usual activities at their own pace. The real problem arises when cardiac output is reduced to such a degree that there is a critical reduction in oxygen availability to the cells. Clinically this often arises when there is hypotension, but clinical signs also include the effects of altered tissue perfusion as shown through the three clinical "windows" of perfusion [3]: altered cutaneous perfusion, altered mentation with disorientation/confusion, and decreased renal perfusion with resultant oliguria. Biochemically, the key indication that this critical level has been reached is the presence of increased blood lactate levels. The usual cutoff value for abnormal blood lactate is set at 2 mEq/L [3], but any value greater than the normal range, i.e., greater than 1.3 to 1.5 mEq/L, is already associated with increased mortality rates [4].

A critical reduction in cardiac output can be due to only one of three mechanisms:

- Severe hypovolemia, for example, in hemorrhage or severe dehydration
- Altered cardiac pump function, i.e., critical reduction in myocardial contractility (e.g., massive myocardial infarction, major arrhythmia [rapid supraventricular tachyarrhythmia or ventricular tachycardia]), or severe valvular disease
- Major obstruction, for example, cardiac tamponade, massive pulmonary embolism, or tension pneumothorax

3

3.3.2 Have Compensatory Mechanisms Already Been Activated?

The activation of mechanisms to compensate for poor tissue oxygenation can indicate whether or not cardiac output is adequate. In the outpatient context, for example, according to the New York Heart classification, the severity of heart failure is assessed by the capacity of exercise of the patient. The less able a patient is to compensate for increased exercise, the greater the degree of heart failure. Similarly in critically ill patients, if compensatory mechanisms have already been activated to a maximum, any worsening of the condition will result in tissue hypoxia.

3.3.2.1 Cardiac-Level Compensation

A first, quite non-specific mechanism to compensate for reduced tissue perfusion is an increase in heart rate. As cardiac output is the product of heart rate and stroke volume, an increased heart rate can compensate for a decrease in stroke volume. The tissues are still perfused but at the price of an increased adrenergic response.

Another compensatory mechanism at the cardiac level is an increase in cardiac size. This is an important compensatory mechanism in heart failure enabling stroke volume to be maintained somewhat by an increased ventricular preload, through the Frank-Starling mechanism. These patients have enlarged ventricles on echocardiographic examination and elevated cardiac filling pressures, which can result in lung and systemic edema.

3.3.2.2 Peripheral-Level Compensation

If DO_2 is reduced, tissues can still maintain oxygen consumption by increasing oxygen extraction, with a reduction in the venous saturation of the hemoglobin. The SvO_2, reflecting the oxygen saturation in the mixed venous blood in the pulmonary artery, can be easily assessed using a pulmonary artery catheter, but these are less widely used than previously. A central venous catheter provides access to blood in the superior vena cava and offers a surrogate for $ScvO_2$. Although $ScvO_2$ is a relatively gross estimate of SvO_2 [5], an inadequate cardiac output is typically associated with an $ScvO_2$ well below 70%.

Therapeutic Implications

Cardiac output is determined by four factors, and treatment of inadequate cardiac output therefore involves optimizing these four aspects: heart rate, preload, afterload, and myocardial contractility. The analogy has been made with the effort needed to increase speed when riding a bicycle [6] (■ Fig. 3.2): pushing harder on the pedals, cycling with the wind from behind, cycling on the road with least resistance, and changing gears.

Heart rate: An increase in heart rate is not very effective unless there is profound bradycardia [7]; otherwise the increase in heart rate is compensated for by a decrease in stroke volume. Moreover, in a patient with inadequate cardiac output, the heart rate may already be increased as a physiological response, so increasing it further is unlikely to bring additional benefit.

Preload: Increasing preload, i.e., the end-diastolic ventricular volume, can increase myocardial contractility by increasing myocardial fiber stretch; this in turn increases cardiac output. Fluid administration should be attempted in all patients with a critical alteration in tissue perfusion (shock) in order to increase preload, even though clinical benefit is unlikely in cases of obstructive shock. Even in cardiogenic shock with pulmonary edema, the acute nature of the lung edema is associated with a relative decrease in blood volume secondary to the extravasation of water into the extracellular fluid. To optimize fluid administration without causing fluid overload and its associated harmful effects, efforts should be taken to determine the patient's likely response to fluid administration. The most effective means of achieving this is by repeated fluid challenges, in which the clinical response is evaluated together with a cardiac filling pressure as a safety measure during the rapid administration of a limited amount of fluid [8]. A passive leg raising test, effectively an "internal" fluid challenge, represents an alternative method of evaluating response, although the procedure is not as simple as it may first seem [9].

Afterload: Afterload represents the forces working to prevent ventricular emptying, effectively represented by systemic vascular resistance. Afterload can be decreased using vasodilators, but this is possible only when the arterial pressure is adequate.

Myocardial contractility: A direct increase in myocardial contractility can be achieved with inotropes. Dobutamine is the first choice for this purpose, and administration of just a few mcg/kg/min can sometimes have dramatic effects, so that infusions should be started at low doses. This is particularly the case when vascular tone is not very high (e.g., in sepsis). Nevertheless there are always risks associated with increased adrenergic stimulation. Importantly, some interventions can act on more than one determinant. For example, phosphodiesterase inhibitors (milrinone, enoximone) or levosimendan can increase myocardial contractility (through an inotropic effect) and reduce ventricular afterload (through a vasodilating effect).

Importantly, the other determinants of DO_2 must not be neglected. Hypoxemia should always be corrected, as it is always associated with a hyperadrenergic response, which adds strain to the heart and increases catabolism. If there is associated anemia, blood transfusion can be considered even when the hemoglobin level is between 7 and 9 g/dL.

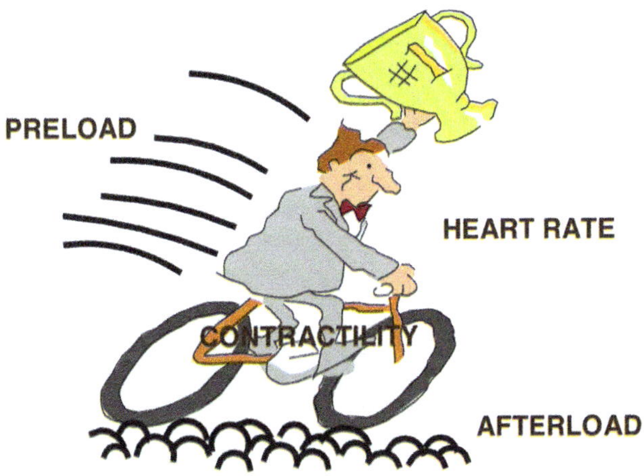

Fig. 3.2 The four determinants of cardiac output, using an analogy to the speed of a bicycle. (Reproduced from [6])

3

Conclusion

Just focusing on cardiac output without considering other variables is insufficient, because any single cardiac output value can be insufficient or excessive, depending on the particular conditions in that patient at that moment in time. If a cardiac output is unable to meet tissue oxygen demand, then it is inadequate. To really assess adequacy, one needs to ask whether the cardiac output is enabling tissue perfusion to be well maintained and whether reserve mechanisms have been activated. This complete analysis will help to determine whether an intervention is needed to increase cardiac output and, if so, what the most appropriate intervention would be.

Take-Home Messages

- There is no "normal" cardiac output value; any cardiac output value can be inadequate or excessive depending on the specific conditions of the individual at the time of measurement.
- Determining whether or not a cardiac output is adequate for a patient must therefore include an assessment of tissue perfusion and the presence of compensatory mechanisms.
- If cardiac output is inadequate, treatments can be aimed at one or more of its four determinants depending on the specific underlying causes and patient status: Preload, afterload, myocardial contractility, and heart rate.

Conflicts of Interest The author has no conflicts of interest to declare.

References

1. Grocott MP, Martin DS, Levett DZ, McMorrow R, Windsor J, Montgomery HE. Arterial blood gases and oxygen content in climbers on Mount Everest. N Engl J Med. 2009;360:140–9.
2. Weiskopf RB, Viele MK, Feiner J, Kelley S, Lieberman J, Noorani M, et al. Human cardiovascular and metabolic response to acute, severe isovolemic anemia. JAMA. 1998;279:217–21.
3. Vincent JL, De Backer D. Circulatory shock. N Engl J Med. 2013;369:1726–34.
4. Nichol AD, Egi M, Pettila V, Bellomo R, French C, Hart G, et al. Relative hyperlactatemia and hospital mortality in critically ill patients: a retrospective multi-Centre study. Crit Care. 2010;14:R25.
5. Chawla LS, Zia H, Gutierrez G, Katz NM, Seneff MG, Shah M. Lack of equivalence between central and mixed venous oxygen saturation. Chest. 2004;126:1891–6.
6. Vincent JL. Understanding cardiac output. Crit Care. 2008;12:174.
7. Tavazzi G, Kontogeorgis A, Guarracino F, Bergsland N, Martinez-Naharro A, Pepper J, et al. Heart rate modification of cardiac output following cardiac surgery: the importance of cardiac time intervals. Crit Care Med. 2017;45:e782–8.
8. Vincent JL, Weil MH. Fluid challenge revisited. Crit Care Med. 2006;34:1333–7.
9. Monnet X, Teboul JL. Passive leg raising: five rules, not a drop of fluid! Crit Care. 2015;19:18.

Determinants of Venous Return

Hollmann D. Aya and Maurizio Cecconi

M. R. Pinsky et al. (eds.), *Hemodynamic Monitoring*, Lessons from the ICU,
https://doi.org/10.1007/978-3-319-69269-2_4

Learning Objectives

After reading this chapter, the reader will learn:

1. Which are the main determinants of venous return and cardiac output?
2. What is the mean systemic filling pressure, what is its importance and what is the gradient of venous return?
3. What is the meaning of central venous pressure in the context of venous return?
4. What is an effective fluid challenge, using Pmsf?

4.1 Introduction

Cardiovascular failure is one of the most common reasons for admission to intensive care units. The main function of the cardiovascular system is the transport of oxygen (O_2) to the tissues. If the concentration of haemoglobin is stable, the main determinant of O_2 transport is the cardiac output (CO).

CO is total volume of blood mobilised by the heart per unit of time, and it is measured in units of flow (L/min). In stable conditions, the cardiovascular system is a close loop system, and the heart can only eject the amount of blood that it receives. Thus, the total volume ejected over a period of time would equal the total volume of blood returning from the venous system. Therefore, venous return equals cardiac output.

In this chapter we will analyse the determinants of venous return, their impact on the cardiovascular physiology and the practical implications that those factors may play a role in the treatment of critically ill patients. The main factors that determine the venous return to the heart from the systemic circulation are:

1. The degree of filling of the circulation
2. The ability of the heart to maintain a low right atrial pressure
3. The resistance to blood flow between the peripheral vessels and the right atrium
4. The resistance to blood flow between the heart and the capillaries

4.2 Blood Volume and Mean Systemic Filling Pressure

The venous system contains about 70% of the total blood volume, whereas the arterial system contains only 13–18% and the capillaries 7% [1, 2]. The venous system is a blood reservoir, able to adjust his capacity according to the haemodynamic conditions. The venous wall is much thinner than the arterial wall, as blood is circulating at low pressure, but it still contains smooth muscle fibres, able to contract and expand according to the haemodynamic situation. During hypovolaemia, sympathetic nervous reflexes cause venoconstriction, sending blood back to the central circulation, increasing preload and increasing cardiac output. Actually, even after 20% of the total blood volume has been lost, the circulatory system functions almost normally because of this variable reservoir function of veins [1].

The heart pumps blood continuously into the aorta keeping the mean arterial pressure high, averaging 80–100 mmHg. This pressure decreases progressively as the blood flows into the systemic circulation, as low as the level of the right atrial pressure (Pra). This fall in pressure is mainly caused by the increasing total cross-sectional area in each level of the vascular tree (◘ Fig. 4.1). When the heart stops, the arterial pressure decreases, and the RAP progressively increases. At certain point, blood will not be flowing, and if the arteri-

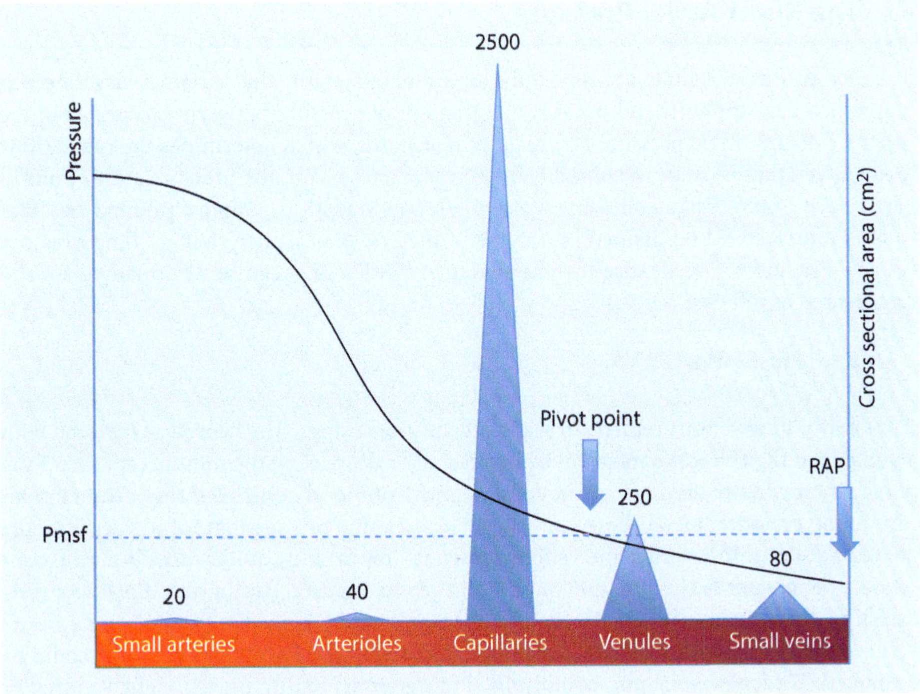

Fig. 4.1 Pressures and cross-sectional area across cardiovascular system. Pmsf mean systemic filling pressure. This is the pressure at all points in the cardiovascular system when the heart stops. During normal circulation, there is a point (pivot point) where the pressure equalises the Pmsf. At that point, the pressure is independent of flow and theoretically localises at the venule territory. The drop in pressure is mainly related to the increase in the total cross-sectional area and the compliance of the vascular wall

oles do not collapse trapping blood in the arterial space, the pressure will be the same in all territories of the circulatory system. This pressure is the *mean systemic filling pressure* (*Pmsf*). This pressure was described by Bayliss and Starling [3], and they figured that somewhere in the circulation, there must be a point where the pressure is not changing when the heart stops. Actually, during a cardiac arrest, the pressure in the small veins (<1 mm) and venules do not change substantially; they are the "pivoting point" of the system (Fig. 4.1) [4]. This pressure is less than the capillary pressure, close to the portal venous pressure and greater than the RAP. Its anatomic location is not necessarily at the same venous branching level in every organ. The importance of this pressure, rather than its anatomical location, is that it provides a quantitative measurement of the intravascular filling status independent from cardiac function: its value is equal to the Pmsf.

Let us imagine the "blood reservoir" as a distensible compartment. The volume required to fill a distensible tube, such as a tyre or a blood vessel, with no pressure rise is called the "unstressed" volume (V_0). Further volume expansion will imply necessarily a pressure rise and an elastic distension of the wall of the tube, which depends on the compliance (C) of the wall. This volume is the "stressed" volume (V_s) and is related to the pressure in the next equation:

$$\text{Pmsf} = V_s / C$$

4

4.3 The Right Atrial Pressure

In order to move a fluid across a tube or tubular system, the variables described in Poiseuille's Law apply. Therefore, it is the gradient of pressure between two points in the system, not any single pressure at any particular point, which determines the rate of flow [5, 6]. Given that most of the blood is in the venous reservoir, the pressure at this point is particularly interesting. Following Poiseuille's Law equation, Guyton pointed out that venous return could be defined by three parameters: the mean systemic filling pressure (Pmsf), Pra and the resistance to venous return (RVR). This can be also mathematically represented as follows:

$$\mathrm{VR} = \left(\mathrm{Pmsf} - \mathrm{Pra}\right) / \mathrm{RVR}$$

Guyton [7] drew venous return curves in recently dead dogs. The heart was replaced with a pump, and the Pra was controlled by increasing or decreasing the minute capacity of the pump. Increasing or decreasing the total quantity of blood controlled the mean circulatory filling pressure. From these curves (Fig. 4.2), one can see that for a given Pra, the greater the Pmsf, the greater the venous return is. Importantly, under isovolumetric conditions, the greater is the Pra, the lower is the venous return. Thus, given this linear relationship, if venous return and Pra can be measured and changed without changes in the volume status, the slope of the line could be calculated (the RVR), and the Pmsf could be estimated. Under isovolaemic conditions, Pra depends mainly on the right ventricular function and its ability to accommodate and pump blood to the pulmonary circulation. Any decrease in the heart function will increase Pra and therefore create congestion in the venous circulation.

A second factor that affects the Pra is the intrathoracic and the pericardial pressure. Under normal circumstances, intrathoracic pressure is negative or equal to the

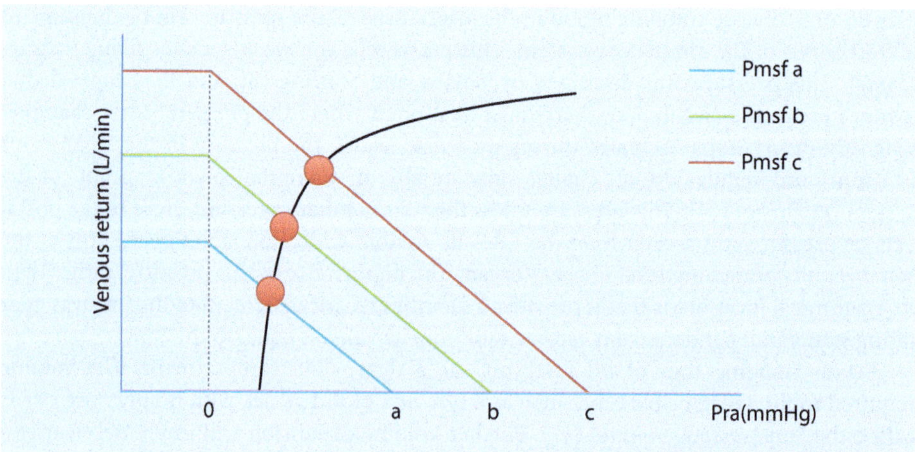

Fig. 4.2 Venous return and Frank-Starling curves. Pmsf mean systemic filling pressure, Pra right atrial pressure. Each venous return curve represents different levels of volume status. To move across a venous return curve, changes in cardiac function are required, without changes in the volume status. The black line represents the Frank-Starling curve for a particular level of cardiac function. In order to move from the blue to the red curve, Pmsf must change from a to c without changes in resistance

atmospheric pressure. Any increase in this pressure that translates in an increase of Pra will result in a decrease of venous return. Similar phenomenon is observed if there is an increase in pericardial pressure, which will increase Pra, and will result in a decrease of venous return.

4.4 Arteriolar Resistance and Metabolic Demand

As the venous system can only transport the amount of volume that arrives from the capillary system, the regulation of the capillary circulation will also determine the venous return. Each tissue in the body has the ability to control its own local blood flow in proportion to its metabolic needs. Rapid changes in vasoconstriction or vasodilation of arterioles, meta-arterioles and precapillary sphincters may happen within seconds to provide adequate local tissue blood flow. The main factors involved in the acute control of local blood flow are:

1. Tissue metabolism: this is by far the most powerful factor. The higher is the local oxygen demand, the higher is the blood flow.
2. Availability of oxygen: whenever there is a deficit of oxygen (hypoxia), there is an increase in local blood flow. Oxygen deficit can occur in several ways, such as (1) failure in oxygenation of blood (ARDS, pneumonia, etc.), (2) failure in transport of oxygen by haemoglobin (CO poisoning) or (3) failure in the ability of tissue to use oxygen (septic shock, cyanide poisoning).
3. Deficit of other nutrients: under special conditions, the lack of glucose, thiamine, niacin and riboflavin can cause vasodilation.

4.5 Control of Venous Tone: Resistance to Venous Return

Certain parts of the venous system are particularly compliant: these include the spleen, the liver, the large abdominal veins and the venous plexus beneath the skin. Splanchnic and cutaneous veins have a high population of α1- and α2-adrenergic receptors, so they are very sensitive to adrenergic stimulation, contrary to skeletal and muscle veins [8]. The control of the venous system has been extensively studied in animal models. There are nerve terminations in the proximity of many small vein smooth muscles [9] but not in the veins of the skeletal muscle [10]. However, circulating catecholamines can induce contraction of venules and veins of the skeletal muscle and mesentery [9, 10]. Thus, probably catecholamines released from the sympathetic nerve termination of the arterial side may pass through the capillary bed and affect the venous system.

Smooth muscles of the veins and arteries do not respond necessarily in the same way to chemical signals. Dihydroergotamine can activate the veins but not the arteries [11]. The venous system primarily has α-adrenergic receptors [12–15]. Stimulation of the β-adrenergic receptors of arterioles cause vasodilation but has little effect on the veins [16, 17]. Angiotensin can increase Pmsf [16, 18]. Isoproterenol, a β-adrenergic agonist, causes a decrease in Pmsf when veins are constricted with angiotensin. On the other hand, vasopressin has very little effect on Pmsf [19] or on vascular capacity once reflex blockade [20] and similar results were reported regarding natriuretic peptides [21].

Nitroglycerin and nitroprusside decrease Pmsf and increase unstressed blood volume but do not change vascular compliance in ganglion-blockade dogs [22]. Verapamil and nifedipine increase venous return by reducing the resistance to venous return without changing the Pmsf, whereas nitroglycerin in small doses can reduce Pmsf without changes in resistance to venous return [23]. Diltiazem reduces both resistance and Pmsf increasing CO [23].

Moderate hypercapnia and hypoxia have little direct non-reflex effect on CO and Pmsf [24]. Severe hypercapnia ($PaCO_2$ to 114 mmHg (15.2 KPa)) caused an increase in Pmsf by 5.5 mmHg, whereas a PaO_2 of 34 mmHg (4.5 KPa) caused an increase in Pmsf by 2.5 mmHg [25].

4.6 Measurement of Pmsf in Humans with Intact Circulation

The Pmsf is not easy to measure in patients with an intact circulation. Schipke et al. [26] performed a fibrillation-defibrillation sequence in 82 patients during cardioverter/defibrillator implantation to measure the Pmsf over 13 s. A true equilibrium pressure was not achieved, and the arterial-central venous pressure difference was 13.2 ± 6.2 mm Hg, and differences still persisted in sequences of 20 s.

Pinsky [27] proposed a model in animals with an intact circulation to construct venous return curves observing the relationship between isovolumetric changes in CO and Pra during intermittent positive pressure recruitment manoeuvres. Pmsf was estimated by calculation of the slope and extrapolation of the Pra value to zero CO. Pmsf calculated was found similar to Pmsf measured during circulatory arrest. Other studies [28–30] have confirmed this linear relationship between VR and Pra and derived Pmsf from the regression equation in animal models with intact circulation. Maas and colleagues [31] applied the same rationale to study the effect of a 12-second inspiratory hold manoeuvre to three different steady-state levels on central venous pressure (CVP), as an estimate of Pra, and blood flow (CO) measured via the pulse contour method during the last 3 s in mechanically ventilated postoperative cardiac patients. This study showed again a linear relationship between changes in CVP and CO, and importantly, Pmsf could be estimated at bedside in intensive care patients with an intact circulation. Obviously this technique is only feasible in fully sedated patients under mechanical ventilation. Keller and colleagues [32] used this method to assess the changes on venous return with passive leg raising (PLR) manoeuvre: they observed nine postoperative cardiac patients at baseline, during PLR and after volume expansion (500 ml of hydroxyethyl starch). They reported a Pmsf at baseline of 19.7 mmHg. This increased to 22 mmHg after PLR and to 26.9 mmHg after volume expansion (VE). Although CO increased after PLR and VE, the gradient of pressure of venous return (difference between Pmsf and CVP) increased by 2 mmHg after PLR and by 5.8 mmHg after VE. This could explain why a PLR test does not consistently increase CO in fluid-responsive patients [33], or even for a fluid challenge, the increase in Pmsf is an essential condition to effectively test the cardiac response.

Parkin and Wright [34] proposed a method for estimating a mean systemic filling pressure analogue (Pmsa) using the mean arterial pressure (MAP), Pra, CO and anthropometric data. Pmsa algorithm is fully described in other publications [35]. In essence, they build a mathematical model that uses the patient's data as predictors of Pmsa. The clinical validity of this approach was tested in ten patients in acute renal failure receiving continuous vein-venous haemofiltration [36]. Fluid replacement therapy was electromechanically controlled to a target value of Pmsa. This method was also used to analyse

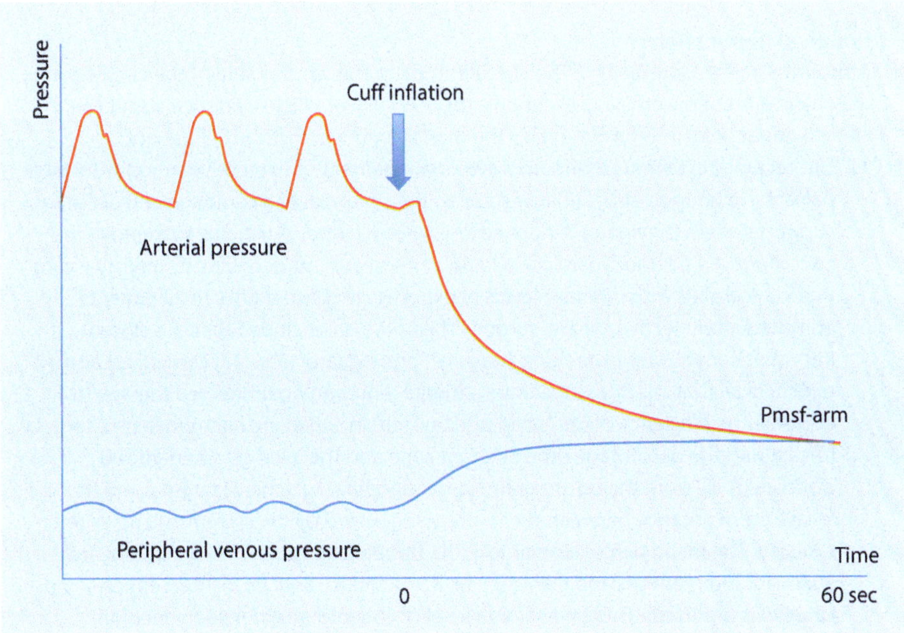

Fig. 4.3 Arterial-venous equilibrium method for measuring Pmsf-arm at bedside with a pneumatic tourniquet

haemodynamic changes after a fluid challenge (250 ml of colloids or crystalloids in 5 min) in patients admitted to intensive care [37]: Pmsa increased similarly in responders and nonresponders, as expected, but interestingly Pra increased more in nonresponders, neutralising the changes in the gradient of pressure of venous return as described by Guyton. Recently, Gupta et al. [38] used Pmsa to investigate the performance of cardiac power (defined as the product of arterial pressure and cardiac output) relative to Pmsa (CP_{vol}). CP_{vol} represents a measurement of cardiac performance adjusted to the vascular tone. According to the authors, values below 0.047 of CP_{vol} have a high sensitivity (97%) and not so high specificity (57.5%) to predict fluid responsiveness.

Anderson [39] proposed a non-invasive technique to measure Pmsf by a rapid occlusion of the circulation in the arm (Pmsf-arm). Once the arterial (Pa) and venous pressures (Pv) in the arm equilibrate, the pressure measured would be Pmsf (Fig. 4.3). Maas et al. [40] compared these three methods in 11 postoperative cardiac surgery patients. Bland-Altman analysis for the difference between Pmsf-arm and Pmsf showed a bias of −1.0 (±3.1) mmHg ($p = 0.06$) and a coefficient of variation (CV) of 15%. Although there was a statistically non-significant bias, one may think that this is actually quite significant considering the small sample size of this study. Regarding the difference between Pmsf and Pmsa, there was a bias of −6.0 (±3.1) mmHg ($p < 0.001$) and a CV of 17%. The three methods were useful to track changes after volume expansion.

The precision of the Pmsf-arm technique has been recently studied [41]. Four repeated measurements were performed in 20 patients after cardiac surgery. Pa and Pv equalised after 60 s of cuff inflation. For a single measurement, the coefficient error (CE) was 5% (±2%), and the least significant change (LSC) was 14% (±5%). Averaging two measurements, the CE improves to 4% (±1%), and the LSC was reduced to 10% (±4%).

4

Practical Implications

Although the measurement of the vascular tone in the venous side of the circulation may have a lot of potential applications, there is still very little evidence about the clinical impact of this information on the management of critically ill patients.

1. Understanding venous return improves management of haemodynamically unstable patients. Rangappa et al. [42] investigated the potential of a computerised decision support system (Navigator™, Applied Physiology, Sidney, Australia) to improve the consistency of haemodynamic evaluation and treatment decisions by intensive care unit clinical staff with different levels of expertise and experience in 20 patients admitted after elective cardiac surgery. The authors concluded that this system improves consistency in decision-making. Sondergaard et al. [43] carried out a small pilot clinical trial in 27 postoperative patients requiring goal-directed therapy to evaluate the efficiency of the Navigator™ system in achieving haemodynamic targets (measuring the percentage time in target zone and the average standardised distance (ASD) from the centre of the target and time to achieve targets) and the level of concordance between the therapy suggested by the system and an expert clinician. The mean percentage time in the target zone was 36.7% for control and 36.5% for intervention, and the ASD was 1.5 in control and 1.6 in intervention (no p value was reported). There was a high level of concordance between decision support recommendation and anaesthetist action (84.3%). The authors concluded that the treatment recommended by the Navigator™ system mirrored that of a senior anaesthetist in the achievement of therapeutic goals. Unfortunately, this study is probably underpowered to show differences in the efficiency measurements, fluid balance or vasoactive medications.
2. The changes in Pmsf can be used to assess systemic compliance and guide the choice between fluids or vasopressors. The current consensus on circulatory shock and haemodynamic monitoring recommends that even in the context of fluid-responsive patients, fluid management should be carefully titrated, especially in the presence of elevated intravascular filling pressures [44]. The similar principle applies to the Pmsf. A fluid challenge can be used to assess fluid responsiveness and also, as spotted by Maas and colleagues [45], to assess systemic compliance. In this study, systemic compliance is reported from 15 postoperative cardiac surgery patients around 64 mL/mmHg. Systemic venous compliance could be very useful information to prioritise treatment: a high compliance after a fluid challenge may indicate the early use of vasoconstrictors instead of infusion of a large amount of fluids. Another study [46] showed that administration of noradrenaline (an α1-adrenergic agonist) increased CO in preload-responsive patients. Noradrenaline increased Pmsf either by reducing venous compliance or by venoconstriction (reduction of venous capacity and shifting unstressed volume to stressed compartment; see ◘ Fig. 4.2). Unfortunately, the authors did not assess the effect of noradrenaline on venous compliance. In the rest of the patients, noradrenaline had predominantly an arterial vasoconstrictive effect, increasing cardiac afterload. This study stressed the importance of monitoring venous tone and CO when using vasopressors.
3. Pmsf can also be used to assess the effect of IV fluid in the circulation, regardless the cardiac response and the efficacy of a fluid challenge. In a recent study about fluid challenges [47], the observation of the Pmsa along with other haemodynamic

variables described the short living effect of this technique and pointed out that the maximal change in CO is about 1 min after the end of IV fluid infusion. Pmsf-arm has been also used to evaluate the minimal volume required to challenge the cardiovascular system. This is a quasi-randomised clinical trial with 80 patients who received between 1 and 4 ml/kg of IV fluids in 5 min. Pmsf-arm only increased significantly in the group of 4 ml/Kg, and the proportion of fluid responders increased significantly from 20% in the group of 1 mL/Kg to 65% in the group of 4 mL/Kg.

4. Since venous return equals CO, in practice CO and CVP changes can provide most of the information about the Guytonian view of the circulation. However, without the understanding how the venous tone works, the values of CVP can be misunderstood. Proof of this is the number of studies that looked at the CVP as a fluid responsiveness predictor [48]. CVP preforms as the meeting point between venous return and the cardiac function: a high CVP can be related to a high Pmsf or a low cardiac function or both. Thus, knowing Pmsf would help clinicians to better understand the haemodynamic status of critically ill patients at bedside.
5. Any cardiovascular intervention in critically ill patients should take into account that the main regulation of cardiac output occurs in the peripheral tissues. Therefore, therapy should also be guided by tissue perfusion signs, and not only by haemodynamic measurements.

Conclusion

The venous system plays an important role in the haemodynamic stability. Most of blood volume is stored and regulated in the venous territory. The mean systemic filling pressure can be now measured, and it is the pressure of the pivot point of the circulation, where the pressure is independent of blood flow. This pressure is the driving pressure of the circulation and affects, along with the cardiac function, venous return. Three methods have been described to measure Pmsf at bedside, in patients with intact circulation. This variable can be now integrated as another piece of information that helps to understand patient's conditions and to guide haemodynamic therapy in accordance to patient's physiology.

Take-Home Message

- Venous return, which is equivalent to cardiac output, is finely controlled at the microcirculatory level in the peripheral tissues. Always remember to put haemodynamics in that context.
- The two main factors that influence the blood flow in peripheral tissues are the metabolic level and the availability of oxygen. These two are also determinants of venous return.
- α1-Adrenergic agonist causes venoconstriction, increasing the availability of blood volume from the venous reservoir to increase cardiac output and blood pressure. This is very useful in the anaesthetic induction of unstable patients, as most anaesthetic drugs may cause profound vasodilation and a severe decrease in venous return.
- In order to do an effective fluid challenge, it is necessary to infuse enough volume to increase Pmsf; otherwise, there is a possibility of a false-negative response. 4 mL/Kg is an adequate dose in most postoperative patients.

Conflict of Interest *Hollmann D. Aya* received financial support for educational programmes and for attending symposia from LiDCO. *Maurizio Cecconi* has received honoraria for speaking at symposia, financial support for educational programmes and honoraria for advisory board from Edwards Lifesciences, LiDCO, Deltex, Applied Physiology, Massimo, Bmeye, Cheetah, and Imacor.

4

References

1. Guyton AC. Textbook of medical physiology. 12th ed. Philadelphia: Elsevier Saunders; 2011.
2. Rothe CF. Reflex control of veins and vascular capacitance. Physiol Rev. 1983;63(4):1281–342.
3. Bayliss WM, Starling EH. Observations on venous pressures and their relationship to capillary pressures. J Physiol. 1894;16(3–4):159–318 7.
4. Rothe CF. Mean circulatory filling pressure: its meaning and measurement. J Appl Physiol (1985). 1993;74(2):499–509.
5. Guyton AC, Lindsey AW, Kaufmann BN, Abernathy JB. Effect of blood transfusion and hemorrhage on cardiac output and on the venous return curve. Am J Phys. 1958;194(2):263–7.
6. Guyton AC, Lindsey AW, Kaufmann BN. Effect of mean circulatory filling pressure and other peripheral circulatory factors on cardiac output. Am J Phys. 1955;180(3):463–8.
7. Guyton AC. Determination of cardiac output by equating venous return curves with cardiac response curves. Physiol Rev. 1955;35(1):123–9.
8. Rowell LB. Human cardiovascular control. New York: Oxford University Press; 1993.
9. Furness JB, Marshall JM. Correlation of the directly observed responses of mesenteric vessles of the rat to nerve stimulation and noradrenaline with the distribution of adrenergic nerves. J Physiol. 1974;239(1):75–88.
10. Marshall JM. The influence of the sympathetic nervous system on individual vessels of the microcirculation of skeletal muscle of the rat. J Physiol. 1982;332:169–86.
11. Mellander S, Nordenfelt I. Comparative effects of dihydroergotamine and noradrenaline on resistance, exchange and capacitance functions in the peripheral circulation. Clin Sci. 1970;39(2):183–201.
12. Appleton CP, Lee RW, Martin GV, Olajos M, Goldman S. Alpha 1- and alpha 2-adrenoceptor stimulation: changes in venous capacitance in intact dogs. Am J Phys. 1986;250(6 Pt 2):H1071–8.
13. Patel P, Bose D, Greenway C. Effects of prazosin and phenoxybenzamine on alpha- and beta-receptor-mediated responses in intestinal resistance and capacitance vessels. J Cardiovasc Pharmacol. 1981;3(5):1050–9.
14. Ruffolo RR Jr. Distribution and function of peripheral alpha-adrenoceptors in the cardiovascular system. Pharmacol Biochem Behav. 1985;22(5):827–33.
15. Shi AG, Ahmad S, Kwan CY, Daniel EE. Characterization of alpha-adrenoceptor subtypes by [3H]prazosin and [3H]rauwolscine binding to canine venous smooth muscle membranes. Can J Physiol Pharmacol. 1989;67(9):1067–73.
16. Hirakawa S, Itoh H, Kotoo Y, Abe C, Endo T, Takada N, et al. The role of alpha and beta adrenergic receptors in constriction and dilation of the systemic capacitance vessels: a study with measurements of the mean circulatory pressure in dogs. Jpn Circ J. 1984;48(7):620–32.
17. Rothe CF, Flanagan AD, Maass-Moreno R. Role of beta-adrenergic agonists in the control of vascular capacitance. Can J Physiol Pharmacol. 1990;68(5):575–85.
18. Lee RW, Lancaster LD, Buckley D, Goldman S. Peripheral circulatory control of preload-afterload mismatch with angiotensin in dogs. Am J Phys. 1987;253(1 Pt 2):H126–32.
19. Pang CC, Tabrizchi R. The effects of noradrenaline, B-HT 920, methoxamine, angiotensin II and vasopressin on mean circulatory filling pressure in conscious rats. Br J Pharmacol. 1986;89(2):389–94.
20. Martin DS, McNeill JR. Whole body vascular capacitance response to vasopressin is mediated by autonomic function. Am J Phys. 1991;261(2 Pt 2):H493–9.
21. Chien Y, Pegram BL, Kardon MB, Frohlich ED. ANF does not increase total body venous compliance in conscious rats with myocardial infarction. Am J Phys. 1992;262(2 Pt 2):H432–6.
22. Ogilvie RI, Zborowska-Sluis D. Effects of nitroglycerin and nitroprusside on vascular capacitance of anesthetized ganglion-blocked dogs. J Cardiovasc Pharmacol. 1991;18(4):574–80.
23. Ito H, Hirakawa S. Effects of vasodilators on the systemic capacitance vessels, a study with the measurement of the mean circulatory pressure in dogs. Jpn Circ J. 1984;48(4):388–404.

24. Rothe CF, Flanagan AD, Maass-Moreno R. Reflex control of vascular capacitance during hypoxia, hypercapnia, or hypoxic hypercapnia. Can J Physiol Pharmacol. 1990;68(3):384–91.
25. Rothe CF, Stein PM, MacAnespie CL, Gaddis ML. Vascular capacitance responses to severe systemic hypercapnia and hypoxia in dogs. Am J Phys. 1985;249(6 Pt 2):H1061–9.
26. Schipke JD, Heusch G, Sanii AP, Gams E, Winter J. Static filling pressure in patients during induced ventricular fibrillation. Am J Physiol Heart Circ Physiol. 2003;285(6):H2510–5.
27. Pinsky MR. Instantaneous venous return curves in an intact canine preparation. J Appl Physiol Respir Environ Exerc Physiol. 1984;56(3):765–71.
28. Versprille A, Jansen JR. Mean systemic filling pressure as a characteristic pressure for venous return. Pflugers Arch. 1985;405(3):226–33.
29. Den Hartog EA, Versprille A, Jansen JR. Systemic filling pressure in intact circulation determined on basis of aortic vs. central venous pressure relationships. Am J Phys. 1994;267(6 Pt 2):H2255–8.
30. Hiesmayr M, Jansen JR, Versprille A. Effects of endotoxin infusion on mean systemic filling pressure and flow resistance to venous return. Pflugers Arch. 1996;431(5):741–7.
31. Maas JJ, Geerts BF, van den Berg PC, Pinsky MR, Jansen JR. Assessment of venous return curve and mean systemic filling pressure in postoperative cardiac surgery patients. Crit Care Med. 2009;37(3):912–8.
32. Keller G, Desebbe O, Benard M, Bouchet JB, Lehot JJ. Bedside assessment of passive leg raising effects on venous return. J Clin Monit Comput. 2011;25(4):257–63.
33. Mahjoub Y, Touzeau J, Airapetian N, Lorne E, Hijazi M, Zogheib E, et al. The passive leg-raising maneuver cannot accurately predict fluid responsiveness in patients with intra-abdominal hypertension. Crit Care Med. 2010;38(9):1824–9.
34. Parkin WG, Wright CA. Three dimensional closed loop control of the human circulation. Int J Clin Monit Comput. 1991;8(1):35–42.
35. Parkin WG, Leaning MS. Therapeutic control of the circulation. J Clin Monit Comput. 2008;22(6):391–400.
36. Parkin G, Wright C, Bellomo R, Boyce N. Use of a mean systemic filling pressure analogue during the closed-loop control of fluid replacement in continuous hemodiafiltration. J Crit Care. 1994;9(2):124–33.
37. Cecconi M, Aya HD, Geisen M, Ebm C, Fletcher N, Grounds RM, et al. Changes in the mean systemic filling pressure during a fluid challenge in postsurgical intensive care patients. Intensive Care Med. 2013;39(7):1299–305.
38. Gupta K, Sondergaard S, Parkin G, Leaning M, Aneman A. Applying mean systemic filling pressure to assess the response to fluid boluses in cardiac post-surgical patients. Intensive Care Med. 2015;41:265.
39. Anderson RM. The gross physiology of the cardiovascular system. 2012 ed. Tucson: Racquet Press; 1993.
40. Maas JJ, Pinsky MR, Geerts BF, de Wilde RB, Jansen JR. Estimation of mean systemic filling pressure in postoperative cardiac surgery patients with three methods. Intensive Care Med. 2012;38(9):1452–60.
41. Aya H, Rhodes A, Fletcher N, Grounds M, Cecconi M, editors. Transient stop-flow arm arterial-venous equilibrium pressure measurement: determination of precision of the technique. Annual Congress of the European Society of Intensive Care Medicine. Barcelona/New York: Springer; 2014.
42. Rangappa R, Sondergaard S, Aneman A. Improved consistency in interpretation and management of cardiovascular variables by intensive care staff using a computerised decision-support system. Crit Care Resusc. 2014;16(1):48–53.
43. Sondergaard S, Wall P, Cocks K, Parkin WG, Leaning MS. High concordance between expert anaesthetists' actions and advice of decision support system in achieving oxygen delivery targets in high-risk surgery patients. Br J Anaesth. 2012;108(6):966–72.
44. Cecconi M, De Backer D, Antonelli M, Beale R, Bakker J, Hofer C, et al. Consensus on circulatory shock and hemodynamic monitoring. Task force of the European Society of Intensive Care Medicine. Intensive Care Med. 2014;40(12):1795–815.
45. Maas JJ, Pinsky MR, Aarts LP, Jansen JR. Bedside assessment of total systemic vascular compliance, stressed volume, and cardiac function curves in intensive care unit patients. Anesth Analg. 2012;115(4):880–7.
46. Maas JJ, Pinsky MR, de Wilde RB, de Jonge E, Jansen JR. Cardiac output response to norepinephrine in postoperative cardiac surgery patients: interpretation with venous return and cardiac function curves. Crit Care Med. 2013;41(1):143–50.
47. Aya HD, Ster IC, Fletcher N, Grounds RM, Rhodes A, Cecconi M. Pharmacodynamic analysis of a fluid challenge. Crit Care Med. 2016;44(5):880–91.
48. Cecconi M, Aya HD. Central venous pressure cannot predict fluid-responsiveness. Evid Based Med. 2014;19(2):63.

Arterial Blood Pressure Regulation

Alexander Kobzik and Michael R. Pinsky

M. R. Pinsky et al. (eds.), *Hemodynamic Monitoring*, Lessons from the ICU,
https://doi.org/10.1007/978-3-319-69269-2_5

5

Learning Objectives

- Mean arterial pressure (MAP) is usually maintained constant as cardiac output varies along a physiologic range of flows by the process of autoregulation.
- Central autoregulatory control reflects stretch receptors in the aortic wall and carotid body called baroreceptors that directly link to brain stem sympathetic and parasympathetic nuclei altering their output.
- Local metabolic demands define local blood flow over the autoregulatory MAP range; thus both hypotension and hypertension represent a failure of normal autoregulation.
- Hypertension to levels above the autoregulatory range causes excess end-organ vascular pressurization leading to end-organ injury from both vascular strain and edema (e.g., type II non-ST elevation myocardial infarction, cerebral edema, acute kidney injury).
- Hypotension represents a failure of normal host adaptive mechanisms and must be associated with end-organ hypoperfusion of some organ tissues relative to their metabolic needs.
- Normal autoregulatory range is shifted rightward and upward with pressure on the *x*-axis in patients with chronic arterial hypertension; thus otherwise normal-but-lower-than-usual blood pressure may cause end-organ hypoperfusion and injury.
- The only way to know that a given MAP is adequate for organ perfusion is to assess organ function. This may be difficult, so surrogates of perfusion like assessment of lactate kinetics and central venous-to-arterial oxygen and carbon dioxide gradients can be used to assess adequacy of blood flow.

5.1 Introduction

The systemic vascular system is highly heterogeneous. Central arterial pressure is kept high owing to both a low central arterial compliance and high outflow resistance in the peripheral arterioles. The primary role of the left ventricle is to eject its stroke volume against these high pressures to keep this central arterial capacitor pressurized. However, most of the blood volume resides in the post-capillary venous circulation, while the majority of the vessel cross-sectional area is dominated by the capillary system [1], as this is where diffusion of gases and exchange of metabolic substrates occur. Tone of the arterial (precapillary) side of the circulation determines relative organ blood flow and perfusion. If downstream blood flow is inadequate to meet the tissue's metabolic demands, local arteriolar and precapillary arteriolar tone decreases so that local blood flow can increase. It is downstream organ oxygenation that determines this tone by direct retrograde vascular endothelial cell signaling via nitric oxide and other endothelium-derived vasodilating factors. Similarly, independent of local metabolic needs, stress and disease states (e.g., adrenal insufficiency, intracranial hypertension) can cause general arterial tone to vary independent of local metabolic demands, resulting in a generalized impairment of the distribution of blood flow within and among organs. Autoregulation can be blunted in sepsis and can be hyperactive in essential hypertension, even if blood pressure is effectively controlled with antihypertensive medication. Importantly, not only is arterial pressure controlled as much as possible, organ blood flow is also controlled even if arterial pressure varies, with the primary goal of sustaining organ blood flow at required levels to sustain their metabolic activity. Thus, arterial pressure autoregulation reflects one of the controlling input processes to sustain blood flow regulation, and the lack thereof is particularly of interest to the intensivist. This chapter will dwell on this important topic from that perspective.

5.2 Blood Pressure Autoregulation and Its Relation to Organ Blood Flow

In normal states, including both at rest and increased metabolic demand (e.g., agitation, hyperpnea, digestion), the human body controls central blood pressure allowing organ-specific regional blood flow autoregulation through multiple mechanisms that tend to match local blood flow to the functional needs of the specific tissue. These central blood pressure-controlling processes can be divided into short-term, intermediate-term, and long-term mechanisms. Though all three are important, the most pertinent for the intensivist is the short-term, rapidly acting mechanism that involves three pathways for control: local ischemia response, baroreceptor feedback, and chemoreceptor feedback. Importantly, changes in arterial tone alone are only part of this complex response. When metabolic need increases, an associated increased global sympathetic tone causes blood flow to be diverted away from less active tissues, and venomotor tone increases to decrease vascular unstressed volume increasing mean systemic pressure and the upstream pressure for venous return and thus increasing cardiac output. This results in an increase in venous return and cardiac output to sustain the increased local blood flow demands without an undue need for increased arterial tone or changes in blood pressure.

Independent of central arterial pressure, local ischemia decreases local arteriolar tone in that ischemic tissue. Two theories prevail as to the mechanism causing this local arterial vasodilation: a vasodilator theory and a lack-of-oxygen theory. The former postulates that a decrease in oxygen availability causes tissue ischemia that increases local adenosine and lactic acid levels. Local release of adenosine and lactic acid causes immediate vasodilation. The other theory is that local tissue ischemia results in arteriolar vasodilation via retrograde endothelial signaling to those feeding arterioles from the ischemic capillaries. Other nutrients implicated in this mechanism include thiamine (e.g., *beriberi* disease), riboflavin, fatty acids, and glucose [1]. Beyond these two mechanisms, nitric oxide, formally known as endothelium-derived relaxing factor [2], contributes to upstream vasodilation once local flow is increased. Increased flow causes shear stress on the local endothelium, causing direct release of nitric oxide to give distal arterioles appropriately increased capacitance [3]. Other plasma substrates involved in local control of vascular tone are electrolytes (e.g., calcium and magnesium), hydrogen ions, carbon dioxide, and other anions such as acetate.

There are exceptions to this local regulation in specific tissues and organs that use blood flow for other purposes. Specifically, renal blood flow is much higher than the metabolic demands of the kidney because the role of the kidneys is to filter solute and intravascular volume control. Thus, renal vein oxygen saturation is usually very high (close to 90%). If an otherwise healthy subject is given a large intravascular fluid bolus, although cardiac output may transiently go up during the active infusion time, blood pressure will remain constant, and renal blood flow and urine output will both go up proportionally. Similarly, the skin increases and decreases its blood flow to sustain a constant internal core temperature independent of dermal metabolic demand. Both skin and renal blood flow above their metabolic need level are highly dependent of arterial input pressure, and systemic hypotension causes marked decreases in skin and renal blood flow.

Hence, these local metabolic demands altering local blood flow occur within the context of systemic blood pressure autoregulation. As long as systemic blood pressure is above some minimal level, local blood flow autoregulation allows tissues to maintain adequate flow to meet their metabolic demand. However, if arterial pressure falls below a level that would allow a totally vasodilated periphery to sustain its blood flow at levels needed to sustain its metabolic needs, then tissue hypoperfusion occurs with its associated ischemic-induced loss of organ-specific function. If hypotension is sustained, organ injury and death ensue. Thus, prevention of systemic hypotension, even for short intervals, is a cardiovascular regulatory priority.

5.3 Systemic Vasomotor Control

As a whole, the nervous system contains many different excitatory and inhibitory signaling systems to maintain a regulated central blood pressure and reginal blood flow. Under normal conditions, the net effect of these signals is one of the partial vasoconstrictions [1]. The central blood pressure control is primarily driven by two fast-acting mechanisms: over seconds by baroreceptors in the aortic arch and carotid sinus and over minutes to hours by left and right atrial stretch receptors and cerebral baroreceptors. When activated, the atrial and cerebral receptors stimulate the release of atrial and brain natriuretic peptides (ANP and BNP, respectively) that not only change renal tubular resorption rate but also arterial tone. Finally, the aldosterone-angiotensin system fine-tunes arterial pressure and effective circulating blood volume on a more chronic (hours to days) time line.

Globally, the rapid response blood pressure control is mediated through the autonomic nervous system, primarily through the sympathetic (and to a lesser extent, parasympathetic) chains that exit the thoracolumbar spinal column. Hypotension stimulates the baroreceptor stretch receptors to increase their output to the brain stem to increase sympathetic output. Stimulation of the sympathetic nerve fibers will lead to arterial vasoconstriction via release of norepinephrine. This sympathetic network affects the arterial system up to, but not including, the precapillary sphincter and capillaries [1]. Moment-to-moment activation of this systemic sympathetic response is primarily driven by the baroreceptor response [4, 5]. These receptors are located in the aortic arch and carotid sinus; when these areas are stretched, afferent inhibitory signals are sent to the sympathetic pathway leading to a decrease in systemic vascular resistance [6]. Conversely, an increase in parasympathetic signaling is noted, commonly demonstrated as bradycardia during carotid massage.

These baroreceptor responses are not generalizable to all disease states. With extrinsic carotid massage, hypotension has been observed without evidence of venodilation. However, models of hemorrhage and negative intravascular pressure (the opposite physiologic stimulus to the carotid sinus) have repeatedly demonstrated venoconstriction, but only in the splanchnic circulation and not the periphery [5].

Other cardiopulmonary pressure-sensitive receptors lie in the atria, the left ventricle, and the lung parenchyma. Animal studies have demonstrated that lack of atrial stretch will lead to arterial vasoconstriction [7], and to a similar effect but through an opposite mechanism, activation of ventricular stretch receptors will lead to vasodilation and bradycardia [8], pulmonary congestion activates juxtapulmonary capillary receptors to induce tachycardia, and inflation of the lungs leads to vasodilation [9]. In summary, experimental models have demonstrated multiple, fast-acting, pressure-related mechanisms of vasomotor control consistent with protective mechanisms to sustain a constant perfusion pressure.

Chemoreceptors located in the aortic and carotid bodies can also modulate sympathetic tone. These chemoreceptor organs are sensitive to lack of arterial oxygen, excess arterial carbon dioxide, and excess arterial hydrogen ion concentration. Detection of any of these three conditions will yield an increase in vasomotor tone. Interestingly, these bodies also respond to decreases in arterial pressure, but they are less sensitive than the aortic arch and carotid sinus.

The central nervous system (CNS) also plays a destabilizing role in arterial pressure regulation when the brain experiences isolated hypoperfusion due to increased intracranial pressure as part of the Cushing reflex [10]. A lack of blood flow to cerebral tissue significant enough to cause ischemia increases local concentration of carbon dioxide, stimulating the medullary vasomotor center, ultimately sending a powerful positive stimulus to the peripheral sympathetic nervous system [1]. This causes systemic hypertension in order to sustain central blood flow in the setting of increased intracranial pressure and reflex bradycardia because the sympathetic output carotid and aortic body baroreceptors are inhibited, whereas parasympathetic output is increased. Furthermore, remainder of the vascular beds is exposed to a very high arterial pressure which often exceeds the autoregulatory range arterial pressure control, causing pressure-dependent hyperperfusion of that tissue-inducing end-organ edema and injury.

Finally, central arterial pressure is not an organ perfusion pressure. Organ perfusion pressure is defined as the input pressure minus the outflow pressure. Arterial input pressure can be lower than mean arterial pressure if arterial resistance beyond the central arterial capacitor is high. For example, hepatic arterial pressure is about 20% lower than mean arterial pressure owing to the high hepatic arterial resistance. Furthermore, cardiac blood flow cannot occur into a contracting heart muscle. Thus, coronary arterial input pressure is closer to diastolic arterial pressure than to mean arterial pressure. In most non-active tissues, the increased resting tone in the arterioles and precapillary sphincters defines a critical closing pressure greater than venous pressure which is the back pressure to organ flow. Importantly, this critical closing pressure is not constant, varies across and among capillary beds and organs, and changes with changes in metabolic activity. Under normal conditions, this allows local blood flow to be tightly controlled so as to maximize flow efficiency. However, as hypotension develops or metabolic activity of the tissue increases, the arteriolar and precapillary tone diminishes such that once fully dilated tissue or outflow venous pressure becomes the back pressure to organ blood flow. For the brain, the outflow pressure is either intracranial pressure or venous pressure in the head, whichever is higher. For the left ventricle, it is left ventricular diastolic pressure or right atrial pressure, whichever is highest. For the intra-abdominal organs, it is either intra-abdominal pressure or central venous pressure, whichever is higher. For the kidneys, it is intracapsular pressure, intra-abdominal pressure, or central venous pressure, whichever is higher. Since all these back pressures can vary independent of each other in disease states, targeting a minimal mean arterial pressure along may not insure adequate organ perfusion pressure among and within organs.

5.4 Disturbance of Normal Blood Pressure Autoregulation

5

In normal physiologic states, even though the above mechanisms aim at keeping blood pressure relatively constant, organ flow is also maintained over a wide range of mean arterial pressures, through the similar feedback mechanisms described above. In extremes of flow regulatory blood pressure, control mechanisms are overwhelmed. This explains the end-organ injury seen with acute, accelerated hypertension (e.g., posterior reversible encephalopathy) and the scattered tissue ischemia seen in states of excess vasodilator-induced hypotension. In the case of significant hypotension, local vasodilation can only provide increased flow with adequate inflow pressures. Thus, when the baroreceptor generalized vasoconstrictor response can no longer augment systemic vascular tone enough to sustain arterial pressure due to inadequate cardiac output, local tissue demands invariably cannot be met by their selective vasodilation; the supply of oxygenated blood is effectively defined by the organ perfusion pressure, and regional tissue vasodilation will either be ineffective or divert flow from another vascular bed in need of flow. These conditions are collectively called circulatory shock and underscore the concept that systemic hypotension is always pathological because it reflects a failure of normal adaptive mechanisms to sustain organ perfusion pressure.

Circulatory shock can be caused by conditions that limit cardiac output due to inadequate blood volume (e.g., hemorrhage), vascular obstruction (e.g., pulmonary emboli), or impaired ventricular pump function (e.g., myocardial infarction). Similarly, circulatory shock can be caused by vasoplegia (e.g., sepsis) even if blood flow is high. But in all these conditions, if hypotension develops, control of local blood flow distribution is impaired and end-organ dysfunction also develops. Circulatory shock, or the syndrome of inadequate organ perfusion, is a state when baroreceptors are maximally stimulated by hypotension. The resultant sympathetic discharge (primarily norepinephrine release) leads to alpha-adrenergic vasoconstriction. Relative flow is then primarily a result of alpha-receptor concentration in the tissue-specific vascular region. The skin and skeletal muscle have the most alpha-receptors, while the coronary arteries have very few and the brain none [11]. Clinically this can be appreciated by skin mottling in states of shock without pathologic vasodilation (e.g., cardiogenic shock), or skin necrosis after infusion of alpha-adrenergic agents, such as norepinephrine [12]. This mechanism of alpha-receptor-mediated preferential vasoconstriction not only allows for preferential blood flow to critical organs but is an essential mechanism of efficient oxygen delivery (DO_2). When DO_2 drops below a critical threshold (DO_2c), local tissue DO_2 becomes pressure-dependent and tissue ischemia usually develops [13].

Sepsis, a form of vasodilatory shock, induces a vasoplegic state wherein despite increased circulating levels of catecholamines (e.g., norepinephrine and epinephrine), arterial vasomotor tone is decreased. Presumably, either alpha-adrenergic receptors on the vasculature becomes unresponsive and require higher levels of catecholamines to increase tone, or local mediators overwhelm the vasoconstrictive capacity of endogenous catecholamines, or both. The exact mechanisms by which this vasoplegia occurs in sepsis are not completely understood but probably include (1) hyperpolarization of the vascular smooth muscle cells rendering them less responsive to changes in transmembrane potential limiting intrinsic contraction; (2) pharmacologic vasodilation by the local presence of excess nitric oxide produced by sepsis-induced activation of inducible nitric oxide synthetase and the local release of other vasoactive mediators related by local inflammatory responses, like bradykinin, prostaglandin, and leukotriene species [12]; and (3) alpha-adrenergic receptor downregulation either due to autodigestion or simple internalization from the associated dysfunctional membrane glycocalyx [11].

On the other end of the spectrum, chronic essential hypertension presents a different autoregulatory challenge. Essential hypertension resets the normal autoregulatory pressure and flow relations upward and to the right with pressure on the *x*-axis (◘ Fig. 5.1). Thus, pressure-dependent low flow below the autoregulatory range will occur in patients with essential hypertension at mean arterial pressures much above the minimal threshold values of otherwise healthy individuals.

Several studies have documented the "J-shaped" curve of cardiovascular and cerebral risk in blood pressure control in patients with essential hypertension [14]. Cerebral blood flow regulation has been demonstrated as having new set points in chronic arterial hypertension [15]. If systemic blood pressure is brought too low by antihypertensive therapy, even though the actual pressures would be in the otherwise normal range (e.g., 120/80 mmHg), there is an increased risk of stroke, renal injury, and myocardial ischemia [16]. Since essential hypertension is one of the most common chronic diseases seen in patients over 40 years of age, understanding this interaction between autoregulation changes and blood flow is important.

A recent clinical trial by Asfar et al. [13] in the control of arterial pressure in septic shock patients using norepinephrine illustrates interaction between the two states of altered or impaired autoregulation, sepsis and essential hypertension. In this study patients with septic shock were treated with mean arterial pressure targets of either 65–75 or 85–95 mmHg, along with usual care. They found that in otherwise normal patients without prior histories of essential hypertension, there was no evidence that targeting a mean arterial pressure of 85–95 mmHg was better at restoring organ blood flow or minimizing risk of death as compared to the lower mean arterial pressure range of 65–75 mmHg. However, patients treated at the high mean arterial pressure range had more arrhythmias, presumably because of the high levels of vasoactive drug infusion they required to sustain

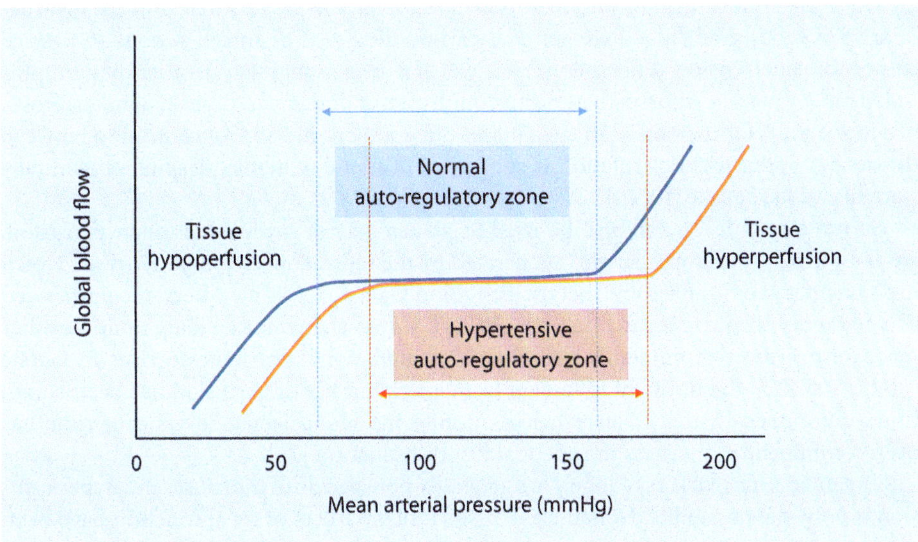

◘ **Fig. 5.1** Effect of varying Mean Arterial Pressure on Global Blood Flow in normal subjects and those with essential hypertension

these higher mean arterial pressure levels. Importantly, in those patients with both septic shock and a history of essential hypertension, targeting the lower mean arterial pressure range was associated with more evidence of renal hypoperfusion (increase in serum creatinine) and injury (need for dialysis).

5.5 Clinical Detection of Inadequate Autoregulation

5

The findings of the study by Asfar et al. mentioned above cannot yet be generalized to all patients in practice, but they are consistent with our understanding of lower limits of autoregulation and thresholds for organ injury. The exact range of arterial blood pressure autoregulation for any given patient cannot be determined exactly at bedside. Measuring the perfusion of specific tissue beds is cumbersome if not impossible for patients in the ICU. Thus the only way to know if a given mean arterial pressure is adequate for tissue is to measure organ function. Even this can be difficult, so surrogates of organ perfusion can be helpful in determining if a measured mean arterial pressure is adequate for the patient at bedside.

Venous oxygen saturation, either a true mixed venous sample from a pulmonary artery catheter (SvO_2) or its surrogate from a central venous catheter in the superior vena cava ($ScvO_2$), can be used as a surrogate marker of organ perfusion. These values represent the amount of oxygen bound to hemoglobin returning to pulmonary circulation after extraction from local tissues. Values below the normal values (70% and 75% for SvO_2 and $ScvO_2$, respectively) are indicative of one of three possible states: arterial hypoxemia, anemia, or decreased blood flow. In the last state, tissues are in contact with hemoglobin molecules longer, allowing for more oxygen extraction. Since venous oxygen saturation has many determinants, a low SvO_2 value by itself does not equate to inadequate autoregulation. In fact, SvO_2 may be high in states of high-output shock associated with tissue hypoperfusion, due to maldistribution of blood flow as commonly seen in sepsis [17].

Concerns regarding high-output hypoperfusion have led to an interest in the measure of arteriovenous gradients of oxygen and carbon dioxide. The mixed venous-to-arterial carbon dioxide tension difference (Pv-aCO_2) has been suggested as a cardiac output-independent marker of tissue bed perfusion. In states of decreased perfusion, anaerobic production of CO_2 increases [18]. An increasing gradient of CO_2 concentration between the venous and arterial circulation is suggestive of tissue ischemia, despite a potentially normal cardiac output [19, 20].

Serum lactate levels can also be used as a surrogate of inadequate organ perfusion. Under normal conditions, lactate is generated by the redox conversion of pyruvate, which itself is generated by anaerobic metabolism. Blood lactate levels have been recommended as a marker of adequate organ resuscitation [21]. However, in disease states, multiple other mechanisms, most prominently beta-agonist stimulation, contribute to rises in lactate production [22]; the utility of following lactate as a marker of perfusion has been sometimes questioned [23, 24]. Nevertheless, monitoring blood lactate levels over time has been recommended to assess the adequacy of resuscitation [25].

Organ-specific markers of injury are generally nonspecific to the cause, and hypoperfusion is only one possibility. Nonetheless, historically markers of renal function have been used to guide perfusion-oriented resuscitation. In states of systemic hypotension and resultant decreased renal blood flow, multiple mechanisms lead to a decrease in glomerular filtration rate and rise in serum creatinine with a decrease in urine output [26]. Unfortunately, a rise in serum creatinine concentration suggestive of injury can be delayed by up to 48 h after injury [27]. Similarly, urine output measurements have been found to be nonspecific [28]. Multiple other markers of early renal injury have been investigated, the most promising of which is the product of urinary concentrations of tissue inhibitor of metalloproteinases (TIMP-2) and insulin-like growth factor-binding protein-7 (IGFBP-7) [29]. It remains to be seen, however, how utilization of this test translates to clinical practice.

Take-Home Messages

Arterial blood pressure is maintained through multiple systemic and local mechanisms. Mean arterial pressure is maintained systemically by multiple rapid-acting mechanisms. Along a wide range of systemic pressures, local vascular beds are able to regulate local perfusion based on metabolic demands. However, disease states associated with marked physiologic stress, with or without a chronic shift of the normal autoregulatory range, can lead to local tissue and systemic organ dysfunction. It is of paramount importance that measuring systemic blood pressure alone does not represent failure or success of autoregulation. Organ hypoperfusion can be appreciated clinically, albeit imperfectly, with the clinical exam, serum biomarkers, blood gas measurements and gradients, and blood lactate levels.

References

1. Guyton AC, Hall JE. Textbook of medical physiology. Philadelphia: W. B. Saunders; 2005.
2. Loscalzo J. The identification of nitric oxide as endothelium-derived relaxing factor. Circ Res. 2013;113:100–3.
3. Tibballs. The role of nitric oxide (formerly endothelium-derived relaxing factor-EDRF) in vasodilatation and vasodilator therapy. Anaesth Intensive Care. 1993;21:759–73.
4. Thrasher T. Baroreceptors and the long-term control of blood pressure. Exp Physiol. 2004;89:331–5.
5. Abboud F, Heistad D, Mark A, Schmid P. Reflex control of the peripheral circulation. Prog Cardiovasc Dis. 1976;18:371–403.
6. Bronk S. Afferent impulses in the carotid sinus nerve I. the relation of the discharge from single end organs to arterial blood pressure. J Cell Compar Physl. 1932;1:113–30.
7. Johnson JA, Moore WW, Segar WE. Small changes in left atrial pressure and plasma antidiuretic hormone titers in dogs. Am J Physiol. 1969;217:210–4.
8. Salisbury P, Cross C, Rieben A. Reflex effects of left ventricular distention. Circ Res. 1960;8:530–4.
9. Ott S. Vasodepressor reflex from lung inflation in the rabbit. Am J Physiol. 1971;221:889–95.
10. Fodstad H, Kelly P, Buchfelder M. History of the cushing reflex. Eur Man Med. 2006;59:1132–7.
11. Bucher M, Kees F, Taeger K, Kurtz A. Cytokines down-regulate α1-adrenergic receptor expression during endotoxemia. Crit Care Med. 2003;31:566.
12. Mentzelopoulos S, Gkizioti S. Vasogenic shock physiology. Open Access Emerg Med. 2011;3:1–6.
13. Asfar P, Meziani F, Hamel J-F, et al. High versus low blood-pressure target in patients with septic shock. N Engl J Med. 2014;370:1583–93.
14. Verdecchia P, Angeli F, Mazzotta G, Garofoli M, Reboldi G. Aggressive blood pressure lowering is dangerous: the J-curve response to aggressive blood pressure lowering is dangerous: the J-curve: con side of the argument. Hypertension. 2014;63:37–40.
15. Strandgaard S, Olesen J, Skinhoj E, Lassen NA. Autoregulation of brain circulation in severe arterial hypertension. Br Med J. 1973;1:507–10.
16. Gifford R. Management of Hypertensive Crises. JAMA. 1991;266:829–35.
17. Robin E, Costecalde M, Lebuffe G, Vallet B. Clinical relevance of data from the pulmonary artery catheter. Crit Care. 2006;10:S3.
18. Mallat J, Lemyze M, Tronchon L, Vallet B, Thevenin D. Use of venous-to-arterial carbon dioxide tension difference to guide resuscitation therapy in septic shock. World J Crit Care Med. 2016;5:47–56.

19. Van Beest P, Lont M, Holman N, Loef B, Kuiper M, Boerma C. Central venous-arterial pCO2 difference as a tool in resuscitation of septic patients. Intens Care Med. 2013;39:1034–9.
20. Chua M, Kuan W. Venous-to-arterial carbon dioxide differences and the microcirculation in sepsis. Ann Transl Med. 2016;4:62.
21. Dellinger P, Levy M, Rhodes A, Annane D, Gerlach H, Opal S, Sevransky J, Sprung C, Douglas I, Jaeschke R. Surviving sepsis campaign: international guidelines for management of severe sepsis and septic shock, 2012. Intensive Care Med. 2013;39:165–228.
22. Ingelfinger J, Kraut J, Madias N. Lactic acidosis. N Engl J Med. 2014;371:2309–19.
23. Kushimoto S, Akaishi S, Sato T, Nomura R, Fujita M, Kudo D, Kawazoe Y, Yoshida Y, Miyagawa N. Lactate, a useful marker for disease mortality and severity but an unreliable marker of tissue hypoxia/hypoperfusion in critically ill patients. Acute Med Surg. 2016;3:293–7.
24. James H, Luchette F, McCarter F, Fischer J. Lactate is an unreliable indicator of tissue hypoxia in injury or sepsis. Lancet. 1999;354:505–8.
25. Vincent JL, Quintairos e Silva A, jr CL, Taccone FS. The value of blood lactate kinetics in critically ill patients: a systematic review. Crit Care. 2016;20:257.
26. Basile D, Anderson M, Sutton T. Pathophysiology of acute kidney injury. Compr Physiol. 2012;2:1303–53.
27. Koyner J. Assessment and diagnosis of renal dysfunction in the ICU. Chest. 2012;141:1584.
28. Prowle J, Liu Y-L, Licari E, et al. Oliguria as predictive biomarker of acute kidney injury in critically ill patients. Crit Care. 2011;15:1–10.
29. Kashani K, Al-Khafaji A, Ardiles T, et al. Discovery and validation of cell cycle arrest biomarkers in human acute kidney injury. Crit Care. 2013;17:1–12.

Pulmonary Circulation

Marco Maggiorini

M. R. Pinsky et al. (eds.), *Hemodynamic Monitoring*, Lessons from the ICU,
https://doi.org/10.1007/978-3-319-69269-2_6

Learning Objectives

The pulmonary circulation is a low-pressure high-flow circuit hidden behind the thorax and therefore difficult to assess. The characteristics of the pulmonary circulation favours gas exchange which is crucial for preserving cell metabolism and hence organ function. In this chapter you will learn about structural and functional characteristics of the pulmonary circulation and its major physiologic differences with the systemic circulation. In addition we will review its haemodynamic properties that are of importance when you assess the interaction between mechanical ventilation and pulmonary circulation or when you treat heart and lung diseases at the bedside. Pulmonary vascular motor tone is crucial to avoid ventilation-perfusion mismatch. On the other hand, elevated pulmonary vascular motor tone may lead to pulmonary hypertension, hence jeopardising right ventricular function. You will learn about the key factors that influence pulmonary vascular motor tone and if elevated over time cause pulmonary vascular remodelling and pulmonary hypertension. At the end we will review the spectrum of pulmonary hypertension in the setting of the intensive care unit.

6.1 Introduction

The discovery of the pulmonary circulation began with the rejection of Galen's and Ibn Sina's (Avicenna's) doctrine, which stated that the liver produces blood that is enriched with air from the lungs and heat from the heart being evaporated or consumed by the other organs of the body. It was the seminal work of Ibn Al-Nafis (1212–1288) in the Arab world and Michael Servetus (1511–1553) and Renaldus Columbus (1516–1559) in the European world that led to the discovery of the pulmonary circulation, as we understand it today. Based on this work, William Harvey (1578–1657) later discovered the "motion of the heart" and the circulation of blood and Marcello Malpighi (1628–1694) the pulmonary capillaries [1–3]. However it took another 300 years until the German physician Julius Kolb (1865) made the first anatomic description of pulmonary vascular disease. He reported on a high-grade pulmonary artery sclerosis with consequent hypertrophy of the right side of the heart found during the autopsy of a 24-year-old male [4]. Nevertheless it took another 80 years to understand the relationship between cardiac and pulmonary physiology. André F. Cournand and Dickinson W. Richards (1945) were the first to report results of a right heart and pulmonary artery catheterisation via a cubital vein [5]. Together with Werner Forssmann, who introduced a urinary catheter into his right heart in 1929 [6], they were jointly awarded with the Nobel Prize in Physiology of Medicine in 1956. The bedside investigation of the pulmonary circulation became only a routine after the cardiologists Harold J. Swan and William Ganz (1970) designed a balloon-tipped pulmonary artery catheter that could be introduced in the pulmonary circulation without fluoroscopy [7]. The use of the pulmonary catheter in the intensive care unit is important for the understanding of the physiology and the pathophysiology of the pulmonary circulation but requires extensive teaching of intensivists. This became evident after the publication of the first reports upon intensivists poor knowledge of the technology [8, 9]. In the present chapter, we will provide the basic knowledge on the physiology and pathophysiology of the pulmonary circulation from the perspective of the clinician taking care of his patient at the bedside in the intensive care unit.

6.2 Structural Characteristics of Pulmonary Vessels

Compared to other organs, the pulmonary circulation is unique due to its flexible structure that is able to meet the needs for gas exchange under different environmental conditions both at rest and during exercise. In the air-filled lung, the configuration of alveoli and capillaries is able to change rapidly in response to alterations of transmural pressure (pressures in the air, arteries and veins). Moreover the pulmonary circulation is able to cope with positive inspiratory pressures (within a certain limit of inspiratory pressure and tidal volume) as they are applied during lung-protective mechanical ventilation.

The pulmonary circulation differs in its shape, structure and compliance from the systemic circulation [10]. The vessels of the systemic circulation can be classified in large conducting arteries and veins that differ from each other in diameter, wall structure and wall thickness. These large vessels connect consecutively to small arteries and veins (with minimal media layer) and capillaries. The muscle layer of the media of the pulmonary arteries and veins is much thinner compared to vessels of the same size of the systemic circulation. This difference reflects the lower pressure in the pulmonary circulation. The difference in blood pressure between the two systems is related to the existence of high-resistance arterioles of the systemic circulation, which are missing in the pulmonary circulation [10]. In their absence much of the pressure in the pulmonary artery is transmitted in a highly pulsatile flow to the permeable precapillary arteries and the alveolar capillaries (◘ Fig. 6.1). Does the hydrostatic pressure transmitted from the pulmonary artery to the precapillary arteries and capillaries exceed their permeability threshold, then pulmonary oedema is formed [11]. This is the mechanism of high-pressure and high-flow pulmonary oedema as it is found at high altitude or consequently to the resection of more than two-thirds of the lung [12].

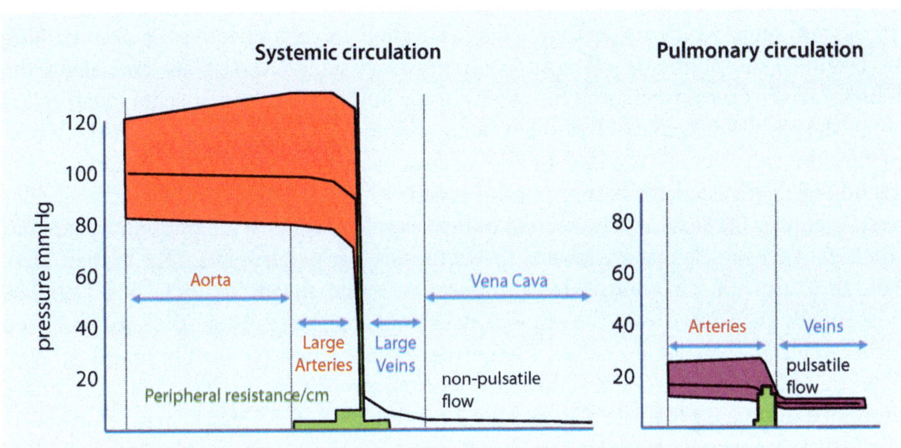

◘ **Fig. 6.1** Functional differences between the systemic and the pulmonary circulation. The pulmonary circulation differs in its shape, structure and compliance from the systemic circulation. The difference in blood pressure between the two is related to the high-resistance arterioles of the systemic circulation that are missing in the pulmonary circulation. In their absence, much of the pressure in the pulmonary artery is transmitted in a highly pulsatile flow to the permeable precapillary arteries, the alveolar capillaries and the pulmonary veins

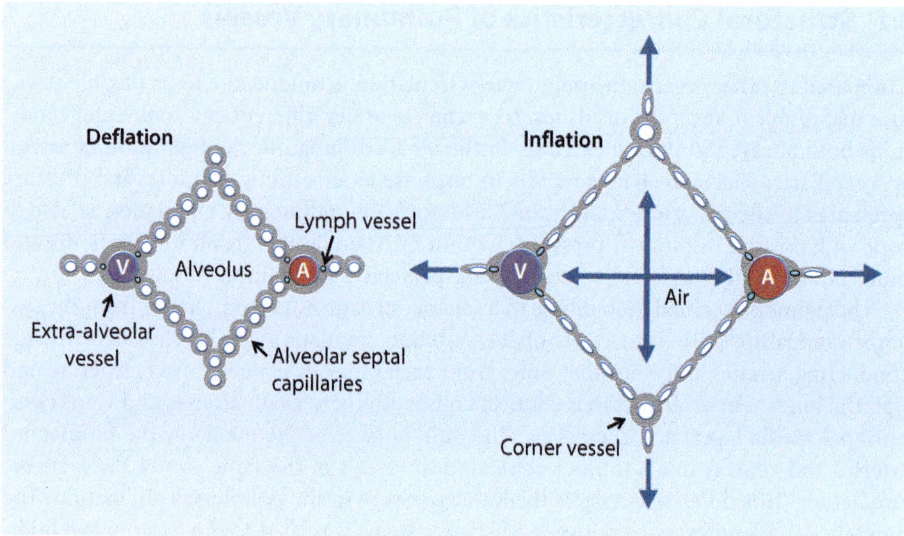

Fig. 6.2 Effect of inflation on alveolar and extra-alveolar vessels. Extra-alveolar vessels, both arteries (A) and veins (V), are surrounded by a sheath of loose connective tissue containing the origin of the pulmonary lymphatics. Alveolar septa insert radial to the sheath of loose connective tissue surrounding extra-alveolar vessels. Consequently the radial pool exercised by the alveolar wall during inspiration results in the creation of a perivascular subatmospheric pressure leading to an increase in extra-alveolar vessel diameter. Corner vessels are located inside the alveolar parenchyma and are therefore not surrounded by a connective tissue sheath. They are protected against high alveolar air pressures and therefore stay open in deflation and inflation. Corner vessels are characteristically found in West zones 1 and 2 and not in zone 3 of the lung

Furthermore and unique for the lung is the presence of extra-alveolar vessels, both arteries and veins, which are surrounded by a sheath of loose connective tissue containing the origin of the pulmonary lymphatics (pulmonary lymph vessels are crucial for the drainage of the excess interstitial fluids within the lung) [13]. Alveolar septa insert radial to the sheath of loose connective tissue surrounding extra-alveolar vessels [14]. Consequently the radial pool exercised by the alveolar wall during inspiration results in the creation of a perivascular subatmospheric pressure leading to an increase in extra-alveolar vessel diameter (Fig. 6.2). The second unique element found in the pulmonary circulation are corner vessels that are located inside the alveolar parenchyma. Due to their location, they are not surrounded by a connective tissue sheath of their one [15, 16]. Functionally they differ from the other alveolar wall capillaries in that they are protected against high alveolar air pressures. Corner vessels are characteristically found in West zones 1 and 2 but not in zone 3 of the lung where all alveolar capillaries are open and have a rounded outline (Fig. 6.3). Under zone 2 conditions, corner vessels may act as shortcuts between precapillary arteries and veins increasing the pulmonary dead space (ventilated but not perfused alveoli) and right-to-left shunt [17, 18]. Importantly, most of the patients undergoing positive pressure ventilation are in zone 2 conditions. In zone 2 the applied PEEP opens collapsed alveoli but may also over-distend opened alveoli at the same time.

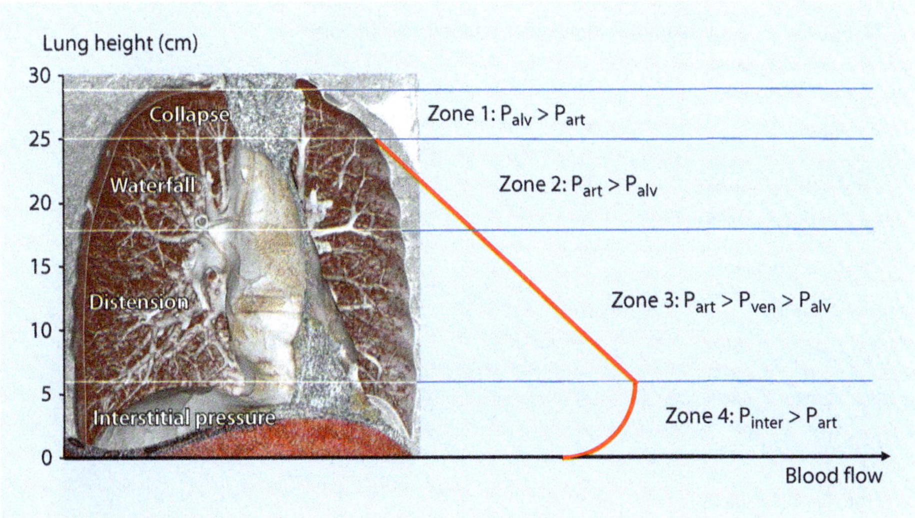

Fig. 6.3 Zonal distribution of perfusion in an upright lung as determined by the interrelationship between arterial, alveolar, venous and interstitial pressure. Gravity-dependent lung perfusion progressively increases from zones 1 and 2 to 3. In zone 1 the flow is limited to the alveolar corner vessels, whereas most alveolar wall capillaries are closed. Zone 2 is similar to zone 1 except that alveolar wall perfusion is increased by patches of open capillaries. In zone 3 alveolar capillaries are all open because venous pressure exceeds alveolar air pressure. In zone 4, the most dependent part of the lung, interstitial pressure exceeds venous pressure, which causes alveolar wall capillaries to close hence perfusion to decrease

6.3 Pulmonary Vascular Function

Compared to the systemic circulation, the pulmonary circulation is a high-flow low-pressure circuit of increased frailty allowing blood gas exchange to occur [12, 19, 20] (Table 6.1). Consequently, the pulmonary circulation is very sensitive to mechanical influences that may cause capillary walls to leak and under extreme conditions to rupture with consecutive leak of plasma, proteins and red blood cells into the interstitial space.

The real filtration pressure in the lung is not the pulmonary artery occlusion pressure (Ppao) but the pulmonary capillary pressure (Pc). Studies using the double-occlusion techniques in animals [21, 22] and the single-occlusion technique in men [12] identified the Pc being approximately 1–4 mmHg above the Pla (left atrial pressure). In the ICU setting, the Pc can be estimated by the analysis of the pulmonary artery curve after arterial occlusion by the balloon at the tip of the pulmonary artery catheter as shown in Fig. 6.4. In healthy individuals, Pc is around 10 mmHg, and the threshold for a hydrostatic leakage in the absence of inflammation is around 18 mmHg. Systemic and local inflammation decreases the hydrostatic threshold for the leak of fluid into the pulmonary interstitium. Plasmatic oncotic pressure and pulmonary lymphatics play a crucial role clearing fluid out of the lung. Based on the measured distribution of resistances in perfused normal lungs, with 60% arterial resistance and 40% capillary-venous resistance, Pc can be estimated from the simple equation of Gaar et al. [23], $Pc = Pla - 0.4 \times (mPpa - Pla)$, where mPpa is mean pulmonary artery pressure. An increase of the capillary-venous resistance has been

Table 6.1 Limits of normal of pulmonary blood flow and pressure

Variables	Mean	Limits of normal
Q L/min	6.4	4.4–8.4
Ppa systolic, mmHg	19	13–26
Ppa diastolic, mmHg	10	6–16
Ppa mean, mmHg	13	7–19
Pcap, mmHg	10	8–12
Ppao, mmHg	9	5–13
Pra, mmHg	5	1–9
PVR, dyn.s.cm^{-5}	50	11–99

From Refs. [12, 19, 20]
These results were obtained in 55 healthy resting volunteers. *Q* flow, *Ppa* pulmonary artery pressure, *Pcap* pulmonary capillary pressure (estimated by arterial occlusion pressure method), *Ppao* pulmonary artery occlusion pressure (wedge pressure), *Pra* right atrial pressure, *PVR* pulmonary vascular resistance

described, i.e. in high-altitude pulmonary oedema (hypoxic venous constriction) [12] and in the late phase of ARDS [24], leading to high capillary filtration pressures.

The pulmonary blood flow generated by the thin-walled right ventricle is driven by the pressure difference between the pulmonary artery (inflow pressure) and the pressure in the left atrium (outflow pressure). Assuming that the flow through the pulmonary circulation behaves as a laminar fluid within rigid straight and cylindrical capillary tubes of Newtonian fluids (Hagen-Poiseuille law), the functional state of the pulmonary circulation can be approximated by a single number, the pulmonary vascular resistance (PVR):

$$\text{PVR} = (\text{mPpa} - \text{Pla}) / \text{cardiac output}$$

The difference (mPpa – Pla) describes the driving pressure of the pulmonary circulation. The PVR is a good indicator of the state of constriction or dilatation of the pulmonary resistive vessels and is useful for detecting changes in the arteriolar vessel calibre due to changes in tone and/or structure. PVR increases with age. This is due to a slight increase in mPpa and more importantly a decrease in cardiac output leading to doubling of the PVR over five decades [25]. Body position affects PVR due to changes in venous return and in the forces exercised over the lung tissue by gravity that result in a de-recruitment of pulmonary vessels (Fig. 6.3). Accordingly haemodynamic measurements of the pulmonary circulation in the critically ill patient should always be performed in a supine position at rest, where a large proportion of the lung is within zone 3 conditions.

The limitation of a single PVR determination is its non-reliability for the evaluation of the functional state of the pulmonary circulation at variable flow rates. The PVR calculation assumes that the relationship between pulmonary artery pressure and cardiac output (Ppa/CO) is linear and crosses the pressure axis at the value of Pla allowing the PVR to be constant and independent of the absolute level of pressure or flow. However, in a number

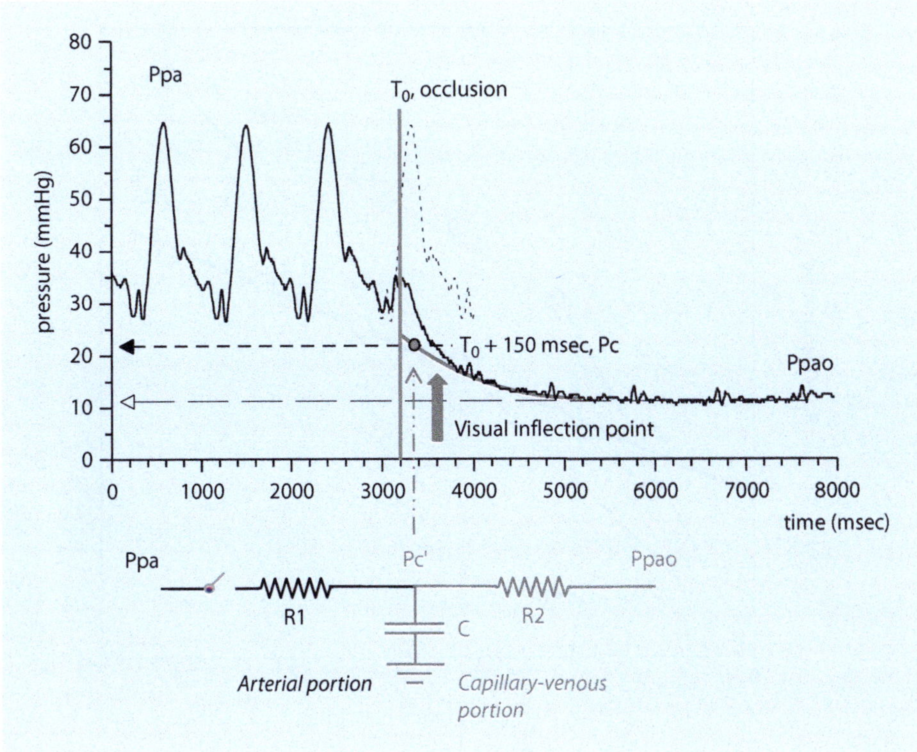

Fig. 6.4 Pulmonary artery pressure (Ppa) trace obtained in a person with high-altitude pulmonary oedema at 4559 m showing a capillary pressure (Pc) of 22 mmHg. The Pc is estimated either by visual inspection of the pressure trace after occlusion of the pulmonary artery with the balloon of the Swan-Ganz catheter (visual inflection point of the curve) or extrapolation of the exponential fitting of the slow component of the pressure decay curve to the moment of occlusion (T_0) plus 150 ms. The inflection point of the pressure decay curve is the intersection point between the rapid and slow part of the curve trace. The first fast component of the curve corresponds to the stop of flow through the resistance of the arteries (R1), whereas the second part of the pressure decay curve corresponds to the emptying of the compliant capillaries (C) through the resistance of the veins (R2). The pressure at the end of the pressure decay curve is the pulmonary artery occlusion pressure (Ppao)

of conditions such as hypoxia, ARDS and other pulmonary as well as cardiac diseases, it has been shown that both the slope and the towards zero-flow extrapolated *y*-axis intercept of the multipoint Ppa/CO plot do increase [26–28] (Fig. 6.5). While the increase in slope of the Ppa/CO relationship can be explained by a decrease of the cumulated surface section area of the pulmonary resistive vessels, the cause for the increase of the extrapolated intercept of the Ppa/CO plot is less clear. As a possible explanation, Permutt et al. proposed a model made of parallel collapsible vessels with various closing pressures which are progressively recruited while cardiac output increases (the waterfall model) [29]. Accordingly the extrapolated pressure intercept is likely to represent the weighed mean of closing pressures, hence under normal conditions Pla. However, in some particular circumstances frequently found in the intensive care settings, the mean closing pressure exceeds left atrial pressure, i.e. the de-recruited upper lung zone 1 [30], pulmonary hypertension in ARDS [28] and left heart failure [27]. This is a tentative explanation for the

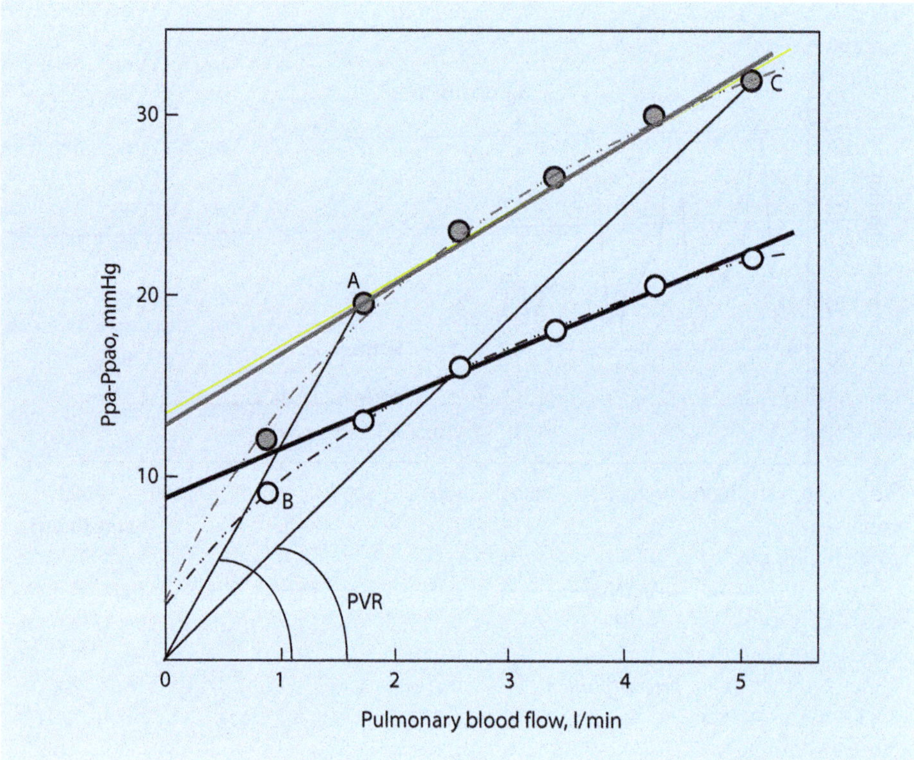

Fig. 6.5 Multipoint transpulmonary artery pressure (Ppa – Ppao)/flow (*Q*) relationship at two levels of pulmonary vascular resistance (PVR). At the flow rates observed in the clinical setting (>2 l/min), the Ppa/*Q* relationship is almost linear to the crossing point of the *y*-axis representing the outflow pressure of the pulmonary circulation (left atrial pressure). Pulmonary hypertension increases the slope and the outflow pressure (*y*-axis intercept) of the pulmonary circulation. The increase in slope is explained by the increase in vascular resistance. The increase in *y*-axis intercept illustrates the emergence of a pulmonary closing pressure which is higher than left atrial pressure (i.e. de-recruited upper lung zone 1 or increased pulmonary venous resistance). The dotted lines represent the curvilinear fitting of the multipoint relationship towards zero flow, which takes into account the natural distensibility of the pulmonary vessels. The thin lines starting from the zero-intercept connecting to B and A and C illustrate the limitation of PVR calculation. From A to B, PVR does not change, while from A to C, PVR decreases in the presence of aggravated pulmonary hypertension, as assessed by higher pressure at a given flow

increase in the towards zero-flow extrapolated *y*-axis intercept of the multipoint Ppa/CO plot in these and other similar conditions.

In the pulmonary circulation, an increase in Pla is transmitted to the Ppa. The PVR equation assumes that this is a 1:1 ratio at any level of cardiac output. However, the PVR equation does not take into account the distensibility of the pulmonary resistive vessels, which cause under steady flow conditions an increase in Pla to be transmitted upstream in a slightly less than 1:1 ratio [31, 32]. In pulsatile flow conditions of the pulmonary circulation, an increase in Pla causes pulmonary perfusion pressure (the difference between systolic pulmonary artery pressure (sPpa) and dPpa) to increase. Accordingly mPpa increases more than Pla causing the transpulmonary pressure gradient (TPG), which is the numerator of the PVR equation (mPpa – Pla), to rise with both an increase in stroke volume and

Pla (Fig. 6.6) [31, 32]. In chronic left heart failure, the TPG is traditionally used to assess the resistive properties of the pulmonary circulation, the upper limit of normal being 12 mmHg. Above this threshold, an "out-of-proportion" increase in mPpa is diagnosed. However, it has been recently reported that the TPG is often higher than 12 mmHg even in patients with purely passive transmission of mPpa [34]. To overcome this problem, it has been proposed to use the diastolic pulmonary artery pressure (dPpa)–Pla gradient (DPG). In fact, in chronic left heart failure with purely passive transmission of the Pla to Ppa, the DPG does not increase, whereas in patients with a remodelling of the pulmonary resistive vessels, DPG increases, because dPpa increases more than Pla (Fig. 6.6). A DPG cut off value of 7 mmHg is proposed for the differential diagnosis between poorly passive and out-of-proportion pulmonary hypertension in left heart disease [33, 35].

6.4 Hypoxic Pulmonary Vasoconstriction

The ability of the pulmonary circulation to react to hypoxia by constriction of the pulmonary arteries and divert blood flow away from poorly oxygenated areas of the lung has been first described by von Euler and Liljestrand [36]. Hypoxic pulmonary vasoconstriction involves mainly resistive arterioles of 1000 mμ in diameter or less but also non-muscular arterioles and pulmonary veins [37–39]. Globally, hypoxic pulmonary vasoconstriction is uneven leading to inhomogeneous distribution of blood flow [40]. Chronic global hypoxic pulmonary vasoconstriction causes remodelling of pulmonary vessels that involves all layers of the vessel wall, including fibroblasts [41]. Structural changes of the vascular wall lead to sustained elevation of Ppa [12, 42]. To resolve normoxia, it takes weeks or months [43, 44]. Hypoxic pulmonary vasoconstriction is enhanced by acidosis, cyclooxygenase inhibition and certain drugs such as the peripheral chemoreceptor stimulator almitrine or low-dose serotonin. On the other hand, hypoxic pulmonary vasoconstriction is inhibited by inhaled nitric oxide. Alkalosis, hypercapnia without associated acidosis, inflammation, endotoxin and intravenous vasodilators such as prostaglandins and nitrates and oral vasodilators such as Ca-channels blockers or phosphodiesterase 5 inhibitors abrogate hypoxic pulmonary vasoconstriction and cause pulmonary shunt to increase [44].

Hypoxic pulmonary vasoconstriction is quasi immediate and evolves in two phases, an initial constrictor response that starts within minutes and a second sustained phase that reaches its plateau within approximately 120 min [45, 46]. Alveolar capillaries have been previously proposed as oxygen sensing with propagation of the hypoxic signal by endothelial membrane depolarisation to upstream arterioles. However, current evidence links preferably oxygen sensing to both pulmonary artery smooth muscle cell mitochondria and nicotinamide adenosine dinucleotide (phosphate) oxidases. A change in reactive oxygen species seems to be important, but there is disagreement whether the signal is an increase or decrease in reactive oxygen species [45, 46]. The second phase of the hypoxic pulmonary vasoconstriction is linked to the endothelium that releases different vasomediators including endothelin-1, prostaglandins and nitric oxide [46]. In hypoxia endothelin-1 synthesis is increased and nitric oxide availability is decreased. Finally, an increase of intracellular Ca^{++} levels further contributes to sustained hypoxic pulmonary vasoconstriction [46].

In the setting of the critically ill patient with acute lung injury, hypoxic pulmonary vasoconstriction is essential to prevent the distribution of blood flow to the nondependent

6

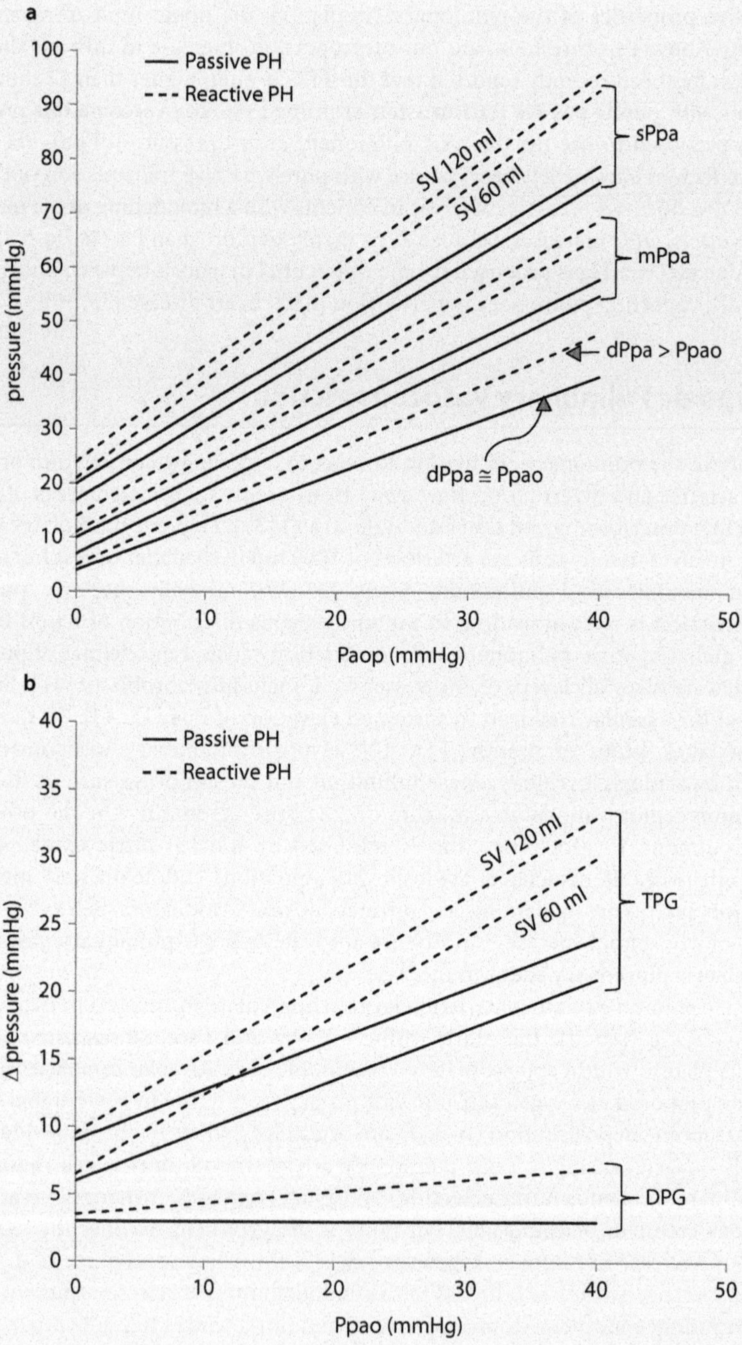
a
Passive PH
Reactive PH
SV 120 ml
SV 60 ml
sPpa
mPpa
dPpa > Ppao
dPpa ≅ Ppao
pressure (mmHg)
Paop (mmHg)
b
Passive PH
Reactive PH
SV 120 ml
SV 60 ml
TPG
DPG
Δ pressure (mmHg)
Ppao (mmHg)

non-ventilated lung regions [47, 48]. Interventions that have been shown to reinforce the effect of hypoxic pulmonary vasoconstriction are prone positioning leading the redistribution of pulmonary blood flow to the nondependent parts of the lung, the inhalation of nitric oxide and the almitrine administration. The simultaneous use of all three measures has a synergistic effect [49].

6.5 Pulmonary Hypertension in the ICU Setting

In healthy persons resting pulmonary artery pressure is on average 14 mmHg, the upper limit being 20 mmHg [25]. However, pulmonary hypertension has been historically defined as a mean mPpa equal or above 25 mmHg at rest as assessed by right heart catheterisation. The clinical significance of mPpa values between 21 and 24 mmHg remains unclear, because these persons were always excluded from clinical trial. However, it may represent a subgroup of persons prone to develop pulmonary hypertension, particularly during exercise and in hypoxia [25, 32]. Pulmonary hypertension is haemodynamically classified in precapillary (Ppao $\leq$ 15 mmHg) and postcapillary (Ppao >15 mmHg) pulmonary hypertension, the latter being further divided in two subgroups, one with an isolated postcapillary hypertension and the other with a combined pre- and postcapillary pulmonary hypertension as shown in ◘ Table 6.2 [33–36]. Based on pathophysiological, clinical and therapeutical considerations, the population with pulmonary hypertension is divided into five major classes: pulmonary arterial hypertension (class 1) which includes patients with veno-occlusive disease and/or pulmonary capillary haemangiomatosis and newborns with persistent pulmonary hypertension; pulmonary hypertension due to left heart disease (class 2); pulmonary hypertension due to lung disease and/or hypoxia (class 3); chronic thromboembolic pulmonary hypertension and other pulmonary obstructions, i.e. malignant cells (class 4); and pulmonary hypertension with unclear and/or multifactorial mechanisms (class 5) [50, 51]. In the intensive care settings of Europe, North America, Australia and New Zealand, the most frequent condition associated with pulmonary hypertension is left heart disease particularly those patients with preserved left ventricular ejection fraction and aortic stenosis. This group is followed by pulmonary hypertension due to lung disease or hypoxia. In developing countries, where worldwide approximately 80% of the affected population lives, pulmonary hypertension is mainly associated with

◘ Fig. 6.6 Effects of pulmonary artery occlusion pressure (Ppao) and stroke volume (SV) on systolic (s), mean (m) and diastolic (d) pulmonary artery pressure (Ppa) in two left heart failure patients, one with passive (continuous line) and the other with "out-of-proportion" (reactive) (dashed line) pulmonary hypertension (PH). If Ppao is directly transmitted to dPpa, there is a disproportional increase in sPpa and mPpa depending on SV, whereas if the dPpa increases more than Ppao, there is an out-of-proportion increase in mPpa and sPpa that is a function of SV (A). In the passive patient, the transpulmonary pressure gradient (TPG) increases depending on SV, but the diastolic pressure gradient (DPG) is independent of both Ppao and SV (continuous line in B). In the reactive left heart failure patient, TPG increases out of proportion, whereas DPG only slightly increases and is independent of SV (dashed line in B). (Adapted from Ref. [33])

Table 6.2 Haemodynamic definitions of pulmonary hypertension at rest

Definition	Characteristics	Clinical groups
Pulmonary hypertension	mPpa ≥25 mmHg	All
Precapillary PH	mPpa ≥25 mmHg Ppao ≤15 mmHg	WHO class 1: pulmonary arterial hypertension WHO class 3: PH due to lung diseases WHO class 4: Chronic thromboembolic PH WHO class 5: PH with unclear and/or multifactorial mechanisms
Postcapillary PH	mPpa ≥25 mmHg Ppao >15 mmHg	WHO class 2: PH due to left heart disease WHO class 5: PH with unclear and/or multifactorial mechanisms
Isolated postcapillary PH	DPG < 7 mmHg PVR ≤ 3 Wood units	
Combined post- and precapillary PH	DPG ≥ 7 mmHg PVR > 3 Wood units[a]	

PH pulmonary hypertension, *mPpa* mean pulmonary artery pressure, *Ppao* pulmonary artery occlusion pressure, *DPG* diastolic pressure gradient (diastolic Ppa – Ppao), *PVR* pulmonary vascular resistance
[a]Units for PVR are Wood units (mmHg * min)/L or dyn.s.cm^{-5} (80 * (mmHg * min)/L). Limits of normal: Wood units (0.25–1.9), dyn.s.cm^{-5} (20–150)

congenital heart disease, rheumatic heart disease and various infection diseases including schistosomiasis and HIV [52]. Pulmonary arterial hypertension and chronic thromboembolic pulmonary hypertension are both rare conditions. Disorders within the pulmonary arterial hypertension group share a similar pulmonary angioproliferative vasculopathy that predominantly affects the precapillary arterioles. A few patients with chronic thromboembolic pulmonary hypertension may present with the involvement of the precapillary arterioles as in class 1; this precludes a surgical treatment of these patients [53].

Treatment options are limited for patients with pulmonary hypertension that arrive at the intensive care unit haemodynamically unstable due to an acutely decompensated cor pulmonale. These patients are at high risk of death [54].

Practical Implications

To understand the physiology and the pathophysiology of the pulmonary circulation, a low-pressure high-pulsatile flow system in close relationship with the alveolar space and the right and the left side of the heart, the clinician at the bedside needs a good and profound understanding of pulmonary right heart catheterisation. Echocardiography adds important information but is not a technology fit for continuous monitoring in the intensive care unit and does not allow the estimation of pulmonary capillary pressure, hence the partitioning between arterial and venous components of pulmonary vascular resistance. Some practical implications for frequent clinical conditions around the assessment of pulmonary haemodynamics in the intensive care settings will be presented.

1. The cardiac output within the pulmonary circulation is generated by the right heart and equals the cardiac output (CO) of the systemic circulation. Changes in venous return and changes in right ventricular afterload (increase in pulmonary vascular resistance) both affect the CO of the pulmonary and the systemic circulation equally according to the formula CO = pressure * resistance. Accordingly, in the pulmonary circulation, an increased PVR, i.e. following hypoxia or pulmonary embolism, increases mPpa as long as CO is maintained by the right ventricle. When the right ventricle fails, the increase in mPpa may be less pronounced, or mPpa is even unchanged due to the decreasing CO. The opposite may be observed during the inhalation of nitric oxide. Under these circumstances, mPpa may not decrease because CO is increasing due to the decrease in right ventricular afterload (PVR). Thus changes in mPpa should always be set in relation with the change in CO (■ Fig. 6.5).
2. Chronic left heart failure is the most frequent cause of pulmonary hypertension in the ICU setting. In this condition remodelling of pulmonary resistive vessels may occur leading to an out-of-proportion increase in mPpa. The use of the pulmonary artery catheter is indispensable to differentiate a purely passive from a reactive (out-of-proportion) increase in mPpa. Since the TPG (mPpa – Ppao) is affected by changes in CO and left atrial pressure, the use of the DPG (dPpa – Ppao) is suggested by the guidelines [51]. In passive transmission of an elevated left atrial pressure, Ppao equals dPpa irrespective of the actual value of Ppao. Hence dPpa can be used as a surrogate marker of Ppao (■ Fig. 6.6). An increased resistance across the resistive arterioles of the pulmonary circulation increases dPpa, but not Ppao, hence the DPG (limit of normal <7 mmHg). Under these circumstances, dPpa cannot be used a surrogate marker of Ppao.
3. Pulmonary hypertension of any class leads to right ventricular failure at the final stage. Dysfunction of the right ventricle causes CO to decrease and right ventricular end-diastolic pressure (RVEDP) to increase, hence right atrial pressure (Pra) to increase. Consequently, in decompensated cor pulmonale, mPpa may decrease due to the CO that decreases while Pra increases. In the decompensated pulmonary hypertension patients of the WHO classes 1, 3 and 4, urgent therapeutic intervention is needed when Pra exceeds Ppao. Monitoring the relationship between Pra and Ppao during the treatment of a decompensated cor pulmonale is crucial for monitoring treatment response. In the healthy person, Pra is 4–5 mmHg lower than Ppao.
4. In the ARDS patient, high levels of PEEP are used to recruit the dependent part of the lungs, hence improving oxygenation. In the dependent part of the lung, the increase in PEEP permutes regions of zone 4 conditions to zone 3 conditions, whereas in the independent part of the lung, regions in zone 3 change into zones 2 and 1 conditions. Consequently, in the dependent part of the lung, pulmonary shunt is decreased, but in the nondependent parts, lung perfusion is increased. After recruitment with PEEP, if the tip of the pulmonary artery catheter is facing merely lung regions in zones 1 and 2, your Ppao will be determined by alveolar pressure (outflow pressure) and not by left atrial pressure [55]. You can solve this issue by decreasing PEEP and turning your patient from supine to prone.

Conclusion

Good and profound understanding of the pulmonary circulation is crucial for the management of the critically ill patient with heart and lung diseases. The pulmonary circulation is a fragile low-pressure, high-pulsatile blood flow circuit conceived for gas exchange. Changes of circuit inlet and outlet pressures, blood flow, alveolar pressure and alveolar gas contents may induce profound alterations within the pulmonary circulation leading potentially to harm and death.

6

Take-Home Message

- The pulmonary circulation is a fragile low-pressure, high-pulsatile flow circuit allowing gas exchange to occur. Fluid clearance out of the alveoli is important to keep them dry. Factors that influence fluid homeostasis and hence gas exchange within the lung negatively are increased capillary pressure, low plasmatic oncotic pressure, high alveolar air pressure and limitation/obstruction of lymphatic drainage of excessive interstitial fluid.
- Hypoxic pulmonary vasoconstriction is essential to deviate blood flow away from poorly oxygenated areas of the lung. Sites of hypoxic pulmonary vasoconstriction are small arteries and postcapillary veins. Chronic hypoxia leads to a remodelling of small pulmonary arteries, capillaries and veins. An increase in the resistance of the small arteries leads to an increase in the slope of the Ppa/CO relationship and PVR. The PVR is useful for detecting changes in arteriolar vessel tone and structure, the limitation being its non-reliability for the evaluation of the functional state of the pulmonary circulation at variable flow rates.
- In the pulsatile flow conditions of the pulmonary circulation, an increase of Pla is transmitted upstream to Ppa. In acute left heart failure, changes in Pla are mirrored by dPpa; hence dPpa can be used as surrogate marker of Pla. In chronic left heart failure, elevated Pla may lead to a remodelling of the resistive pulmonary artery vessels. In these patients, dPpa is higher than Pla and therefore cannot be used as a surrogate marker of Pla.

Pulmonary hypertension is defined as an mPpa equal or above 25 mmHg. Pulmonary hypertension is classified as precapillary if Ppao is $\leq$15 mmHg and postcapillary if $>$15 mmHg. The latter is further classified into an isolated postcapillary pulmonary hypertension if the DPG is $<$7 mmHg and an out-of-proportion postcapillary pulmonary hypertension if the DPG $\geq$ 7 mmHg.

References

1. ElMaghawry M, Zanatta A, Zampieri F. The discovery of pulmonary circulation: from Imhotep to William Harvey. Glob Cardiol Sci Pract. 2014;2014(2):103–16.
2. West JB. Marcello Malpighi and the discovery of the pulmonary capillaries and alveoli. Am J Physiol Lung Cell Mol Physiol. 2013;304(6):L383–90.
3. West JB. Ibn al-Nafis, the pulmonary circulation, and the Islamic Golden Age. J Appl Physiol (1985). 2008;105(6):1877–80.
4. van Wolferen SA, Grünberg K, Vonk Noordegraaf A. Diagnosis and management of pulmonary hypertension over the past 100 years. Respir Med. 2007;101(3):389–98.

5. Cournand A, Riley RL, Breed ES, Baldwin ED, Richards DW, Lester MS, et al. Measurement of cardiac output in man using the technique of catheterization of the right auricle or ventricle. J Clin Invest. 1945;24(1):106–16.
6. Forssmann DW. Die Sondierung des Rechten Herzens. Klin Wochenschr. 1929;8(45):2085–7.
7. Swan HJ, Ganz W, Forrester J, Marcus H, Diamond G, Chonette D. Catheterization of the heart in man with use of a flow-directed balloon-tipped catheter. N Engl J Med. 1970;283(9):447–51.
8. Iberti TJ, Fischer EP, Leibowitz AB, Panacek EA, Silverstein JH, Albertson TE. A multicenter study of physicians' knowledge of the pulmonary artery catheter. Pulmonary Artery Catheter Study Group. JAMA. 1990;264(22):2928–32.
9. Gnaegi A, Feihl F, Perret C. Intensive care physicians' insufficient knowledge of right-heart catheterization at the bedside: time to act? Crit Care Med. 1997;25(2):213–20.
10. O'Rourke MF. Arterial function in health and disease. London: Churchill Livingston; 1982.
11. Drake RE, Smith JH, Gabel JC. Estimation of the filtration coefficient in intact dog lungs. Am J Phys. 1980;238(4):H430–8.
12. Maggiorini M, Mélot C, Pierre S, Pfeiffer F, Greve I, Sartori C, et al. High-altitude pulmonary edema is initially caused by an increase in capillary pressure. Circulation. 2001;103(16):2078–83.
13. Drake RE, Scott RL, Gabel JC. Relationship between weight gain and lymph flow in dog lungs. Am J Phys. 1983;245(1):H125–30.
14. Howell JB, Permutt S, Proctor DF, Riley RL. Effect of inflation of the lung on different parts of pulmonary vascular bed. J Appl Physiol. 1961;16:71–6.
15. Lamm WJ, Kirk KR, Hanson WL, Wagner WW Jr, Albert RK. Flow through zone 1 lungs utilizes alveolar corner vessels. J Appl Physiol (1985). 1991;70(4):1518–23.
16. Lamm WJ, Obermiller T, Hlastala MP, Albert RK. Perfusion through vessels open in zone 1 contributes to gas exchange in rabbit lungs in situ. J Appl Physiol (1985). 1995;79(6):1895–9.
17. Conhaim RL, Rodenkirch LA. Functional diameters of alveolar microvessels at high lung volume in zone II. J Appl Physiol (1985). 1998;85(1):47–52.
18. Topulos GP, Brown RE, Butler JP. Increased surface tension decreases pulmonary capillary volume and compliance. J Appl Physiol (1985). 2002;93(3):1023–9.
19. Naeije R, Mélot C, Mols P, Hallemans R. Effects of vasodilators on hypoxic pulmonary vasoconstriction in normal man. Chest. 1982;82(4):404–10.
20. Mélot C, Naeije R, Hallemans R, Lejeune P, Mols P. Hypoxic pulmonary vasoconstriction and pulmonary gas exchange in normal man. Respir Physiol. 1987;68(1):11–27.
21. Hakim TS, Maarek JM, Chang HK. Estimation of pulmonary capillary pressure in intact dog lungs using the arterial occlusion technique. Am Rev Respir Dis. 1989;140(1):217–24.
22. Maarek JM, Hakim TS, Chang HK. Analysis of pulmonary arterial pressure profile after occlusion of pulsatile blood flow. J Appl Physiol (1985). 1990;68(2):761–9.
23. Gaar KA J, Taylor AE, Owens LJ, Guyton AC. Pulmonary capillary pressure and filtration coefficient in the isolated perfused lung. Am J Phys. 1967;213(4):910–4.
24. Nunes S, Ruokonen E, Takala J. Pulmonary capillary pressures during the acute respiratory distress syndrome. Intensive Care Med. 2003;29(12):2174–9.
25. Kovacs G, Olschewski A, Berghold A, Olschewski H. Pulmonary vascular resistances during exercise in normal subjects: a systematic review. Eur Respir J. 2012;39(2):319–28.
26. Naeije R, Chesler N. Pulmonary circulation at exercise. Compr Physiol. 2012;2(1):711–41.
27. Naeije R, Lipski A, Abramowicz M, Lejeune P, Mélot C, Antoine M, et al. Nature of pulmonary hypertension in congestive heart failure. Effects of cardiac transplantation. Am J Respir Crit Care Med. 1994;149(4 Pt 1):881–7.
28. Zapol WM, Snider MT. Pulmonary hypertension in severe acute respiratory failure. N Engl J Med. 1977;296(9):476–80.
29. Permutt S, Bromberger-Barnea B, Bane HN. Alveolar pressure, pulmonary venous pressure, and the vascular waterfall. Med Thorac. 1962;19:239–60.
30. West JB, Dollery CT, Naimark A. Distribution of blood flow in isolated lung; relation to vascular and alveolar pressures. J Appl Physiol. 1964;19:713–24.
31. Linehan JH, Haworth ST, Nelin LD, Krenz GS, Dawson CA. A simple distensible vessel model for interpreting pulmonary vascular pressure-flow curves. J Appl Physiol (1985). 1992;73(3):987–94.
32. Naeije R, Vanderpool R, Dhakal BP, Saggar R, Saggar R, Vachiery JL, et al. Exercise-induced pulmonary hypertension: physiological basis and methodological concerns. Am J Respir Crit Care Med. 2013;187(6):576–83.

33. Naeije R, Vachiery JL, Yerly P, Vanderpool R. The transpulmonary pressure gradient for the diagnosis of pulmonary vascular disease. Eur Respir J. 2013;41(1):217–23.
34. Gerges C, Gerges M, Lang MB, Zhang Y, Jakowitsch J, Probst P, et al. Diastolic pulmonary vascular pressure gradient: a predictor of prognosis in "out-of-proportion" pulmonary hypertension. Chest. 2013;143(3):758–66.
35. Guazzi M, Naeije R. Pulmonary hypertension in heart failure: pathophysiology, pathobiology, and emerging clinical perspectives. J Am Coll Cardiol. 2017;69(13):1718–34.
36. Von Euler US, Liljestrand G. Observation of the pulmonary arterial pressure in the cat. Acta Physiol Scand. 1946;12:301–20.
37. Mothely HL, Cournand A, et al. The influence of short periods of induced acute anoxia upon pulmonary artery pressures in man. Am J Phys. 1947;150(2):315–20.
38. Nagasaka Y, Bhattacharya J, Nanjo S, Gropper MA, Staub NC. Micropuncture measurement of lung microvascular pressure profile during hypoxia in cats. Circ Res. 1984;54(1):90–5.
39. Schwenke DO, Pearson JT, Umetani K, Kangawa K, Shirai M. Imaging of the pulmonary circulation in the closed-chest rat using synchrotron radiation microangiography. J Appl Physiol (1985). 2007;102(2):787–93. Epub 2006 Oct 12. Pubmed PMID: 17038493.
40. Dehnert C, Risse F, Ley S, Kuder TA, Buhmann R, Puderbach M, et al. Magnetic resonance imaging of uneven pulmonary perfusion in hypoxia in humans. Am J Respir Crit Care Med. 2006;174(10):1132–8.
41. Stenmark KR, Tuder RM, El Kasmi KC. Metabolic reprogramming and inflammation act in concert to control vascular remodeling in hypoxic pulmonary hypertension. J Appl Physiol (1985). 2015;119(10):1164–72.
42. Dorrington KL, Clar C, Young JD, Jonas M, Tansley JG, Robbins PA. Time course of the human pulmonary vascular response to 8 hours of isocapnic hypoxia. Am J Phys. 1997;273(3 Pt 2):H1126–34.
43. Penaloza D, Arias-Stella J. The heart and pulmonary circulation at high altitudes: healthy highlanders and chronic mountain sickness. Circulation. 2007;115(9):1132–46.
44. Wilkins MR, Ghofrani HA, Weissmann N, Aldashev A, Zhao L. Pathophysiology and treatment of high-altitude pulmonary vascular disease. Circulation. 2015;131(6):582–90.
45. Sylvester JT, Shimoda LA, Aaronson PI, Ward JP. Hypoxic pulmonary vasoconstriction. Physiol Rev. 2012;92(1):367–520.
46. Sommer N, Strielkov I, Pak O, Weissmann N. Oxygen sensing and signal transduction in hypoxic pulmonary vasoconstriction. Eur Respir J. 2016;47(1):288–303.
47. Brimioulle S, Lejeune P, Naeije R. Effects of hypoxic pulmonary vasoconstriction on pulmonary gas exchange. J Appl Physiol (1985). 1996;81(4):1535–43.
48. Brimioulle S, Julien V, Gust R, Kozlowski JK, Naeije R, Schuster DP. Importance of hypoxic vasoconstriction in maintaining oxygenation during acute lung injury. Crit Care Med. 2002;30(4):874–80.
49. Richard JC, Janier M, Lavenne F, Berthier V, Lebars D, Annat G, et al. Effect of position, nitric oxide, and almitrine on lung perfusion in a porcine model of acute lung injury. J Appl Physiol (1985). 2002;93(6):2181–91.
50. Hoeper MM, Bogaard HJ, Condliffe R, Frantz R, Khanna D, Kurzyna M, et al. Definitions and diagnosis of pulmonary hypertension. J Am Coll Cardiol. 2013;62(25 Suppl):D42–50.
51. Galiè N, Humbert M, Vachiery JL, Gibbs S, Lang I, Torbicki A, et al. ESC Scientific Document Group. 2015 ESC/ERS guidelines for the diagnosis and treatment of pulmonary hypertension: The Joint Task Force for the Diagnosis and Treatment of Pulmonary Hypertension of the European Society of Cardiology (ESC) and the European Respiratory Society (ERS): endorsed by: Association for European Paediatric and Congenital Cardiology (AEPC), International Society for Heart and Lung Transplantation (ISHLT). Eur Heart J. 2016;37(1):67–119.
52. Hoeper MM, Humbert M, Souza R, Idrees M, Kawut SM, Sliwa-Hahnle K, et al. A global view of pulmonary hypertension. Lancet Respir Med. 2016;4(4):306–22.
53. Kim NH, Delcroix M, Jenkins DP, Channick R, Dartevelle P, Jansa P, et al. Chronic thromboembolic pulmonary hypertension. J Am Coll Cardiol. 2013;62(25 Suppl):D92–9.
54. Jentzer JC, Mathier MA. Pulmonary hypertension in the intensive care unit. J Intensive Care Med. 2016;31(6):369–85.
55. Teboul JL, Andrivet P, Ansquer M, Besbes M, Rekik N, Lemaire F, et al. A bedside index assessing the reliability of pulmonary occlusion pressure during mechanical ventilation with positive end-expiratory pressure. J Crit Care. 1992;7:22–9.

The Pulse: An Essential Vital Sign

Paul E. Marik

M. R. Pinsky et al. (eds.), *Hemodynamic Monitoring*, Lessons from the ICU,
https://doi.org/10.1007/978-3-319-69269-2_7

Leaning Objectives

The objectives of this chapter are to review the pathophysiology, causes, and approach to the treatment of both sinus tachycardia and sinus bradycardia in ICU patients.

7.1 Introduction

It is by no accident that the four vital signs, namely, blood pressure, heart rate, respiratory rate, and temperature, are called *vital signs*. Yet, many clinicians do not appreciate the importance of these *vital* signs nor how to interpret them. The blood pressure (mean arterial pressure—MAP) and heart rate are the most important of the vital signs, while the temperature is the "least vital" of all the vital signs. Any patient with an abnormal vital sign is at an increased risk of death. The risk of death is compounded by derangements of multiple vital signs [1]. In addition, the trends in the vital signs are vitally important in tracking a patient's progress.

7.2 Physiology of Heart Rate

All cardiac myocytes in the embryonic heart have pacemaker properties. Some myocytes synthesize large amounts of contractile proteins to become "working" myocardium. Others retain pacemaking ability and generate impulses spontaneously; the mammalian heart region that ordinarily generates impulses at the greatest frequency is the sinoatrial (SA) node; it is the natural pacemaker of the heart. The SA node is the phylogenetic remnant of the sinus venosus of lower vertebrate hearts. In humans it is about 8 mm long and 2 mm thick. It lies in the groove where the superior vena cava joins the right atrium.

The autonomic nervous system controls various aspects of cardiac function, including the frequency at which the heart beats. However, cardiac function does not require intact nervous pathways as a completely denervated heart (a cardiac transplant recipient) can adapt well to stressful situations. Ordinarily, the frequency of pacemaker firing is controlled by the activity of both divisions of the autonomic nervous system. Increased sympathetic nervous activity, through the release of norepinephrine, raises the heart rate principally by increasing the slope of the pacemaker potential. This mechanism of increasing heart rate operates during physical exertion, anxiety, and certain illnesses, such as febrile infectious diseases. Increased vagal activity, through the release of acetylcholine, diminishes the heart rate by hyperpolarizing the pacemaker cell membrane and by reducing the slope of the pacemaker potential.

7.3 Tachycardia

Cardiac output (CO) is a function of heart rate (HR) and stroke volume (SV); Cardiac output = heart rate × stroke volume, with an increase in heart rate being the most important mechanism of increasing cardiac output. Tachycardia, defined as a heart rate > 100/min, therefore occurs in situations of increased oxygen demand with the need for an increased cardiac output or in conditions associated with decreased SV. Tachycardia also occurs in situations of increased sympathetic tone, i.e., anxiety and fight-flight response. Stroke volume may be reduced due to decreased preload (volume depletion) or impaired systolic heart function. Since tachycardia reduces diastolic time during which ventricular filling occurs, stroke volume may decrease at high heart rates; this however only becomes clinically significant in patients with diastolic dysfunction who have impaired diastolic filling. This implies that unless the patient has predominant diastolic dysfunction, slowing the heart rate (e.g., with a beta-blocker) will reduce cardiac output and oxygen delivery.

There is decreased responsiveness to beta-adrenergic receptor stimulation and decreased reactivity to baroreceptors and chemoreceptors with aging. Fibrosis and calcification of the fibrous skeleton of the heart, composed of the annular rings and fibrous trigones, together with calcification of the bases of the aortic cusps develop. These changes contribute to the high incidence of sick sinus syndrome, atrial arrhythmias and bundle branch blocks. In younger persons, cardiac output is increased predominantly by increasing heart rate in response to beta-adrenergic stimulation. With aging there is a relative "hyposympathetic state" in which the heart becomes less responsive to sympathetic stimulation, possible secondary to declining receptor function. The aging heart, therefore, increases cardiac output predominantly by increasing ventricular filling (preload) and stroke volume rather by an increase in heart rate.

Sinus tachycardia is always an ominous sign, and its cause must always be determined. A presenting heart rate >105/min and a sustained heart rate >90/min in patients with hemodynamic compromise are associated with an increased risk of death [2, 3]. The higher the heart rate, the more life-threatening the situation, and a tachycardia >110/min in an elderly patient is a very worrying sign. Tachycardia is most commonly due to a low stroke volume and/or a hypermetabolic state with an increased oxygen demand and in most instances represents an appropriate compensatory response. However, the clinical context and derangements of the other vital signs are important in assessing the implications of a tachycardia. Tachycardia in combination with hypotension (SBP < 110 or MAP < 75 mmHg) and a high respiratory rate (>20/min) is a deadly trio [1]. A tachycardia in the setting of left- (systolic heart failure) or right-sided heart failure (e.g., pulmonary embolism) [4] is a particularly foreboding sign being indicative of severely diminished stroke volume. It is important to emphasize that in almost all circumstance, one should treat the underlying cause (if possible) of the tachycardia and not the tachycardia itself. Always determine the cause of a sinus tachycardia (echocardiogram, stroke volume determination, etc.) and never treat an unexplained sinus tachycardia with a beta-blocker. The higher the heart rate, the more life-threatening the situation, and a tachycardia >110/min in an elderly patient is a very ominous sign. ICU patients with cardiac risk factors and a persistent tachycardia (HR > 95/min) are at an increased risk of having an acute cardiac event [5].

The role of a short-acting cardioselective beta-blocker (esmolol) in resuscitated septic shock patients who remain tachycardiac is controversial. While Morelli et al. demonstrated a benefit from this approach [6], this study has a number of limitations, including the fact that all patients required high inotropic support with levosimendan and that the overall mortality was very high, which may have concealed a potential detrimental impact of beta-blockade. This approach may be of benefit in patients with demonstrated diastolic dysfunction; however, this therapy is best attempted under continuous cardiac output monitoring.

Inappropriate sinus tachycardia is defined as a sinus heart rate >100 bpm at rest (with a mean 24-h heart rate >90/min not due to primary causes) [7, 8]. Patients are primarily young women, and clinical symptoms range from intermittent palpitations to general multisystem complaints.

The more common causes of sinus tachycardia in the ICU setting include:

- Hypovolemia
- Blood loss (hemorrhagic shock)
- Myocardial dysfunction
- Sepsis
- Fever
- Hypoxemia
- Anxiety/delirium/agitation
- Substance withdrawal; alcohol, opiates, etc.
- Alcohol intoxication
- Thyrotoxicosis
- Pulmonary embolism
- Severe anemia
- Drug induced; dopamine, epinephrine, etc.
- Drug toxicity with sympathomimetic agents (cocaine, amphetamines), synthetic cannabinoids, etc.

7.4 Bradycardia

Sinus bradycardia is defined as a heart rate less than 60 beats/min. Patients with a sinus bradycardia usually have a rate between 45 and 59 beats/min, but on rare occasion it may be as slow as 35 beats/min. Sinus bradycardia is often benign and does not necessarily indicate sinus node dysfunction. In the ICU, sinus bradycardia is most commonly due to a drug reaction, but it may occur in patients with intrinsic disease of the conducting tissues of the heart. Bradycardia may also occur with hypothermia, hypothyroidism, and raised intracranial pressure. The most commonly implicated drugs include beta-blockers, calcium channel blockers, dexmedetomidine, propofol, clonidine, and digoxin. Dexmedetomidine, an alpha-2 receptor agonist, decreases the production and response to catecholamines and leads to bradycardia from these sympatholytic effects. Propofol induces bradycardia by blocking calcium and potassium channels in cardiac cells. While propofol and dexmedetomidine alone have a relatively low incidence of bradycardia when combined with other AV nodal blocking medications, the risk of bradycardia increases substantially [9].

7.4.1 Treatment

Asymptomatic bradyarrhythmias do not carry a poor prognosis, and in general no therapy is indicated. Recommended initial therapy for bradycardia inducing end organ perfusion problems is atropine. Atropine is an anticholinergic medication with parasympatholytic properties leading to enhanced SA node automaticity and AV node conduction. The initial intravenous dose of atropine is 0.5–1.0 mg, which can be repeated every 5 min to a total dose of 0.04 mg/kg (3 mg for the average adult). Dopamine and isoproterenol are alternative agents in patients who have responded poorly to atropine. Dopamine is the preferred catecholamine for symptomatic bradycardia refractory to atropine. Glucagon may be beneficial in the treatment of bradycardia associated with β-blocker or calcium channel blocker toxicity. An initial intravenous dose of 0.05–0.15 mg/kg is recommended. Emergency cardiac pacing is indicated for patients with hemodynamically unstable bradycardia, especially for patients who have failed medical therapy. The presence of syncope, heart failure, or other symptoms accompanying bradycardias is an indication for pacemaker implantation.

Take-Home Messages

- Sinus tachycardia, defined as a heart rate >100/min is an ominous prognostic sign in the critically ill and injured patient.
- The underlying cause of the tachycardia must be determined in all cases, with treatment directed at the underlying cause. Treatment with a beta-blocker may be a hazardous complication.
- Sinus bradycardia, defined as a heart rate <60/min, is usually a benign rhythm that occurs most commonly due to an adverse drug reaction.

Conflicts of Interest None of the authors have any real or potential conflicts of interest with regards to this manuscript.

References

1. Bleyer AJ, Vidya S, Russell GB, et al. Longitudinal analysis of one million vital signs in patients in an academic medical center. Resuscitation. 2011;82:1387–92.
2. Parker MM, Shelhamer JH, Natanson C, et al. Serial cardiovascular variables in survivors and nonsurvivors of septic shock: heart rate as an early predictor of prognosis. Crit Care Med. 1987;15:923–9.
3. Vellinga NA, Boerma C, Koopmans M, et al. International study on microcirculatory shock occurrence in acutely ill patients. Crit Care Med. 2015;43:48–56.
4. Qaddoura A, Digby G, Kabali C, et al. The value of electrocardiography for prognostication of acute pulmonary embolism: a systematic review and meta-analysis [abstract]. J Am Coll Cardiol. 2016;67:830.
5. Sander O, Welters ID, Foex P, et al. Impact of prolonged elevated heart rate on incidence of major cardiac events in critically ill patients with a high risk of cardiac complications. Crit Care Med. 2005;33:81–8.
6. Morelli A, Ertmer C, Westphal M, et al. Effect of heat rate control with esmolol on hemodynamic and clinical outcomes in patients with septic shock. A randomized clinical trial JAMA. 2013;310:1683–91.
7. Sheldon RS, Grubb BP, Olshansky B, et al. 2015 Heart Rhythm Society expert consensus statement on the diagnosis and treatment of postural tachycardia syndrome, inappropriate sinus tachycardia, and vasovagal syncope. Heart Rhythm. 2015;12:e41–63.
8. Shen WK. How to manage patients with inappropriate sinus tachycardia. Heart Rhythm. 2005;2:1015–9.
9. Handler J. Adverse effects using combined rate-slowing antihypertensive agents. J Clin Hyperten. 2011;13:529–32.

Autonomic Dysfunction in Shock

Gareth L. Ackland

M. R. Pinsky et al. (eds.), *Hemodynamic Monitoring*, Lessons from the ICU,
https://doi.org/10.1007/978-3-319-69269-2_8

Learning Objectives

Circulatory shock is accompanied, and likely to be preceded, by profound alterations in autonomic function. In stable conditions, sympathetic and parasympathetic limbs of the autonomic nervous system work in a highly coordinated manner, by virtue of physical and biochemical afferent signals being transduced into coordinated neural activity to maintain homeostasis in multiple organs innervated by specialized autonomic nerves. In this chapter, we assess how normal autonomic activity is regulated and the practical implications of how perturbation of the autonomic nervous system fuels further detrimental changes in shock. We will also highlight how autonomic regulation of cardiovascular and extra-cardiovascular physiology contributes to circulatory shock and define autonomic dysfunction practically in a clinical context.

8.1 Introduction

8

The autonomic system, comprising sympathetic and parasympathetic limbs, plays a crucial role in the homeostatic control of the cardiovascular system. Key neurotransmitters and receptors mediating each limb are summarized in ◘ Fig. 8.1. In healthy subjects, physiological variability in heart rate and blood pressure is controlled by the interplay between the two limbs of autonomic system: parasympathetic and sympathetic system. Contrary to established physiological teaching, advances in autonomic experimental techniques have shed new light on the conventional model of opposing autonomic limbs [1].

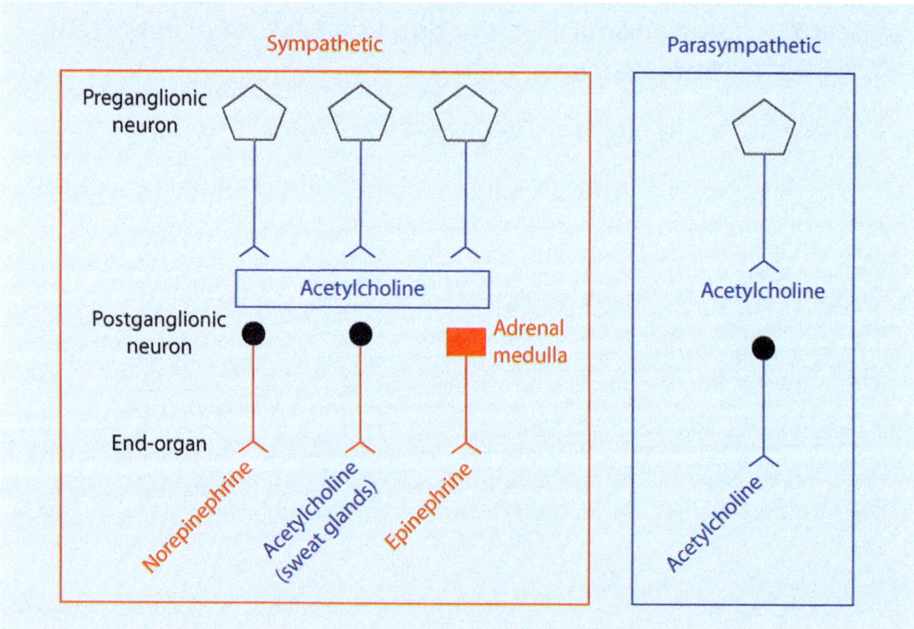

◘ **Fig. 8.1** Basic anatomic organization of neurotransmitters of the autonomic nervous system

Optimal cardiac output requires the simultaneous co-activation of both autonomic limbs, which permits both a longer time for ventricular filling and more efficient contraction of the myocardium [2, 3]. The maintenance of cardiovascular variability in response to routine physiological perturbation is mediated by two key physiological reflexes: the arterial baroreflex and peripheral chemoreflex.

8.2 Arterial Baroreflex

The arterial baroreflex mechanism buffers acute fluctuations in blood pressure [4]. The afferent limb of the baroreflex transduces changes in arterial pressure within the aortic arch and carotid sinus into electrical signals, relayed to the brainstem via aortic and glossopharyngeal nerves. These electrical signals are integrated by neurons within the brainstem, principally the nucleus tractus solitarius. Even small increases in blood pressure result in increased parasympathetic activity which, via the vagus nerve, slows the heart. Conversely, falls in arterial blood pressure lead to central neural activation of the sympathetic nervous system and consequent catecholamine release (epinephrine and norepinephrine). Reduced baroreceptor sensitivity is associated with excess morbidity [5] and increased mortality in critical illness [6].

8.3 Chemoreflex

Respiratory autonomic control is regulated by central and peripheral chemoreceptors, the latter of which are located in the carotid and aortic bodies. Changes in partial pressure of oxygen and carbon dioxide are transduced into neural signals [7]. Through central integration of this information initially within the nucleus tractus solitarii in the brainstem and other higher respiratory centres, changes in ventilation alter efferent autonomic neural signals acting on a diverse array of target organs. Peripheral chemoreceptors influence cardiovascular regulation directly, through hypoxia causing increased heart rate and sympathetic vasoconstrictor nerve activity within skeletal muscle vascular beds, which contributes to the progression of chronic cardiac failure [8]. Acute hypoxia results in resetting of the arterial baroreflex to higher pressures and higher levels of heart rate and muscle sympathetic nerve activity [9]. These effects occur without altering arterial baroreflex sensitivity and are also independent of breathing rate and tidal volume. Thus, autonomic regulation of cardiovascular and respiratory function is very likely to interact during acute shock states. Indeed, peripheral chemoreceptors play a role beyond that of detecting changes in ventilation, since they also sense a broad range of metabolic and inflammatory molecules [10]. Inflammatory mediators robustly increase peripheral chemoreceptor discharge, which is likely to an important reason why respiratory rate is such a strongly predictive clinical parameter for detecting sepsis [11]. Moreover, feedback from the lungs, through hyperventilation driven by hypoxia, acidosis and/or inflammation, also impacts on efferent autonomic activity. Loss of chemoreflex [12] and baroreceptor sensitivity [6] is associated with increased mortality in critical illness [13].

8.4 Autonomic Variability: An Intrinsic Feature of Health

The successful maintenance of homeostasis, from cells through to the whole organism, requires dynamic interaction between multiple control systems leading to highly complex, variable patterns that are not reflected by static clinical measures such as heart rate and arterial pressure [14]. The maintenance of autonomic variability is a crucial element contributing to this dynamic control of homeostasis, reflecting the ability of afferent, central and efferent autonomic components to detect, and act upon, subtle physiological alterations [15]. While often related to cardiovascular homeostasis, a wealth of recent data shows that the autonomic nervous system also regulates the biological activity of other cell types, including immune cells [16, 17]. Of direct relevance to shock states, both limbs of the autonomic nervous system alter release of inflammatory mediators through the immunomodulatory actions of epinephrine (sympathetic), acetylcholine and vasoactive intestinal peptide (parasympathetic). Although beyond the scope of this chapter, the extra-cardiovascular regulation of inflammation may very well contribute to the magnitude, persistence and/or reversibility of shock states (Fig. 8.2).

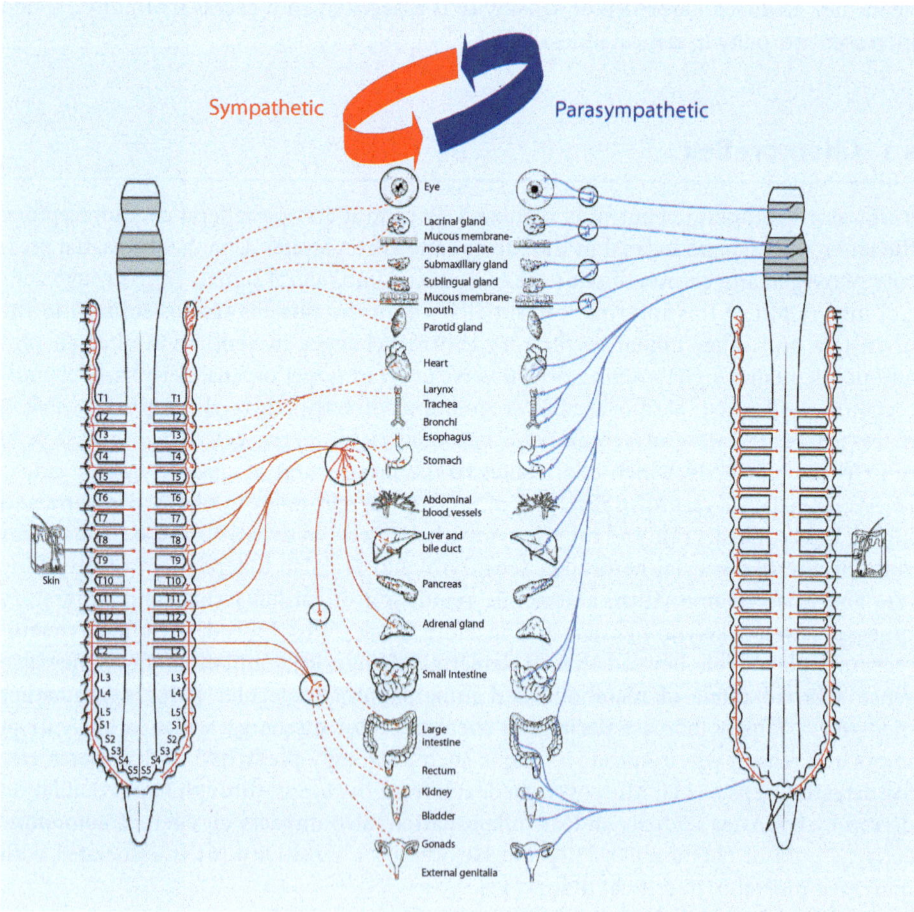

Fig. 8.2 Physiologic interaction at the organ level between sympathetic and parasympathetic components of the autonomic nervous system.

8.5 Key Features of Autonomic Dysfunction in Shock (Circulatory Failure)

Profound changes in autonomic function accompany shock, although the type of shock (cardiogenic, haemorrhagic, septic) may impact upon the precise autonomic phenotype. The autonomic profile of redistributive shock, such as that occurs under general anaesthesia, is further complicated by the peripheral and central actions of pharmacological agents [18]. Human (clinical) studies in humans at the onset of septic or haemorrhagic shock are understandably rare and challenging, so the confounding influence of therapy/sedation needs to be taken into account when understanding the autonomic changes that accompany shock. This means that much of our human physiological understanding of autonomic changes in "pure" shock states is derived from sophisticated physiological experiments where lower body negative pressure is used to produce controlled hypotensive shock [19]. However, it is worth bearing in mind that in patients most susceptible to acquiring infections (e.g. cardiac failure), pre-existing autonomic dysfunction is common and likely to exacerbate the early features of the shock state through cardiovascular and non-cardiovascular mechanisms [20]. Regardless of the model or clinical type of shock, the most ubiquitous autonomic feature of shock is the dramatically heightened activation of the sympathetic nervous system, leading to increased release of catecholamines which spill over into the circulation [21, 22]. Central neural processing of afferent signals further coordinates the emergent neuroendocrine release of vasopressin and angiotensin, amongst other neurohormones, to counteract relative hypovolaemia. Experimental data demonstrate, through direct measurement of neural activity, that sympathetic increases in renal, hepatic, adrenal, splenic and cardiac vascular beds occur during the early phases of shock [23]. Even at very modest levels of hypovolaemia (absolute or redistributive) when heart rate and arterial blood pressure remain unchanged, a baroreflex-mediated increase in muscle sympathetic nerve activity serves to compensate for acute hypovolaemic changes. Non-hypotensive hypovolaemia reduces the diameter of both major arteries containing the stretch-sensitive aortic and carotid arterial baroreceptors, the deactivation of which drives heightened sympathetic drive and parasympathetic withdrawal [24].

8.6 Autonomic Dysfunction and Cardiovascular Collapse

After the onset of shock, in the absence or presence of clinical intervention, circulatory collapse may develop. This most likely occurs as a result of the acute impairment of arterial baroreflex control, rather than loss of sympathetic vasomotor activity. Once coherence between arterial blood pressure and sympathetic nerve activity is lost, profound vasodilation and decreased systemic vascular resistance occur [24]. Other physiological stressors that are common features of acute critical illness, including pain, anxiety and sympatholytic anaesthetic/analgesic agents disrupt autonomic coherence in clinically unpredictable ways. A similar phenomenon is attributable to circulatory collapse following pathological cardiovagal reflex activity [25], where the sudden attenuation of baroreflex function occurs before haemodynamic decompensation. The often unpredictable, sudden circulatory collapse that ensues once shock is established may be underpinned by individual differences in autonomic function. Multiple experimental studies demonstrate highly variable individual differences in the ability of healthy humans to tolerate central hypovolemia. This observation is likely to be even more pertinent in patients at risk of shock who frequently have pre-existing comorbidity associated with autonomic impairment [5, 26]. Genetic variability has been linked to toleration of shock [27], as well as differences in the release of vasoactive hormones [28], baroreflex gain of sympathetic nerve activation [29] and speed of onset of increased sympathetic neural activity [30]. Myocardial cell injury is readily induced by excessive sympathetic activity during shock [31], and thus persistent sympathetic activation may limit cardiac output through this secondary mode of insult.

8.7 Autonomic Dysfunction as a Feature of Persistent Shock

The traditional notion of autonomic impairment is exemplified by abnormal responses to the Valsalva manoeuvre and neurological syndromes characterized by paradoxical hypotension or hypertension. Contrary to these clinically defined phenotypes, a far more sophisticated, biologically relevant model has developed with the understanding of how adrenoreceptor expression is regulated. Signalling mechanisms following G-protein-coupled receptor activation (e.g. beta-adrenoreceptor) require dynamic regulatory mechanisms that enable rapid adaptation to meet cellular demands. Within minutes of agonist activation, the process of desensitization of GPCRs begins. In the heart, catecholamines bind to β1 and β2- GPCRs leading to conformational changes in GPCR structure that trigger the dissociation of heterotrimeric G-proteins into α and βγ subunits. In turn, this activates signalling via various downstream proteins. Deactivation of GPCR-elicited signalling is essential for efficient receptor-mediated signalling, requiring GRKs to desensitize the receptor to agonist stimulation. GRKs (chiefly GRK2 AND 5 in the heart) firstly phosphorylate the active receptor to enable binding of β-arrestin, which subsequently may lead to clathrin-induced endocytosis, reactivation or degradation of the receptor. GTPases promote G-protein trimer reformation, which reprimes the GPCR in readiness for further agonist stimulation. When the balance between activation and deactivation is disrupted, cardiac dysfunction develops. In clinical practice, this phenomenon is manifest by acutely raised sympathetic drive (as seen at the onset of septic shock [32]) leading to "cardiac uncoupling" where there is a functional disconnection between sympathetic autonomic function and the physiological response of the cardiac myocyte [33]. Moreover, experimental models, and translational studies, demonstrate that baroreflex dysfunction is associated with reduced cardiac contractility. Reduced baroreceptor sensitivity leads to unrestrained release of (higher) angiotensin. High levels of plasma angiotensin generate injurious release of reactive oxygen species through activation of nicotinamide adenine dinucleotide phosphate oxidase subunit 2 leading to reduced cardiac contractility [26]. This cardiac dysfunction is associated with the upregulation of G-protein-coupled receptor kinase expression in cardiomyocytes [26]. Persistent exposure to elevated sympathetic activity, and hence endogenous catecholamine release, is a core feature of critical illness following shock even after apparently successful resuscitation. For example, prolonged bed rest is likely to contribute to persistent autonomic baroreflex dysfunction [34].

Practical Implications

Although the measurement of autonomic function may have a lot of potential applications, there are several inherent challenges in capturing processing and interpretation these data. Furthermore, pre-existing autonomic impairment is common in surgical patients with a similar clinical profile as those who develop critical illness for different reasons. This suggests that a more detailed understanding of these patients' autonomic physiology may help us understand rational, targeted treatments either to prevent, or reverse, shock. However, there is still very little evidence about the clinical impact of this information on the management of critically ill patients. For example, heart rate variability has been explored in the critical care setting (including in the early stages of septic shock and traumatic hypovolaemia), but has not been widely adopted because of technical limitations and lack of outcome data. Dynamic tests of beta-adrenoreceptor responsivity appear to hold most promise [35–38], where the cardiometabolic response to catecholamine infusion appears to identify a relationship between beta-adrenoreceptor signalling/physiology and outcome. Across several studies, the failure of patients to respond to β-1 adrenoreceptor agonists is strongly predictive of outcome. Even where many patients required treatment with vasopressors for persistent circulatory shock, graded dobutamine challenge revealed that preserved cardiac responsivity to dobutamine stimulation was more frequently present in survivors. Early studies, using an intravenous infusion of dobutamine at 10 microg/kg/min for 1 h after resuscitation, demonstrated that survivors were far more likely to increase oxygen consumption by more than 15%. In a study where the majority of patients continued to require pressor support, dobutamine not only increased oxygen delivery and consumption in responders but also exerted a significant metabolic effect as reflected by a greater temperature increase. Thus, an intact cardiometabolic response following a dobutamine "stress test" is consistent with the idea that disruption of beta-adrenoreceptor physiology is pivotal in determining outcome from shock. Further evidence is provided by experimental models of baroreflex dysfunction and clinical measurement of spontaneous baroreflex sensitivity, which further support the hypothesis that disruption of beta-adrenoreceptor recycling underlies the development, and persistence, of circulatory shock.

8.8 Clinical Interventions

The developing interest in critical care of controlling heart rate with beta-blockers [39], novel sedative agents [40] and early mobilization [41] is likely to exert profound effects on autonomic control. For the reasons outlined previously, the benefits of many of these apparently unconnected interventions may centre on reversing the detrimental effects of prolonged sympathetic activation on receptor recycling mechanisms.

Conclusion

Shock and critical illness induce profound alterations in autonomic function. Several core features of shock may largely be explained by the pre-existence, or rapid development, of autonomic impairment. The longer-term implications of this are likely to mirror outcomes in cardiovascular disease, where extremes of autonomic impairment are independently predictive of survival.

Take-Home Messages

- Multiple drugs used in the ICU may mask or provoke features of autonomic dysfunction. Cardiovascular therapy needs to take this into account the whole clinical picture and not just focus on numerical targets.
- Static measures of heart rate and blood pressure do not reflect underlying autonomic compromise. Rapid changes in patient position, or painful/stimulatory interventions, may evoke unpredictable, exaggerated or even ablated changes in heart rate/blood pressure.
- Tachycardia may reflect a number of underlying pathophysiological features that are typical of critical illness. The clinical exclusion of triggers for tachycardia, such as pain, hypovolaemia and adequate sedation, does not mean that persistently high heart rates are benign.
- In established critical illness, recurrent episodes of postural hypotension, intermittent pressor requirement, dysrhythmias (including atrial fibrillation) and/or persistent tachycardia should prompt consideration of more in-depth cardiovascular interrogation. Transthoracic echocardiography offers a rapid evaluation of cardiorespiratory physiology that may assist in ruling out primary autonomic abnormalities if pathological alterations are evident.

8

References

1. Paton JF, Boscan P, Pickering AE, Nalivaiko E. The yin and yang of cardiac autonomic control: Vago-sympathetic interactions revisited. Brain Res Brain Res Rev. 2005;49(3):555–65.
2. Machhada A, Marina N, Korsak A, Stuckey DJ, Lythgoe MF, Gourine AV. Origins of the vagal drive controlling left ventricular contractility. J Physiol. 2016;594(14):4017–30.
3. Machhada A, Trapp S, Marina N, Stephens RCM, Whittle J, Lythgoe MF, et al. Vagal determinants of exercise capacity. Nat Commun. 2017;8:15097.
4. Wehrwein EA, Joyner MJ. Regulation of blood pressure by the arterial baroreflex and autonomic nervous system. Handb Clin Neurol. 2013;117:89–102.
5. Toner A, Jenkins N, Ackland GL, POM-O Study Investigators. Baroreflex impairment and morbidity after major surgery. Br J Anaesth. 2016;117(3):324–31.
6. Sharshar T, Gray F, de la Grandmaison GL, Hopklnson NS, Ross E, Dorandeu A, et al. Apoptosis of neurons in cardiovascular autonomic centres triggered by inducible nitric oxide synthase after death from septic shock. Lancet. 2003;362(9398):1799–805.
7. Kara T, Narkiewicz K, Somers VK. Chemoreflexes – physiology and clinical implications. Acta Physiol Scand. 2003;177(3):377–84.
8. Toledo C, Andrade DC, Lucero C, Schultz HD, Marcus N, Retamal M, et al. Contribution of peripheral and central chemoreceptors to sympatho-excitation in heart failure. J Physiol. 2017;595(1):43–51.
9. Querido JS, Wehrwein EA, Hart EC, Charkoudian N, Henderson WR, Sheel AW. Baroreflex control of muscle sympathetic nerve activity as a mechanism for persistent sympathoexcitation following acute hypoxia in humans. Am J Physiol Regul Integr Comp Physiol. 2011;301(6):R1779–85.

10. Ackland GL, Kazymov V, Marina N, Singer M, Gourine AV. Peripheral neural detection of danger-associated and pathogen-associated molecular patterns. Crit Care Med. 2013;41(6):e85–92.
11. Singer M, Deutschman CS, Seymour CW, Shankar-Hari M, Annane D, Bauer M, et al. The third international consensus definitions for sepsis and septic shock (sepsis-3). JAMA. 2016;315(8):801–10.
12. Schmidt H, Muller-Werdan U, Nuding S, Hoffmann T, Francis DP, Hoyer D, et al. Impaired chemoreflex sensitivity in adult patients with multiple organ dysfunction syndrome – the potential role of disease severity. Intensive Care Med. 2004;30(4):665–72.
13. Schmidt H, Müller-Werdan U, Hoffmann T, Francis DP, Piepoli MF, Rauchhaus M, et al. Autonomic dysfunction predicts mortality in patients with multiple organ dysfunction syndrome of different age groups*. Crit Care Med. 2005;33(9):1994–2002.
14. Ernst G. Heart-rate variability-more than heart beats? Front Public Health. 2017;5:240.
15. Thayer JF, Lane RD. The role of vagal function in the risk for cardiovascular disease and mortality. Biol Psychol. 2007;74(2):224–42.
16. Elenkov IJ, Wilder RL, Chrousos GP, Vizi ES. The sympathetic nerve – an integrative interface between two supersystems: the brain and the immune system. Pharmacol Rev. 2000;52(4):595–638.
17. Andersson U, Tracey KJ. Reflex principles of immunological homeostasis. Annu Rev Immunol. 2012;30:313–35.
18. Neukirchen M, Kienbaum P. Sympathetic nervous system: evaluation and importance for clinical general anesthesia. Anesthesiology. 2008;109(6):1113–31.
19. Wolthuis RA, Bergman SA, Nicogossian AE. Physiological effects of locally applied reduced pressure in man. Physiol Rev. 1974;54(3):566–95.
20. van de Borne P, Montano N, Pagani M, Oren R, Somers VK. Absence of low-frequency variability of sympathetic nerve activity in severe heart failure. Circulation. 1997;95(6):1449–54.
21. Chan JY, Ou CC, Wang LL, Chan SH. Heat shock protein 70 confers cardiovascular protection during endotoxemia via inhibition of nuclear factor-kappaB activation and inducible nitric oxide synthase expression in the rostral ventrolateral medulla. Circulation. 2004;110(23):3560–6.
22. de Montmollin E, Aboab J, Mansart A, Annane D. Bench-to-bedside review: Beta-adrenergic modulation in sepsis. Crit Care. 2009;13(5):230.
23. Ninomiya I, Nisimaru N, Irisawa H. Sympathetic nerve activity to the spleen, kidney, and heart in response to baroceptor input. Am J Phys. 1971;221(5):1346–51.
24. Floras JS, Butler GC, Ando SI, Brooks SC, Pollard MJ, Picton P. Differential sympathetic nerve and heart rate spectral effects of nonhypotensive lower body negative pressure. Am J Physiol Regul Integr Comp Physiol. 2001;281(2):R468–75.
25. Ocon AJ, Medow MS, Taneja I, Stewart JM. Respiration drives phase synchronization between blood pressure and RR interval following loss of cardiovagal baroreflex during vasovagal syncope. Am J Physiol Heart Circ Physiol. 2011;300(2):H527–40.
26. Ackland GL, Whittle J, Toner A, Machhada A, Del Arroyo AG, Sciuso A, et al. Molecular mechanisms linking autonomic dysfunction and impaired cardiac contractility in critical illness. Crit Care Med. 2016;44(8):e614–24.
27. Klemcke HG, Joe B, Rose R, Ryan KL. Life or death? A physiogenomic approach to understand individual variation in responses to hemorrhagic shock. Curr Genomics. 2011;12(6):428–42.
28. Convertino VA, Sather TM. Vasoactive neuroendocrine responses associated with tolerance to lower body negative pressure in humans. Clin Physiol. 2000;20(3):177–84.
29. Wijeysundera DN, Butler GC, Ando S, Pollard M, Picton P, Floras JS. Attenuated cardiac baroreflex in men with presyncope evoked by lower body negative pressure. Clin Sci (Lond). 2001;100(3):303–9.
30. Convertino VA, Rickards CA, Ryan KL. Autonomic mechanisms associated with heart rate and vasoconstrictor reserves. Clin Auton Res. 2012;22(3):123–30.
31. Ellison GM, Torella D, Karakikes I, Purushothaman S, Curcio A, Gasparri C, et al. Acute beta-adrenergic overload produces myocyte damage through calcium leakage from the ryanodine receptor 2 but spares cardiac stem cells. J Biol Chem. 2007;282(15):11397–409.
32. Annane D, Trabold F, Sharshar T, Jarrin I, Blanc AS, Raphael JC, et al. Inappropriate sympathetic activation at onset of septic shock: a spectral analysis approach. Am J Respir Crit Care Med. 1999;160(2):458–65.
33. Norris PR, Ozdas A, Cao H, Williams AE, Harrell FE, Jenkins JM, et al. Cardiac uncoupling and heart rate variability stratify ICU patients by mortality: a study of 2088 trauma patients. Ann Surg. 2006;243(6):804–12; discussion 812–4.

34. Hughson RL, Shoemaker JK. Autonomic responses to exercise: deconditioning/inactivity. Auton Neurosci. 2015;188:32–5.
35. Kumar A, Schupp E, Bunnell E, Ali A, Milcarek B, Parrillo JE. Cardiovascular response to dobutamine stress predicts outcome in severe sepsis and septic shock. Crit Care (London, England). 2008;12(2):R35.
36. Vallet B, Chopin C, Curtis SE, Dupuis BA, Fourrier F, Mehdaoui H, et al. Prognostic value of the dobutamine test in patients with sepsis syndrome and normal lactate values: a prospective, multicenter study. Crit Care Med. 1993;21(12):1868–75.
37. Rhodes A, Lamb FJ, Malagon I, Newman PJ, Grounds RM, Bennett ED. A prospective study of the use of a dobutamine stress test to identify outcome in patients with sepsis, severe sepsis, or septic shock. Crit Care Med. 1999;27(11):2361–6.
38. Jellema WT, Groeneveld AB, Wesseling KH, Thijs LG, Westerhof N, van Lieshout JJ. Heterogeneity and prediction of hemodynamic responses to dobutamine in patients with septic shock. Crit Care Med. 2006;34(9):2392–8.
39. Morelli A, Ertmer C, Westphal M, Rehberg S, Kampmeier T, Ligges S, et al. Effect of heart rate control with esmolol on hemodynamic and clinical outcomes in patients with septic shock: a randomized clinical trial. JAMA. 2013;310(16):1683–91.
40. Cruickshank M, Henderson L, MacLennan G, Fraser C, Campbell M, Blackwood B, et al. Alpha-2 agonists for sedation of mechanically ventilated adults in intensive care units: a systematic review. Health Technol Assess. 2016;20(25):v–xx, 1–117
41. Schweickert WD, Pohlman MC, Pohlman AS, Nigos C, Pawlik AJ, Esbrook CL, et al. Early physical and occupational therapy in mechanically ventilated, critically ill patients: a randomised controlled trial. Lancet. 2009;373(9678):1874–82.

Oxygen Delivery

Eleonora Duscio, Francesco Vasques, Federica Romitti, Francesco Cipulli, and Luciano Gattinoni

M. R. Pinsky et al. (eds.), *Hemodynamic Monitoring*, Lessons from the ICU,
https://doi.org/10.1007/978-3-319-69269-2_9

Learning Objectives

- Oxygen delivery and its determinants, how to measure them and how to interpret their possible derangements.
- Recognize oxygen delivery impairment before energy crisis and cellular damage develop.
- Recognize any impairment of energy production even if oxygen delivery is still adequate.
- "Supernormal" values theory and early goal-directed therapy (EGDT).

9.1 Introduction

Oxygen plays an essential role in aerobic life, acting as final acceptor of electrons in mitochondria from which energy, as ATP, is supplied to the whole organism. We may recognize three primary essential steps for oxygen utilization: first, the transport of oxygen-rich gas mixture from the ambient to the lung by ventilation and then its transfer from alveoli to blood; second, the transport of oxygenated blood to tissues; and, third, oxygen reduction to water in mitochondria. Oxygen movement from inspired gas toward mitochondria is possible thanks to pressure gradients: oxygen partial pressure is indeed 150 mmHg in the inspired gas and between 4 and 25 mmHg in its final destination, the mitochondria. After the oxygen has been delivered to tissues, the mixed venous blood returns to alveoli, and another cycle of oxygen transport and utilization begins. Mixed venous blood contains an amount of oxygen that represents oxygen that has been delivered but not consumed and can be considered as a sort of reserve. Although the term oxygen transport, strictly speaking, should refer to all the processes through which oxygen is transferred from inhaled gas to the final place of utilization, in the intensive care literature, it usually refers only to the hemodynamic phase. In this chapter, we will analyze primarily the hemodynamic phase of oxygen transport, and we will give some hints about oxygen utilization. It should not be forgotten, indeed, that in several conditions which may be common in intensive care patients, primarily sepsis and septic shock, the real problem is not only in the hemodynamic phase of oxygen delivery but also the oxygen utilization. This step relates to all the processes occurring in mitochondria where oxygen, acting as final acceptor of the electron cascade, makes possible the high levels of aerobic energy production.

9.2 Oxygen Transport

Oxygen transfer from lung to blood requires an adequate ventilation-perfusion ratio of terminal lung units. Ventilation is the process that provides fresh oxygen in an amount equal to the oxygen that is extracted from blood. Once in the blood, oxygen combines immediately to hemoglobin, and only a small amount of it remains in blood in a dissolved form. These two forms of oxygen transport, the dissolved one (measured as oxygen partial pressure, PO_2) and the combined one (measured as hemoglobin saturation, SO_2), together represent the total oxygen blood content, and their relationship is best described by hemoglobin dissociation curve.

9.2.1 Oxygen Bound to Hemoglobin

Before analyzing oxygen dissociation curve, it is necessary to know which is the maximum capability of hemoglobin to carry oxygen. At a hypothetical hemoglobin saturation of 100%, each mole of hemoglobin is able to carry four moles of oxygen. Given a molecular weight of hemoglobin of 64,500 Da, corresponding to a molar weight of 64,500 g, the total oxygen bound at 0 °C should be 22.4 L of oxygen for each hemoglobin mole equal to 89.6 oxygen liters in total [1]. In the Eq. 9.1, k represents the volume of oxygen that is transported by a single gram of completely saturated hemoglobin and is referred as hemoglobin carrying capacity.

$$k = \frac{89,600\,\mathrm{L}}{64,500\,\mathrm{g}} = 1.389\,\mathrm{mL/g} \tag{9.1}$$

The hemoglobin carrying capacity is 1.39 mL/g; this means that each gram of completely saturated hemoglobin is able to bind 1.39 mL of oxygen. Surprisingly, however, the literature provides different coefficients, ranging from 1.32 to 1.39, which is due to the different molecular weights that are attributed to the hemoglobin molecule as a result of the existence of several hemoglobin subtypes with their own molecular weights. The amount of oxygen carried by hemoglobin is easily computed using Eq. 9.2.

$$\mathrm{cHbO_2}\left(\mathrm{mL/dL}\right) = 1.39 \times \mathrm{Hb} \times \mathrm{SO_2} \tag{9.2}$$

The hemoglobin oxygen binding capacity depends on the possible structural changes that the hemoglobin molecules undergo in different conditions. This hemoglobin behavior is graphically explained by hemoglobin dissociation curve (Fig. 9.1). The sigmoid shape of the curve comes from changes in protein structure caused by progressive oxygen binding as the more oxygen is bound by the hemoglobin, the more hemoglobin affinity for oxygen increases [2]. This is true until hemoglobin has reached its maximum binding capacity that corresponds to the plateau part of the curve. At this point even big changes in blood PO_2 will produce only a small difference in oxygen saturation. There are many other factors that affect hemoglobin affinity for oxygen determining a shift of the curve toward the right or the left (i.e., decreasing or increasing its oxygen affinity). These factors include pH, temperature, carbon dioxide (CO_2) tension, and the concentration of 2,3-diphosphoglycerate. In the presence of low concentration of 2,3-DPG, lower CO_2 tension, high pH levels, and low temperature, the hemoglobin curve shift toward the left. This phenomenon is translated in a reduction in hemoglobin affinity for oxygen and an increased oxygen dissociation. In the opposite conditions (high 2,3-DPG, higher CO_2, low pH, and high temperature), the curve will shift to the right. The value that better describes this behavior is the P_{50} which represents the partial oxygen pressure at which the hemoglobin saturation is 50%. For example, if P_{50} increases from its normal value (26 mmHg in standard condition, i.e., pH 7,4, $PaCO_2$ 40 mmHg, 37 °C), the Hb dissociation curve shifts to the left, meaning that in order to obtain the same oxygen saturation of 50%, oxygen partial pressure must increase. These changes in hemoglobin oxygen affinity produce relevant consequences both on the arterial side, where oxygen is loaded and CO_2 is released, and on the capillary side, where oxygen is delivered and CO_2 is charged.

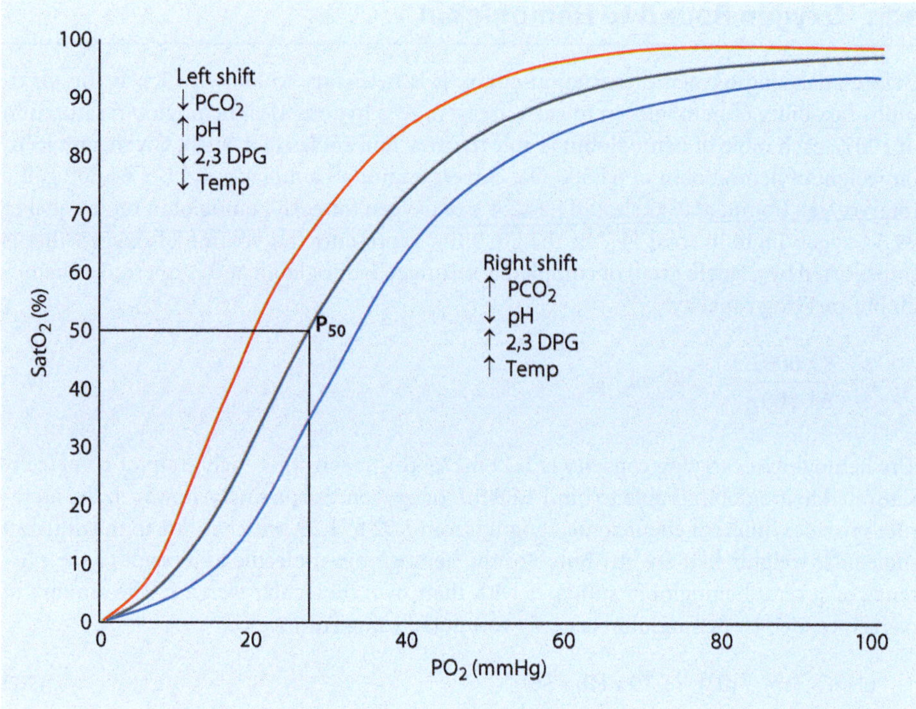

Fig. 9.1 Hemoglobin dissociation curve. The table displays an arterial hemoglobin dissociation curve at PCO_2 40 mmHg, pH 7.4, normal values of 2,3-DPG (5 mmol/L circa), and blood temperature 37 °C (black line). An increase in PCO_2, 2,3-DPG, or temperature or a decrease in pH produces a shift of the curve to the right (blue line). A decrease in PCO_2, 2,3-DPG, or temperature or an increase in pH produces a shift of the curve to the left (blue line)

The sigmoid shape of the curve and its affinity has been extensively studied in the 1970s, and several equations are available in order to compute hemoglobin oxygen saturation starting from oxygen partial pressure and correcting for pH, base excess, temperature, and PCO_2 [3]. The best known of these equations is the one developed by Kelman in 1966 [4]: this equation uses seven different coefficients in order to generate a curve. Most of these models, however, have intrinsic biases coming from the fact that they have been built not considering the possible presence of "abnormal" types of hemoglobin, such as methemoglobin, sulfhemoglobin, and fetal hemoglobin. Furthermore, their reliability decreases at low PO_2 levels and with most of the conditions that may cause a shift in the curve position. All these scenarios are quite common in clinical practice while referring to critical care patients and even more common while analyzing different kind of blood such as the arterial and the venous one. This means that results provided by different authors may be very similar when regarding to arterial blood, but great discrepancy may be observed when these equations are used to compute venous saturation. This problem comes from the fact that every single body district has his own hemoglobin dissociation curve: in other words, each given PO_2 corresponds to a hemoglobin saturation in each blood compartment. Therefore, when there is the need to compute other variables (i.e., oxygen content) starting from saturation, it is far better to rely on saturation measurements instead of computed ones [3].

9.2.2 Dissolved Oxygen

A small part of the oxygen transported by the blood is dissolved both in plasma and in red cells. The concentration of oxygen present as molecular oxygen unbound in blood, according to Henry's law of gases, depends on the partial pressure of oxygen in the gas phase.

$$C = k \times P \quad (9.3)$$

where *C* is gas dissolved concentration, *P* is gas partial pressure in gas phase, and *k* is a fixed constant that represents the solubility for each gas, temperature, and solvent. The equilibrium is reached when an equal number of oxygen molecules go from gas to blood and vice versa. Talking about oxygen and blood, at a body temperature of 37 °C, oxygen solubility coefficient equals to 0.00314 $mL \cdot dL^{-1} \cdot mmHg^{-1}$; this means that each mmHg of PO_2 corresponds to 0.003 mL of oxygen for each deciliter of blood.

Therefore, the amount of oxygen dissolved in blood (csO_2) is

$$csO_2 \left(mL / dL\right) = 0.003 \times PaO_2 \quad (9.4)$$

Considering a normal PaO_2 of 100 mmHg, the amount of oxygen dissolved in the arterial blood will be 0.3 mL/dL, a volume that represents only 1.5% of the total arterial oxygen content, and that could reasonably be negligible in clinical calculations.

9.2.3 Oxygen Total Content

After this brief discussion, we are able to talk about oxygen blood content in its totality as the sum of oxygen transported by hemoglobin and free blood oxygen:

$$cO_2 = cHbO_2 + csO_2 \quad (9.5)$$

$$cO_2 \left(mL / dL\right) = 1.39 \times Hb \times SO_2 + 0.003 \times PaO_2 \quad (9.6)$$

Normal arterial oxygen content value (cO_2), considering a pH equal to 7.4, a temperature of 37 °C, base excess (BE) equal to zero, a PO_2 of 100 mmHg, and Hb of 14 mL/dL, is about 20 mL/dL.

9.3 Blood Oxygen Measurement Techniques

Blood gas analysis represents a fundamental tool in clinical practice. It is an accessible, reliable, and rapid instrument that could guide the clinician in the management of most of the clinical settings starting from respiratory diseases going to hemodynamic impairment passing through metabolic issues. In this chapter, we will discuss oxygen-related parameters of blood gas analysis and pulse oximetry; these values can come from a direct measurement made by blood gas analyzer or from a computation (◘ Table 9.1).

Table 9.1 Blood gas analyzer parameters DO_2 related

Parameter	Method
PO_2 (mmHg)	Measured (polarography)
HHb (g/dL)	Measured (spectral analysis)
O_2Hb (g/dL)	Measured (spectral analysis)
COHb (g/dL)	Measured (spectral analysis)
MetHb (g/dL)	Measured (spectral analysis)
tHb (g/dL)	Computed from the above values
HHb (%)	*HHb/tHb*100*
COHb (%)	C*OHb/tHb*100*
MetHb (%)	Met*Hb/tHb*100*
SO_2 (%)	$O_2Hb/(O_2Hb + HHb)$ (Eq. 9.7)
O_2Hb (%)	$O_2Hb/tHb*100$
cSO_2 (%)	Computed from PO_2 and corrected for PCO2, BE, and pH (see text for details)

In this table we briefly summarize blood gas analysis parameters related to DO_2 and how they are obtained. Note that there are three ways to compute $cHbO_2$: 1,39*Hb*SO_2 (1); 1,39*Hb*O_2Hb% (2); 1,39*Hb*cSO_2 (3). The reliability of the values obtained varies depending on the clinical condition, but we recommend not to use the third one (see text for details)

PO_2 oxygen partial pressure, *HHb* deoxyhemoglobin, *O_2Hb* oxyhemoglobin, *COHb* carboxyhemoglobin, *MetHb* methemoglobin, *tHb* total hemoglobin, *SO_2* hemoglobin oxygen saturation, *cSO_2* computed hemoglobin oxygen saturation, *BE* base excess

9

9.3.1 Oxygen Blood Partial Pressure (Polarography)

This technique was firstly described by Clark in 1956 [5]. Clark's sensor, using amperometry principles, is able to quantify oxygen concentration in biological fluids. The system can be simplified as composed by an anode, a cathode, and an oxygen-permeable membrane between the sample and the electrolyte solution. Thanks to the oxygen-permeable membrane, the oxygen concentration quickly equilibrates between electrolyte solution and the sample, and when a potential difference is applied to the conductor, the electricity current that passes through the system will be directly proportional to the oxygen concentration of the system. Many factors regarding the collection and conservation of blood samples could affect the accuracy of the measurement such as temperature, analysis delay, and even syringe type. Therefore, attention to the pre-analytic phase is needed in order to maintain this measurement accuracy.

9.3.2 Oxygen Blood Saturation ($SatO_2$)

Modern blood gas analyzer measures Hb oxygen saturation using spectral analysis of the hemoglobin released from a sample of hemolyzed arterial blood. Indeed, using dedicated wavelengths for different hemoglobin species (oxyhemoglobin, HbO_2; reduced hemoglobin, HHb; carboxyhemoglobin, COHb; and methemoglobin, MetHb), modern blood gas analyzer is able to measure total hemoglobin (tHb), (Eq. 9.7).

$$tHb = HHb + O_2Hb + COHb + MetHb \tag{9.7}$$

After the machine has measured the concentrations of hemoglobin subtypes, it gives three values related to hemoglobin oxygen saturation (HbO_2, SO_2, and cSO_2) using the following equations (Table 9.1).

$$HbO_2(\%) = \frac{cHbO_2}{HHb + O_2Hb + COHb + MetHb} \tag{9.8}$$

$$SO_2(\%) = \frac{cHbO_2}{cHbO_2 + cHHb} \tag{9.9}$$

Or:

$$SO_2(\%) = \frac{cHbO_2}{tHb - (COHb + MetHb)} \tag{9.10}$$

The last value is computed oxygen saturation (cSO2). This value comes (as previously discussed) from one of the available equations that compute hemoglobin oxygen saturation as a function of PO_2, pH, base excess, temperature, and PCO_2 [3].

It must be noted that among all the detected hemoglobin species, COHb and MetHb are not involved in oxygen transport as they are not able to bind oxygen. In normal conditions, considering a negligible amount of COHb and MetHb, HbO_2 and SO_2 values should overlap. However, in some pathological conditions (e.g., carbon oxide intoxication), HbO_2 and SO_2 will be significantly different. In this particular condition, a patient may have a normal SO_2 (or a SpO_2) and arterial oxygen partial pressure (PaO_2), but the effective oxygen saturation may be extremely low. This condition is brought by a very low value of HbO_2 and high levels of COHb.

9.3.3 Pulse Oximetry (SpO_2)

Pulse oximetry is a noninvasive and simple technique that allows, using spectral analysis, continuous measurement of hemoglobin oxygen saturation at the bedside. The two wavelengths commonly used are at 660 nm and at 940 nm. These two different wavelengths are able to distinguish between reduced hemoglobin and oxyhemoglobin, as the first one adsorbs the first wavelength (660 nm) ten times more than O_2Hb, while the opposite happens with the 940 nm wavelength. The pulse oximetry probe emits these two different wavelengths through the cutaneous vascular bed, and the system analyzes the pulsatile characteristics of arterial blood flow neglecting all the background stationary signals coming from tissues, venous blood, and the non-pulsatile arterial blood. A limitation of the traditional two wavelengths pulse oximetry is the capability of measuring only O_2Hb and HHb, assuming a blood concentration of COHb and MetHb of zero. In the presence of these two altered hemoglobin forms, SpO_2 becomes less reliable as COHb causes a falsely high level of SpO_2, and MetHb in significant concentrations forces SpO_2 result toward 85% regardless of real hemoglobin saturation [6]. Some modern pulse oximeters, using a more wave lengths, are able to measure both COHb and MetHb [7].

9.4 Cardiac Output

Once oxygen has been transferred to the blood, bound or unbound to hemoglobin, the cardiocirculatory function is of crucial importance to the delivery of oxygen to the peripheral tissues. Cardiac output (CO) represents the volume of blood that is ejected by the heart each minute and is generally measured as the product between heart rate (HR) and stroke volume (SV):

$$CO(L/min) = HR \times SV \tag{9.11}$$

Cardiac output is the most important determinant of oxygen delivery, and its modulation represents the best compensatory mechanism in bioenergetic crises. Cardiac output is modulated by the autonomic nervous system and by many chemical and mechanical stimuli. Among chemical factors, PO_2, PCO_2, and pH are key factors in the hemodynamic response to tissue hypoperfusion and hypoxia [8]. Indeed, a decrease in oxygen arterial content is promptly compensated by an increase in cardiac function. The opposite usually doesn't happen, as normal arterial saturation (very near to 100%) lies on the plateau portion of hemoglobin dissociation curve and hemoglobin concentration cannot change in acute if sudden impairment of hemodynamic function happens.

9

Cardiac output can be measured using several methods. The more common are briefly summarized in ◘ Table 9.2 and recently reviewed by Laher [9].

9.5 Oxygen Delivery (DO_2) and Extraction

Oxygen delivery is the oxygen volume transferred from lungs to the tissues in 1 min time. Therefore, it may be represented as

$$DO_2(mL/min) = caO_2 \times CO \tag{9.12}$$

In normal conditions at rest (CO equal to 5 L/min, $SatO_2$ 100%, and PaO_2 100 mmHg), therefore, the volume of oxygen transferred from lungs to peripheral tissues is about 1000 mL/min. If tissue oxygen consumption is, at rest, about 250 mL/min, the oxygen amount that returns to the lung will be 750 mL/min. This means that only 25% of oxygen is extracted by the tissues. Oxygen extraction ratio (O_2ER) can be expressed as

$$O_2ER(\%) = \frac{VO_2}{DO_2} \times 100 \tag{9.13}$$

Therefore, oxygen that remains in mixed venous blood corresponds to 75% of total oxygen that has been delivered. This percentage corresponds approximately to normal mixed venous blood hemoglobin saturation (SvO_2). SvO_2 can be precisely computed as an oxygen fraction function, using the equation below:

$$SvO_2(\%) = SaO_2 \times \left(1 - \frac{VO_2}{DO_2}\right) \tag{9.14}$$

Table 9.2 Principal cardiac output monitoring techniques

Method	Vascular access	Principle	Pros	Cons	Timing
Swan Ganz catheter	Pulmonary artery cannulation	Thermodilution	Gold standard	Invasiveness	Intermittent
Transthoracic echocardiography	None	Ultrasound and Doppler effect	Noninvasive, measurement of cardiac output and other cardiac parameters	Operator dependency, variable quality echocardiographic windows in ICU patients	Intermittent
Transesophageal echocardiography	None	Ultrasound and Doppler effect	Direct measurement of cardiac output and cardiac structures	Minimally invasive, operator dependent	Intermittent
Calibrated pulse contour analysis	Arterial and venous access	Thermodilution plus pulse contour analysis	Measurement of CO plus other variables	Minimally invasive	Intermittent and continuous
Uncalibrated pulse contour analysis	Arterial access	Pulse contour analysis	Measurement of CO plus other variables	Minimally invasive, inaccuracy in unstable patients or during use of vasoactive drugs	Continuous

Every situation that causes a decrease in SaO_2 or an increase in oxygen extraction will result in a decrease in the saturation of the mixed venous blood.

This approach underlines the importance of measuring SvO_2 as an indicator of the balance between oxygen delivery and oxygen consumption. Equation 9.15 can be rewritten as.

$$SvO_2 = SaO_2 - \frac{VO_2\,(L/min)}{CO\,L/min} \times \frac{1}{0.00139 \times Hb\,(g/L)} \tag{9.15}$$

This equation makes explicit the importance of SvO_2 monitoring. Indeed, abnormal values of SvO_2 (below 0.65) indicate a change in Hb levels or a worsening in the relationship linking arterial saturation (SaO_2), tissue metabolism (VO_2), and hemodynamics (CO). Therefore, it is important to keep in mind that a decrease in SvO_2 does not specify which of its determinants is altered but that one or more of them are out of range. An altered SvO_2 dictates a detailed search of the underlying causes, and each of them may be life threatening. If mixed venous blood sampling is not possible, central venous blood saturation ($ScvO_2$) is an acceptable surrogate even if, depending on the clinical condition, it may be higher or lower than SvO_2 [10].

9.6 Step Toward Energetic Crisis

In patients suffering from conditions that may affect oxygen transport, appropriate monitoring during the course of the disease should indicate if one of the following conditions is developing:

1. Energy production is adequate to the patient needs.
   The definition of adequate oxygen supply does not depend on a given amount of hemoglobin, cardiac output, or oxygen saturation but may only be defined in clinical practice by indirect methods. In other words, in different conditions a cardiac output of 3.6 L or more could be equally adequate to satisfy the energy needs, as well as a PO_2 of 90, 100, or 120 mmHg or an oxygen saturation of 90% or 100%. Defining the best PO_2, the best cardiac output or the best hemoglobin level, ignoring their association with the energetic needs is, in our view, not only useless but potentially dangerous. What should help the clinician to identify if there is a problem in satisfying the energy needs of the system is the identification of the compensatory mechanisms.

2. Energy production is still adequate but compensatory mechanisms are operating.
   It is well known for decades that oxygen consumption, when plotted as a function of oxygen transport remains constant until a critical point, which may vary, depending on the underlying disease [11]. Below this critical point, oxygen consumption starts to decrease while lactate starts to increase (◘ Fig. 9.2).

   All compensatory mechanisms are operating to maintain the aerobic energy production constant in the range of oxygen supply that goes from normal values to the critical point. The decrease in oxygen consumption and the increase in lactate levels are signal of the energy crisis. The most sensitive indicator of oxygen transport is the central venous saturation.

   ◘ Figure 9.3 displays the relative weight of each of the determinants of SvO_2 as they decrease in a 10% step from the initial value, while other factors remain constant. As shown, arterial saturation changes (SaO_2) are linearly related to the changes in SvO_2. As the SaO_2 is easily measured by pulse oximetry, changes in SvO_2 due to changes in SO_2 may be easily estimated considering their proportional relationship. It is interesting to note that a 10% change in hemoglobin or cardiac output produces exactly the same change in venous saturation. Therefore, the decrease in SvO_2 clearly indicates that some of the oxygen transport mechanisms are impaired but not necessarily indicates that energy crisis is taking place. Physical activity, even in normal individuals, is associated with an increase in oxygen consumption, i.e., energy demand. In this situation, the hemodynamic response to the augmented energy demand is represented by an increase in cardiac output and a decrease in venous oxygen saturation. In intensive care patients however, in whom muscle activity is near to zero, a change in SvO_2 requires a diagnosis of the underlying causes. While the meaning of a decrease in SvO_2 is well established, the pathophysiological meaning of an increased SvO2 is less evident. Theoretically, whatever increase in cardiac output exceeding the energy requirement should produce an increase in SvO_2. The most likely explanation, however, although not clearly defined quantitatively, is that high SvO_2 is the result of one of these conditions indistinguishable from each other:

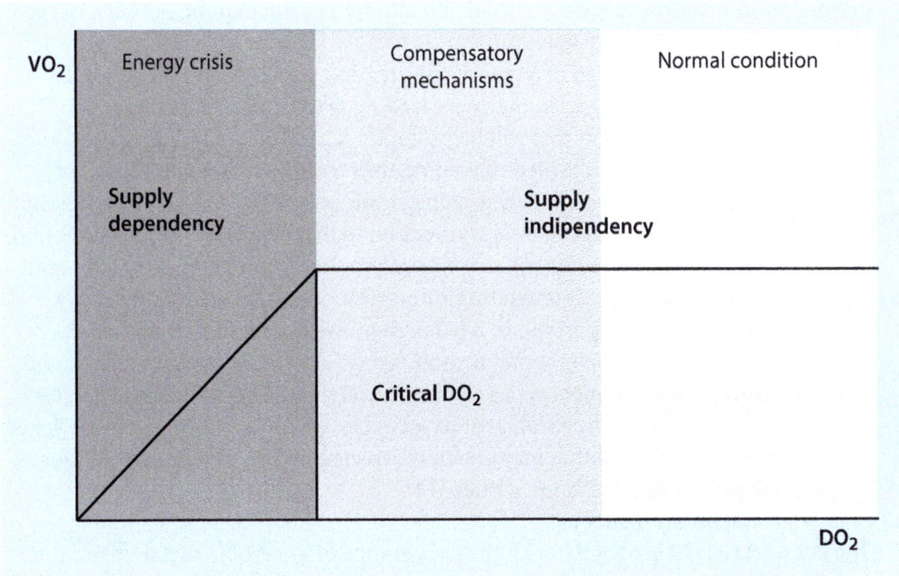

Fig. 9.2 Critical oxygen delivery. Table shows oxygen consumption trend when oxygen supply is impaired. In "supply independency phase," system responds to a decrease in oxygen delivery with an increase in oxygen extraction in order to maintain a normal value of oxygen consumption. When a critical value of oxygen delivery is reached, oxygen consumption becomes oxygen delivery dependent and starts to decrease (energy crisis). VO_2 oxygen consumption, DO_2 oxygen delivery

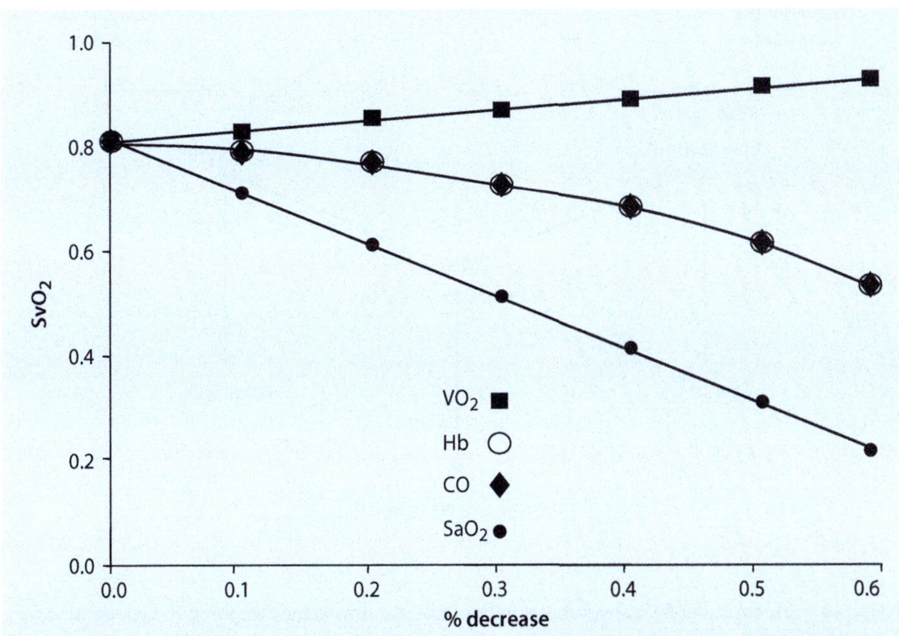

Fig. 9.3 Relative "weight" of mixed venous saturation determinants. This table shows in a graphical way the impact of a decrease (with 10% steps) in VO_2, Hb, CO, and SaO_2 on SvO_2. Data coming from institutional database, unpublished. SvO_2 mixed venous blood oxygen saturation, VO_2 oxygen consumption, Hb hemoglobin concentration, CO cardiac output, SaO_2 arterial oxygen saturation

peripheral shunting or respiratory chain alterations and uncoupling between oxygen consumption and energy production.

Another important signal of a precritical situation comes from the kidney. In mammalians, a hemodynamic impairment leading at the end to tissue hypoxia dictates a flow redistribution that will be promptly sensed by the kidney that will activate all its mechanisms devoted to volume conservation. The main players of kidney response are renin-angiotensin-aldosterone system (RASS) and vasopressin. These mediators are responsible for a contraction in urine output and a Na retention that will be easily recognized by urinary electrolytes inversion (low urinary Na and relatively high urinary K). Although this kidney response may seem not directly related to the oxygen transport but to a reflex response to pressure changes coming from baroceptors, we believe that hemodynamic in general cannot be separated from the oxygen transport concept as all our hemodynamic apparatus evolved just with the function of providing sufficient oxygen delivery to tissues. A complete set of hemodynamic impairment that may anticipate tissue hypoxia or be its actual cause is shown in ◻ Fig. 9.4 adapted from Schrier [12].

3. Energy production is inadequate.
The energy crisis likely begins with the appearance of anaerobic metabolism. It is possible that it may occur at different times in different organs, but a rapid rise in

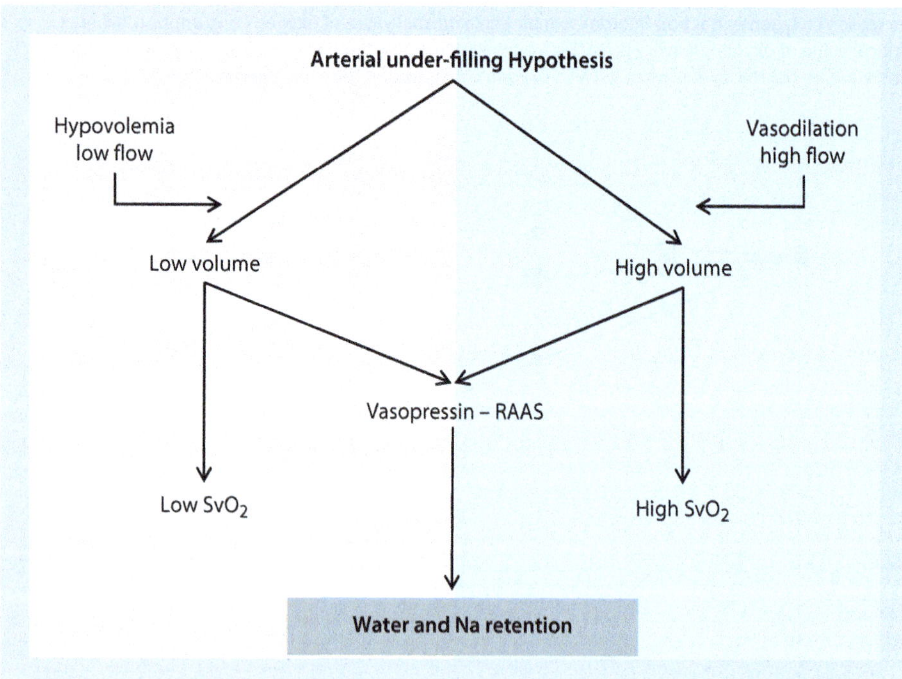

◻ **Fig. 9.4** Arterial under-filling hypothesis. In this table we show kidney response to hypoperfusion. Hypovolemia and low flow (i.e., hemorrhage and heart failure) cause decrease in kidney perfusion and oxygenation, with activation of RASS, vasopressin release, increase in O_2ER, and consequent SvO_2 decrease (on the left). Vasodilatation and high flow (i.e., cirrosis and sepsis) are conditions in which "high volume" is associated to a relatively hypoperfused kidney (right) with consequent activation of the same mechanisms lactate is an unquestionable sign, when associated with problems of oxygen transport/utilization, of a life-threatening condition. When oxygen delivery is severely impaired and reaches its critical value, a further increase in oxygen extraction is not possible. In this situation, at cellular level, tissue hypoxia, through hypoxia inducible factors (HIFs), activates a series of emergency mechanisms to maintain energy production [13]. This include an increased production of glycolytic enzymes and a decreased production of the enzymes necessary for Krebs cycle preparing cellular metabolism to the production of energy through anaerobic metabolism.

The energy production by anaerobic glycolysis, however, is only 5–6% of the one associated with aerobic metabolism. One mole of glucose (180 g) produces two moles of lactate and two moles of ATP. As the lactate is the final acceptor of electrons, in absence of oxygen 2 moles of ATP is the total amount of energy that is produced compared to the 32/36 moles of ATP produced during aerobic metabolism.

Some of the mechanisms operating during an overt energy crisis reflect in part what has been observed in hibernated animals. These animals decrease dramatically their energy requirement by decreasing protein synthesis and increasing enzymes half-life. They develop channel arrest and decrease proton movement through the ATPase as well as the electron transport in the respiratory chain and the proton leaks through the mitochondrial membranes. In humans, the oxygen supply dependency is a pale representation of the mechanism operating in hibernating animals and consists in similar systems for saving energy primarily through a decrease in protein synthesis. Unfortunately, this energy sparing condition may last only few hours after which irreversible changes in mitochondria may occur with final apoptosis and, in particular conditions, necrosis. Therefore, when the energetic crisis appears, we know that only few hours are available for correction and an immediate diagnosis of the underlying causes and a prompt intervention to correct them is needed.

Summarizing, the largely accepted view of oxygen transport impairment is the following:

- A decrease in tissue oxygenation is compensated at least in part by a greater oxygen release from hemoglobin and increase in oxygen extraction.
- When tissue partial oxygen pressure and oxygen concentration reach critical levels (which are clinically difficult to be defined), lactate production increases while oxygen consumption is partially decreased.
- When energy is insufficient, despite all the compensatory mechanisms, cellular dysfunction and damage begin: protein synthesis decreases, reactive oxygen species increases, and hypoxic damages, including necrosis and apoptosis, unavoidably follow.

There are conditions, however, which may occur in intensive care in which the decrease in oxygen consumption is not due to the decrease of transport to tissues but instead to the oxygen utilization. This may happen, as an example, if the complex molecules of the respiratory chain are structurally altered as may occur in sepsis. In addition, it is also possible that in some conditions, the underlying mechanism is the uncoupling between oxygen consumption and ATP production. This may occur in all the conditions which may impair proton concentration in the intermembrane space of the mitochondria. In this case the electrons flow down to the molecular oxygen to form water regularly, but the concentration of protons in the intermembrane space is decreased by the presence of intermediates (uncoupling agents) which shuttle the protons from inside to outside the membrane.

Therefore, three conditions of tissue dysoxia may be recognized which require different interventions and attention:

- Classical decrease in oxygen transport to tissues typically represented by hemodynamic impairment, hypoxemia, or anemia
- Respiratory chain impairment with decrease in ATP production
- Presence of uncoupling agents which dissociates oxygen consumption from energy production

Of note all the three conditions may present together at different extent in severe sepsis, and it is worth to underline that what really matters is not the oxygen transport "per se" but the energy production.

9.7 Oxygen Transport and Goal-Directed Therapy

A remarkable part of intensive care is devoted directly or indirectly to the control of oxygen transport and to the prevention of its impairment or to its correction when altered. When oxygen transport is impaired because of cardiac failure or volume depletion as in hemorrhage, the causes of tissue hypoxia are clear, and the correction is straightforward to renovate CO and circulating volume. The issue is less clear when other severe conditions as sepsis are involved.

Indeed the issue of oxygen transport originated a lot of debates and controversies after Shoemaker, one of the giants of intensive care, promoted the concept of "supernormal" oxygen delivery [14]. This was defined as a cardiac index greater than 4.5 L/min/m^2, an oxygen delivery greater than 600 mL/min/m^2, and an oxygen consumption greater than 170 mL/min/m^2. Shoemaker's observations derived from his experience in high-risk surgical patients in whose targeting therapies in order to reach "supernormal values" showed to improve clinical outcome. Early trials suggested that an increase in oxygen delivery would prevent organ failures and improve survival rates in such patients [15, 16]. The concept of "supernormal values," firstly developed in a particularly subset of patients, was immediately translated to other conditions up to ICU general population. However when the hypothesis of "supernormal" oxygen delivery was tested in clinical trials on general ICU population, no benefits were observed and these two trials signed the end of "supernormal" values [17, 18].

Ten years later Rivers found an impressive improvement in survival applying to severe sepsis and septic shock patients an approach targeted primarily to a central venous saturation of 70% and a MAP greater than 65 mmHg, defined as early goal-directed therapy (EGDT) [19]. The early goal-directed therapy became immediately popular and produced in intensive care physicians an increased attention to hemodynamics. Ten years later, three studies together retested Rivers' hypothesis and compared patients with severe sepsis and septic shock treated with normal care or treated following Rivers' goals [20–22]. No benefits could be demonstrated, and this lead to the implicit conclusion that $Scvo_2$ monitoring is useless. These studies rose a series of discussion which still persist, but we believe that these results should be discussed after two considerations:

- Beyond all the unavoidable differences in study populations, it must be noted that the success of supernormal values were obtained in patients treated before the intensive care, i.e., in the perioperative period by Shoemaker et al. and in emergency room by Rivers et al.

- Baseline Svo_2 in Rivers' study was extremely low (around 50%), while it was higher around 70% in all the studies performed in intensive care, meaning that Rivers' patients were sicker.

We believe anyway that, in patients with septic shock, time of intervention plays a crucial role, but we also believe that the negative results of these trials should switch the attention to the fact that in patients with sepsis or septic shock, the problem is not always related to oxygen transport to periphery per se but also to its final utilization. In our opinion this is what all the recent studies have suggested, and the logical conclusion is not that Svo_2 monitoring is useless but that the problems of most septic patients is not the oxygen transport.

Practical Implications

DO_2 monitoring should be performed in all those patients at risk of "energy crisis." This kind of patients include those in which one or more DO_2 determinants are at risk of impairment as cardiovascular, hemorrhagic, and patients with respiratory insufficiency but also those patients in which, even if DO_2 is still satisfactory, there is a difficulty in oxygen utilization, such as septic patients (see ◘ Fig. 9.4).

In all these patients urinary output, mixed venous saturation (or central venous saturation if a pulmonary catheter is not in place), urinary electrolytes, and, at the end, lactate represent very informative tools in identifying a situation in which compensatory mechanisms are activated and energy crisis is about to show.

A mixed venous saturation under 65% (or a negative trend), urinary output contraction, reversal in urinary electrolytes (Na lower than K), and a positive lactate trend dictate an accurate evaluation of DO_2 determinants.

Take-Home Messages

- Oxygen delivery is a parameter that is important to consider in critical patients management. What is of crucial importance, anyway, is not oxygen delivery per se but the early identification of all those parameters that are indirect signals of an insufficient oxygen supply or, lately, of an energetic crisis.
- Oxygen delivery concept should go beyond the simple result of the computation of cardiac output times oxygen content and should be thought in a more comprehensive way starting from pulmonary gas exchange and ventilation and arriving to mitochondria's utilization.
- Sepsis and septic shock are conditions in which a discrepancy between DO_2 and VO_2 is more evident.

References

1. Gattinoni L, Pesenti A, Matthay M. Understanding blood gas analysis. Intensive Care Med. 2018;44(1):91–3.
2. Adair GS. The hemoglobin system: VI. The oxygen dissociation curve of hemoglobin. J Biol Chem. 1925;63(2):529–45.
3. Breuer HW, Groeben H, Breuer J, Worth H. Oxygen saturation calculation procedures: a critical analysis of six equations for the determination of oxygen saturation. Intensive Care Med. 1989;15(6):385–9.

4. Kelman GR. Digital computer subroutine for the conversion of oxygen tension into saturation. J Appl Physiol. 1966;21(4):1375–6.
5. Clark LCJ. Monitor and control of blood and tissue oxygen tensions. ASAIO J. 1956;2(1):41–8.
6. Sinex JE. Pulse oximetry: principles and limitations. Am J Emerg Med. 1999;17(1):59–67.
7. Barker SJ, Curry J, Redford D, Morgan S. Measurement of carboxyhemoglobin and methemoglobin by pulse oximetry: a human volunteer study. Anesthesiology. 2006;105(5):892–7.
8. Shepherd AP, Granger HJ, Smith EE, Guyton AC. Local control of tissue oxygen delivery and its contribution to the regulation of cardiac output. Am J Phys. 1973;225(3):747–55.
9. Laher AE, Watermeyer MJ, Buchanan SK, Dippenaar N, Simo NCT, Motara F, et al. A review of hemodynamic monitoring techniques, methods and devices for the emergency physician. Am J Emerg Med. 2017;35(9):1335–47.
10. Reinhart K, Rudolph T, Bredle DL, Hannemann L, Cain SM. Comparison of central-venous to mixed-venous oxygen saturation during changes in oxygen supply/demand. Chest. 1989;95(6):1216–21.
11. Schumacker PT, Cain SM. The concept of a critical oxygen delivery. Intensive Care Med. 1987;13(4): 223–9.
12. Schrier RW, Howard RL. Unifying hypothesis of sodium and water regulation in health and disease. Hypertension. 1991;18(5 Suppl):III164–8.
13. Bunn HF, Poyton RO. Oxygen sensing and molecular adaptation to hypoxia. Physiol Rev. 1996;76(3):839–85.
14. Shoemaker WC, Appel PL, Kram HB, Waxman K, Lee TS. Prospective trial of supranormal values of survivors as therapeutic goals in high-risk surgical patients. Chest. 1988;94(6):1176–86.
15. Boyd O, Grounds RM, Bennett ED. A randomized clinical trial of the effect of deliberate perioperative increase of oxygen delivery on mortality in high-risk surgical patients. JAMA. 1993;270(22):2699–707.
16. Tuchschmidt J, Fried J, Astiz M, Rackow E. Elevation of cardiac output and oxygen delivery improves outcome in septic shock. Chest. 1992;102(1):216–20.
17. Hayes MA, Timmins AC, Yau EH, Palazzo M, Hinds CJ, Watson D. Elevation of systemic oxygen delivery in the treatment of critically ill patients. N Engl J Med. 1994;330(24):1717–22.
18. Gattinoni L, Brazzi L, Pelosi P, Latini R, Tognoni G, Pesenti A, et al. A trial of goal-oriented hemodynamic therapy in critically ill patients. SvO2 Collaborative Group. N Engl J Med. 1995;333(16):1025–32.
19. Rivers E, Nguyen B, Havstad S, Ressler J, Muzzin A, Knoblich B, et al. Early goal-directed therapy in the treatment of severe sepsis and septic shock. N Engl J Med. 2001;345(19):1368–77.
20. Mouncey PR, Osborn TM, Power GS, Harrison DA, Sadique MZ, Grieve RD, et al. Trial of early, goal-directed resuscitation for septic shock. N Engl J Med. 2015;372(14):1301–11.
21. Pro CI, Yealy DM, Kellum JA, Huang DT, Barnato AE, Weissfeld LA, et al. A randomized trial of protocol-based care for early septic shock. N Engl J Med. 2014;370(18):1683–93.
22. ARISE Investigators; ANZICS Clinical Trials Group, Peake SL, Delaney A, Bailey M, Bellomo R, et al. Goal-directed resuscitation for patients with early septic shock. N Engl J Med. 2014;371(16):1496–506.

Mitochondrial Function

Mervyn Singer

M. R. Pinsky et al. (eds.), *Hemodynamic Monitoring*, Lessons from the ICU,
https://doi.org/10.1007/978-3-319-69269-2_10

Learning Objectives

- To explain how mitochondria produce energy substrate (ATP)
- To describe how mitochondrial function is perturbed in pathological conditions
- To cover various techniques for monitoring mitochondrial function

10.1 Introduction

The mitochondrion is the powerhouse of the cell, utilizing over 90% of the body's oxygen consumption predominantly towards generation of ATP, the energy currency of the cell. Failure of adequate delivery of oxygen to the tissues (hypoxia) and/or utilization of oxygen (dysoxia) towards ATP production may be sufficient to compromise cell metabolism. It is thus incumbent upon the clinician to identify this insufficiency as early as possible in order to initiate effective treatments that can reverse, or at least, attenuate, the consequences of tissue hypoxia and/or dysoxia that is manifest clinically as organ dysfunction. This chapter will briefly review mitochondrial physiology and pathophysiology and discuss monitoring modalities that can assess mitochondrial function either directly or indirectly.

10.2 The Physiology of Mitochondrial Function

Apart from erythrocytes, all other cells in the body possess mitochondria. Though usually associated with ATP production, mitochondria play other crucial roles in maintaining cell and organism housekeeping and functionality such as calcium regulation, hormone production and apoptotic death pathways. These aspects will not be discussed further.

Mitochondria are 1–3 microns in diameter though they vary in size and shape both between different organs and even within anatomically different parts of the same organ. Numbers vary from relatively few to as many as several thousands in heavily metabolic cells such as hepatocytes and cardiomyocytes. Most of the DNA encoding mitochondrial proteins sit within the nucleus, with the 900 or so gene products imported from the cytoplasm for subsequent incorporation into the varied mitochondrial structures. However, uniquely for another organelle, the mitochondrion also possesses 37 genes with its own machinery for producing RNA (24 genes) and protein subunits (13 genes). These are generally considered to originate from probacteria incorporated into cells to produce eukaryotic cells capable of utilizing oxygen for metabolic processes.

The mitochondrion consists of outer and inner membranes, separated by an intermembrane space, and these enclose the cristae (infolding of the inner membrane) and matrix. The cristae enable a huge expansion of the surface area of the mitochondrial membrane; Rich estimated that the average human possesses 14,000 m^2 of inner membrane [1]. The matrix contains many ribosomes and enzymes, including those constituting the citric acid (Krebs') cycle.

The outer membrane is a protein-lipid structure similar in composition to the plasma membrane. It contains specialized transporters that can transfer ADP into, and ATP out of, the organelle. The inner membrane contains the five protein complexes that make up the electron transport chain: nicotinamide adenine dinucleotide (NADH) dehydrogenase (Complex I), succinate dehydrogenase (Complex II), ubiquinone-cytochrome *c* oxidoreductase (Complex III), cytochrome oxidase (Complex IV) and ATP synthase (Complex V)

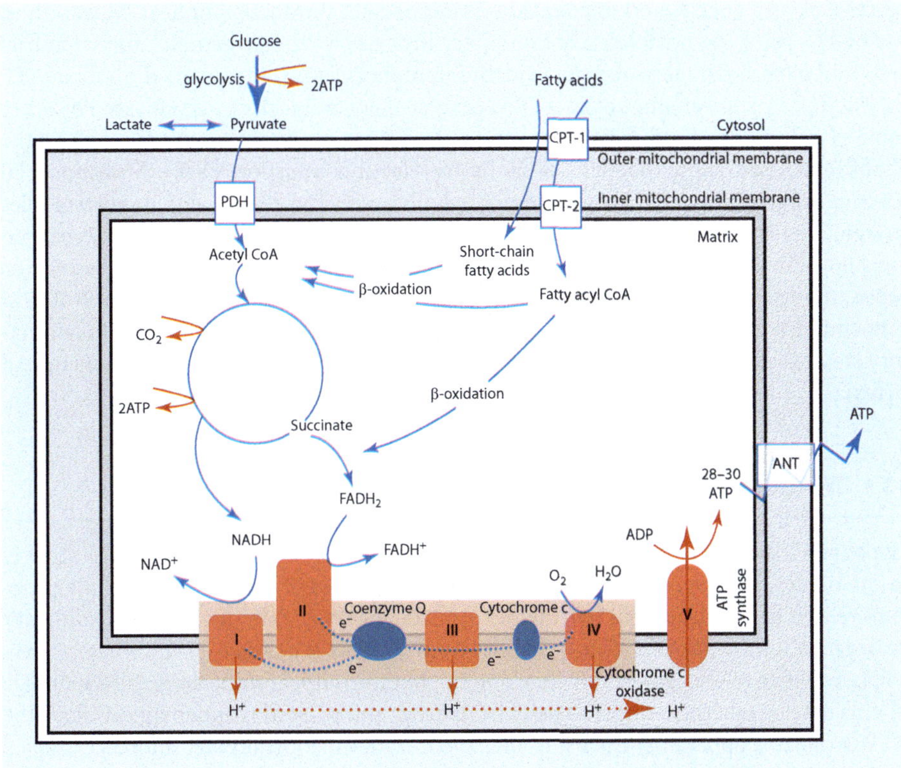

Fig. 10.1 Mitochondrial respiration. PDH pyruvate dehydrogenase, CPT-1,-2 carnitine palmitoyl transferase-1,-2, ATP adenosine triphosphate, ADP adenosine diphosphate, NADH nicotinamide adenine dinucleotide, $FADH_2$ flavin adenine dinucleotide, ANT adenine nucleotide translocase

which phosphorylates ADP to ATP. In addition, the chain has two small electron carriers, ubiquinone (coenzyme Q10) and cytochrome *c* (Fig. 10.1).

The Krebs' cycle donates electrons to the electron transport chain, predominantly to Complex I (via NADH) but also to Complex II (via succinate to $FADH_2$) in a ratio of 3:1. The Krebs' cycle is 'refuelled' by provision of acetyl-CoA from both pyruvate (the end product of glycolysis) and fatty acid oxidation. This electron donation oxidizes the energy-rich molecules NADH (to NAD^+) and FAD (flavin adenine dinucleotide) to $FADH_2$. As the electrons pass down the chain, protons pass across the inner mitochondrial membrane from Complexes I, III and IV, generating a membrane potential of approximately 200 mV. Molecular oxygen is the final electron acceptor at Complex IV, and this single enzyme is responsible for the bulk of the body's oxygen consumption. The electrochemical gradient provides the energy to drive ATP synthase to phosphorylate ADP into ATP. Rich further estimated that the transmembrane proton flux is of the order of 3×10^{21} protons per second with ATP being reformed at a rate of around 9×10^{20} molecules per second, equivalent to a turnover rate of ATP of 65 kg per day [1]. A typical adult male would consume around 380 l of oxygen daily, and this would require 2×10^{19} molecules of cytochrome oxidase.

This utilization is primarily directed towards production of ATP, the energy substrate used for cellular metabolic processes ('coupled respiration'), but also for generation of reactive oxygen species and uncoupled respiration with production of heat. Most cells in the body – with the notable exception of erythrocytes – rely on 'aerobic' mitochondrial respiration (through the process of oxidative phosphorylation) to provide the bulk of ATP production. A smaller amount of ATP is generated anaerobically by glycolysis. For every mole of glucose oxidized, a net of 2 moles of ATP are produced by glycolysis, 2 by the Krebs' cycle and approximately 28–30 by the electron transport chain. Mitochondrial reactive oxygen species (ROS) are relevant in both health and disease with important roles in signalling and modulation of respiration. Approximately 1% of mitochondrial oxygen consumption is used for ROS generation in health. This rises in disease states such as sepsis, though the extent is uncertain. Similarly, uncoupling can account for up to 50% of mitochondrial oxygen consumption in skeletal muscle [2]; how this changes in inflammatory states such as sepsis is unknown, but it may plausibly contribute to the production of pyrexia.

10.3 Mitochondrial Dysfunction in Disease States

Hypoxia is a state of oxygen-limited respiration, imposed by an imbalance between supply to the tissues and the cellular respiratory demand. Causes of low delivery include problems related to cardiac output (*circulatory hypoxia*), haemoglobin (*anaemic hypoxia*) and/or oxygenation (*hypoxic hypoxia*). Distinct from hypoxia is *dysoxia*, a state whereby oxygen is available to the cells in sufficient amount but the mitochondria are unable to utilize it. This may be related to direct toxicity from drugs and poisons that damage or block the ATP-producing apparatus. The list is long and includes metformin that inhibits Complex I, dinitrophenol that increases uncoupling, and poisons such as cyanide and carbon monoxide that inhibit Complex IV. Even antibiotics can affect mitochondrial function – bactericidal antibiotics can damage the membrane and affect membrane potential, while bacteriostatic antibiotics can compromise biogenesis (formation of new mitochondria). Deficiency of crucial cofactors such as thiamine can affect glycolysis and the Krebs' cycle, causing beriberi. There may be also damage or inhibition of the electron transport chain by excess levels of endogenous mediators, notably reactive oxygen species and nitrogen species including nitric oxide. Nitric oxide can reversibly inhibit Complex IV by directly competing with oxygen for the same binding site. A similar effect is seen with the other endogenous gaseous mediators, carbon monoxide and hydrogen sulphide. A longer-lasting inhibition can be achieved by nitric oxide or its metabolites such as peroxynitrite through nitrosylation or nitration of all the respiratory complexes, notably Complexes I and IV. Other mechanisms leading to mitochondrial dysfunction include decreased transcription of genes encoding mitochondrial proteins, as seen in sepsis, and hormonal influences that may depress metabolism and mitochondrial activity, such as low thyroid levels seen in critical illness as the low T3/sick euthyroid syndrome.

10.4 Mitochondrial Monitoring Modalities

A variety of techniques can assess in vivo mitochondrial function either directly or indirectly. Some are currently available as bedside monitors whereas others, such as magnetic resonance spectroscopy, require transfer of the patient to a specialized facility. It is important to stress that surrogate measures such as plasma lactate or whole body oxygen consumption are not specific for mitochondrial function and may also be affected by other factors.

10.4.1 Lactate and Lactate/Pyruvate (L:P) Ratio

Lactate is a by-product of glycolysis. Glucose is metabolized to pyruvate which is then taken up into the mitochondria and converted via pyruvate dehydrogenase to acetyl-CoA. Any remaining pyruvate goes into equilibrium with lactate, using the bidirectional lactate dehydrogenase. Lactate can be produced in excess if there is an accelerated rate of glycolysis and/or a downstream block exists in the Krebs' cycle or electron transport chain. There may also be problems with lactate utilization, e.g. liver failure or released from infarcted tissue.

Glycolysis can be accelerated either as part of a compensatory response to cellular oxygen limitation, in an attempt to increase ATP production where oxidative phosphorylation is compromised ('anaerobic glycolysis'). Alternatively, oxygen may be available, but glycolysis is stimulated by excess catecholamines ('aerobic glycolysis'). Teleologically, aerobic glycolysis is an adaptive response to ongoing stress whereby muscle lactate is produced in excess and released into the circulation for utilization as an important fuel substrate by other organs including the heart, brain, liver and kidney. Within the brain, lactate derived from astrocytes provides an important energy substrate for neurons [3]. A downstream block within the mitochondria, related to a failure of normal functioning of the Krebs' cycle (e.g. due to thiamine deficiency) or to the electron transport chain (e.g. lack of substrate/oxygen availability due to tissue hypoxia or to inhibition/damage related to cyanide poisoning, sepsis and excess nitric oxide production), will also result in an increase in pyruvate and thus lactate.

The L:P ratio correlates with the cytoplasmic ratio of reduced NADH to oxidized NAD^+ as pyruvate + NADH + $H^+ \longleftrightarrow$ lactate + NAD^+. The L:P ratio can thus be used as a surrogate measure of the cytosolic oxidoreduction state. During tissue hypoxia, where the L:P ratio is increased, reduced forms of oxidoreduction coenzymes such as NADH and $FADH_2$ predominate.

Blood lactate monitors are widely available as both laboratory and point-of-care devices; these utilize the lactate oxidase reaction. Pyruvate is more unstable, and measurement requires more sophisticated laboratory equipment. In conjunction with an elevated lactate (>2 mmol/l), a lactate/pyruvate (L:P) ratio > 25 suggests a disorder of the respiratory chain complex or the Krebs' cycle and can be observed in the critically ill. In conjunction with an elevated lactate, an L:P ratio < 25 suggests a defect in pyruvate metabolism. Abnormal concentrations of lactate, pyruvate and the L:P ratio are not however diagnostic for any single disorder and must be interpreted in context with the patient's presenting history, clinical features and other laboratory tests.

Tissue lactate, pyruvate and the L:P ratio can be measured by microdialysis using fine catheters implanted into tissue beds such as the brain, subcutaneous tissue, muscle, kidney and liver [4]. A very slow rate (usually well below 1 microlitre/min) of perfusate fluid is pumped through the catheters, and the dialysate is collected for analysis. This slow perfusion allows equilibration across the catheter membrane of lactate and pyruvate present in the interstitial fluid with the perfusion fluid. Samples are collected into microvials that can be analysed at the bedside by an online device or sent for measurement in a laboratory.

10.4.2 Arterial Ketone Body Ratio (AKBR)

The ratio of arterial blood acetoacetate to β-hydroxybutyrate is considered to reflect the hepatic ketone body ratio and thus hepatic mitochondrial redox potential (NAD^+/NADH), which is itself an indicator of hepatic energy charge. Both these ketones are produced almost exclusively by the liver, from whence they are released into the circulation for utilization (oxidation) as an energy substrate by various organs such as the brain, heart, muscle and kidney. A decrease in AKBR correlates with increasing liver dysfunction. The ratio is >1 in health but <1 in liver disease states and falling progressively with increasing severity. The patient needs to be adequately glucose loaded. Although, multiple publications were produced in the 1980s and 1990s [5], this concept has waned in popularity and is now rarely used.

10.4.3 Oxygen Consumption (Whole Body/Organ/Cell Level)

Oxygen is predominantly (90–95%) used within the body by mitochondria, with a small proportion consumed by non-mitochondrial processes and oxygen-dependent enzymes (e.g. oxidases). The main utilization of oxygen within the mitochondrion is for ATP production by cytochrome oxidase (Complex IV); however oxygen is also required for production of reactive oxygen species, of which the mitochondrial is the main producer in the body, and heat through uncoupled respiration. Importantly, the proportions by which these processes alter during critical illness are not known so assumptions that a maintained oxygen consumption equates to adequate ATP production may be misguided. A significant amount of oxygen consumption may be diverted towards heat production (contributing to pyrexia) and to generation of reactive oxygen species.

Whole-body oxygen consumption can be calculated in several ways, usually by variants of the Fick principle whereby total uptake of a substance (in this case, oxygen) equals the product of the blood flow and the arterial-venous concentration difference (gradient) of the oxygen. Knowledge is thus required of the cardiac output and the contents of oxygen in arterial and mixed venous (i.e. pulmonary arterial or right ventricular outflow) blood sampled or monitored from catheters in the corresponding locations.

Arterial oxygen content is the product of haemoglobin (Hb), arterial oxygen saturation (SaO_2) and 1.34 (ml of oxygen bound by 1 g Hb). The small amount of oxygen dissolved in plasma can be essentially excluded at normal atmospheric pressures. The oxygen content of mixed venous blood (product of Hb, mixed venous oxygen saturation and 1.34) is subtracted from the arterial oxygen content, thus providing the arteriovenous difference which, multiplied by cardiac output, provides a measure of oxygen consumption. This approach excludes oxygen consumed within the lung. The normal resting value of oxygen delivery is approximately 1000 ml/min and consumption 250 ml/min. Low values of oxygen consumption may relate to inadequate supply of oxygen to the tissues (as reflected by low values of cardiac output, Hb and/or SaO_2) or to decreased utilization due to direct mitochondrial toxicity or dysfunction. In the former case, mixed venous oxygen saturation is low (normal range 70–75%), and in the latter, it is supranormal. High values of venous oxygen saturation may also be seen with large right-to-left peripheral vascular shunts. The contribution of microvascular shunting towards generating high values of mixed venous oxygen saturation in pathological conditions such as sepsis is uncertain.

An alternative approach using the same Fick principle is respiratory indirect calorimetry measuring the oxygen concentration in inspired and expired gases, using in-line oxygen sensors and minute ventilation. Oxygen consumption is the difference between (inspired gas volume × fractional oxygen) and (expired gas volume × fractional oxygen). This can be measured using a metabolic cart with a canopy or hood in spontaneously breathing individuals or through the ventilator circuit during mechanical ventilation. Care must be taken to correct for temperature, humidification, barometric pressure and ventilator flow by circuits as significant errors may be introduced [6].

At the organ level, oxygen consumption can be calculated by measuring organ blood flow and the oxygen content within the arterial supply and venous drainage of that organ.

Tissues (e.g. muscle) or cells (including white blood cells) can be taken from the patient and oxygen consumption measured ex vivo in respirometers. The tissue is placed into fluid inside a closed chamber of known volume with an integral oxygen sensor. The rate of fall of oxygen tension within the chamber, corrected for the weight of tissue or number of cells, enables computation of oxygen consumption. An advantage of this ex vivo approach is that the tissue can be exposed to different substrates, activator inhibitors and uncouplers of the electron transport chain and ATP synthase. This enables assessment of the proportion of oxygen consumed by coupled and uncoupled mitochondrial respiration and by non-mitochondrial processes, as well as maximal respiratory capacity [7].

10.4.4 Microvascular Oxyhaemoglobin Saturation

Misleadingly called 'tissue oxygen saturation' (StO_2), this technique uses near-infrared spectroscopy (NIRS) to provide continuous, noninvasive monitoring of microvascular haemoglobin oxygen saturation [8]. The concept utilizes the relative transparency of tissue to light in the near-infrared (700–1300 nm) range, the oxygenation-dependent light-absorbing characteristics of haemoglobin, and the Beer-Lambert law. Using several wavelengths, the relative changes in oxy- and deoxyhaemoglobin concentration can be displayed continuously. While haemoglobin is assumed to be the main chromophore in biological tissue that absorbs light in this NIR region, there will also be components drawn from oxy- and deoxy-myoglobin that cannot be separated out using currently available monitoring techniques.

Although similar in many ways to pulse oximetry, the main difference lies in what is being sampled. Pulse oximetry monitors the percentage of oxygenated haemoglobin within arterial blood, whereas NIRS measures changes in oxy- and deoxyhaemoglobin in the microvasculature (arterioles, capillaries, venules) within the tissue under investigation. The most commonly used site is the thenar eminence on the thumb; however multiple factors may affect measurements [9]. The normal range in healthy volunteers is thus very wide (67–97%) [10], so without knowing a stable healthy baseline value, a low value may or may not be indicative of poor perfusion. Attempts to use other sites, e.g. deltoid and masseter, have been disappointing.

Greater utility can be gained from this technique by a more dynamic assessment involving limb vascular occlusion. The rate of fall in oxygen saturation on arterial occlusion signifies local oxygen consumption, whereas the rate of recovery signal on release of the occlusion indicates microvascular regulation. A significant reduction in oxygen consumption with accompanying microvascular dysregulation was found in septic shock patients [11].

10.4.5 Tissue Oxygen Tension

Tissue oxygen tension (PtO_2) represents the local balance between oxygen supply and utilization. There is a normal range for different tissues which varies depending on their individual blood supply and metabolic activity. So, for example, resting muscle PtO_2 values are considerably higher than those seen in the liver and renal cortex [12]. A fall in PtO_2 occurs when oxygen delivery cannot meet local metabolic needs (e.g. hypoxia), and the converse is seen either when (i) oxygen delivery is excessive, (ii) metabolic need is suppressed (e.g. hypothermia) or (iii) mitochondrial utilization of oxygen is impaired (e.g. resuscitated sepsis). Laboratory studies indicate that falls in PtO_2 are more sensitive than global markers such as haemodynamics, arterial lactate or base deficit in detecting early hypoxia [13, 14].

PtO_2 can be monitored in real time by implanting oxygen sensors into tissue. The initial oxygen sensors were based on voltage changes measured by Clark electrodes, but newer sensors utilize materials (e.g. platinum, ruthenium) that fluoresce or phosphoresce on exposure to flashes of light with the decay half-life of the fluorescence/phosphorescence being inversely related to the local oxygen tension according to the Stern-Vollmer equation. Advantages of the newer sensors are their 'plug-and-play capability' as in vivo calibration is not required and their increasing accuracy at lower oxygen tensions. To date, there has been relatively limited use in critically ill and perioperative patients including monitoring in the muscle, brain and conjunctiva [15–17]. However, bladder wall PtO_2 monitoring utilizing a modified Foley bladder catheter to allow sensor introduction into the bladder will soon be trialled in patients.

10.4.6 Mitochondrial Redox State

Mitochondrial redox state, either the ratio of reduced NADH to oxidized NAD^+ or oxidized to reduced cytochrome oxidase (CCO), can be monitored noninvasively using the phenomenon of autofluorescence. NADH and oxidized CCO fluoresce when excited by ultraviolet illumination, whereas, conveniently, NAD^+ and reduced CCO are not. By monitoring shifts in autofluorescence intensity, in vivo changes in mitochondrial redox state can be interrogated in real time within living tissue. The necessary assumption is that the total pool of NADH/NAD+ and oxidized/reduced CCO remains the same; in the short term, this is highly likely. As the redox state primarily depends upon availability of mitochondrial oxygen, a monitor responding to redox state can be considered directly responsive to hypoxia.

NADH carries electrons generated in the redox reactions of the Krebs' cycle and glycolysis to Complex I of the electron transport chain (ETC) (Fig. 10.1). The ability of NADH to offload electrons to the ETC, and so drive the electrochemical gradient across the inner mitochondrial membrane used to synthesize ATP, is contingent on the presence of sufficient oxygen to accept donated electrons. If the mitochondrial oxygen tension is insufficient, a backlog occurs within the ETC. Below a certain threshold, the rate of the Krebs' cycle reactions that generate NADH will exceed the rate of the reverse reactions generating NAD^+. The redox balance tilts from its resting equilibrium towards a reduced state so the NADH fluorescence intensity increases. A similar situation pertains for cytochrome oxidase which under normal conditions is in the oxidized state. A reduction in oxygen availability results in a shift towards the reduced CCO; however, as it is the oxidized form that fluoresces, the signal intensity here will decrease.

Importantly, oxidative (aerobic) respiration can continue at near-maximal capacity, even at subnormal partial pressures of oxygen within the mitochondria, as the K_m for oxygen – the Michaelis constant, where the concentration of substrate which permits the enzyme to achieve half its maximal activity (V_{max}) – of cytochrome oxidase is extremely low [18]. When mitochondrial oxygen supply is significantly compromised, there is a rapid change in NADH or cytochrome oxidase state from equilibrium towards reduction. This provides a ratiometric value rather than an absolute measure but nevertheless can still indicate when oxygen supply limits respiration and the cell becomes 'unhappy'. This may delineate the lower bounds of physiological tolerance and provide an objective target for "permissive resuscitation" indicating, for that tissue at least, whether deranged physiology is being tolerated. This likely varies from organ to organ so a suitable canary organ that is readily accessible for routine clinical practice would need to be identified.

10.4.7 Mitochondrial Oxygen Tension

Mik and colleagues have developed a technique for measuring mitochondrial PO_2 in the epidermal skin layer [19, 20]. It utilizes endogenous protoporphyrin IX (PpIX) which is only located within the mitochondria as an intramitochondrial oxygen-sensitive dye. Topical application of its precursor, 5-aminolevulinic acid (ALA), in a cream to the skin increases the PpIX concentration, and application of a green laser flashlight results in a red delayed fluorescence that is quenched in an oxygen-dependent manner. Applying the Stern-Vollmer equation therefore enables a calculation of mitochondrial PO_2. The signal obtained by this technique is indeed likely to represent an index of mitochondrial PO_2 as it can be ablated by topical administration of cyanide, an inhibitor of the electron transport chain. Whether the absolute values obtained are accurate remains open for debate as values obtained are higher than those obtained by other techniques for interstitial 'tissue' PO_2 and those assumed for mitochondrial PO_2 by mathematical modelling. Nevertheless, it likely offers a means of monitoring change over time. Another use is to perform a dynamic challenge by occluding local blood flow (e.g. with a proximal blood pressure cuff) and measuring the oxygen disappearance rate, which should be directly related to mitochondrial oxygen consumption.

Downsides of the approach include the need to apply the topical ALA cream for several hours prior to measurement to enable PpIX levels to increase and the need to cover the skin as the application of high-intensity excitation light to the ALA can induce phototoxicity. While it has been used to measure values in the heart and liver in animal models, ALA is not licenced for intravenous use in patients, so it is currently restricted to epidermal monitoring.

Take-Home Messages

- Production of sufficient energy substrate (ATP) by mitochondria is integral to adequate functioning of virtually all cell types within the body.
- Monitoring of mitochondrial functionality and tissue oxygenation provides important windows into determining the adequacy of organ perfusion and 'cell happiness' during critical illness.
- Several techniques – either direct measures or surrogates – are available to be performed at the bedside.

References

1. Rich P. Chemiosmotic coupling: the cost of living. Nature. 2003;421:583.
2. Rolfe DF, Brown GC. Cellular energy utilization and molecular origin of standard metabolic rate in mammals. Physiol Rev. 1997;77(3):731–58.
3. Mächler P, Wyss MT, Elsayed M, Stobart J, Gutierrez R, Faber-Castell von A, et al. In vivo evidence for a lactate gradient from astrocytes to neurons. Cell Metab. 2016;23:94–102.
4. de Lima Oliveira M, Kairalla AC, Fonoff ET, Martinez RC, Teixeira MJ, Bor-Seng-Shu E. Cerebral microdialysis in traumatic brain injury and subarachnoid hemorrhage: state of the art. Neurocrit Care. 2014;21:152–62.
5. Ozawa K, Aoyama H, Yasuda K, Shimahara Y, Nakatani T, Tanaka J, et al. Metabolic abnormalities associated with postoperative organ failure: a redox theory. Arch Surg. 1983;118:1245–51.
6. Black C, Grocott MP, Singer M. Metabolic monitoring in the intensive care unit: a comparison of the Medgraphics Ultima, Deltatrac II, and Douglas bag collection methods. Br J Anaesth. 2015;114:261–8.
7. Pesta D, Gnaiger E. High-resolution respirometry: OXPHOS protocols for human cells and permeabilized fibers from small biopsies of human muscle. Methods Mol Biol. 2012;810:25–58.
8. Jobsis FF. Noninvasive, infrared monitoring of cerebral and myocardial oxygen sufficiency and circulatory parameters. Science. 1977;198:1264–7.
9. Annane D. Thenar tissue oxygen saturation monitoring: noninvasive does not mean simple or accurate! Crit Care Med. 2011;39:1828–9.
10. Crookes BA, Cohn SM, Bloch S, Amortegui J, Manning R, Li P, et al. Can near-infrared spectroscopy identify the severity of shock in trauma patients? J Trauma. 2005;58:806–13.
11. De Blasi R, Palmisani S, Alampi D, Mercieri M, Romano R, Collini S, et al. Microvascular dysfunction and skeletal muscle oxygenation assessed by phase-modulation near-infrared spectroscopy in patients with septic shock. Intensive Care Med. 2005;31:1661–8.
12. De Santis V, Singer M. Tissue oxygen tension monitoring of organ perfusion: rationale, methodologies, and literature review. Br J Anaesth. 2015;115:357–65.
13. Dyson A, Simon F, Seifritz A, Zimmerling O, Matallo J, Calzia E, et al. Bladder tissue oxygen tension monitoring in pigs subjected to a range of cardiorespiratory and pharmacological challenges. Intensive Care Med. 2012;38:1868–76.
14. Dyson A, Ekbal N, Stotz M, Barnes S, Carré J, Tully S, et al. Component reductions in oxygen delivery generate variable haemodynamic and stress hormone responses. Br J Anaesth. 2014;113:708–16.
15. Naumann CP, Ruetsch YA, Fleckenstein W, Fennema M, Erdmann W, Zäch GA. pO2 profiles in human muscle tissue as indicator of therapeutical effect in septic shock patients. Adv Exp Med Biol. 1992;317:869–77.
16. Dings J, Meixensberger J, Jäger A, Roosen K. Clinical experience with 118 brain tissue oxygen partial pressure catheter probes. Neurosurgery. 1998;43:1082–95.
17. Kram HB, Appel PL, Fleming AW, Shoemaker WC. Conjunctival and mixed-venous oximeters as early warning devices of cardiopulmonary compromise. Circ Shock. 1986;19:211–20.
18. Cooper CE, Davies NA, Psychoulis M, Canevari L, Bates TE, Dobbie MS, et al. Nitric oxide and peroxynitrite cause irreversible increases in the Km for oxygen of mitochondrial cytochrome oxidase: in vitro and in vivo studies. Biochim Biophys Acta. 2003;1607:27–34.
19. Mik EG. Measuring mitochondrial oxygen tension: from basic principles to application in humans. Anesth Analg. 2013;117:834–46.
20. Ince C, Mik EG. Microcirculatory and mitochondrial hypoxia in sepsis, shock, and resuscitation. J Appl Physiol. 2016;120:226–35.

Perioperative Haemodynamics

Katherine McAndrew, Maurizio Cecconi, and Andrew Rhodes

M. R. Pinsky et al. (eds.), *Hemodynamic Monitoring*, Lessons from the ICU,
https://doi.org/10.1007/978-3-319-69269-2_11

Learning Objectives

The perioperative period can be one of the most vulnerable times for surgical patients, particularly those who have a number of co-morbidities. The additive effects of general anaesthesia, mechanical ventilation and the trauma of surgery itself, unless carefully managed, have the potential to compromise haemodynamic stability. This requires careful consideration and a proactive management approach.

11.1 Introduction

Cardiovascular physiology is perfectly developed to ensure the metabolic requirements of the body are met in most circumstances by increasing (or decreasing) the delivery of nutrients and oxygen in accordance with needs. This complex interplay between metabolic requirements, cardiovascular pump function and venous and arterial tone can be easily seen in the perioperative period where a variety of stressing insults can risk altering this homeostasis adversely with negative impacts for the patient. This is especially the case in frail elderly patients with complex co-morbid conditions presenting for surgery where at times their baseline physiological state is at best marginal and can easily be tipped over into an acute state that the body cannot cope with.

In the perioperative setting, a patient is subjected to stressors from a variety of sources relating to the surgical procedure and the anaesthetic management. During this period, the body's oxygen requirements need to increase to deal with the significant stress response and to help the patient recover and heal from the surgical trauma [1]. If the body is unable to increase its cardiac output, the oxygen requirements may not be met, and the patient develops tissue dysoxia and cellular dysfunction. This phenomenon, previously described as an acquired oxygen debt, has been associated with organ failure and death in patients unable to meet these demands for whatever reason [2, 3].

The association between this perioperative oxygen flux and the resultant complications was originally described by Shoemaker in the 1970s who identified the key variables impacting patient outcome as being cardiac index, oxygen delivery and oxygen consumption [2]. This body of research has helped ensuring high-risk patients are admitted to intensive care units postoperatively where they can be invasively monitored and have their haemodynamics manipulated as will be described in this chapter.

This chapter aims to provide an overview on the haemodynamic considerations to be made when anaesthetising patients and the impact of mechanical ventilation, and this should provide insights into how haemodynamics can be manipulated in the intra- and postoperative settings.

11.2 Baseline Physiology

As the population gets older in the Western world, it is becoming more common for patients with complex medical conditions to present for surgery [4]. The prevalence of hypertension, diabetes mellitus, chronic respiratory illnesses and heart failure is all more common than in previous years and leads to challenging physiologic states for the perioperative period. On top of this, patients presenting for surgery are often debilitated by the condition that the surgery is designed to cure, and many will come into the operative environment with mild vascular volume deficits and changing levels of maintenance drug therapies due to them not being continued up and through the perioperative period. While the exact mechanisms are not completely known, it is understood that the surgical stress is associated with the development of complications, which can develop in regions distant to the surgical site (i.e. a pneumonia in a postoperative hip replacement). The development of postoperative surgical complications is associated with in-hospital mortality, higher length of stay, higher costs and long-term mortality [5–7].

The Frank-Starling mechanism describes the process by which the heart is able to accommodate and eject the blood returned to it, despite variable venous return (VR). The increased preload, or venous return, increases the stretch of the cardiac myocyte. The resulting increase in sarcomere length leads to an increased force of contraction with the desired result being an increased volume of blood ejected from the heart [8].

The venous system is not a passive conduit for blood to return to the heart. It is an adjustable reservoir that is able to modify blood flow according to changing metabolic requirements. The veins contain almost 70% of the total blood volume, much higher than that contained in either the arteries (13–18%) or capillaries (7%). In addition, anatomically the veins are very different to the arteries with a much higher compliance than arterial walls. The veins are essentially a blood reservoir that keeps 70% of the circulating blood volume in a distensible compartment.

According to Guyton, the majority of blood is kept in an 'unstressed' compartment of the body vasculature where volume and pressure are essentially independent of one another. But a small proportion (about 1/5) is kept within a 'stressed' compartment where increases in volume directly lead to increases in mean pressure [9]. This is called the *mean systemic filling pressure (Pmsf)* and is the pressure related to the intravascular volume and the mean systemic capacity of the system.

The heart pumps blood continuously into the aorta which therefore has a high pressure, averaging 80–100 mmHg. As the blood flows into the systemic circulation, the mean pressure reduces progressively until it gets to the right heart (whose pressure can be described by the central venous pressure or right atrial pressure (Pra)). If the heart was to stop for any reason, the arterial pressure would fall, and the Pra would progressively increase until a certain point when there is no blood motion. At this point, the pressure at every single point of the circulatory system would be the same. This point equals to the value of the Pmsf.

The rate of blood flow is determined by the difference in pressure between two points of the cardiovascular system and not by any single pressure at any point. Given that most of blood is in the venous reservoir, the pressure at this point is particularly interesting. Venous return is defined by three parameters: the Pmsf, the right atrial pressure (Pra) and the resistance to venous return (RVR). This can be also mathematically represented as follows:

$$\mathrm{VR} = \left(\mathrm{Pmsf} - \mathrm{Pra}\right) / \mathrm{RVR}$$

The gradient of pressure between Pmsf and Pra is directly proportional to the venous return. Guyton et al. described venous return curves changing the Pra under isovolumetric conditions. As during steady conditions, cardiac output (CO) and venous return are equal; Pmsf plays an important role on the regulation of CO [9].

Guyton described the concept that the left ventricular cardiac output is closely maintained and controlled by manipulations in venous tone and return [9]. Any condition that leads to alterations in venous tone and therefore venous return to the right heart would be expected to lead to alterations in left ventricular (LV) output and therefore systemic haemodynamics. There are many stressors of the venous system present during surgery under general anaesthesia so it should not be a surprise to understand that drops in cardiac output in combination with systemic falls in arterial blood pressure are a common consequence of induction of anaesthesia and maintenance of intermittent positive pressure ventilation. There is some emerging evidence that keeping the systemic haemodynamics at the preoperative state is beneficial to the patients, but this does require an understanding of cardiovascular physiology and in complex patients the monitoring of these variables to identify the changes.

11.3 Haemodynamics and General Anaesthesia

The physiological alterations that result from induction of general anaesthesia are well known. The impacts on the cardiovascular system include reductions in both venous and arterial tone, myocardial depression, decreased cardiac output and hypotension. The different drugs used have specific patterns of change on this system, and to a certain extent, an in-depth understanding of these impacts can help the clinician choose an appropriate agent for any given situation.

It is the role of the anaesthetist to anticipate the haemodynamic fluctuations observed intraoperatively to ensure adequate perfusion to the vital organs is maintained during this stressful time. In the 1950s, Finnerty investigated the effects of inducing cerebral ischaemia by intravenous administration of hexamethonium and/or tilting on cerebral haemodynamics and metabolism [10]. It was noted that the degree of fall in mean arterial pressure which resulted in cerebral ischaemia varied from 29 to 80 mmHg depending on individual patient characteristics. More modern drugs have far less of an impact than this but still need to be used with caution in patients who may not tolerate such swings in physiological status quo.

Propofol is widely used as an induction agent due to a number of desirable characteristics such as rapid onset and recovery. The cardiovascular depressant effects, mediated by peripheral mechanisms such as depression of myocardial contractility, vasodilation and inhibition of the sympathetic nervous system, are well tolerated in healthy subjects [11]. Hypotension post induction of general anaesthesia is strongly associated with age over 50 years, hypotension preoperatively and use of propofol as a hypnotic agent. Propofol use can be problematic in high-risk patients with intrinsic cardiac disease or multi-organ system disease [12]. In addition, the cardiovascular effects of propofol can be worsened in patients who are concomitantly taking angiotensin-converting enzyme (ACE) inhibitors. Propofol has been shown to increase endothelial production and release of nitric oxide (NO). Malinowska-Zaprzalka postulated that the haemodynamic compromise seen when these agents are used together could be due to an additive effect on NO release [13], that results in both systolic and diastolic blood pressures being significantly lowered following propofol induction in patients chronically treated with enalapril compared to normotensive patients [13]. Recent evidence has suggested that increased NO bioavailability may account for the enhanced hypotensive effects of propofol in ACE inhibitor-treated patients [14].

The risk of induction of anaesthesia in hypertensive patients has been widely described [15]. From the increased arterial pressure during laryngoscopy [16] to the equally deleterious hypotension following premedication, the patient is at risk of myocardial ischaemia, transient left ventricular failure and arrhythmia [17]. While Finnerty noted the increased sensitivity to low mean arterial pressure (MAP), others have described the greater absolute intraoperative blood pressure decreases among patients who had persistent hypertension compared to those with a well-controlled blood pressure. However, in order for labile blood pressure to be associated with postoperative cardiac complications, the drop in blood pressure needs to be significant and long lasting (50% of usual value or to 33% for at least 10 min) [11, 18].

11.4 Mechanical Ventilation

General anaesthesia is combined with intermittent positive pressure ventilation (IPPV) and neuromuscular relaxation. The impacts of this intervention on the cardiovascular system can be significant, primarily by changing lung volume and intrathoracic pressure.

IPPV induces cyclic changes to the flow into the ventricles. Mechanically insufflating the lungs decreases preload and increases afterload in the right ventricle (RV). The RV preload reduction is a result of the increased pleural pressure, and the increase in RV afterload relates to the inspiratory increase in transpulmonary pressure [19]. These effects combined lead to a reduced RV stroke volume particularly at the end of the inspiratory period. This inspiratory reduction in RV ejection results in decreased left ventricular (LV) filling following a phase lag of two to three heartbeats because of the protracted pulmonary transit time [20]. Hence, the LV preload reduction may induce a decrease in LV stroke volume which is at its minimum during the expiratory period [19].

The effects of positive end-expiratory pressure (PEEP) on LV preload are complex and dependent on systemic venous return, RV output and LV filling, and as such, increased levels of PEEP may potentiate detrimental consequences for venous return and RV afterload, resulting in reduced cardiac output. As these effects are also mediated by increased lung volumes, it is important to be aware that these increased lung volumes cannot only produce detrimental lung injury but will also necessitate close haemodynamic monitoring to avoid compromising cardiac output [21, 22].

11.5 Manipulation of Haemodynamics

11.5.1 Volume Status During the Perioperative Period

The volume of fluid therapy administered during the perioperative period has been correlated with outcome, and increased mortality is associated with very high and very low volumes used [23]. A recent trial from the ANZICS trials group confirmed this by randomising 3000 patients to either a restrictive or liberal intravenous fluid regime during and up to 24 h after surgery and found that the restrictive regime conferred little benefit and the suspicion of some harm to the patients (increased infections and requirement for renal replacement therapy) [24]. It seems clear that, especially in the highest-risk patients, giving the right amount of intravenous fluids (not too much and not too little) is of paramount importance and can often only be achieved with a thorough understanding of the underlying haemodynamics, and this often requires sophisticated haemodynamic monitoring.

Differing approaches to fluid therapy are frequently seen, but what needs to be consistent is that patients receive fluids targeted to their individual requirements. These should effectively challenge their physiology, and overall responsiveness should be assessed via appropriate monitoring only following volumes which are likely to increase Pmsf [25].

To achieve the desired increase in 'stressed' volume that will result in sarcomere stretch, an appropriate fluid challenge should be administered. A wide disparity in practice has been observed with crystalloids such as 0.9% saline and Hartmann's being used in around three quarters of fluid challenges. The average volume given as a challenge is 500 ml [26]. Aya et al. studied fluid challenges using volumes of 1, 2, 3 and 4 ml/kg over 5 min in postsurgical patients and demonstrated that 4 ml/kg was the most reliable volume to stress the cardiac system and demonstrate a response [27].

Clinical examination and cardiac monitoring can assist the clinician in predicting whether a fluid challenge will be effective. High pulse pressure variation, vena cava collapsibility and dynamic passive leg raising correlate with effective fluid challenge [28]. Myatra et al. demonstrated how reviewing the impact of a transient increase in tidal volume from 6 to 8 ml/kg in ventilated patients can also predict fluid responsiveness [29].

11.5.2 Goal-Directed Therapy

Haemodynamic monitoring techniques can be used in protocolised practices aiming to augment cardiac output specifically in high-risk, postoperative patients. This concept is widely described as 'optimisation' or 'goal-directed therapy'.

11

Major surgery is associated with a significant stress response which allows the body to heal and recover from the surgical trauma [1]. Dysoxia and cellular dysfunction may arise if the body is unable to increase its cardiac output in response to this increased demand, and any patient who falls into this category is at high risk of complications, organ failure and death [2, 3].

Optimisation strategies aim to ensure the circulatory status is adequate during the perioperative period, and it does this by targeting the key variables of cardiac index, oxygen delivery and oxygen consumption. Hence, they specifically aim to augment the haemoglobin level, the arterial oxygen saturation of haemoglobin (S_pO_2) and the cardiac index in order to optimise the oxygen delivery.

The evidence for the particular targets originate from the research by Shoemaker et al., who hypothesised that aiming for supranormal physiological parameters would decrease morbidity and mortality, and he described targets of cardiac output >4.5 L/min/m^2 and oxygen delivery >600 ml/min/m^2 [2]. In recent years most strategies of GDT studies used volume optimisation approaches alone, targeting optimal stroke volume by fluid challenge techniques or by targeting fluid responsiveness variables.

The targeting of stroke volume and/or cardiac index requires monitoring of it, which can be done using many of the methods described elsewhere. Once measured, if it is perceived to be too low, then it is initially increased by intravenous fluid filling. Many patients may have a heart rate and blood pressure within a normal range, but the aim of the fluid administration is to increase preload and therefore stroke volume and cardiac output to these supranormal targets. If this is still not achieved, then the use of an appropriate cardiovascular agents that will improve cardiac output, such as dobutamine, can be used in suitable patients [25]. A number of trials have shown that this method of optimising cardiac output is associated with reduced mortality, less complications and an overall reduction in length of hospital stay [30–32]. More recent trials such as OPTIMISE and POEMAS, both large randomised control trials looking at GDT outcomes in high-risk patients undergoing major abdominal surgery, have not demonstrated the same benefits [33, 34]. A possible explanation for this discrepancy is that patient care throughout the perioperative period has greatly improved. Expert-led preoperative assessment ensures patients are at a physiological peak prior to the procedure, and advancements in anaesthesiology and cardiac monitoring throughout surgery mean that patients are in better physiological conditions throughout the surgical and postoperative periods [35].

Conclusion

The physiological disturbances associated with major surgery are complex. Clinicians need to have an in-depth understanding of cardiovascular physiology, the changes associated with their medical interventions and how these interact with complex premorbid disease states. If this understanding is in place, then appropriate therapies can be selected to give patients the best chance of surviving their surgical stress.

Take-Home Messages

- Haemodynamic alterations are very common in the perioperative period.
- Poor haemodynamic control is associated with adverse patient outcomes.
- Understanding of haemodynamic changes in patients with complex cardiovascular disease may require advanced haemodynamic monitoring.
- Haemodynamic therapy is best titrated against haemodynamic endpoints that are monitored.
- Appropriately titrated therapy can reduce adverse outcomes in this patient group.

References

1. Desborough JP. The stress response to trauma and surgery. Br J Anaesth. 2000;85(1):109–17.
2. Shoemaker WC, Appel PL, Kram HB. Role of oxygen debt in the development of organ failure sepsis, and death in high-risk surgical patients. Chest. 1992;102(1):208–15.
3. Older P, Hall A, Hader R. Cardiopulmonary exercise testing as a screening test for perioperative management of major surgery in the elderly. Chest. 1999;116(2):355–62.
4. Shrime MG, Bickler SW, Alkire BC, Mock C. Global burden of surgical disease: an estimation from the provider perspective. Lancet Glob Health. 2015;3(Suppl 2):S8–9.
5. Ebm C, Cecconi M, Sutton L, Rhodes A. A cost-effectiveness analysis of postoperative goal-directed therapy for high-risk surgical patients. Crit Care Med. 2014;42(5):1194–203.
6. Khuri SF, Henderson WG, DePalma RG, Mosca C, Healey NA, Kumbhani DJ, et al. Determinants of long-term survival after major surgery and the adverse effect of postoperative complications. Ann Surg. 2005;242(3):326–41. discussion 41-3
7. Rhodes A, Cecconi M, Hamilton M, Poloniecki J, Woods J, Boyd O, et al. Goal-directed therapy in high-risk surgical patients: a 15-year follow-up study. Intensive Care Med. 2010;36(8):1327–32.
8. Patterson SW, Piper H, Starling EH. The regulation of the heart beat. J Physiol. 1914;48(6):465–513.
9. Guyton AC. Determination of cardiac output by equating venous return curves with cardiac response curves. Physiol Rev. 1955;35(1):123–9.

10. Finnerty FA Jr, Witkin L, Fazekas JF. Cerebral hemodynamics during cerebral ischemia induced by acute hypotension. J Clin Invest. 1954;33(9):1227–32.
11. Smith I, White PF, Nathanson M, Gouldson R. Propofol. An update on its clinical use. Anesthesiology. 1994;81(4):1005–43.
12. Oliveira-Paula GH, Pinheiro LC, Ferreira GC, Garcia WNP, Lacchini R, Garcia LV, et al. Angiotensin converting enzyme inhibitors enhance the hypotensive effects of propofol by increasing nitric oxide production. Free Radic Biol Med. 2018;115:10–7.
13. Malinowska-Zaprzalka M, Wojewodzka M, Dryl D, Grabowska SZ, Chabielska E. Hemodynamic effect of propofol in enalapril-treated hypertensive patients during induction of general anesthesia. Pharmacol Rep. 2005;57(5):675–8.
14. Linz W, Wiemer G, Gohlke P, Unger T, Scholkens BA. Contribution of kinins to the cardiovascular actions of angiotensin-converting enzyme inhibitors. Pharmacol Rev. 1995;47(1):25–49.
15. Aronson S, Boisvert D, Lapp W. Isolated systolic hypertension is associated with adverse outcomes from coronary artery bypass grafting surgery. Anesth Analg. 2002;94(5):1079–84, table of contents.
16. Xue FS, Zhang GH, Sun HT, Li CW, Liu KP, Xu YC, et al. Blood pressure and heart rate changes during fibreoptic orotracheal intubation: a comparison of children and adults. Eur J Anaesthesiol. 2007;24(1):39–45.
17. Manne VS, Paluvadi VR. Attenuation of cardiovascular response to direct laryngoscopy and intubation, comparative study of lignocaine, nifedipine, and placebo during general anesthesia. Anesth Essays Res. 2017;11(1):47–51.
18. Prys-Roberts C, Meloche R, Foex P. Studies of anaesthesia in relation to hypertension. I. Cardiovascular responses of treated and untreated patients. Br J Anaesth. 1971;43(2):122–37.
19. Michard F, Teboul JL. Using heart-lung interactions to assess fluid responsiveness during mechanical ventilation. Crit Care. 2000;4(5):282–9.
20. Luecke T, Pelosi P. Clinical review: positive end-expiratory pressure and cardiac output. Crit Care. 2005;9(6):607–21.
21. Pinsky MR, Desmet JM, Vincent JL. Effect of positive end-expiratory pressure on right ventricular function in humans. Am Rev Respir Dis. 1992;146(3):681–7.
22. Suter PM, Fairley B, Isenberg MD. Optimum end-expiratory airway pressure in patients with acute pulmonary failure. N Engl J Med. 1975;292(6):284–9.
23. Bellamy MC. Wet, dry or something else? Br J Anaesth. 2006;97(6):755–7.
24. Myles PS, Bellomo R, Corcoran T, Forbes A, Peyton P, Story D, et al. Restrictive versus liberal fluid therapy for major abdominal surgery. N Engl J Med. 2018;378:2263.
25. Bennett VA, Cecconi M. Perioperative fluid management: from physiology to improving clinical outcomes. Indian J Anaesth. 2017;61(8):614–21.
26. Cecconi M, Hofer C, Teboul JL, Pettila V, Wilkman E, Molnar Z, et al. Fluid challenges in intensive care: the FENICE study: a global inception cohort study. Intensive Care Med. 2015;41(9):1529–37.
27. Aya HD, Rhodes A, Chis Ster I, Fletcher N, Grounds RM, Cecconi M. Hemodynamic effect of different doses of fluids for a fluid challenge: a quasi-randomized controlled study. Crit Care Med. 2017;45(2):e161–e8.
28. Aditianingsih D, George YW. Guiding principles of fluid and volume therapy. Best Pract Res Clin Anaesthesiol. 2014;28(3):249–60.
29. Myatra SN, Prabu NR, Divatia JV, Monnet X, Kulkarni AP, Teboul JL. The changes in pulse pressure variation or stroke volume variation after a "tidal volume challenge" reliably predict fluid responsiveness during low tidal volume ventilation. Crit Care Med. 2017;45(3):415–21.
30. Cecconi M, Corredor C, Arulkumaran N, Abuella G, Ball J, Grounds RM, et al. Clinical review: goal-directed therapy-what is the evidence in surgical patients? The effect on different risk groups. Crit Care. 2013;17(2):209.
31. Hamilton MA, Cecconi M, Rhodes A. A systematic review and meta-analysis on the use of preemptive hemodynamic intervention to improve postoperative outcomes in moderate and high-risk surgical patients. Anesth Analg. 2011;112(6):1392–402.
32. Pearse R, Dawson D, Fawcett J, Rhodes A, Grounds RM, Bennett ED. Early goal-directed therapy after major surgery reduces complications and duration of hospital stay. A randomised, controlled trial [ISRCTN38797445]. Crit Care. 2005;9(6):R687–93.
33. Pearse RM, Harrison DA, MacDonald N, Gillies MA, Blunt M, Ackland G, et al. Effect of a perioperative, cardiac output-guided hemodynamic therapy algorithm on outcomes following major gastrointestinal surgery: a randomized clinical trial and systematic review. JAMA. 2014;311(21):2181–90.

34. Pestana D, Espinosa E, Eden A, Najera D, Collar L, Aldecoa C, et al. Perioperative goal-directed hemodynamic optimization using noninvasive cardiac output monitoring in major abdominal surgery: a prospective, randomized, multicenter, pragmatic trial: POEMAS Study (PeriOperative goal-directed thErapy in Major Abdominal Surgery). Anesth Analg. 2014;119(3):579–87.
35. De Hert S, Imberger G, Carlisle J, Diemunsch P, Fritsch G, Moppett I, et al. Preoperative evaluation of the adult patient undergoing non-cardiac surgery: guidelines from the European Society of Anaesthesiology. Eur J Anaesthesiol. 2011;28(10):684–722.

Hemodynamics and Extracorporeal Circulation

Maxime Coutrot, Alain Combes, and Nicolas Bréchot

M. R. Pinsky et al. (eds.), *Hemodynamic Monitoring*, Lessons from the ICU,
https://doi.org/10.1007/978-3-319-69269-2_12

Learning Objectives

Veno-arterial extracorporeal membrane oxygenation (VA-ECMO) is increasingly used as first-line therapy for refractory cardiogenic shock [1–3]. It can be easily and rapidly implanted at patient's bedside, even outside of the hospital thanks to mobile ECMO units [4, 5]. It combines biventricular cardiac and respiratory support, with a device delivering high and stable blood flow. With the improvement of biomaterials and technologies, ECMO can now stay in place several days or even weeks, as a bridge to "decision" that includes recovery, transplantation, long-term mechanical circulatory support, or withdrawal in case of futility [1, 6, 7].

It should however be mentioned that VA-ECMO alters the hemodynamics of implanted patients, depending on the type of cannulation, ECMO blood flow, and patient's spontaneous residual ejection. In this chapter, we will discuss hemodynamic changes during VA-ECMO in the macro- and microcirculation, in relation with cannulation site and the interactions between ECMO and patients' cardiovascular system.

12.1 Principles of VA-ECMO Circulatory Support

12

The VA-ECMO circuit includes drainage and return cannulas, a centrifugal pump, and a membrane oxygenator (◘ Figs. 12.1 and 12.2). For peripheral femoro-femoral cannulation, the multiperforated drainage cannula is placed at the entry of the right atrium (RA) through the femoral and inferior cava veins and connected to the drainage (venous) line (◘ Fig. 12.2, mark 1). The blood is drained in the circuit by the centrifugal pump (◘ Fig. 12.2, mark 3), passes through the membrane lung (◘ Fig. 12.2, mark 4), and is reinjected retrogradly in the aorta through the return (arterial) cannula (◘ Fig. 12.2, mark 2) placed in the iliac artery. Peripheral VA-ECMO (PVA-ECMO) thus allows biventricular support, bypassing the heart of the patient. Additionally, the membrane lung provides blood oxygenation and decarboxylation, which are determined by ECMO and sweep gas flows (◘ Fig. 12.2, mark 5), and membrane FiO_2 (◘ Fig. 12.2, mark 6). Alternatively, the axillary route can be used for the return cannula, particularly in case of peripheral arterial disease. For central intrathoracic cannulation, the drainage cannula is placed directly in the right atrium (RA) and the return cannula in the ascending aorta. Central cannulation can also be used for mono-ventricular or biventricular support, depending on patient's condition: RA to pulmonary artery for right ventricular support and/or left atrium to the aorta, for left ventricular support.

Pump speed (◘ Fig. 12.2, mark 8) is set on the ECMO device controller (◘ Fig. 12.2, mark 7), which also displays the resulting ECMO blood flow (◘ Fig. 12.2, mark 9), and in the latest-generation machine circuit pressures, hematocrit and blood oxygen saturation. Target ECMO blood flow is 2–3 $L/min/m^2$, to reverse clinical and biological signs of circulatory shock [1, 8, 9].

12.2 Macrohemodynamics Under VA-ECMO

Pressure-volume loops describe left ventricular function (◘ Fig. 12.3a), with (1) isovolumic contraction, (2) ejection, (3) isovolumic relaxation, and (4) filling of the heart. End-systolic pressure-volume relationship (ESPVR) follows a linear relation with a slope depending on myocardial contractility. End-diastolic pressure-volume relationship (EDPVR) is curvilinear, with its slope increasing as end-diastolic volume increases and

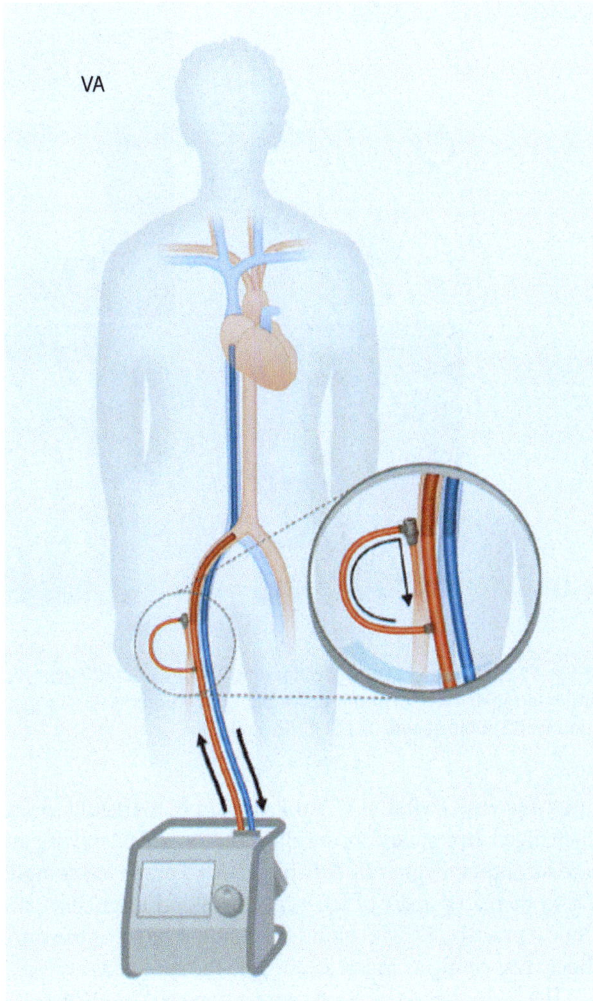

■ **Fig. 12.1** Schematic representation of peripheral VA-ECMO inserted in a patient, with venous drainage line in blue and arterial return line in red

depending on relaxation and compliance properties of the heart. Arterial impedance might also alter myocardial performance, modifying pressure-volume loop aspect. A rise in total peripheral resistance (part of cardiac afterload against which the heart contracts) will be responsible for a rightward shift of ESPVR and EDPVR, increasing LV end-systolic pressure as well as LV end-systolic volume (■ Fig. 12.3d). The failing heart combines a decrease in myocardial contractility and in diastolic relaxation, which is transduced by a rightward shift of the pressure-volume loop (■ Fig. 12.3a). LV end-diastolic as well as end-systolic pressure and volume are increased, while stroke volume is decreased (■ Fig. 12.3a).

12.2.1 Hemodynamics Under PVA-ECMO

PVA-ECMO, which provides retrograde blood flow in the aorta, is responsible for a marked increase in cardiac afterload, which further shifts rightward the pressure-volume loop of the failing heart (■ Fig. 12.3a). As ECMO flow increases, LV end-systolic and end-diastolic pres-

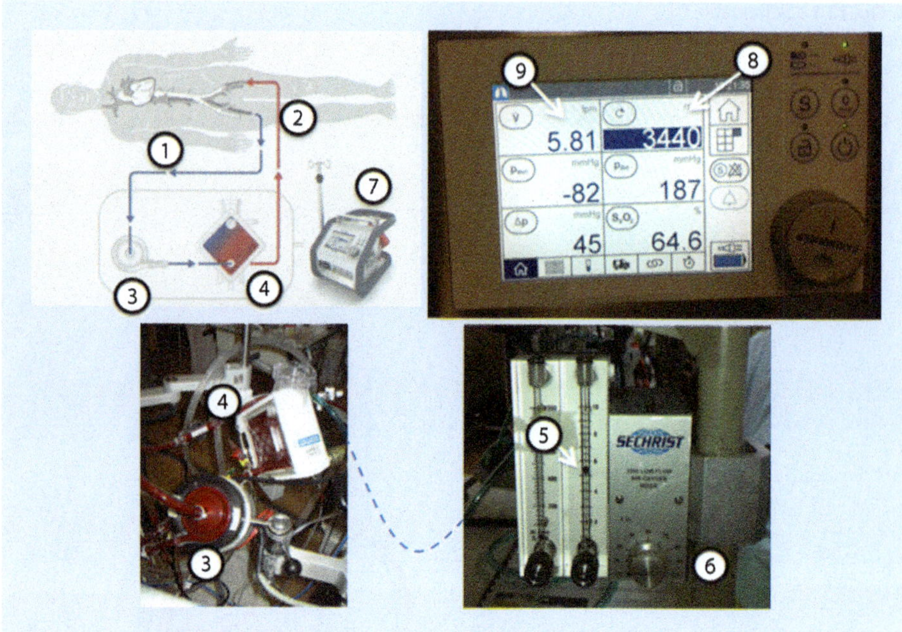

Fig. 12.2 Representation of different parts of VA-ECMO circuit, with (1) drainage (venous) line, (2) return (arterial) line, (3) centrifugal pump, (4) membrane, (5) sweep gas flow, (6) membrane FiO_2, (7) console, (8) pump speed, (9) ECMO flow rate

12

sures increase, while LV stroke volume markedly decreases, as contractility remains unchanged. In conclusion, despite rescuing peripheral organs, PVA-ECMO further decreases cardiac output. Higher ECMO blood flows may even completely abolish heart ejection, leading to increased risks of left ventricle blood stagnation and thrombosis (Fig. 12.3b). In clinical practice, ECMO blood flow should be set at the minimal level to allow correction of shock, respecting as much as possible the spontaneous ejection of the native heart.

The major risk associated to elevation of LV end-diastolic pressure is pulmonary edema, which occurs in around 30–50% of PVA-ECMO patients [1, 8, 10, 11]. The risk is higher for chronic heart failure patients, as adaptive mechanisms to heart failure are responsible for a switch rightward of the pressure-volume loop, with LV end-diastolic pressure already elevated. Patients with a very low spontaneous LV ejection under ECMO are also at risk, as decreasing contractility is also responsible for a further switch rightward of pressure-volume loop [10]. Ways to control the risk of pulmonary edema under ECMO are as follows:

1. Increasing contractility. This will allow the pressure-volume loop to translate leftward, with an increase in EDPVR slope and a decrease in LV end-diastolic pressure and volume (Fig. 12.3c). It explains why inotropes are usually maintained under ECMO for patients at high risk for pulmonary edema.
2. Decreasing the afterload (i.e., total peripheral resistance). As shown in Fig. 12.3d, for a specific contractility (i.e., for a given and constant ESPVR slope), decreasing total peripheral resistance will decrease LV end-systolic and end-diastolic pressure and volume and will increase stroke volume.
3. Furosemide to increase diuresis, as decreasing LV preload will also decrease LV end-diastolic pressure and LV end-diastolic volume.

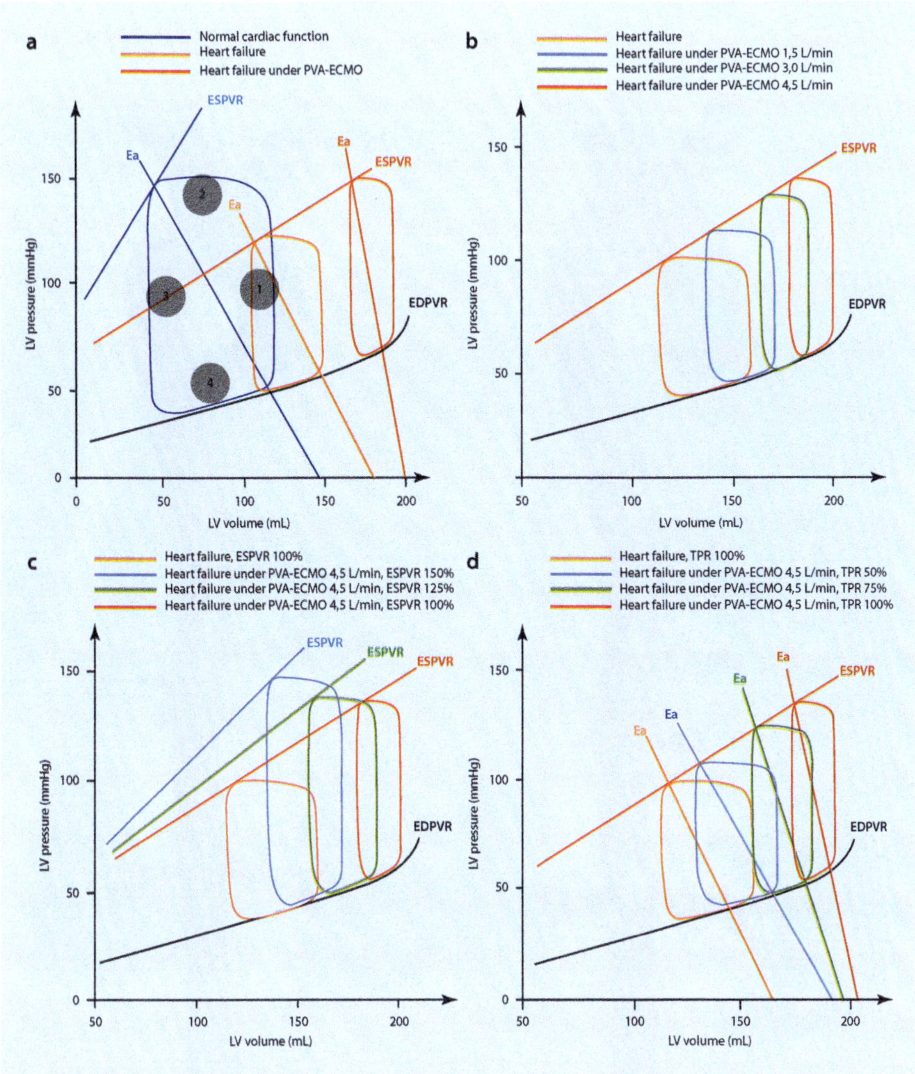

Fig. 12.3 Schematic representation of left ventricle pressure-volume loop **a** during normal conditions, heart failure and heart failure assisted with peripheral VA-ECMO, **b** with increasing peripheral VA-ECMO blood flow, **c** under peripheral VA-ECMO with increasing contractility, **d** under peripheral VA-ECMO with decreasing total peripheral resistance. Ae arterial elastance, EDPVR end-diastolic pressure-volume relationship, ESPVR end-systolic pressure-volume relationship, PVA-ECMO peripheral veno-arterial ECMO, TPR total peripheral resistance. (Adapted from Burkhoff et al. [26])

12.2.2 Harlequin Syndrome

During PVA-ECMO, blood flow ejected by the patient's heart mixes with the retrograde PVA-ECMO flow in the aorta (Fig. 12.4). The level where these two flows mix in the aorta depends on the ratio between native heart spontaneous ejection (itself depending on contractility, preload, and afterload conditions) and PVA-ECMO flow. When spontaneous

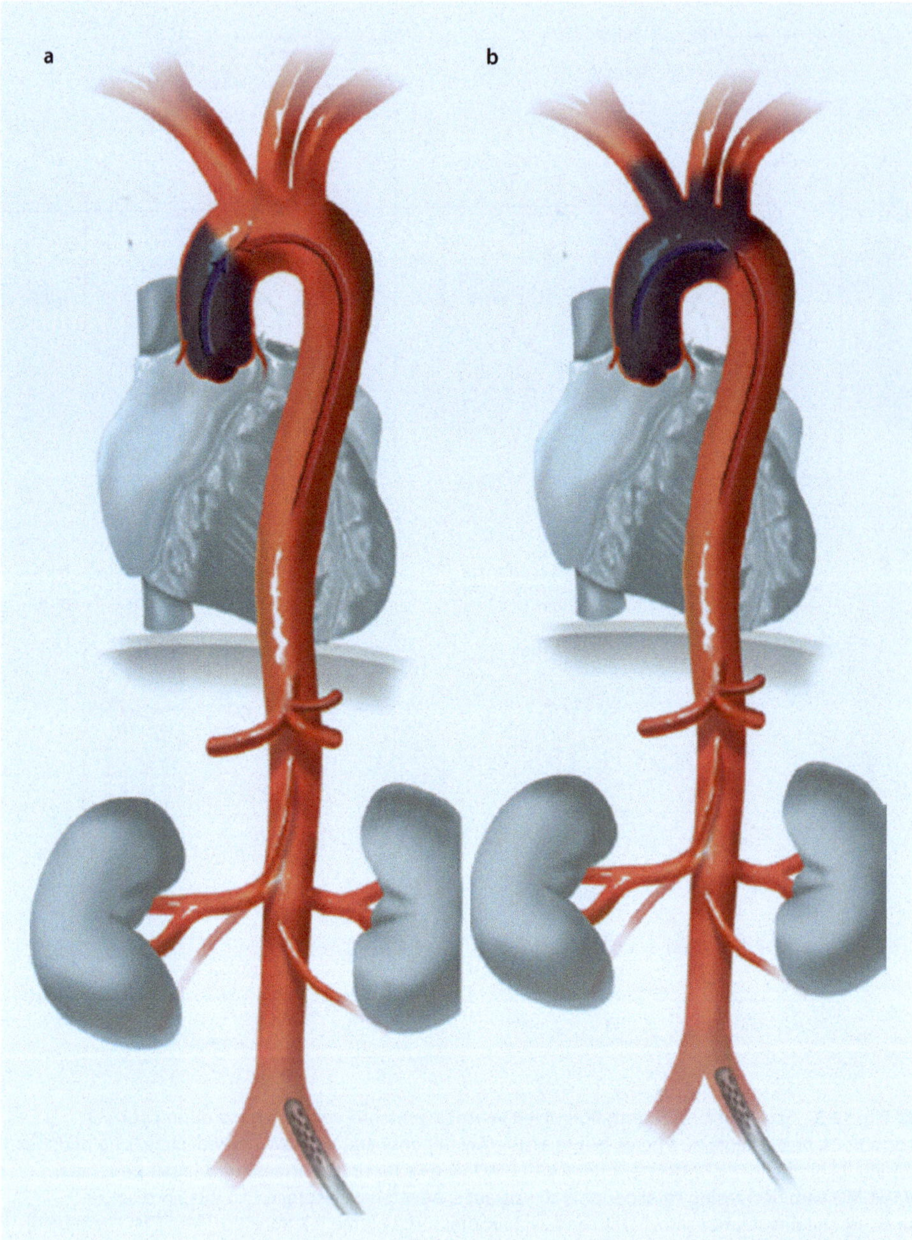

Fig. 12.4 Schematic representation of competing between PVA-ECMO blood flow and patient's spontaneous residual ejection, with reducing PVA-ECMO blood flow from **a** to **b**. (Adapted from Wong et al. [27])

12

ejection is abolished, all circulation is supported by PVA-ECMO flow. The more the stroke volume increases (after recovery and/or inotropic drug infusion and/or PVA-ECMO flow decrease), the more the mixing zone will be far away from the aortic valve. If severe respiratory failure is associated with circulatory failure, this can lead to severe hypoxemia in territories vascularized by the proximal part of the aorta, while the lower parts of the body remain fully oxygenated. Upper body oxygenation could theoretically be corrected by decreasing heart contractility (discontinuing inotropic drugs infusion) and stroke volume by increasing ECMO flow, but this would further impair myocardial recovery and pulmonary edema. The best option will be to switch to veno-arteriovenous cannulation, with blood returned to the femoral artery and the internal jugular vein [12].

12.3 Central VA-ECMO

Central VA-ECMO use is limited by a higher morbidity compared to PVA-ECMO. The need for sternotomy is associated with a higher risk of bleeding and infections, and the risk of stroke is more pronounced [13]. It can be an option in case of severe peripheral arterial disease, or for prolonged circulatory support, particularly in post-cardiotomy patients in whom a sternotomy has already been performed. Double central cannulation (RA-right pulmonary artery+ LV-aorta) is preferred to RA-aorta cannulation for long-term support, to preserve pulmonary circulation and lung vascularization. Compared to PVA-ECMO, central cannulation allows (◘ Fig. 12.5) (1) a decrease of LV afterload, as the return flow has a more physiological anterograde direction in the aorta, and (2) a better LV unloading. Direct positioning of the drainage cannula in the RA allows indeed a more efficient drainage of both inferior and superior cava veins. Better RV unloading decreases LV preload, decreasing LV end-diastolic pressure and volume. The risk of pulmonary edema is therefore significantly decreased compared with peripheral cannulation (◘ Fig. 12.5).

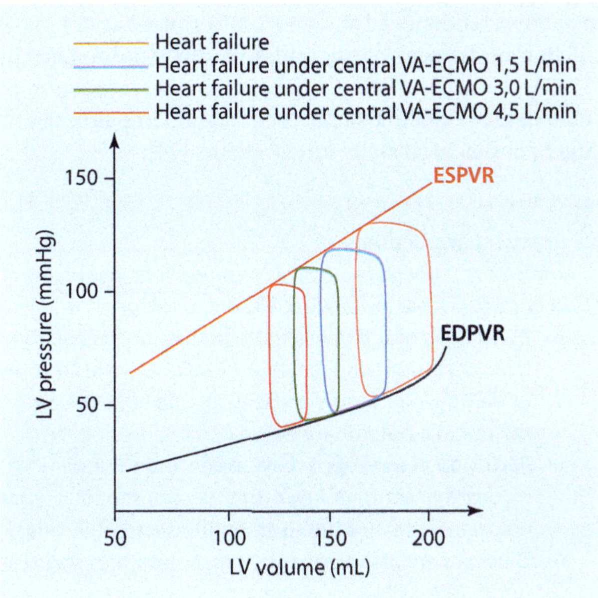

◘ **Fig. 12.5** Schematic representation of left ventricle pressure-volume loop during various flows under central VA-ECMO

12.4 Microcirculation Under ECMO

12.4.1 Impact of VA-ECMO on the Microcirculation

Although severe cardiogenic shock patients exhibit clear signs of microcirculation impairment [14, 15], data reporting the effects of ECMO in this setting are scarce and report conflicting results. In 14 neonates on VA-ECMO for acute respiratory distress associated with myocardial dysfunction, functional capillary density significantly improved after ECMO treatment [16]. On the contrary, in 24 adults suffering from refractory cardiogenic shock, sublingual microvascular dysfunction did not correct after VA-ECMO initiation. However, non-survivor patients had more pronounced microcirculation impairments under assistance compared to survivors [17]. In another study in 13 patients under VA-ECMO, recovery of sublingual microvascular dysfunction was associated with successful weaning from ECMO [18]. Thus, the exact effect of extracorporeal circulation on microcirculation remains an area for future investigations.

12.4.2 Effects of Continuous Versus Pulsatile Flow

12

While unloading the heart and increasing LV afterload, VA-ECMO will further decrease LV stroke volume, reducing blood flow pulsatility. More severe patients are exhibiting a nonpulsatile laminar blood flow under ECMO. The potential deleterious effects of nonpulsatile blood flow are subject to debate. Based on experimental studies, it has been advocated that continuous blood flow could be responsible for an increase in systemic vascular resistance and a decrease in peripheral organ perfusion, as well as increased endothelial activation and coagulation disorders [19, 20]. In several open randomized studies conducted by one group in patients operated for coronary artery bypass, intra-aortic balloon pumping during CEC was associated with a reduction in postoperative organ dysfunctions and coagulation disorders. However, these effects were not replicated in another randomized study in 100 coronary artery bypass patients. Likewise, microcirculation assessment during pulsatile cardiopulmonary bypass led to conflicting results [21–23]. Under VA-ECMO, although an observation in one patient suggested that IABP could improve sublingual microcirculation impairment, this effect was not confirmed in a larger physiological study in 12 patients [24].

Practical Implication

From these pathophysiological considerations, key points for hemodynamic management of patients assisted with VA-ECMO are as follows:

- PVA-ECMO blood flow should be the lowest allowing correcting peripheral tissue hypoperfusion. Minimal PVA-ECMO flow will limit the increase in afterload due to ECMO, thus limiting the rise in LV end-diastolic pressure and reducing the risk of hydrostatic pulmonary edema.
- Perfusion of inotropes may be continued under PVA-ECMO. It will increase myocardial contractility, promote spontaneous left ventricle ejection, and ultimately prevent blood stagnation and pulmonary edema.
- Diuretics are also frequently prescribed to prevent and treat pulmonary edema under PVA-ECMO.

- Intra-aortic balloon pump (IABP), with deflation during systole decreasing LV afterload, may also be helpful in combination to PVA-ECMO to prevent pulmonary edema [25].
- The risk of Harlequin syndrome should be assessed when cardiac function improves, with pulse oximetry and blood gazes analyzed from blood drained from right arm arteries (as far as possible from ECMO blood flow).
- Daily echocardiography must be performed to detect LV thrombosis, to assess residual cardiac function and to adjust inotropes, if needed, and to evaluate cardiac recovery allowing ECMO weaning.

Conclusion

VA-ECMO is increasingly used during refractory cardiogenic shock. Understanding the complex interactions between VA-ECMO and patient's cardiovascular function is crucial for optimal care. VA-ECMO settings should be tailored to each patient-specific cardiovascular function and hemodynamic status to maximize the benefits of mechanical circulatory support with minimal adverse effects.

Take-Home Messages

- PVA-ECMO and central VA-ECMO are two modalities of mechanical circulatory support that have very distinct hemodynamic consequences.
- Hemodynamic status under PVA-ECMO, resulting from the interaction of VA-ECMO flow in one hand, and the patient residual cardiovascular function on the other hand, is also influenced by VA-ECMO flow, preload, and afterload and inotrope and vasopressor infusion.
- PVA-ECMO increases LV afterload, worsening residual stroke volume and increasing risks of pulmonary edema and blood stagnation in cardiac cavities. These risks can be lowered by setting the lowest possible ECMO blood flow, maintaining inotropes and diuretics, and eventually combining IABP to ECMO support.

References

1. Combes A, Leprince P, Luyt C-E, Bonnet N, Trouillet J-L, Léger P, et al. Outcomes and long-term quality-of-life of patients supported by extracorporeal membrane oxygenation for refractory cardiogenic shock. Crit Care Med. 2008;36(5):1404–11.
2. Abrams D, Combes A, Brodie D. Extracorporeal membrane oxygenation in cardiopulmonary disease in adults. J Am Coll Cardiol. 2014;63(25):2769–78.
3. Abrams D, Combes A, Brodie D. What's new in extracorporeal membrane oxygenation for cardiac failure and cardiac arrest in adults? Intensive Care Med. 2014;40(4):609–12.
4. Beurtheret S, Mordant P, Paoletti X, Marijon E, Celermajer DS, Léger P, et al. Emergency circulatory support in refractory cardiogenic shock patients in remote institutions: a pilot study (the cardiac-RESCUE program). Eur Heart J. 2013;34(2):112–20.
5. Arlt M, Philipp A, Voelkel S, Camboni D, Rupprecht L, Graf B-M, et al. Hand-held minimised extracorporeal membrane oxygenation: a new bridge to recovery in patients with out-of-centre cardiogenic shock☆☆☆. Eur J Cardiothorac Surg [Internet]. 2011. [cited 2017 Dec 21]; Available from: https://academic.oup.com/ejcts/article-lookup/doi/10.1016/j.ejcts.2010.12.055.

6. Dangers L, Bréchot N, Schmidt M, Lebreton G, Hékimian G, Nieszkowska A, et al. Extracorporeal membrane oxygenation for acute decompensated heart failure. Crit Care Med. 2017;45(8):1359–66.
7. Tarzia V, Bortolussi G, Bianco R, Buratto E, Bejko J, Carrozzini M, et al. Extracorporeal life support in cardiogenic shock: impact of acute versus chronic etiology on outcome. J Thorac Cardiovasc Surg. 2015;150(2):333–40.
8. Demondion P, Fournel L, Golmard J-L, Niculescu M, Pavie A, Leprince P. Predictors of 30-day mortality and outcome in cases of myocardial infarction with cardiogenic shock treated by extracorporeal life support. Eur J Cardiothorac Surg. 2014;45(1):47–54.
9. Schmidt M, Tachon G, Devilliers C, Muller G, Hekimian G, Bréchot N, et al. Blood oxygenation and decarboxylation determinants during venovenous ECMO for respiratory failure in adults. Intensive Care Med. 2013;39(5):838–46.
10. Bréchot N, Demondion P, Santi F, Lebreton G, Pham T, Dalakidis A, et al. Intra-aortic balloon pump protects against hydrostatic pulmonary oedema during peripheral venoarterial-extracorporeal membrane oxygenation. Eur Heart J Acute Cardiovasc Care. 2017. https://doi.org/10.1177/2048872617711169.
11. Madershahian N, Liakopoulos OJ, Wippermann J, Salehi-Gilani S, Wittwer T, Choi Y-H, et al. The impact of intraaortic balloon counterpulsation on bypass graft flow in patients with peripheral ECMO. J Card Surg. 2009;24(3):265–8.
12. Napp LC, Kühn C, Hoeper MM, Vogel-Claussen J, Haverich A, Schäfer A, et al. Cannulation strategies for percutaneous extracorporeal membrane oxygenation in adults. Clin Res Cardiol Off J Ger Card Soc. 2016;105(4):283–96.
13. Kanji HD, Schulze CJ, Oreopoulos A, Lehr EJ, Wang W, MacArthur RM. Peripheral versus central cannulation for extracorporeal membrane oxygenation: a comparison of limb ischemia and transfusion requirements. Thorac Cardiovasc Surg. 2010;58(8):459–62.
14. De Backer D, Creteur J, Dubois M-J, Sakr Y, Vincent J-L. Microvascular alterations in patients with acute severe heart failure and cardiogenic shock. Am Heart J. 2004;147(1):91–9.
15. Van Genderen ME, Lima A, Akkerhuis M, Bakker J, van Bommel J. Persistent peripheral and microcirculatory perfusion alterations after out-of-hospital cardiac arrest are associated with poor survival*. Crit Care Med. 2012 Aug;40(8):2287–94.
16. Top APC, Ince C, van Dijk M, Tibboel D. Changes in buccal microcirculation following extracorporeal membrane oxygenation in term neonates with severe respiratory failure. Crit Care Med. 2009;37(3):1121–4.
17. Kara A, Akin S, dos Reis MD, Struijs A, Caliskan K, van Thiel RJ, et al. Microcirculatory assessment of patients under VA-ECMO. Crit Care [Internet]. 2016. [cited 2018 Jan 3];20(1). Available from: http://ccforum.biomedcentral.com/articles/10.1186/s13054-016-1519-7.
18. Akin S, dos Reis MD, Caliskan K, Soliman OI, Guven G, Struijs A, et al. Functional evaluation of sublingual microcirculation indicates successful weaning from VA-ECMO in cardiogenic shock. Crit Care [Internet]. 2017. [cited 2018 Jan 3];21(1). Available from: http://ccforum.biomedcentral.com/articles/10.1186/s13054-017-1855-2.
19. Hornick P, Taylor K. Pulsatile and nonpulsatile perfusion: the continuing controversy. J Cardiothorac Vasc Anesth. 1997;11(3):310–5.
20. Elhadj S, Mousa SA, Forsten-Williams K. Chronic pulsatile shear stress impacts synthesis of proteoglycans by endothelial cells: effect on platelet aggregation and coagulation. J Cell Biochem. 2002;86(2):239–50.
21. O'Neil MP, Fleming JC, Badhwar A, Guo LR. Pulsatile versus nonpulsatile flow during cardiopulmonary bypass: microcirculatory and systemic effects. Ann Thorac Surg. 2012;94(6):2046–53.
22. Elbers PWG, Wijbenga J, Solinger F, Yilmaz A, van Iterson M, van Dongen EPA, et al. Direct observation of the human microcirculation during cardiopulmonary bypass: effects of pulsatile perfusion. J Cardiothorac Vasc Anesth. 2011;25(2):250–5.
23. Bienz M, Drullinsky D, Stevens L-M, Bracco D, Noiseux N. Microcirculatory response during on-pump versus off-pump coronary artery bypass graft surgery. Perfusion. 2016;31(3):207–15.
24. Petroni T, Harrois A, Amour J, Lebreton G, Brechot N, Tanaka S, et al. Intra-aortic balloon pump effects on macrocirculation and microcirculation in cardiogenic shock patients supported by venoarterial extracorporeal membrane oxygenation*. Crit Care Med. 2014;42(9):2075–82.
25. Sauren LDC, Reesink KD, Selder JL, Beghi C, van der Veen FH, Maessen JG. The acute effect of intra-aortic balloon counterpulsation during extracorporeal life support: an experimental study. Artif Organs. 2007;31(1):31–8.

26. Burkhoff D, Sayer G, Doshi D, Uriel N. Hemodynamics of mechanical circulatory support. J Am Coll Cardiol. 2015;66(23):2663–74.
27. Wong JK, Smith TN, Pitcher HT, Hirose H, Cavarocchi NC. Cerebral and lower limb near-infrared spectroscopy in adults on extracorporeal membrane oxygenation. Artif Organs. 2012;36(8):659–67.

Clinical Assessment and Measurements

Contents

Clinical Assessment of Hemodynamic Instability

Jan Bakker

M. R. Pinsky et al. (eds.), *Hemodynamic Monitoring*, Lessons from the ICU,
https://doi.org/10.1007/978-3-319-69269-2_13

Learning Objectives

In this chapter the reader will learn the relevance of three simple-to-use windows using simple techniques to assess acute circulatory failure at the bedside. The three windows of circulatory failure represent the brain, the skin, and the kidney where the tools of listening, feeling, and observing can be rapidly used to assess the status of the patient. The reader will appreciate after having read the chapter that any abnormality found using these tools represents a serious warning signal that necessitates further investigations and follow-up.

13.1 Introduction

Hemodynamic instability is a frequent reason for ICU admission and is associated with significant morbidity and mortality. Many decades have been spent on the origin, the naming, and definitions of shock or circulatory failure. Despite the fact that our understanding of the physiology of this syndrome far exceeds that of our predecessors, they already stated in 1861 that it may be better to be able to recognize shock than define it [1]. This is also reflected in our current guidelines, where it is stressed that early recognition and adequate treatment are of paramount importance to prevent organ damage and improve outcome. In the early phase, the availability of hemodynamic data is usually limited. Although changes in blood pressure and heart rate are frequently seen as key features in hemodynamic instability, and used frequently in the definition of circulatory failure, they are not specific nor sensitive in many clinical circumstances. As stated by the famous American trauma surgeon Samuel Gross in the Civil War: "It is not necessary to describe minutely the symptoms of shock, as the nature of the case is apparent at first sight from the excessive pallor of the countenance, the weakened or absent pulse, the confused state of mind, the nausea or nausea and vomiting, and the excessive bodily prostration" [1]. As in many cases hemodynamic monitoring is not (yet) available, we will focus in this chapter on the clinical recognition in a patient with acute circulatory failure, and it will be a history that is repeating itself given the revival of peripheral perfusion assessment in clinical practice (◘ Table 13.1).

13.2 Historical Perspective

As observation and treatment of circulatory shock were also limited in the days before (complex) hemodynamic monitoring became available, it makes sense to review the early descriptions of the syndrome. The first use of the word shock originates from the 1743 English translation of a French manuscript on gunshot wounds published 2 years earlier. Already in this publication, it was stated that although blood was still flowing in the major arteries, it was suspended in the smaller capillaries leading to the clinical symptoms of cold sweat and pale extremities [2]. Six months after Lord Nelson died in the Battle of Trafalgar (1805), Benjamin West painted The Death of Nelson based on recollections of over 50 survivors resulting in a painting on what might have been, not of the circumstances as they happened [3]. In the painting, the bright red faces of the soldiers clearly stand out from the dying Lord Nelson's pale face (◘ Fig. 13.1). One hundred years after the first use of the term shock, Johann Scherer described the first measurements of increased lactate levels in patients who had died from shock [4]. In the first cases, he described women dying of, what we now would call, septic shock with symptoms of altered mental status, delirium, cold, clammy and mottled skin, and dark urine. These symptoms became the windows of shock of modern intensive care [5].

Table 13.1 Table Clinical assessment of peripheral perfusion

Window	Parameter	Limitation
Brain	Mental state	Only available in non-sedated patients Needs a communicable level of consciousness to detect confusion, delirium, etc. Traumatic brain injury may add to the change in mental state irrespective of the circulatory state
Skin	Temperature	Influenced by environmental temperature like outside temperature in trauma patients and room temperature in hospitalized patients Subjective with unknown inter-/intra-rater variability
	Color	Limited in dark skin colors Limited in patients with significant occlusive vascular disease (diabetes, arteriosclerosis)
	Capillary refill time	Press the nailbed of the patient's finger (usually the second or third finger) between your thumb (which is on the nailbed) and index finger so that the blood is pushed out (white nailbed). Do this for 5 seconds, and count the number of seconds it takes for the color of the nailbed to return to the original color
Kidney	Urine production	Not available in patients without kidney function (dialysis patients) Takes time to observe limited urine output

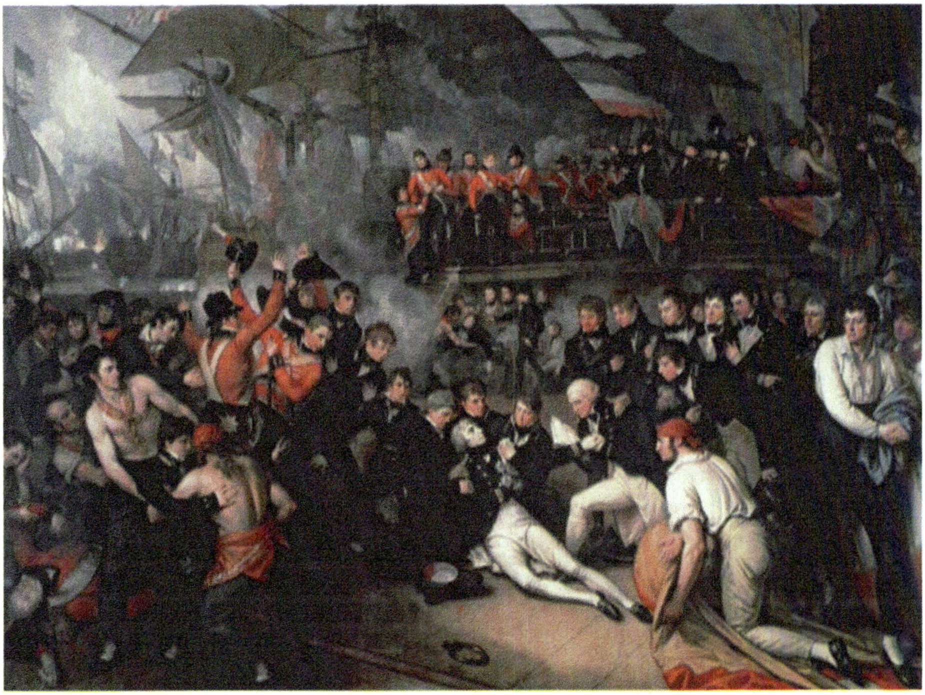

Fig. 13.1 Painting of the death of Lord Nelson, painted 6 months after his death

13.3 Circulatory Failure

An important function of the circulation is to supply the organs with adequate amounts of oxygen and nutrients to maintain their function. Although the supply of oxygen is a factor of the oxygen content of the blood (hemoglobin and arterial oxygen saturation), the main element is blood flow (cardiac output). Together with regional changes in vasomotor tone, the output of the left ventricle results in tissue perfusion coupled to the metabolic needs of the tissues.

In case of loss of significant tissue perfusion, the sympathetic nervous system gets activated. The aim of this response is twofold: first to increase venous return by decreasing venous capacitance to preserve cardiac output and second to maintain blood pressure to ensure vital organ perfusion pressure (heart and brain). Increased sympathetic tone results in increased heart rate (activated beta-receptors), generalized vasoconstriction, increased secretions of sweat glands (activated alpha-receptors), and increased glucose metabolism (activated by alpha-receptors) resulting in the symptoms known for centuries: increased heart rate, cold sweaty and/or mottled skin, decreased urine production, and increased lactate levels. In the following we will discuss the parameters most frequently used to assess the abnormal peripheral circulation in patients with hemodynamic instability.

13.4 Clinical Assessment of Circulatory Failure

In this chapter we focus on the three clinical windows of circulatory failure: the brain, the skin, and the kidney [5]. For this we need only basic skills: listen, feel, and observe. These tools are fast and cheap and don't require monitoring devices. Abnormalities diagnosed with these tools indicate additional measurements and follow-up (Fig. 13.2).

13.4.1 Brain

Changes in mental state occur early in the course of circulatory failure. Like in the case of the 23-year-old Eva Rumpel, in the first publication of lactate measurements, who became delirious first while finally losing consciousness [4]. Already in the early descriptions of a shock state, it was referred to as a state of the nervous system with early signs described as general indifference, apathetic and disoriented to even agitated [1, 6]. Recent developments in scoring systems have revealed that changes/fluctuations in mental status and/or attention, the presence of disorganized thinking, and an altered level of consciousness relate to abnormal brain function [7].

When using clinical observation, almost 25% of the patients with sepsis have symptoms of alterations in mental status [8]. However, when using more profound diagnostic tools, almost all sepsis patients have abnormalities [9].

In general, it is believed that changes in the cerebral oxygen delivery and changes in microcirculatory perfusion play an important role in the deterioration of function. In hemorrhagic shock both cardiac output and low blood pressure contribute to the changes in cerebral perfusion and function [10–12]. Although in septic shock the cardiac output is often preserved, loss of autoregulatory mechanisms due to iNOS activation may result in

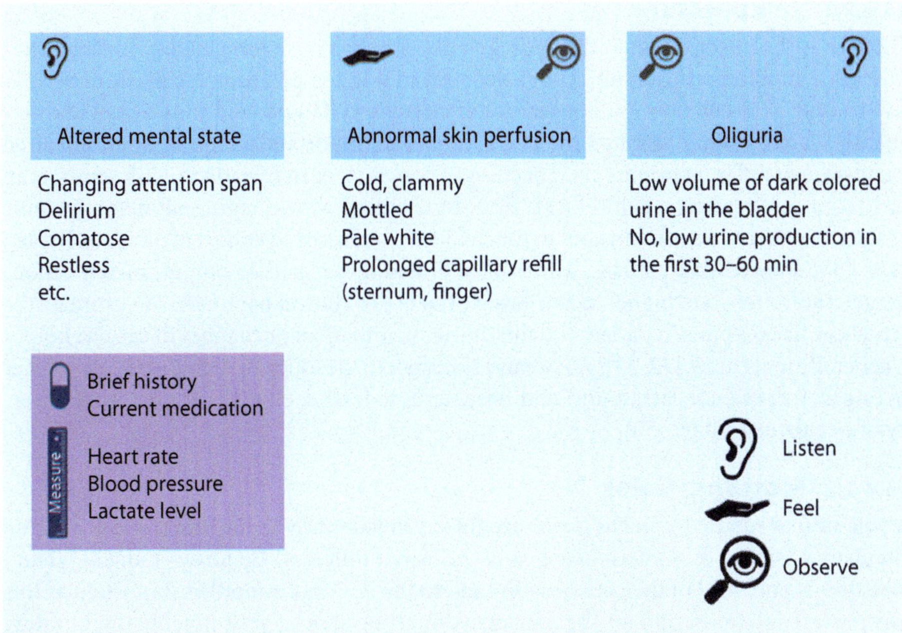

Fig. 13.2 The three windows of acute circulatory failure and the basic skills to use them

microcirculatory perfusion abnormalities that lead to loss of adequate perfusion and function [13–16]. On the other hand, the inflammatory response to infection in itself leads to changes in mental state [17] sometimes referred to as the sickness syndrome [18] but currently usually referred to as sepsis-associated encephalopathy where changes in metabolism may result in an abnormal mental state in these patients [19].

Like many clinical signs described in the realm of circulatory failure, a change in mental state is neither sensitive nor specific [1]. Nevertheless, a patient presenting with a sudden (hours) change in cerebral function should be carefully examined for possible circulatory failure, whereas an abnormal mental state in a patient with clear circulatory failure may be a warning signal of a patient reaching the limits of compensatory mechanisms being at the brink of circulatory arrest [10, 20].

13.4.2 Skin

One of the first mechanisms to preserve tissue perfusion of the vital organs (heart, brain) is to decrease perfusion of the non-vital organs (e.g., skin, kidney) mediated by the activation of the sympathetic nervous system present in both shock related to severe decreases in blood flow as well as to sepsis-related circulatory failure [21, 22]. This may result in decreased perfusion of the skin that can be monitored by several clinical symptoms. In this section we only discuss the assessment of skin perfusion using a clinical exam without the use of devices which bears subjectivity; all of these parameters have been related to similar abnormalities using objective measures of skin perfusion [23–28].

13.4.2.1 Temperature

The skin is the major organ in thermoregulation and has no autoregulatory mechanisms; a decrease in skin perfusion results in a decrease in skin temperature. A shift from peripheral to central circulation is a key feature of circulatory failure, and thus a cool and frequently clammy skin has long time been seen as an important symptom of an impaired circulation of different origins [1]. Therefore, a cool skin, even in patients with sepsis, is an early sign of circulatory failure [29]. Few studies have shown abnormal hemodynamic profiles in patients with a skin cool to touch [30, 31]. In a mixed cohort of patients, Kaplan et al. [30] showed that patients with cool skin had lower cardiac output, mixed venous oxygen saturation, and higher lactate levels. The use of clinical parameters to estimate the actual cardiac output of a patient (qualitative or quantitative) or changes in cardiac output is generally inaccurate [32, 33]. A (sweaty) skin cool to the touch may thus indicate further testing of, for instance, lactate and acid-base status to further objectify the presence/severity of circulatory failure [30].

13.4.2.2 Mottling: Color

A pale skin or mottled skin has been recognized already early in the descriptions of acute circulatory failure. In modern acute care, this is not different. Coudroy et al. [34] found that almost one third of the patients admitted to the ICU had a mottled skin whereas this was present in almost 50% of the patients with septic shock. Most notably the mottling was present on the day of admission. In a study in septic shock patients, Ait-Oufella et al. [35] reported an incidence of up to 70% of the patients. Extensive mottling is a sign the patient is in grave danger of an early death. Ait-Oufella et al. [35] also found that patients with the most severe mottling were more likely to die already on the first day of admission. Therefore, extensive skin mottling should be regarded as a medical emergency irrespective of the blood pressure.

13 The mechanisms involved are poor distribution of blood flow (microcirculatory weak units) [36, 37], loss of autoregulation [38], and nitric oxide synthase metabolites [39]. Although mottling-like areas may also present during diffuse intravascular coagulation (DIC), this is a separate clinical picture that also does not respond to regular resuscitation measures and not to vasodilators (see later). The difference between the two can be easily unmasked as the mottling from DIC is not responsive to pressure on the skin. When infused with a very small dose of nitroglycerine, the mottled areas in DIC won't respond. Only the outer perimeter of the lesions might turn red but the core area not, which is clearly different from the mottling due to circulatory failure (see ◘ Fig. 13.3a, b).

13.4.2.3 Capillary Refill Time

The CRT is a fast and simple procedure that can be performed in all situations even in the prehospital setting [40]. It reflects the time it takes for the color of the nailbed to return to its original color when blanched by applying direct pressure to the nailbed (◘ Table 13.2 table of pictograms). The concept was first introduced early after the Second World War as an assessment of wounded soldiers [41] using qualitative descriptions like "definite slow-

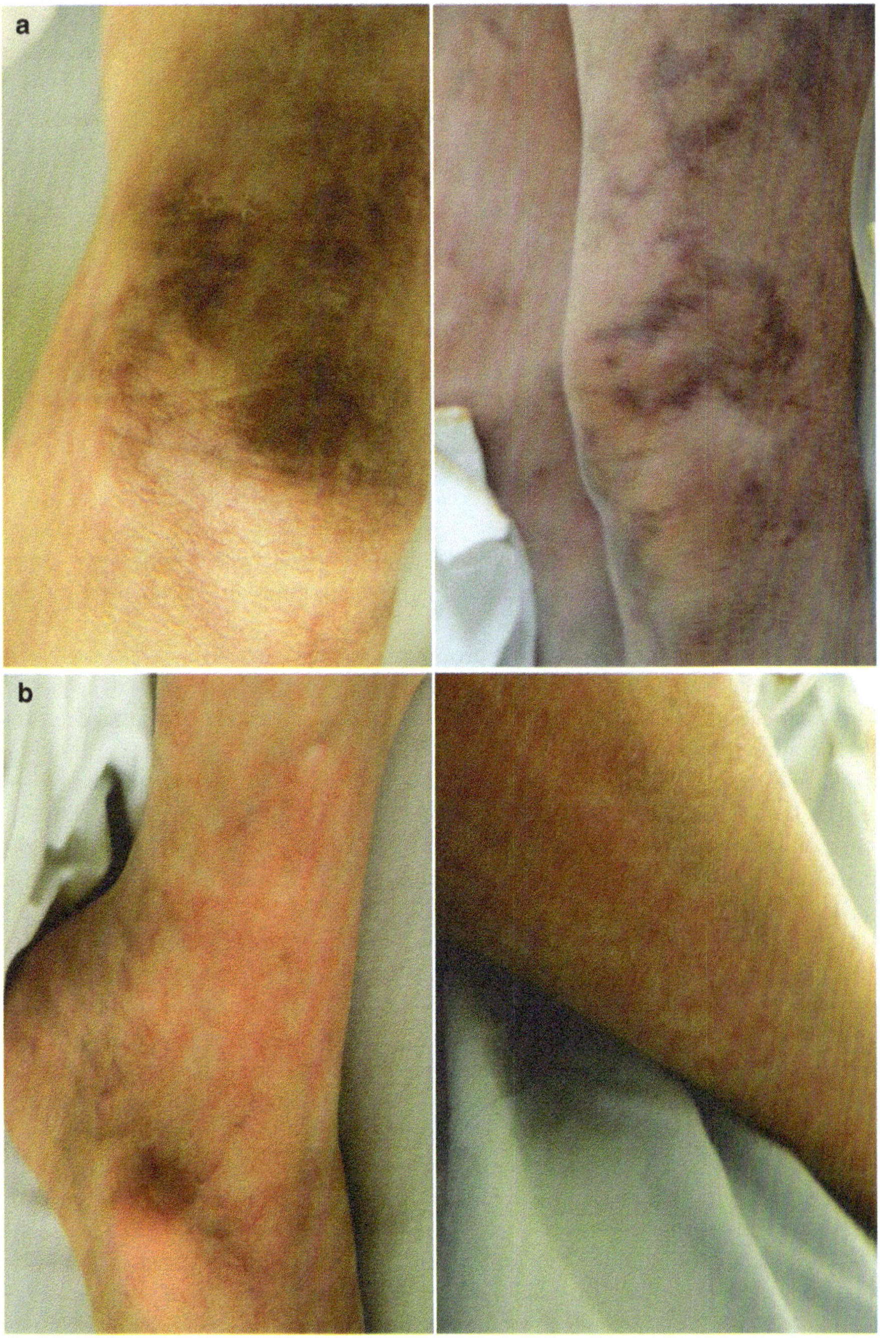

Fig. 13.3 Pre- and post-nitroglycerin bolus in a patient with septic shock. An elderly patient with pneumococcal septic shock was admitted to the ICU after initial treatment (fluids, mechanical ventilation, antibiotics, vasopressor) in the emergency room. Following additional fluid resuscitation while reaching a mean arterial pressure of 65 mmHg with norepinephrine at 0.8 mcg/kg.min, his legs persistently showed extensive mottling (**a**, mottling score, 4). He was then treated with a slow bolus of 0.05 mg nitroglycerin upon the peripheral perfusion rapidly increased to a bright red color **b**. The bolus infusion was followed up by a continuous infusion of 2 mg/h

Table 13.2 Table of pictograms

	*Listen* to a short medical history. Listen to what the patient has to say. Notice inconsistencies in, for instance, data/time/place (relate to the history, i.e., dementia). Confused, delirious, anxious, and agitated Ask for recent urine production, diarrhea, and vomiting
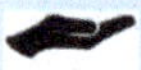	*Feel* the temperature of the extremities with the dorsal side of your hand. Move from the distal part of the extremities to the proximal part. Note the extension of the cold skin. Feel if the skin is sweaty (cold) Make sure you know from the patient's history (if possible) that the cool skin is unusual Do a capillary refill time on the index finger
	*Look* at the color of the skin of the legs, arms, and ears. Notice a pale-white color or mottling. Notice the extension of the mottling on the legs. Make sure you know from the patient's history (if possible) that the color is unusual. Observe the production of urine and its color

ing" and "very sluggish" to indicate moderate and severe shock, respectively. It was introduced in its current form (measuring in seconds) by Champion et al. [42, 43] as part of the triage of trauma patients.

CRT has been shown to be related to more objective measurements of (skin) perfusion like toe-to-central temperature [27] and the temperature difference between a distal finger and the proximal skin of the arm [23]. CRT is confounded by external factors that decrease skin temperature [24, 25].

The normal range is still being debated; however it is related to several factors like age and sex of the patient and influenced by ambient temperature and light [25, 44, 45]. Although originally a cutoff of 2 s has been used by many, in a large study in healthy volunteers, a cutoff of 3.5 s (95th percentile) was reported [44]. Studies using a higher cutoff (4–5 s) have shown good associations with outcome parameters [23, 24, 46–48].

Although the intra-/interobserver variability has been questioned by some studies [49], even advocating its routine use should be reconsidered [50]; studies in well-trained ICU personnel have shown excellent variability [48, 51]. This might also be subject to bias, as prior to the actual measurement, the doctor/nurse may already be prone to a specific result by the status of the patient. This is supported by a study where nurses were asked to assess CRT and the normality of the CRT using a recorded video of a CRT measurement in patients without circulatory failure [52]. Using different levels of expertise to measure CRT and apply it throughout the treatment of the patient may not be adequate. In a recent study by Alsma et al. [50] on the use of CRT, medical specialists performed better than residents and medical students.

The CRT is usually one of the first parameters to normalize during resuscitation [46, 53] where there are no meaningful relationships reported between CRT and hemodynamics [51, 54] or changes in CRT and changes in hemodynamics [24, 51] although relationships with lactate levels have been reported [23, 55]. The latter should however be valued with caution as the time constant of lactate and CRT is very different [46]. However, an important relationship between CRT and a perfusion parameter of the gut, spleen, liver, and kidney has been reported [56]. Although the latter study was a more exploratory study, it may also represent an important link between persistent abnormal peripheral circulation in patients who seem to be adequately resuscitated and the ongoing development of organ failure [23, 24, 48, 57]. The normalization of perfusion parameters, including peripheral parameters, may therefore be even more important than global systemic parameters [58].

The use of CRT, and possible other clinical characteristics of circulatory failure, clearly requires a meaningful context as using this as a universal screening tool in every patient has limited value [50]. From the studies available, it seems that CRT is most useful in the assessment of patients with circulatory failure [49].

13.4.3 Kidney

Already in early publications, it was noted that patients with severe circulatory failure produced little dark urine [4]. Although the activation of the SNS in circulatory failure intends to preserve blood flow to vital organs, the kidney is one of the organs to shut down first. One of the main functions of the kidney, filtering blood and removing waste and excess fluids, is thus an early sign of an impaired perfusion of the kidneys, and thus urine output is seen as a key marker of circulatory failure in many guidelines [59–61] and also as an endpoint of early resuscitation [61] with a cutoff level of 0.5 mL/kg h. Although this cutoff level is used universally to characterize acute circulatory failure and as a resuscitation target, there is limited evidence for this. In fact, renal injury may be associated with polyuria [62, 63].

Interestingly, healthy doctors are more likely to be oliguric than their patients while having zero risk of renal failure [64]. Also, in patient studies, this threshold has been challenged. In a recent study, the use of 0.5 mL/kg h was challenged in patients undergoing major surgery. In a study by Mizota et al. [65], a threshold of 0.3 mL/kg h was found to indicate risk of acute kidney injury, where Puckett et al. [66] found that using 0.2 mL/kg•h was safe in similar patients. In patients with septic shock, a 3–5 h duration of oliguria (0.5 mL/kg•h) was found to be a threshold for acute kidney injury [67].

It therefore seems that the insult to the kidney is, in many cases, of more importance than its symptom. Although in cases of hemorrhage and low cardiac output due to tamponade, restoration of cardiac output results in a fast restoration of urine output, this is not the case in sepsis even when renal blood flow has been restored [68, 69]. In a recent study in patients with early septic shock and post-cardiac surgery patients, the septic shock patients had significantly lower urine output despite similar macro-hemodynamics [70]. Although in this study parameters of peripheral perfusion were not reported, it complements the study by Brunauer et al. [56] who reported decreased renal perfusion despite adequate initial resuscitation based on macro-hemodynamic parameters in septic shock patients. The reason for this dissociation is multifactorial as many factors relate to the decrease in renal function [71] in sepsis. However, it's unlikely that tubular injury is an important factor [72]; therefore the term acute tubular necrosis should be avoided to address renal dysfunction in acute circulatory failure.

A decrease in urine output or its absence remains an alarming signal in patients with acute circulatory failure and should prompt assessment and resuscitation.

Key Points

- Simple and fast methods are available to assess the status of a patient with possible circulatory dysfunction.
- When using basic skills like listen, feel, and observe, powerful warning signs can rapidly be identified.
- These warning signs mandate additional assessments and follow-up.
- Persistent warning signs following initial resuscitation may represent persistent inadequacy of organ perfusion.
- Persistent warning signs after initial resuscitation are associated with increased mortality even early in the phase of resuscitation.
- The effects of common resuscitation strategies (i.e., fluid resuscitation, vasopressors, or vasodilators) should take into account the assessment of peripheral circulation.
- Currently insufficient evidence is available to promote any of these clinical signs of acute circulatory failure to definite endpoints.

13.5 Relation to Outcome Parameters

All of the clinical parameters of circulatory failure have been associated with increased morbidity and mortality.

Changes in mental state in patients with sepsis have shown to be related to outcome and an independent predictor of mortality [8, 9, 17, 73, 74]. In septic shock, brain dysfunction is associated with multiple lesions on MRI scanning and an associated poor outcome [73]. Persistent abnormalities in cerebral function following circulatory failure have also been associated with worse outcome parameters especially in combination with direct injury to the brain [75]. Abnormal skin perfusion has long been related to a worse outcome when compared to patients with normal skin perfusion. A cool and clammy skin has been associated with increased mortality in patients with cardiogenic shock [76]. A cool skin to the touch has been associated with progressive organ failure in a mixed group of patients with circulatory failure [23]. Mottling and prolonged CRT have all been related to increased morbidity and mortality in a mixed group of patients [23, 24, 35, 40, 48, 51, 77]. In the prehospital setting of trauma patients, a prolonged CRT was associated with the need for lifesaving interventions (odds ratio 17) [40]. Ait-Oufella et al. [35] found a significant association between the extent of skin (leg) mottling and mortality in patients with septic shock. In patients with (almost) complete mottling of the legs, the odds ratio for day 14 mortality was 74 while the hemodynamics were not related to mortality in these patients. Skin mottling has also been associated with day 28 mortality [78]. Persistent mottling in critically ill patients is an independent predictor of mortality that seems to be independent of the severity of illness and organ failure scores [34]. Although the presence of decreased urine output using a threshold of 0.5 mL/kg·h is unlikely to represent a specific and sensitive parameter to diagnose and treat acute circulatory failure, the presence of low urine output still represents a risk for renal failure and associated mortality [63, 76, 79]. In a study on post-ischemic oliguria due to aortic cross-clamping, increasing levels of oliguria were associated with increasing mortality [63]. In general, the need for renal replacement therapy is a consistent predictor of mortality in many causes of acute circulatory failure [80].

Clinical Use

A few basic statements can be made at the end of this chapter.

First, the clinical signs described in this chapter all represent a warning signal for the clinician in every patient in a context of acute illness.

Second, although none are specific or sensitive, they warrant further clinical investigation and follow-up.

Finally, improvements in the clinical manifestations of acute circulatory failure can be seen as a success of the resuscitation effort.

In several studies it has been shown that improvements in peripheral perfusion occur more rapidly than other parameters frequently used to indicate inadequate tissue perfusion (i.e., lactate) and that they may represent a more accurate marker of initial success of the resuscitation [46, 81]. In addition, specific therapies can rapidly improve peripheral perfusion parameters in patients with acute circulatory failure even when initial resuscitation has failed to normalize peripheral perfusion parameters [26]. The infusion of nitroglycerin can rapidly improve profound mottling in patients with acute circulatory failure (◘ Fig. 13.3) even in small dosages [26]. Its use in clinical practice during the early resuscitation of patients with acute circulatory failure has been associated with improved outcome when used in a complex resuscitation protocol [82].

Whether oliguria should be respected as renal success or as renal failure is still open for discussion [83]. However, current practice shows urine output to be both an indication for fluid resuscitation as well as an endpoint of fluid resuscitation [84]. However, ongoing fluid resuscitation in an effort to restore urine output seems a flawed goal as there is frequently a dissociated response between the renal response and the macro-hemodynamic response [85], and ample data exist to suggest the opposite [86–89] especially when the source of the circulatory failure has not been controlled [68, 90]. Although oliguria remains an alarming signal, immediate restoration of urine output doesn't need to be a clinical goal [67]. Fluid restriction, following initial resuscitation, seems to be safe especially when peripheral perfusion is normal [47, 88] where some even advocate that further fluid resuscitation is not warranted [85].

Thus, at the moment clear studies to promote normality of peripheral perfusion parameters as endpoints of resuscitation in patients with acute circulatory failure are lacking [91]. For this, the recently completed study comparing lactate-guided resuscitation versus CRT-guided resuscitation in patients with septic shock could help to further optimize the use of these parameters in clinical practice [92].

Take-Home Messages

- A patient presenting to you with an acute illness and having abnormal symptoms viewed from the three windows of acute circulatory failure is at an increased risk of dying.
- Abnormalities in peripheral perfusion are not specific nor sensitive but require immediate assessment of the circulatory status.
- When in doubt about the validity of the abnormal window views, do additional assessments (measure lactate, blood gases, organ function parameters, etc.).
- Always follow up on the course of the abnormalities found when viewing the three windows. When symptoms do not improve or disappear, be vigilant about your initial assessment, adequacy of diagnosis, and/or treatment.

References

1. Millham FH. A brief history of shock. Surgery. 2010;148(5):1026–37.
2. Riede U, Sandritter W, Mittermayer C. Circulatory shock: a review. Pathology. 1981;13(2):299–311.
3. The death of Nelson, 1806. Wikipedia. https://en.wikipedia.org/wiki/The_Death_of_Nelson_(West_painting)#/media/File:Death_of_Nelson.jpg. Accessed 11 Apr 2018.
4. Kompanje EJ, Jansen TC, van der Hoven B, et al. The first demonstration of lactic acid in human blood in shock by Johann Joseph Scherer (1814–1869) in January 1843. Intensive Care Med. 2007;33(11):1967–71.
5. Vincent JL, Ince C, Bakker J. Clinical review: circulatory shock - an update: a tribute to Professor Max Harry Weil. Crit Care. 2012;16(6):239.
6. Kovach AG. The function of the central nervous system after haemorrhage. J Clin Pathol Suppl (R Coll Pathol). 1970;4:202–12.
7. Ely EW, Truman B, Shintani A, et al. Monitoring sedation status over time in ICU patients: reliability and validity of the Richmond Agitation-Sedation Scale (RASS). JAMA. 2003;289(22):2983–91.
8. Sprung CL, Peduzzi PN, Shatney CH, et al. Impact of encephalopathy on mortality in the sepsis syndrome. The Veterans Administration Systemic Sepsis Cooperative Study Group. Crit Care Med. 1990;18(8):801–6.
9. Ebersoldt M, Sharshar T, Annane D. Sepsis-associated delirium. Intensive Care Med. 2007;33(6):941–50.
10. Kovach AG, Sandor P. Cerebral blood flow and brain function during hypotension and shock. Annu Rev Physiol. 1976;38:571–96.
11. MacKenzie ET, Farrar JK, Fitch W, et al. Effects of hemorrhagic hypotension on the cerebral circulation. I. Cerebral blood flow and pial arteriolar caliber. Stroke. 1979;10(6):711–8.
12. Gregory PC, McGeorge AP, Fitch W, et al. Effects of hemorrhagic hypotension on the cerebral circulation. II. Electrocortical function. Stroke. 1979;10(6):719–23.
13. Schweighofer H, Rummel C, Mayer K, et al. Brain function in iNOS knock out or iNOS inhibited (l-NIL) mice under endotoxic shock. Intensive Care Med Exp. 2014;2(1):24.
14. Rosengarten B, Hecht M, Wolff S, et al. Autoregulative function in the brain in an endotoxic rat shock model. Inflamm Res. 2008;57(11):542–6.
15. Taccone FS, Scolletta S, Franchi F, et al. Brain perfusion in sepsis. Curr Vasc Pharmacol. 2013;11(2):170–86.
16. Taccone FS, Su F, Pierrakos C, et al. Cerebral microcirculation is impaired during sepsis: an experimental study. Crit Care. 2010;14(4):R140.
17. Eidelman LA, Putterman D, Putterman C, et al. The spectrum of septic encephalopathy. Definitions, etiologies, and mortalities. JAMA. 1996;275(6):470–3.
18. Tracey KJ. Reflex control of immunity. Nat Rev Immunol. 2009;9(6):418–28.
19. Sprung CL, Cerra FB, Freund HR, et al. Amino acid alterations and encephalopathy in the sepsis syndrome. Crit Care Med. 1991;19(6):753–7.
20. Baethmann A, Kempski O. The brain in shock. Secondary disturbances of cerebral function. Chest. 1991;100(3 Suppl):205S–8S.
21. Schadt JC, Ludbrook J. Hemodynamic and neurohumoral responses to acute hypovolemia in conscious mammals. Am J Phys. 1991;260(2 Pt 2):H305–18.
22. Dunser MW, Hasibeder WR. Sympathetic overstimulation during critical illness: adverse effects of adrenergic stress. J Intensive Care Med. 2009;24(5):293–316.
23. Lima A, Jansen TC, Van Bommel J, et al. The prognostic value of the subjective assessment of peripheral perfusion in critically ill patients. Crit Care Med. 2009;37(3):934–8.
24. van Genderen ME, Lima A, Akkerhuis M, et al. Persistent peripheral and microcirculatory perfusion alterations after out-of-hospital cardiac arrest are associated with poor survival. Crit Care Med. 2012;40(8):2287–94.
25. Lima A, van Genderen ME, Klijn E, et al. Peripheral vasoconstriction influences thenar oxygen saturation as measured by near-infrared spectroscopy. Intensive Care Med. 2012;38(4):606–11.
26. Lima A, van Genderen ME, van Bommel J, et al. Nitroglycerin reverts clinical manifestations of poor peripheral perfusion in patients with circulatory shock. Crit Care. 2014;18(3):R126.
27. Bourcier S, Pichereau C, Boelle PY, et al. Toe-to-room temperature gradient correlates with tissue perfusion and predicts outcome in selected critically ill patients with severe infections. Ann Intensive Care. 2016;6(1):63.

28. Lima A, van Bommel J, Sikorska K, et al. The relation of near-infrared spectroscopy with changes in peripheral circulation in critically ill patients. Crit Care Med. 2011;39(7):1649–54.
29. Thompson MJ, Ninis N, Perera R, et al. Clinical recognition of meningococcal disease in children and adolescents. Lancet. 2006;367(9508):397–403.
30. Kaplan LJ, McPartland K, Santora TA, et al. Start with a subjective assessment of skin temperature to identify hypoperfusion in intensive care unit patients. J Trauma. 2001;50(4):620–7.
31. Schey BM, Williams DY, Bucknall T. Skin temperature as a noninvasive marker of haemodynamic and perfusion status in adult cardiac surgical patients: an observational study. Intensive Crit Care Nurs. 2009;25(1):31–7.
32. Hiemstra B, Eck RJ, Keus F, et al. Clinical examination for diagnosing circulatory shock. Curr Opin Crit Care. 2017;23(4):293–301.
33. Grissom CK, Morris AH, Lanken PN, et al. Association of physical examination with pulmonary artery catheter parameters in acute lung injury. Crit Care Med. 2009;37(10):2720–6.
34. Coudroy R, Jamet A, Frat JP, et al. Incidence and impact of skin mottling over the knee and its duration on outcome in critically ill patients. Intensive Care Med. 2015;41(3):452–9.
35. Ait-Oufella H, Lemoinne S, Boelle PY, et al. Mottling score predicts survival in septic shock. Intensive Care Med. 2011;37(5):801–7.
36. Lehr HA, Bittinger F, Kirkpatrick CJ. Microcirculatory dysfunction in sepsis: a pathogenetic basis for therapy? J Pathol. 2000;190(3):373–86.
37. Ince C, Sinaasappel M. Microcirculatory oxygenation and shunting in sepsis and shock. Crit Care Med. 1999;27(7):1369–77.
38. Johnson PC. Autoregulation of blood flow. Circ Res. 1986;59(5):483–95.
39. Zhou M, Wang P, Chaudry IH. Endothelial nitric oxide synthase is downregulated during hyperdynamic sepsis. Biochim Biophys Acta. 1997;1335:182–270.
40. Holcomb JB, Niles SE, Miller CC, et al. Prehospital physiologic data and lifesaving interventions in trauma patients. Mil Med. 2005;170(1):7–13.
41. Beecher HK, Simeone FA, et al. The internal state of the severely wounded man on entry to the most forward hospital. Surgery. 1947;22(4):672–711.
42. Champion HR, Sacco WJ, Carnazzo AJ, et al. Trauma score. Crit Care Med. 1981;9(9):672–6.
43. Champion HR, Sacco WJ, Hannan DS, et al. Assessment of injury severity: the triage index. Crit Care Med. 1980;8(4):201–8.
44. Anderson B, Kelly AM, Kerr D, et al. Impact of patient and environmental factors on capillary refill time in adults. Am J Emerg Med. 2008;26(1):62–5.
45. Brown LH, Prasad NH, Whitley TW. Adverse lighting condition effects on the assessment of capillary refill. Am J Emerg Med. 1994;12(1):46–7.
46. Hernandez G, Pedreros C, Veas E, et al. Evolution of peripheral vs metabolic perfusion parameters during septic shock resuscitation. A clinical-physiologic study. J Crit Care. 2012;27(3):283–8.
47. van Genderen ME, Engels N, van der Valk RJ, et al. Early peripheral perfusion-guided fluid therapy in patients with septic shock. Am J Respir Crit Care Med. 2015;191(4):477–80.
48. van Genderen ME, Paauwe J, de Jonge J, et al. Clinical assessment of peripheral perfusion to predict postoperative complications after major abdominal surgery early: a prospective observational study in adults. Crit Care. 2014;18(3):R114.
49. Pickard A, Karlen W, Ansermino JM. Capillary refill time: is it still a useful clinical sign? Anesth Analg. 2011;113(1):120–3.
50. Alsma J, van Saase J, Nanayakkara PWB, et al. The power of flash mob research: conducting a nationwide observational clinical study on capillary refill time in a single day. Chest. 2017;151(5): 1106–13.
51. Ait-Oufella H, Bige N, Boelle PY, et al. Capillary refill time exploration during septic shock. Intensive Care Med. 2014;40(7):958–64.
52. Brabrand M, Hosbond S, Folkestad L. Capillary refill time: a study of interobserver reliability among nurses and nurse assistants. Eur J Emerg Med. 2011;18(1):46–9.
53. Hernandez G, Luengo C, Bruhn A, et al. When to stop septic shock resuscitation: clues from a dynamic perfusion monitoring. Ann Intensive Care. 2014;4(30).
54. Bailey JM, Levy JH, Kopel MA, et al. Relationship between clinical evaluation of peripheral perfusion and global hemodynamics in adults after cardiac surgery. Crit Care Med. 1990;18(12):1353–6.
55. Morimura N, Takahashi K, Doi T, et al. A pilot study of quantitative capillary refill time to identify high blood lactate levels in critically ill patients. Emerg Med J. 2015;32(6):444–8.

56. Brunauer A, Kokofer A, Bataar O, et al. Changes in peripheral perfusion relate to visceral organ perfusion in early septic shock: a pilot study. J Crit Care. 2016;35:105–9.
57. Lima A, van Bommel J, Jansen TC, et al. Low tissue oxygen saturation at the end of early goal-directed therapy is associated with worse outcome in critically ill patients. Crit Care. 2009;13
58. Dunser MW, Takala J, Brunauer A, et al. Re-thinking resuscitation: leaving blood pressure cosmetics behind and moving forward to permissive hypotension and a tissue perfusion-based approach. Crit Care. 2013;17(5):326.
59. Cecconi M, De Backer D, Antonelli M, et al. Consensus on circulatory shock and hemodynamic monitoring. Task force of the European Society of Intensive Care Medicine. Intensive Care Med. 2014;40(12):1795–815.
60. Mebazaa A, Tolppanen H, Mueller C, et al. Acute heart failure and cardiogenic shock: a multidisciplinary practical guidance. Intensive Care Med. 2016;42(2):147–63.
61. Rhodes A, Evans LE, Alhazzani W, et al. Surviving sepsis campaign: international guidelines for management of sepsis and septic shock: 2016. Intensive Care Med. 2017;43(3):304–77.
62. Hsu CH, Preuss HG, Argy WP, et al. Prolonged tubular malfunction following acute oliguric renal failure. Nephron. 1974;13(4):342–8.
63. Stone HH, Fulenwider JT. Renal decapsulation in the prevention of post-ischemic oliguria. Ann Surg. 1977;186(3):343–55.
64. Solomon AW, Kirwan CJ, Alexander ND, et al. Urine output on an intensive care unit: case-control study. BMJ. 2010;341:c6761.
65. Mizota T, Yamamoto Y, Hamada M, et al. Intraoperative oliguria predicts acute kidney injury after major abdominal surgery. Br J Anaesth. 2017;119(6):1127–34.
66. Puckett JR, Pickering JW, Palmer SC, et al. Low versus standard urine output targets in patients undergoing major abdominal surgery: a randomized noninferiority trial. Ann Surg. 2017;265(5):874–81.
67. Leedahl DD, Frazee EN, Schramm GE, et al. Derivation of urine output thresholds that identify a very high risk of AKI in patients with septic shock. Clin J Am Soc Nephrol. 2014;9(7):1168–74.
68. van Genderen ME, Klijn E, Lima A, et al. Microvascular perfusion as a target for fluid resuscitation in experimental circulatory shock. Crit Care Med. 2014;42(2):E96–E105.
69. Langenberg C, Wan L, Egi M, et al. Renal blood flow in experimental septic acute renal failure. Kidney Int. 2006;69(11):1996–2002.
70. Skytte Larsson J, Krumbholz V, Enskog A, et al. Renal blood flow, glomerular filtration rate, and renal oxygenation in early clinical septic shock. Crit Care Med. 2018;46(6):e560–6.
71. Schrier RW, Wang W. Acute renal failure and sepsis. N Engl J Med. 2004;351(2):159–69.
72. Lerolle N, Nochy D, Guerot E, et al. Histopathology of septic shock induced acute kidney injury: apoptosis and leukocytic infiltration. Intensive Care Med. 2010;36(3):471–8.
73. Sharshar T, Carlier R, Bernard F, et al. Brain lesions in septic shock: a magnetic resonance imaging study. Intensive Care Med. 2007;33(5):798–806.
74. Young GB, Bolton CF, Archibald YM, et al. The electroencephalogram in sepsis-associated encephalopathy. J Clin Neurophysiol. 1992;9(1):145–52.
75. Maas AIR, Menon DK, Adelson PD, et al. Traumatic brain injury: integrated approaches to improve prevention, clinical care, and research. Lancet Neurol. 2017;16(12):987–1048.
76. Hasdai D, Holmes DR Jr, Califf RM, et al. Cardiogenic shock complicating acute myocardial infarction: predictors of death. GUSTO Investigators. Global Utilization of Streptokinase and Tissue-Plasminogen Activator for Occluded Coronary Arteries. Am Heart J. 1999;138(1 Pt 1):21–31.
77. Lima A, Beelen P, Bakker J. Use of a peripheral perfusion index derived from the pulse oximetry signal as a noninvasive indicator of perfusion. Crit Care Med. 2002;30(6):1210–3.
78. de Moura EB, Amorim FF, da C, Santana AN, et al. Skin mottling score as a predictor of 28-day mortality in patients with septic shock. Intensive Care Med. 2016;42(3):479–80.
79. Kellum JA, Sileanu FE, Murugan R, et al. Classifying AKI by urine output versus serum creatinine level. J Am Soc Nephrol. 2015;26(9):2231–8.
80. Ostermann M, Chang RW. Acute kidney injury in the intensive care unit according to RIFLE. Crit Care Med. 2007;35(8):1837–43; quiz 1852
81. Lara B, Enberg L, Ortega M, et al. Capillary refill time during fluid resuscitation in patients with sepsis-related hyperlactatemia at the emergency department is related to mortality. PLoS One. 2018;12(11):e0188548.
82. Jansen TC, van Bommel J, Schoonderbeek FJ, et al. Early lactate-guided therapy in intensive care unit patients a multicenter, open-label, randomized controlled trial. Am J Respir Crit Care Med. 2010;182(6):752–61.

83. Thurau K, Boylan JW. Acute renal success. The unexpected logic of oliguria in acute renal failure. Am J Med. 1976;61(3):308–15.
84. Cecconi M, Hofer C, Teboul JL, et al. Fluid challenges in intensive care: the FENICE study: a global inception cohort study. Intensive Care Med. 2015;41(9):1529–37.
85. Schortgen F, Schetz M. Does this critically ill patient with oliguria need more fluids, a vasopressor, or neither? Intensive Care Med. 2017;43(6):907–10.
86. Vellinga NA, Ince C, Boerma EC. Elevated central venous pressure is associated with impairment of microcirculatory blood flow in sepsis: a hypothesis generating post hoc analysis. BMC Anesthesiol. 2013;13:17.
87. Legrand M, Dupuis C, Simon C, et al. Association between systemic hemodynamics and septic acute kidney injury in critically ill patients: a retrospective observational study. Crit Care. 2013;17(6):R278.
88. Hjortrup PB, Haase N, Wetterslev J, et al. Effects of fluid restriction on measures of circulatory efficacy in adults with septic shock. Acta Anaesthesiol Scand. 2017;61(4):390–8.
89. Boyd JH, Forbes J, Nakada TA, et al. Fluid resuscitation in septic shock: a positive fluid balance and elevated central venous pressure are associated with increased mortality. Crit Care Med. 2011;39(2): 259–65.
90. Bickell WH, Wall MJ, Pepe PE, et al. Immediate versus delayed fluid resuscitation for hypotensive patients with penetrating torso injuries. N Engl J Med. 1994;331:1105–9.
91. Ait-Oufella H, Bakker J. Understanding clinical signs of poor tissue perfusion during septic shock. Intensive Care Med. 2016;42(12):2070–2.
92. Hernández G, Cavalcanti AB, Ospina-Tascón G, et al. Early goal-directed therapy using a physiological holistic view: the ANDROMEDA-SHOCK—a randomized controlled trial. Ann Intensive Care. 2018;8(1):52.

Assessment of the Microcirculation

Daniel De Backer

M. R. Pinsky et al. (eds.), *Hemodynamic Monitoring*, Lessons from the ICU,
https://doi.org/10.1007/978-3-319-69269-2_14

Learning Objectives

- To understand what is microcirculation and what are the determinants of microvascular perfusion
- To address the interest and limitations of techniques used to evaluate the microcirculation
- To illustrate the typical microcirculatory alterations encountered in critically ill patients
- To understand the critical role of microcirculatory alterations in the development of organ dysfunction

14.1 Introduction

While tissue perfusion is one of our main targets for hemodynamic resuscitation, classical hemodynamic monitoring only provides indirect evidence of tissue perfusion. Many patients with circulatory failure present alterations in tissue perfusion despite optimization of systemic hemodynamics. While impaired distribution of blood flow has to be considered, microcirculatory alterations have also been implicated. Microcirculatory alterations have been demonstrated in various experimental models. However, the identification of microcirculatory alterations in critically ill patients has long been difficult due to the lack of adequate technology. Recent advances in technology have nevertheless allowed the evaluation of microcirculation in patients. Microvascular dysfunction has first been reported in patients with sepsis and septic shock [1] but was later reported in many other conditions encountered in critically ill patients. In this chapter, we will discuss the specificities of the microcirculation, the evidence for microvascular alterations, and the tools that can be used to assess the microcirculation.

14.2 Anatomical Structure of the Microcirculation

The microcirculation is composed of vessels smaller than 100 microns and is composed of arterioles, capillaries, and venules. The most usual architecture is the branched tree aspect, with arterioles dividing at several branch points into smaller ones, up to capillaries, which collect in venules, themselves collecting in larger venules. The role of arterioles is basically to distribute blood flow to the different parts of the organ, adapting the flow to local metabolism. The larger arterioles are called resistive arterioles, as they experience a large drop in pressure between entry and exit of these vessels. Distal arterioles and capillaries are the places where oxygen exchange with the tissues takes place. As oxygen diffuses from red blood cell flowing in capillaries, the diffusion distance becomes the limiting factor. Hence, at the microcirculatory level, the density of perfused vessels is more relevant for tissue oxygenation than the velocity at which red blood cells are flowing in perfused capillaries.

Organs like the kidney and gut have different microvascular architectures, associated with precapillary shunting or countercurrent exchange, which make these organs more vulnerable to hypoxia than other organs.

The control of microvascular perfusion is influenced by local factors, with backward communication through different channels, allowing adaptation of perfusion to local metabolism.

Another important factor for oxygen delivery at the microcirculatory level is capillary hematocrit. As the volumic effect of the plasma layer at the surface of vascular endothelium is proportionally greater at capillary level than in large vessels, the capillary hematocrit is much lower than the systemic one. In addition, hematocrit is lower in side branch vessels than in straight vessels, due to the kinetic inertia of red blood cells. Accordingly, capillary hematocrit is difficult to predict from measurements of systemic hematocrit.

All these factors make it difficult to predict microvascular perfusion and tissue oxygen delivery from measurements of systemic hemodynamics. Also, therapeutic interventions aiming at increasing systemic oxygen delivery may fail to increase delivery of oxygen at the microcirculatory level.

14.3 Microvascular Alterations in Disease

14.3.1 Sepsis

In a landmark paper published in 2002, De Backer et al. [1] demonstrated that the sublingual microcirculation of patients with sepsis and septic shock was markedly altered compared to that of healthy volunteers and ICU controls. Septic patients experienced a decrease in density of perfused vessels, due to a combined increase in stopped flow as well as in intermittently perfused vessels, with perfused vessels in close vicinity to perfused vessels (◘ Fig. 14.1). These alterations were only observed in vessels smaller than 20 microns, representing mostly capillaries. A key factor of these microcirculatory alterations is heterogeneity inside the observed field but also between several fields closed by a few microns. Importantly, these abnormalities were not fixed, as topical administration of acetylcholine fully normalized the sublingual microcirculation of these septic patients. These results have been reproduced in more than 40 papers from different teams around the world.

What is the relevance of these alterations? In experimental models, zones of impaired microvascular perfusion are co-localized with areas of hypoxia and even cell deaths [2]. In humans, this is more complicated to demonstrate, but improvements in microvascular perfusion are associated with improvement in lactate levels. Several studies have shown that sublingual microcirculatory alterations are associated with outcome [1, 3, 4]. Among the microcirculatory variables associated with outcome, perfused capillary density and proportion of perfused capillaries were positively associated with survival, while heterogeneity index was inversely related with survival [1, 3–5]. On the contrary, the velocity of red blood cells in perfused vessels did not differ between survivors and non-survivors [6], illustrating that diffusion and not convection is crucial for tissue oxygenation. Thus microvascular alterations are associated in the pathophysiology of organ dysfunction and death.

What could be the potential mechanisms responsible for these alterations? Experimental models of sepsis highlighted that several mechanisms are implicated, including endothelial dysfunction, impaired backward communication, impaired sensitivity to vasoconstrictive and vasodilating substances, glycocalyx alterations, and adhesion of circulating cells [7].

Are these alterations related to alterations in systemic hemodynamics? The relation between microvascular perfusion and arterial pressure or cardiac output is, at best, loose [8, 9]. Microvascular alterations are similar in low- and high-cardiac-output septic patients [10]. Hence these cannot be detected by looking at systemic hemodynamics. Can systemic hemodynamics be neglected? Obviously not, microvascular perfusion cannot be sustained if a minimal cardiac output or blood pressure is not obtained, but this value is quite

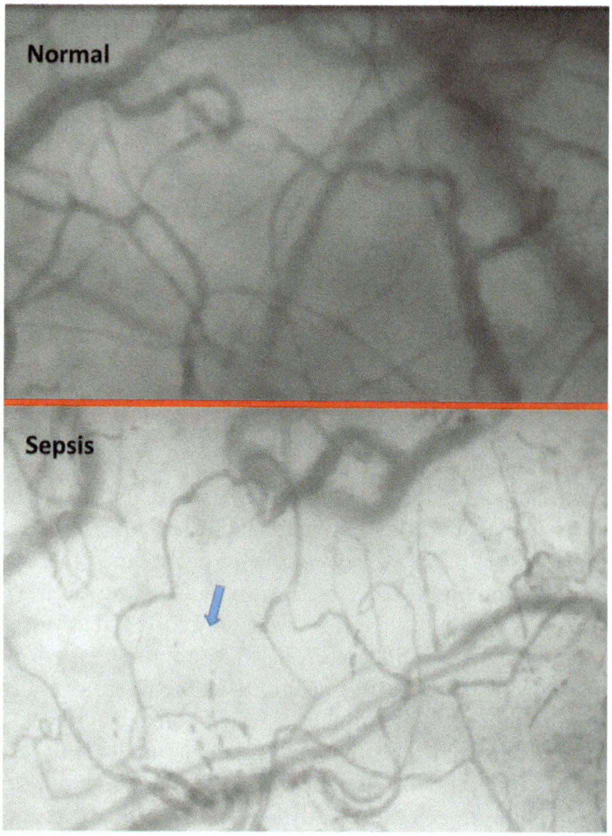

Fig. 14.1 Examples of microvideoscopic evaluation of sublingual microcirculation. SDF images recorded in a control patient (normal) and in a patient with septic shock (sepsis). The blue arrow denotes a not-perfused area

variable among individuals so that it is quite difficult to identify a clear cutoff value. For this reason, increasing perfusion pressure and cardiac output are both associated with a variable and unpredictable response [8, 11].

14.3.2 Microvascular Dysfunction in Other Conditions

Microvascular alterations relatively similar (even though often less severe) to those reported in septic shock have also been observed in other conditions. In patients with cardiogenic shock, microvascular density and perfusion of capillaries are decreased, together with an increase in perfusion heterogeneity [12, 13]. These alterations are associated with outcome [12, 13].

In patients resuscitated from trauma, the severity and duration of microvascular perfusion are associated with organ dysfunction [14]. Similarly, high-risk surgical patients presenting postoperative complications had more severe and more prolonged perioperative microvascular dysfunction than their counterpart with uncomplicated course [15].

Microvascular dysfunction has also been observed in eclampsia [16] or after cardiac arrest [17].

14.4 How to Assess the Microcirculation

As reported above, microvascular alterations cannot be detected by classical hemodynamic monitoring. At best, these can be suggested in a patient with cardiac output and arterial pressure values within targets and a high venous oxygen saturation (SvO_2) presenting clinical signs of hypoperfusion or with increased lactate levels. Biomarkers such as lactate may indicate tissue hypoxia, but the origin of it cannot be located in the microcirculation. In addition, lactate decrease may take time once perfusion is restored.

Clinical signs may appear attractive. Skin mottling, capillary refill time, and skin temperature are excellent indices of skin microvascular perfusion [18]. These are easily measured and often inexpensive. In addition, skin perfusion alterations have been associated with outcome [19, 20]. Unfortunately, these clinical signs are only approaching skin microvascular perfusion and are very influenced by local conditions (ambient temperature) or patient condition (peripheral arterial disease, Raynaud phenomenon, etc.) or vasopressor use. In addition, the skin microvasculature may not reflect more central microvascular areas, especially as skin vasoconstriction is an important physiological response helping to preserve perfusion to more vital organs. Hence, skin microvascular perfusion assessment is very helpful as a triage tool but lacks specificity. Chasing normalization of skin microvascular perfusion thus carries the risk of overtreating some patients or even diverting blood flow from vital organ to skin perfusion (as it may occur with some vasodilatory agents).

14.4.1 Direct Visualization of the Microcirculation

Two different handheld microscopes are currently used to visualize the microcirculation in critically ill patients (sidestream dark-field (SDF) and incident dark-field (IDF) imaging) [21]. Basically, these illuminate the field using light reflection from deeper layers, and vessels are visualized because light is absorbed at the selected wavelength by the hemoglobin contained in the red blood cells. These microscopes are mostly applied on the sublingual area (■ Fig. 14.1), as skin is covered by a thick epithelium rendering difficult visualization of the microcirculation. The sublingual microcirculation has the advantage of being relatively central and at core temperature, being less influenced by ambient temperature and peripheral vasoconstriction. Unfortunately, it is difficult to apply these devices on the sublingual area in non-intubated patients. In addition great care should be taken to discard secretions and to limit pressure artifacts. Recommendations on image acquisition and analysis have recently been published [21]. Microcirculatory images are mostly analyzed by offline manual analysis using a grid to count the vessels. Eyeballing is feasible and reliable for evaluation of simple variables. Software-assisted analysis is becoming available.

14.4.2 Indirect Assessment of Microvascular Perfusion

14.4.2.1 Vasoreactivity Tests

Due to the heterogeneity of microvascular perfusion in disease, microcirculation cannot be evaluated directly by laser Doppler or oxygen sensors. Indeed, these measure perfusion or oxygenation in a relatively large volume (at least 1 mm^3) which contains many vessels including arterioles, capillaries, and venules. Accordingly, the measured value represents the average of flow/PO_2 in the various vessels and fails to take into account the non-perfused vessels. However, microcirculation can be indirectly evaluated by the estimation of vasoreactivity after a transient occlusion. Analysis of changes in blood flow/O_2 saturation during a brief episode of forearm ischemia enables quantification of microvascular reserve. Several indices can be measured, but the ascending slope, or recovery slope, is the easiest to measure and is the most reproducible.

Iontophoresis [22] and thermal challenge [23], both coupled with laser Doppler, can both be used to evaluate skin response to various vasodilatory drugs or to standardized heating, respectively. Compared to transient occlusion, these have the advantage to explore more central skin areas and not to be sensitive to peripheral vasoconstriction which occurs in response to disease as well as to vasopressor administration.

14.4.2.2 PCO_2 Gradients

Tissue PCO_2 increases in low flow conditions. In order to get rid of the influence of arterial PCO_2, the tissue to arterial PCO_2 gradient, or PCO_2 gap, is computed. Measurements of tissue PCO_2 have been used to reflect microvascular perfusion in sublingual or even gastric area. Unfortunately, these techniques are no more available.

Venoarterial gradients in PCO_2 can be used to indirectly evaluate microvascular perfusion [24]. Venous PCO_2 is measured on venous blood gas obtained in central venous or pulmonary artery catheter, simultaneous to an arterial blood gas. As PCO_2 can diffuse longer distances than PO_2, accumulation of PCO_2 in non-perfused areas is slowly diffusing to drainage veins (Fig. 14.2) so that the venoarterial PCO_2 gradient also increases in case of microcirculatory alterations, even though less significantly than in tissue itself. Venoarterial PCO_2 gradients have to be interpreted in conjunction with venous O_2 saturation: the increased venoarterial PCO_2 gradient mostly represents an altered cardiac output when venous O_2 saturation is low, while it mostly represents microvascular alterations when venous O_2 saturation is normal or elevated [25].

14.5 Limitations

One of the most important limitations is that we are looking at the microcirculation in one organ expecting that it may represent the microcirculation of other organs. While the process leading to endothelial dysfunction is affecting the microcirculation in the various organs (it has nicely been demonstrated in experimental setting that in sepsis the microcirculation is similarly affected in all organs, including the brain, liver, and kidney), some anatomical specificities or local factors can make some organs even more sensitive than others. Accordingly, it is usually considered that the microcirculatory alterations detected in the sublingual area likely reflect the minimal alterations that can be observed in other organs, while other organs may present more severe alterations or respond differently to therapeutic interventions due to local factors.

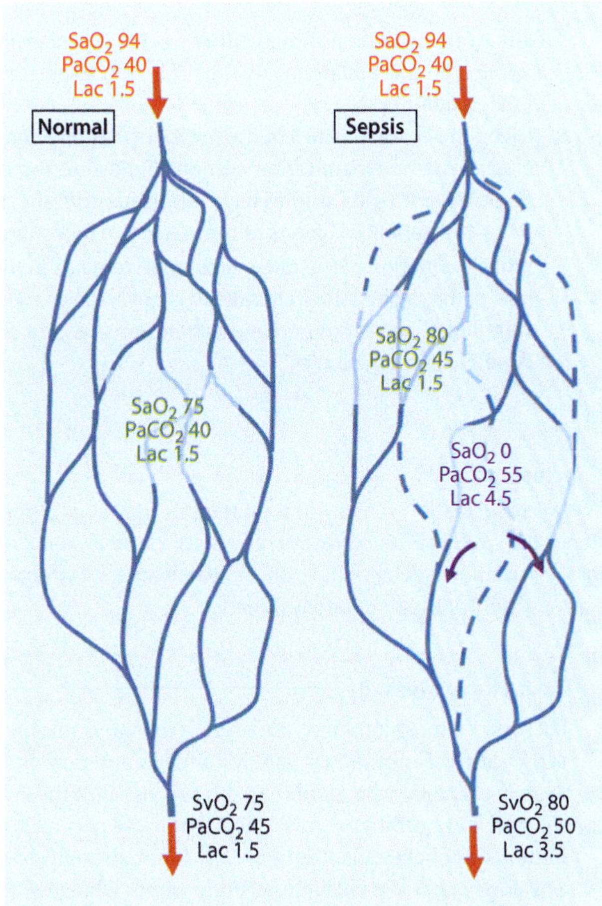

Fig. 14.2 Relationship between venoarterial PCO_2 gradients and microvascular alterations. In normal conditions, most areas are adequately perfused and thus oxygenated. Metabolic requirements are met and there is no flow stagnation. CO_2 production is rapidly washed out, and venoarterial PCO_2 gradient is minimal. In septic conditions, the microcirculation is heterogeneous, with areas that are poorly perfused in close vicinity to well-perfused areas. In the not-perfused areas, there is CO_2 increase due to flow stagnation and indirect anaerobic CO_2 generation due to buffering of H^+ generated by ATP hydrolysis. Interestingly, CO_2 diffuses longer distances than O_2 so that it can reach drainage venules. In the well-perfused areas, flow becomes excess, so that venous SO_2 of this area is in excess, contributing to the high SvO_2. Hence, the venular side of the diseased microcirculation is characterized by a high SvO_2, PCO_2, and lactate

Practical Implications

1. The microcirculation is a critical determinant of organ perfusion. Once a satisfactory cardiac output and arterial pressure are generated, microcirculatory alterations become the primary determinant of tissue perfusion.
2. Microcirculatory alterations have been demonstrated mostly in sepsis but also in severe heart failure, trauma, and high-risk surgery. These alterations are characterized by a decrease in density of perfused vessels and heterogeneity of areas close by a few microns.
3. Microcirculatory alterations cannot be detected by classical hemodynamic tools. The link between arterial pressure/cardiac output and microvascular perfusion is at best relatively loose.
4. Clinical evaluation of the microcirculation is often not contributing as dissociation from peripheral to more central circulation is often observed.

5. The microcirculation should either be directly measured (handheld microscopes applied on the sublingual area) or indirectly evaluated by measuring venoarterial PCO_2 gradients.
6. Given the characteristics of the microcirculation alterations, these often fail to classical hemodynamic interventions (fluids/inotropic agent/vasopressor agents). While experimental studies have reported promising results with some interventions, the beneficial effects of these need to be confirmed in the clinical area.
7. While evaluation of the microcirculation remains in the research area, comprehension of microcirculatory alterations is nevertheless very important for the understanding of persistent perfusion alterations despite correction of alterations in systemic hemodynamics.

Conclusions

The microcirculation is a key determinant of tissue perfusion, and microcirculatory alterations often persist after correction of systemic alterations. Even though investigation of the microcirculation still belongs to the research area, it is important to understand these may exist and contribute to organ dysfunction.

Take-Home Message

Microcirculatory alterations are present in many critically ill patients, and especially in sepsis, and contribute to organ dysfunction and poor outcome.
Even if it is not always feasible to directly visualize these alterations nor to manipulate these, it is important to understand that these may exist in order either to ensure better control of sepsis source or to prevent attempts to increase tissue perfusion by pushing further the systemic hemodynamics while the microcirculation fails to respond to these interventions.

References

1. De Backer D, Creteur J, Preiser JC, Dubois MJ, Vincent JL. Microvascular blood flow is altered in patients with sepsis. Am J Respir Crit Care Med. 2002;166(1):98–104.
2. Wu L, Mayeux PR. Effects of the inducible nitric-oxide synthase inhibitor L-N(6)-(1-iminoethyl)-lysine on microcirculation and reactive nitrogen species generation in the kidney following lipopolysaccharide administration in mice. J Pharmacol Exp Ther. 2007;320(3):1061–7.
3. De Backer D, Donadello K, Sakr Y, Ospina-Tascon GA, Salgado DR, Scolletta S, et al. Microcirculatory alterations in patients with severe sepsis: impact of time of assessment and relationship with outcome. Crit Care Med. 2013;41(3):791–9.
4. Hernandez G, Boerma EC, Dubin A, Bruhn A, Koopmans M, Edul VK, et al. Severe abnormalities in microvascular perfused vessel density are associated to organ dysfunctions and mortality and can be predicted by hyperlactatemia and norepinephrine requirements in septic shock patients. J Crit Care. 2013;28(4):538–14.
5. Sakr Y, Dubois MJ, De Backer D, Creteur J, Vincent JL. Persistant microvasculatory alterations are associated with organ failure and death in patients with septic shock. Crit Care Med. 2004;32:1825–31.
6. Edul VS, Enrico C, Laviolle B, Vazquez AR, Ince C, Dubin A. Quantitative assessment of the microcirculation in healthy volunteers and in patients with septic shock. Crit Care Med. 2012;40:1443–8.

7. De Backer D, Donadello K, Taccone FS, Ospina-Tascon G, Salgado D, Vincent JL. Microcirculatory alterations: potential mechanisms and implications for therapy. Ann Intensive Care. 2011;1(1):27.
8. De Backer D, Creteur J, Dubois MJ, Sakr Y, koch M, Verdant C, et al. The effects of dobutamine on microcirculatory alterations in patients with septic shock are independent of its systemic effects. Crit Care Med. 2006;34(2):403–8.
9. Ospina-Tascon G, Neves AP, Occhipinti G, Donadello K, Buchele G, Simion D, et al. Effects of fluids on microvascular perfusion in patients with severe sepsis. Intensive Care Med. 2010;36(6):949–55.
10. Edul VS, Ince C, Vazquez AR, Rubatto PN, Espinoza ED, Welsh S, et al. Similar microcirculatory alterations in patients with normodynamic and hyperdynamic septic shock. Ann Am Thorac Soc. 2016;13(2):240–7.
11. Dubin A, Pozo MO, Casabella CA, Palizas F Jr, Murias G, Moseinco MC, et al. Increasing arterial blood pressure with norepinephrine does not improve microcirculatory blood flow: a prospective study. Crit Care. 2009;13(3):R92.
12. De Backer D, Creteur J, Dubois MJ, Sakr Y, Vincent JL. Microvascular alterations in patients with acute severe heart failure and cardiogenic shock. Am Heart J. 2004;147:91–9.
13. den Uil CA, Lagrand WK, van der EM, Jewbali LS, Cheng JM, Spronk PE, et al. Impaired microcirculation predicts poor outcome of patients with acute myocardial infarction complicated by cardiogenic shock. Eur Heart J. 2010;31:3032–9.
14. Tachon G, Harrois A, Tanaka S, Kato H, Huet O, Pottecher J, et al. Microcirculatory alterations in traumatic hemorrhagic shock. Crit Care Med. 2014;42(6):1433–41.
15. Jhanji S, Lee C, Watson D, Hinds C, Pearse RM. Microvascular flow and tissue oxygenation after major abdominal surgery: association with post-operative complications. Intensive Care Med. 2009;35(4):671–7.
16. Ospina-Tascon GA, Nieto Calvache AJ, Quinones E, Madrinan HJ, Valencia JD, Bermudez WF, et al. Microcirculatory blood flow derangements during severe preeclampsia and HELLP syndrome. Pregnancy Hypertens. 2017;10:124–30.
17. Donadello K, Favory R, Salgado-Ribeiro D, Vincent JL, Gottin L, Scolletta S, et al. Sublingual and muscular microcirculatory alterations after cardiac arrest: a pilot study. Resuscitation. 2011;82(6):690–5.
18. Ait-Oufella H, Bakker J. Understanding clinical signs of poor tissue perfusion during septic shock. Intensive Care Med. 2016;42(12):2070–2.
19. Ait-Oufella H, Lemoinne S, Boelle PY, Galbois A, Baudel JL, Lemant J, et al. Mottling score predicts survival in septic shock. Intensive Care Med. 2011;37(5):801–7.
20. Hernandez G, Pedreros C, Veas E, Bruhn A, Romero C, Rovegno M, et al. Evolution of peripheral vs metabolic perfusion parameters during septic shock resuscitation. A clinical-physiologic study. J Crit Care. 2012;27(3):283–8.
21. Ince C, Boerma EC, Cecconi M, De Backer D, Shapiro NI, Duranteau J, et al. Second consensus on the assessment of sublingual microcirculation in critically ill patients: results from a task force of the European Society of Intensive Care Medicine. Intensive Care Med. 2018;44:281.
22. Kubli S, Boegli Y, Ave AD, Liaudet L, Revelly JP, Golay S, et al. Endothelium-dependent vasodilation in the skin microcirculation of patients with septic shock. Shock. 2003;19:274–80.
23. Orbegozo D, Mongkolpun W, Stringari G, Markou N, Creteur J, Vincent JL, et al. Skin microcirculatory reactivity assessed using a thermal challenge is decreased in patients with circulatory shock and associated with outcome. Ann Intensive Care. 2018;8(1):60.
24. Ospina-Tascon GA, Umana M, Bermudez WF, Bautista-Rincon DF, Valencia JD, Madrinan HJ, et al. Can venous-to-arterial carbon dioxide differences reflect microcirculatory alterations in patients with septic shock? Intensive Care Med. 2016;42(2):211–21.
25. Perner A, Gordon AC, De Backer D, Dimopoulos G, Russell JA, Lipman J, et al. Sepsis: frontiers in diagnosis, resuscitation and antibiotic therapy. Intensive Care Med. 2016;42(12):1958–69.

SvO_2/$ScvO_2$

Zsolt Molnar and Marton Nemeth

M. R. Pinsky et al. (eds.), *Hemodynamic Monitoring*, Lessons from the ICU,
https://doi.org/10.1007/978-3-319-69269-2_15

Learning Objectives

- The primary goal of hemodynamic optimization is to restore and maintain the balance between oxygen supply (DO_2) and consumption (VO_2) in critically ill patients. There is increasing evidence that patients may benefit from a multimodal individualized approach as compared to protocolized therapy, when predefined hemodynamic goal or goals are targeted. For this purpose, monitoring actual tissue oxygenation/metabolism of a given patient is a very important piece in this hemodynamic puzzle.
- Mixed venous oxygen saturation (SvO_2) and its surrogate, central venous oxygen saturation ($ScvO_2$), are two easily determined blood gas-driven parameters that can mirror changes of the relationship between DO_2 and VO_2.
- This article summarizes the physiological rationale, current knowledge, and some aspects of the clinical applications of SvO_2/$ScvO_2$ and also highlights some of the most important pitfalls of their interpretation at the bedside.

15.1 Introduction

Physical examination plays a very important role in the evaluation of critically ill patients. Certain features such as skin color, capillary refill, mentation, urine output, and pulse quality can tell us a lot about the patient's hemodynamic status. However, some very important features remain hidden even from the most experienced observer or become obvious only at their extremes. These are bicarbonate and lactate levels, hydrogen ion concentrations (i.e., pH), and the balance between oxygen delivery and consumption. Although for detailed monitoring invasive hemodynamic measurements are required, these are not available in every patient. However, arterial and central venous catheters are part of routine monitoring of the intensive care patient, and a simple blood gas measurement can reveal important physiological processes, which cannot be detected otherwise. In the coming chapter, we are going to discuss the rationale and clinical implication of the venous oxygen saturation.

15.2 Physiological Notes

Tissue oxygenation is the net product of oxygen delivery and oxygen consumption, which can be described by the following formulae:

$$DO_2 = CO \times CaO_2$$

$$DO_2 = CO \times \left(Hb \times 1.34 \times SaO_2 + 0.003 \times PaO_2\right)$$

$$VO_2 = CO \times \left(CaO_2 - CvO_2\right)$$

$$VO_2 = CO \times \left[\left(Hb \times 1.34 \times SaO_2 + 0.003 \times PaO_2\right) - \left(Hb \times 1.34 \times SvO_2 + 0.003 \times PvO_2\right)\right]$$

$$\text{Oxygen extraction}\left(O_2ER\right) = VO_2 / DO_2$$

$$O_2ER : \left(SaO_2 - SvO_2\right) / SaO_2$$

If SaO_2 is taken as 1, as under normal circumstances the hemoglobin is almost fully saturated with oxygen, and the other hemodynamic variables are kept constant, then:

$$O_2ER \approx 1 - SvO_2$$

where DO_2 is oxygen delivery; C, cardiac output; Hb, hemoglobin; SaO_2, arterial oxygen saturation; PaO_2, partial pressure of oxygen in the arterial blood; CaO_2, arterial oxygen content; VO_2, oxygen consumption; SvO_2, mixed venous oxygen saturation; and CvO_2, mixed venous oxygen content.

Taking a 75 kg healthy adult man when resting, the relationship between DO_2 and VO_2 can be estimated as:

$$\text{Oxygen delivery}: CO = 70\ \text{ml} \times 70/\text{min} \sim 5000\ \text{ml}/\text{min}$$

$$CaO_2 = (150\ \text{g}/\text{L} \times 1.34\ \text{ml} \times 1.00) + (0.003 \times 100\ \text{mmHg}) \sim 200\ \text{ml}/\text{L}$$

$$DO_2 \sim 1000\ \text{ml}/\text{min}$$

$$\text{Oxygen consumption}: CO = 70\ \text{ml} \times 70/\text{min} \sim 5000\ \text{ml}/\text{min}$$

$$CvO_2 = (150\ \text{g}/\text{L} \times 1.34\ \text{ml} \times 0.75) + (0.003 \times 40\,\text{mmHg}) \sim 150\ \text{ml}/\text{L}$$

$$VO_2 = 5\ \text{l}/\text{min} \times (200\ \text{ml}/\text{L} - 150\ \text{ml}/\text{L}) \sim 250\ \text{ml}/\text{min}$$

$$\text{Oxygen extraction}: O_2ER: 250\ \text{ml}/\text{min}/1000\ \text{ml}/\text{min} \times 100 = 25\%$$

The main difference between the equations of DO_2 and VO_2 is the oxygen content (CaO_2 vs. CvO_2), especially the venous oxygen saturation (this can either be mixed venous, SvO_2, or central venous, $ScvO_2$). Therefore, it can be useful to assess the imbalance between DO_2 and VO_2 in the critically ill. The potential causes of an imbalance between DO_2 and VO_2 and the basic therapeutic interventions are summarized in ◘ Fig. 15.1.

15.3 Interpreting Venous Saturations

When DO_2 is decreasing, oxygen consumption can be maintained – due to an increase in O_2ER – for a considerable period of time. However, without intervention, compensatory mechanisms will become exhausted, and beyond that critical point, VO_2 becomes DO_2 dependent (◘ Fig. 15.2). Till this critical point, venous saturations should decrease proportionally to that of DO_2. On the steep part of the curve, cells switch to anaerobic metabolism; hence, lactate production increases. If urgent interventions are delayed, tissue hypoxia and organ dysfunction can develop.

It is important to note that during resuscitation – i.e., on the steep or DO_2-dependent part of the curve – when interventions are applied to increase DO_2, there is also an increase of VO_2; hence, there is little if any change in venous oxygen saturations, which may remain "low" and will only increase dramatically when VO_2 becomes DO_2 independent (i.e., when the patient reaches the flat part of the curve shown in ◘ Fig. 15.2).

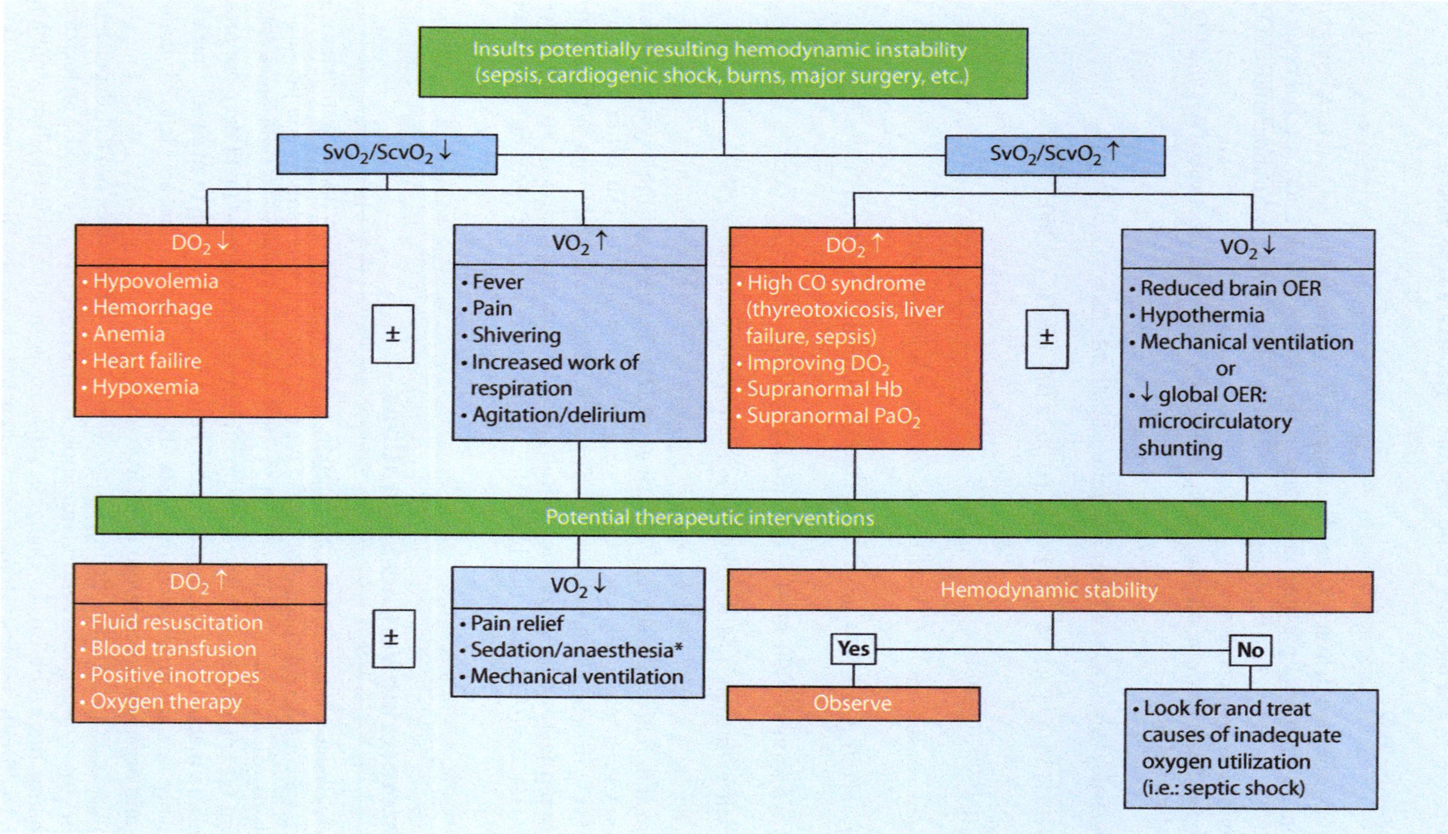

Fig. 15.1 The relationship between venous saturations and DO_2 and VO_2. DO_2 oxygen delivery, VO_2 oxygen consumption, OER oxygen extraction ratio. * – Although sedation can decrease VO_2, however, this should be a delicate option as this may also cause decreased cardiac output; hence, it may worsen the situation by decreasing DO_2. For further explanation, see main text

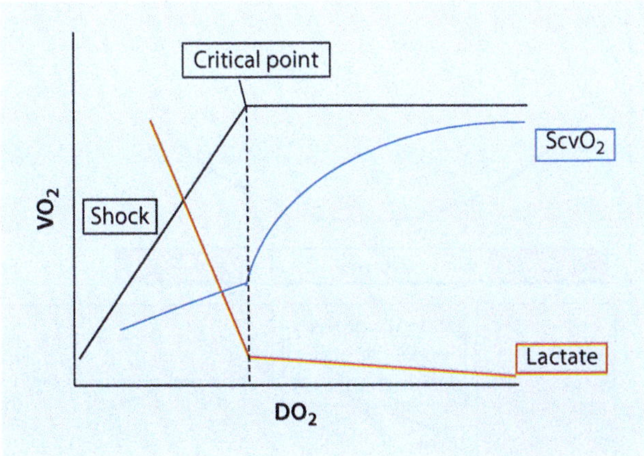

Fig. 15.2 Relationship between oxygen delivery and consumption. DO_2 oxygen delivery, VO_2 oxygen consumption, $ScvO_2$ central venous oxygen saturation. For details, see main text. Of note, this is a simplified diagram to show the rough tendency how these parameters are related. However, due to the irregular redistribution of blood flow as a compensatory mechanism to centralize circulation, certain organs may start anaerobic metabolism earlier than others; therefore, lactate may increase sooner and can be detected in the serum as compared to what is indicated in this figure as the "critical point." Regarding $ScvO_2$, its decrease and increase during resuscitation may not be that dramatic, as it depends on the relationship between VO_2 and DO_2. If VO_2 increases parallel with DO_2, this should cause hardly any change in $ScvO_2$ during resuscitation. However, if DO_2 increases faster than VO_2, then $ScvO_2$ will also increase rapidly

Another problem when interpreting venous saturations is that "high" values can indicate improvement but may also indicate inadequate oxygen uptake [1]. Similar to fluid therapy, this is also reflected in morbidity and mortality, as both high and low venous saturations are accompanied by increased morbidity and mortality (Fig. 15.3). Therefore, despite the high values, further interventions may be required (fluid resuscitation, positive inotropic agents, etc.).

Under these circumstances, when venous oxygen saturations are difficult to interpret, the central venous-to-arterial pCO_2 gap [2] and/or detailed invasive hemodynamic monitoring may serve as complementary tools to assess the hemodynamic status [3]. These will be discussed in other chapters.

15.4 SvO_2 or $ScvO_2$?

Nowadays, measurement of SvO_2 has become a rarity in the everyday clinical practice, because for sampling, a pulmonary artery catheter must be placed, which is a time-consuming, complicated procedure with significant risks [4]. On the contrary, central venous catheters are part of routine monitoring; hence, central venous oxygen saturation ($ScvO_2$) measurement is readily available. It has been shown that oxygen saturation measured in the superior vena cava is a good alternative of SvO_2 [5].

Accurate measurement requires that the tip of the catheter is positioned at the superior vena cava a couple of centimeters above the right atrium. The normal value of $ScvO_2$ ranges between 67% and 77% which is 5–8% higher compared to SvO_2 [6]. Although the absolute values are not interchangeable, their trends show good correlation in various disease states [7].

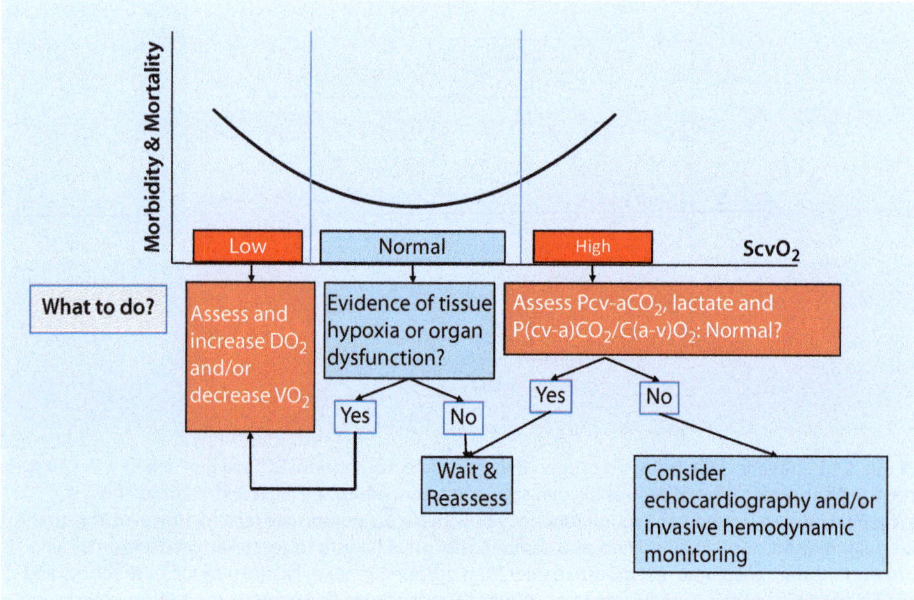

Fig. 15.3 The relationship between $ScvO_2$ and morbidity and mortality. DO_2 oxygen delivery, VO_2 oxygen consumption, $ScvO_2$ central venous oxygen saturation, $Pcv\text{-}aCO_2$ central venous-to-arterial CO_2 gap, $C(a\text{-}v)O_2$ arterial and venous oxygen content difference. This figure indicates that regardless of the actual value of $ScvO_2$, whether it is considered low, normal, or high, careful assessment of the full clinical picture is necessary to best interpret results and to commence appropriate interventions in time

However, as $ScvO_2$ reflects the oxygen consumption mainly of organs draining blood into the superior vena cava, one has to take into account that the biggest consumer of those is the brain. Therefore, during circumstances when brain oxygen uptake is affected (i.e., anesthesia, diffuse brain damage, etc.), $ScvO_2$ may be misleading or at least difficult to interpret.

Nevertheless, by and large these two parameters can be discussed in a similar manner; therefore, to avoid unnecessary citations of both, in the coming paragraphs, we will mainly quote $ScvO_2$, which is the most readily available of the two, unless indicated otherwise.

15.5 The Current Place of $ScvO_2$ in Clinical Practice

15.5.1 $ScvO_2$ in Sepsis and Septic Shock

Sepsis is a life-threatening organ dysfunction caused by a dysregulated host response to infection [8]. Organ dysfunction is most likely the result of inadequate tissue perfusion causing cellular hypoxia. Therefore, treatment strategies that are aimed to restore tissue perfusion by improving the balance between DO_2 and VO_2 may prevent the development of organ dysfunction syndrome and thus improve the outcome of septic patients.

Rivers and colleagues reported in a landmark paper that in patients with severe sepsis, early goal-directed intervention guided by continuous monitoring of $ScvO_2$, central venous pressure, and mean arterial pressure (MAP), with target values of CVP 8–12 mmHg, MAP > 65 mmHg, and $ScvO_2 > 70\%$, reduced mortality from 46.5% to 30.5% at the 28th day [9].

Consequent studies applying early goal-directed therapy (EGDT) with these clinical endpoints suggested that incorporation of $ScvO_2$ in the treatment algorithm and compliance with the algorithm are beneficial in septic patients [10–12]. On the contrary, two large randomized trials, the ProCESS and the ARISE trials, could not show any benefit of the "protocol-based standard therapy" and "usual care" groups. They found no significant difference in 90-day mortality, 1-year mortality, or the need for organ support [13, 14].

The controversy around the usefulness of the "Rivers' EGDT protocol" has been going on for years. Detailed evaluation of these studies is well beyond the scope of this chapter. However, there are some other issues worth discussing in this context.

During the aforementioned studies, "low" $ScvO_2$ was a warning sign that intervention is needed; however, recent data suggest that high $ScvO_2$ values may also have adverse outcomes in septic patients [15]. Due to impaired oxygen utilization, normal or supraphysiological $ScvO_2$ values may thus represent an inability of the cells to extract oxygen or microcirculatory shunting in sepsis [16]. This underscores that some of these patients can be fluid responsive; in other words, their DO_2 can be further increased despite high $ScvO_2$ [1]. In patients with $ScvO_2 > 70\%$ complimentary parameters, such as elevated venous-to-arterial CO_2 gap (dCO_2) (>6 mmHg), serum lactate levels could help the clinicians to identify tissue hypoxia. In a retrospective analysis, septic patients with physiological $ScvO_2$ and abnormal dCO_2 mortality were significantly higher compared to patients with physiological values (56.1% vs. 16.1%; $p < 0.001$) [17].

15.5.2 $ScvO_2$ in Cardiogenic Shock

Based on the previous physiological notes, it follows a simple logic that acute heart failure which caused low cardiac output, irrespective from the underlying pathophysiology, can cause VO_2/DO_2 imbalance that could be detected by low $ScvO_2$ [18].

Indeed, it has been shown in one of the earliest papers in this field that after myocardial infarction in patients with heart failure and cardiogenic shock, SvO_2 was 43%, while in patients with heart failure without shock, it was 56% compared to patients without heart failure with an SvO_2 of 70% [19].

Treatment effectiveness may also be supported by changes in $ScvO_2$. When cardiogenic shock patients were treated with fluids and inotropes, improvement of DO_2 resulted in an increase in SvO_2 suggesting better tissue oxygenation [20]. It may also be useful in patients with cardiogenic shock requiring the support by intra-aortic balloon counter pulsation. In a study, intra-aortic balloon pump assist ratio was decreased gradually from 1:1 to 1:3. In the weaning failure group decreased support was accompanied by a drop in $ScvO_2$, while it remained constant in the successful group [21].

Even in patients with chronic heart failure, $ScvO_2$ has important predictive values. In these patients, the $ScvO_2$ can be chronically low. However, during acute decompensation, major cardiac events were observed in 81% of patients with $ScvO_2 \leq 60\%$ at 24 h, while it was only 13% in patients with higher $ScvO_2$ [22].

15.5.3 $ScvO_2$ to Predict Successful Extubation

During the weaning procedure, there can be an increase of VO_2 due to the increased respiratory muscle activity and increased alertness. If DO_2 is inadequate, then an imbalance can occur between the VO_2/DO_2. Theoretically, this can be picked up by low or at least decreasing $ScvO_2$ values. In a recent clinical trial, *a* > 4% drop in $ScvO_2$ after a 30-min spontaneous breathing trial indicated extubation failure with high sensitivity and specificity [23].

15.5.4 $ScvO_2$ as a Physiological Transfusion Trigger

One of the most common causes of impaired DO_2 in critically ill patients is anemia requiring red blood cell transfusions [24]. Large multicenter trials (TRICC, TRISS) suggest that patients with hemoglobin levels above 10 mg/dl usually do not require transfusion, while red blood cell administration is usually beneficial if the hemoglobin level is below 7 mg/dl [25, 26]. However, there is a gray zone between 7 and 9.5 mg/dl where physicians have to rely on clinical signs like mental status, tachycardia, tachypnea, blood pressure, and diuresis.

In this gray zone, $ScvO_2$ may offer an easily obtainable tool to detect a low hemoglobin-related altered O_2ER and hence may serve as a physiological trigger for blood transfusion [27]. It was found during hemorrhage in animal and human experimental models that $ScvO_2$ may be useful for the identification of patients with occult or ongoing clinically significant blood loss [28]. In a human study, acute isovolemic anemia of hemoglobin of 50 g/l in conscious healthy resting humans did not produce hemodynamic instability, but oxygen imbalance was accompanied by a significant drop in SvO_2 [29]. These results were reinforced by a retrospective analysis of a prospective observational study in which $ScvO_2$ was found to be a good indicator of transfusion [30]. The results of our animal study on isovolemic hemodilution gave further evidence that anemia-induced change in VO_2/DO_2 showed significant negative correlation with changes of $ScvO_2$ [31].

15.6 $ScvO_2$ and Major/High-Risk Surgery

15

In addition to the acutely ill, the high-risk surgical patients may also develop an imbalance between VO_2 and DO_2 in the perioperative period. Therefore, monitoring $ScvO_2$ may have a rationale during both the intraoperative and postoperative management.

It has been shown that low $ScvO_2$ values are good indicators of complications and poor prognosis in the postoperative period [27]. We reported in a small, single-center prospective randomized study that an $ScvO_2$-assisted intraoperative hemodynamic optimization resulted in less organ dysfunction and better outcome after major abdominal surgery [32]. This was in accord with the results of an earlier single-center study, where patients in the $ScvO_2$-directed group had fewer postoperative complications and had shorter length of hospital stay compared to patients in the control group [28].

However, there are some special considerations when interpreting $ScvO_2$ in the perioperative setting. Firstly, in an anesthetized, mechanically ventilated patient, "normal" values of $ScvO_2$ are 5–10% higher (i.e., 75–80%) than in an awake or sedated intensive care patient or in a normal subject. Secondly, it is important to note that while fluid therapy on the one hand improves cardiac output, on the other hand, it can also cause hemodilution.

In our experimental stroke volume-guided hemorrhage and fluid resuscitation animal model, $ScvO_2$ normalized at the end of resuscitation but returned to a significantly lower level (with a mean of 5%) due to the hemodilution which caused significant drop in hemoglobin levels [33].

Goal-directed therapy is also a controversial issue in surgical patients. However, according to a recent meta-analysis, while goal-directed therapy had no significant effect in the low-risk surgical population, both mortality and morbidity were significantly better in the goal-directed group among the high-risk subgroups [34]. In our view, $ScvO_2$ is an important element of this complex perioperative multimodal monitoring-based concept, including advanced hemodynamic monitoring and assessment of VO_2/DO_2, what we call the individualized, multimodal approach [35].

15.7 Pitfalls of $ScvO_2$

$ScvO_2$ is the net result of the complex physiological and pathophysiological interactions of DO_2 and tissue VO_2. Low values strongly suggest inadequate DO_2; however, in patients with chronic heart failure, chronic anemia, etc., with a "compensated" state, low levels should be considered as "normal" but at least accepted. Not acknowledging this may result in unnecessary and potentially harmful interventions like overzealous fluid resuscitation.

The interpretation of "high" values of $ScvO_2$ is even more challenging. Under physiological circumstances, dissolved oxygen is negligible in DO_2. In an elegant trial on mechanically ventilated ICU patients, after increasing FiO_2 from 40% to 100%, PaO_2 increased from 100 mmHg to almost 400 mmHg: Without any change in cardiac output or hemoglobin, $ScvO_2$ rose from 71% to 84% [36]. Therefore, and this holds true for all the above mentioned examples, relatively stable conditions are desirable for the appropriate assessment. When there are too many changes occurring within a relatively short period time, this can make interpretation of $ScvO_2$ even more difficult.

During circumstances when brain oxygen uptake is affected (i.e., anesthesia, diffuse brain damage, etc.), $ScvO_2$ may be misleading or at least difficult to interpret. Data are lacking, but for these special situations, multimodal monitoring of depth of anesthesia (bispectral index, entropy) and brain oxygen consumption (near-infrared spectroscopy) may be useful and also another step to individualize our treatment for the given patient's actual needs..

Practical Implications

Venous oxygen saturation can be determined from either obtaining blood from the pulmonary artery (SvO_2) or from the superior vena cava ($ScvO_2$). Both can provide useful information about the balance between VO_2 and DO_2 and may also help monitoring the effectiveness of hemodynamic stabilization.

1. In sepsis, impaired oxygen utilization can result in normal or supraphysiological $ScvO_2$ values, which may represent the inability of cells to extract oxygen most likely due to microcirculatory shunting [16]. In the complex pathology of sepsis, treating one single parameter – Let it be $ScvO_2$, lactate, MAP, cardiac output, or else – Can certainly be misleading. Putting easily obtainable clinical and laboratory data including arterial and venous blood gas-driven parameters into context may help to recognize oxygen debt early and may also help to identify those patients

who will require advanced invasive hemodynamic monitoring [3]. This also forms the basis of multimodal, individualized patient management.
2. It has been shown by several studies that in acute left ventricular failure, low SvO_2/$ScvO_2$ is an important sign of severe imbalance in the VO_2/DO_2 relationship, and this parameter also has an important prognostic value [19, 22].
3. Following the changes of SvO_2/$ScvO_2$ over time may be used for weaning patients from cardiac support both pharmacological and assist devices [21], and during spontaneous breathing trials, changes may also provide a good prognosticating factor for extubation success or failure [23].
4. In otherwise stable but anemic patients, SvO_2/$ScvO_2$ may serve as physiologic transfusion trigger [30, 31], although no precise recommendation can be made.
5. In high-risk surgical patients, intraoperative evaluation of $ScvO_2$ can be a very useful tool both for diagnosing and monitoring VO_2/DO_2 imbalance as described in other clinical scenarios, as part of the multimodal monitoring approach [35].

Conclusion

Assessing oxygen consumption requires detailed hemodynamic assessment, which is not always feasible. Measurement of venous oxygen saturations – especially $ScvO_2$ – may serve as a simple, easily and readily available tool for assessing oxygen debt at the bedside. When interpreting the cellular well-being of the high-risk intensive care or surgical patient, $ScvO_2$ can play a very useful role. On its own it can be an important alarming signal of inadequate oxygen delivery, but to see the full picture, it should be incorporated into the complex of the hemodynamic puzzle.

Take-Home Messages

- Venous oxygen saturations are important tools to assess VO_2/DO_2 at the bedside.
- $ScvO_2$ is an easily obtainable and useful alternative of SvO_2.
- Low venous saturations should be considered as an important alarming signal of VO_2/DO_2 imbalance, and causes of low DO_2 – Such as hypovolemia, heart failure, bleeding, anemia, and hypoxemia – Should be looked for.
- High or even normal venous saturations should be interpreted with caution especially in patients who require moderate or high level of hemodynamic support, as they may indicate impaired oxygen uptake.
- In general, but especially under circumstances when interpretation of venous saturation is not straightforward, instead of targeting a given value of SvO_2/$ScvO_2$ (i.e., 65–70%), complimentary parameters, such as venous-to-arterial CO_2 gap, lactate levels, echocardiography, and/or invasive hemodynamic monitoring provided indices, should be put into context in order to individualize hemodynamic support.

15.8 Case Studies

Clinical Case 1

A 35-year-old man suffered acute myocardial infarction. During percutaneous coronary angioplasty, he developed cardiogenic shock and required continuous infusion of norepinephrine (NE) and endotracheal intubation. At the end of the intervention, due to the persistent shock, intra-aortic balloon pump (IABP) was placed to support coronary flow. On arrival to the ICU, he required 75 μg/min NE to maintain a blood pressure of 98/51(73) mmHg. He was ventilated at 60% FiO_2, 10 of PEEP, in BiPAP mode.

The IABP was set to a 1:1 support mode and a control arterial and central venous blood gases were taken.

	Arterial blood gas	Central venous blood gas
pH	7.41	7.35
pCO_2 (mmHg)	42	53 (Pcv-aCO_2-gap: 11)
pO_2 (mmHg)	103	46
BE (mmol/L)	1.3	–
HCO_3 (mmol/L)	26.0	–
SO_2 (%)	98	77
Lactate (mmol/L)	1.4	1.3

These results indicate remarkable oxygenation, ventilation, and acid-base homeostasis, as far as pH, HCO_3, and lactate are concerned. However, central venous blood gas results, taken at the same time, revealed a completely different picture.

$ScvO_2$ could be considered as "normal" or "high." However, the elevated CO_2 gap suggests that cardiac output may be low. An echocardiography was performed, which revealed poor left ventricular function (EF, 35%) with dilated ventricles (135 mL). The IABP was then stopped for 5 min and blood gases were repeated.

	Arterial blood gas	Central venous blood gas
pH	7.39	7.36
pCO_2 (mmHg)	44	51 (Pcv-aCO_2-gap: 7)
pO_2 (mmHg)	87	46
BE (mmol/L)	10.8	–
HCO_3 (mmol/L)	26.0	–
SO_2 (%)	97	81
Lactate (mmol/L)	1.3	1.3

Interpretation

Stopping the IABP for 5 min caused an increase in $ScvO_2$ by 4% and a decrease in CO_2 gap to 7 mmHg, indicating a possible improvement in cardiac output. For more information, invasive hemodynamic monitoring was commenced with transpulmonary thermodilution, which revealed elevated end-diastolic volume (GEDVI) of 1043 ml/m^2 (normal, 600–800 ml/m^2) and increased extravascular lung water (EVLWI) of 21 ml/kg (normal, less than 10 ml/kg), indicating gross fluid overload; hence, fluid removal was decided, initially with furosemide, and then later with continuous veno-venous hemofiltration.

Conclusion

Arterial blood gas analysis on its own is not enough to assess the hemodynamic situation – in fact it may show a false-positive picture – unless there is already severe metabolic acidosis with low pH, HCO_3, and high lactate levels. Including the central venous blood gas results in the assessment, an early warning sign was revealed indicating that the patient is still unstable, and further information and intervention may be required.

Clinical Case 2

An 83-year-old woman with urinary tract infection was treated on a medical ward and was asked to be reviewed due to respiratory distress and hypotension. On assessment she looked frail, she was tachypneic (30/min), and her blood pressure was 90/40(57) mmHg. The attending ICU resident immediately started oxygen supplementation via face mask and after inserting a large bore (14G) peripheral venous catheter ordered a fluid bolus of 500 mL balanced crystalloid solution to be infused. At the same time, an arterial blood gas was sent to the ICU.

	Arterial blood gas
pH	7.19
pCO_2 (mmHg)	28
pO_2 (mmHg)	64
BE (mmol/L)	−16.4
HCO_3 (mmol/L)	10.5
SO_2 (%)	88
Lactate (mmol/L)	6.9

Based on these results, the patient was immediately transferred to the ICU.

15 By the time of arrival, her blood pressure and oxygenation already improved, and she felt better in general. An indwelling arterial catheter was inserted into the left radial artery, and another blood gas was taken. In the meantime she received another bolus of 500 mL crystalloid.

	Arterial blood gas
pH	7.27
pCO_2 (mmHg)	27
pO_2 (mmHg)	92
BE (mmol/L)	−13.1
HCO_3 (mmol/L)	12.5
SO_2 (%)	96
Lactate (mmol/L)	3.7

These results indicate improvement, but metabolic acidosis is still present; hence, a central venous catheter was inserted into the right internal jugular vein, and in the meantime a transthoracic echocardiography was also performed. The latter revealed good ventricular function and small ventricular diameters; therefore, fluid administration was continued, and another 500 mL of bolus crystalloid was administered. The patient's blood pressure hasn't changed and remained anuric; hence, norepinephrine was also commenced into a peripheral vein at a rate of 5 µg/min. After inserting the central venous catheter, arterial and central venous blood gases were taken at the same time.

	Arterial blood gas	Central venous blood gas
pH	7.38	7.34
pCO_2 (mmHg)	39	52 ($Pcv\text{-}aCO_2$-gap: 13)
pO_2 (mmHg)	130	25
BE (mmol/L)	−5.1	–
HCO_3 (mmol/L)	20.5	–
SO_2 (%)	98	49
Lactate (mmol/L)	2.4	2.2

Interpretation

According to these results, there is still an imbalance between VO_2 and DO_2 as indicated by low $ScvO_2$, and the grossly elevated CO_2 gap also suggests the inadequacy of flow (cardiac output). Therefore, fluid resuscitation was continued, and after another two boluses of 500 mL of crystalloid, the patient's condition eventually improved, and both macrohemodynamics (blood pressure, urine output) and blood gases normalized.

Conclusion

Despite dramatic improvement in arterial blood gases, lactate, respiratory, and macrohemodynamic indices, central venous blood gas results revealed that serious hemodynamic instability is still present indicated by very low $ScvO_2$ and very high CO_2 gap. Putting both blood gases into context helped the decision to continue fluid resuscitation, which ended with positive results; hence, advanced monitoring and further intervention became unnecessary.

Clinical Case 3

A 67-year-old man required acute surgery due to a perforated colon diverticulum. From his previous medical history, controlled hypertension and mild ischemic heart disease are worth mentioning. In the postoperative period, he required some vasopressor support for 24 h, but by day 3 his condition improved, he felt well, he was without any pain, all vital signs were stable, and he started eating and drinking the day before; hence, he was considered as ready to be discharged. The only abnormal finding was a hemoglobin of 7.2 g/dL. These were his blood gases:

	Arterial blood gas	Central venous blood gas
pH	7.34	7.32
pCO_2 (mmHg)	46	52 ($Pcv\text{-}aCO_2$-gap: 6)
pO_2 (mmHg)	84	43

	Arterial blood gas	Central venous blood gas
BE (mmol/L)	−0.6	–
HCO_3 (mmol/L)	26.5	–
SO_2 (%)	98	73
Lactate (mmol/L)	1.9	2.0

Interpretation

Based on the stable macrocirculation, well-established oral intake of food and drinks, the normal $ScvO_2$, lactate, and CO_2 gap, we decided not to transfuse this patient. He was then discharged, and following him up, his hemoglobin started to increase gradually and did not require blood transfusion during his hospital stay.

Conclusion

Although most transfusion guidelines would recommend transfusing an elderly patient with previous medical history of ischemic heart disease, especially in the early postoperative period with a hemoglobin of 7.2 g/dL, but putting all available data into context, there was no evidence that this degree of anemia caused any instability to this particular patient; therefore, transfusion had no physiological indication; hence, it was put on hold, and transfusion – with all its potential side effects – was eventually avoided.

References

1. Velissaris D, Pierrakos C, Scolletta S, Backer D, Vincent JL. High mixed venous oxygen saturation levels do not exclude fluid responsiveness in critically ill septic patients. Crit Care. 2011;15:R177.
2. Weil MH, Rackow EC, Trevino R, Grundler W, Falk JL, Griffel MI. Difference in acid-base state between venous and arterial blood during cardiopulmonary resuscitation. N Engl J Med. 1986;315:153–6.
3. Møller MH, Cecconi M. Venous-to-arterial carbon dioxide difference: an experimental model or a bedside clinical tool? Intensive Care Med. 2016;42:287–9.
4. Evans DC, Doraiswamy VA, Prosciak MP, Silviera M, Seamon MJ, Rodriguez Funes V, et al. Complications associated with pulmonary artery catheters: a comprehensive clinical review. Scand J Surg. 2009;98:199–208.
5. Dueck MH, Klimek M, Appenrodt S, Weigand C, Boerner U. Trends but not individual values of central venous oxygen saturation agree with mixed venous oxygen saturation during varying hemodynamic conditions. Anesthesiology. 2005;103:249–57.
6. Reinhart K, Kuhn HJ, Hartog C, Bredle DL. Continuous central venous and pulmonary artery oxygen saturation monitoring in the critically ill. Intensive Care Med. 2004;30:1572–8.
7. Reinhart K, Rudolph T, Bredle DL, Hannemann L, Cain SM. Comparison of central-venous to mixed-venous oxygen saturation during changes in oxygen supply/demand. Chest. 1989;95:1216–21.
8. Singer M, Deutschman CS, Seymour CW, Shankar-Hari M, Annane D, Bauer M, et al. The third international consensus definitions for sepsis and septic shock (sepsis-3). JAMA. 2016;315:801–10.
9. Rivers E, Nguyen B, Havstad S, Ressler J, Muzzin A, Knoblich B, et al. Early goal-directed therapy in the treatment of severe sepsis and septic shock. N Engl J Med. 2001;345:1368–77.
10. Trzeciak S, Dellinger RP, Abate NL, Cowan RM, Stauss M, Kilgannon JH, et al. Translating research to clinical practice: a 1-year experience with implementing early goal-directed therapy for septic shock in the emergency department. Chest. 2006;129:225–32.
11. Jones AE, Shapiro NI, Roshon M. Implementing early goal-directed therapy in the emergency setting: the challenges and experiences of translating research innovations into clinical reality in academic and community settings. Acad Emerg Med. 2007;14:1072–8.
12. Rhodes A, Phillips G, Beale R, Cecconi M, Chiche JD, De Backer D, et al. The surviving sepsis campaign bundles and outcome: results from the International Multicentre Prevalence Study on Sepsis (the IMPreSS study). Intensive Care Med. 2015;41:1620–8.

13. ProCESS Investigators, Yealy DM, Kellum JA, Huang DT, Barnato AE, Weissfeld LA, et al. A randomized trial of protocol-based care for early septic shock. N Engl J Med. 2014;370:1683–93.
14. ARISE Investigators, ANZICS Clinical Trials Group, Peake SL, Delaney A, Bailey M, Bellomo R, et al. Goal-directed resuscitation for patients with early septic shock. N Engl J Med. 2014;371:1496–506.
15. Pope JV, Jones AE, Gaieski DF, Arnold RC, Trzeciak S, Shapiro NI, Emergency Medicine Shock Research Network (EMShockNet) Investigators. Multicenter study of central venous oxygen saturation ($ScvO_2$) as a predictor of mortality in patients with sepsis. Ann Emerg Med. 2010;55:40–6.
16. Ince C, Sinaasappel M. Microcirculatory oxygenation and shunting in sepsis and shock. Crit Care Med. 1999;27:1369–77.
17. Du W, Liu DW, Wang XT, Long Y, Chai WZ, Zhou X, et al. Combining central venous-to-arterial partial pressure of carbon dioxide difference and central venous oxygen saturation to guide resuscitation in septic shock. J Crit Care. 2013;28:1110.
18. Muir AL, Kirby BJ, King AJ, Miller HC. Mixed venous oxygen saturation in relation to cardiac output in myocardial infarction. Br Med J. 1970;4:276–8.
19. Goldman RH, Braniff B, Harrison DC, Spivack AP. The use of central venous oxygen saturation measurements in a coronary care unit. Ann Intern Med. 1968;68:1280–7.
20. Creamer JE, Edwards JD, Nightingale P. Hemodynamic and oxygen transport variables in cardiogenic shock secondary to acute myocardial infarction, and response to treatment. Am J Cardiol. 1990;65:1297–300.
21. Hsin HT, Chen LY, Lin PC, Shieh JS, Ao CV. Central venous oxygen saturation ($ScVO_2$) facilitates the weaning of intra-aortic balloon pump in acute heart failure related to acute myocardial infarction. Int J Cardiol. 2013;168:4568–70.
22. Gallet R, Lellouche N, Mitchell-Heggs L, Bouhemad B, Bensaid A, Dubois-Randé JL, et al. Prognosis value of central venous oxygen saturation in acute decompensated heart failure. Arch Cardiovasc Dis. 2012;105:5–12.
23. Teixeira C, da Silva NB, Savi A, Vieira SR, Nasi LA, Friedman G, et al. Central venous saturation is a predictor of reintubation in difficult-to-wean patients. Crit Care Med. 2010;38:491–6.
24. Luciano Gattinoni MD, Davide Chiumello MD. Anemia in the intensive care unit: how big is the problem? Transfusion Alternatives Transfusion Med. 2002;4:118–20.
25. Hébert PC, Wells G, Blajchman MA, Marshall J, Martin C, Pagliarello G, et al. A multicenter, randomized, controlled clinical trial of transfusion requirements in critical care. Transfusion Requirements in Critical Care Investigators, Canadian Critical Care Trials Group. N Engl J Med. 1999;340:409–17.
26. Holst LB, Haase N, Wetterslev J, Wernerman J, Guttormsen AB, Karlsson S, et al. Lower versus higher hemoglobin threshold for transfusion in septic shock. N Engl J Med. 2014;371:1381–91.
27. Collaborative Study Group on Perioperative ScvO2 Monitoring. Multicentre study on peri- and postoperative central venous oxygen saturation in high-risk surgical patients. Crit Care. 2006;10:R158.
28. Pearse R, Dawson D, Fawcett J, Rhodes A, Grounds RM, Bennett ED. Changes in central venous saturation after major surgery, and association with outcome. Crit Care. 2005;9:R694–9.
29. Weiskopf RB, Viele MK, Feiner J, Kelley S, Lieberman J, Noorani M, et al. Human cardiovascular and metabolic response to acute, severe isovolemic anemia. JAMA. 1998;279:217–21.
30. Kobayashi M, Ko M, Irinoda T, Meguro E, Hayakawa Y, et al. Clinical usefulness of continuous central venous oxygen saturation measurement for postoperative management of patients following transthoracic esophagectomy for carcinoma. Esophagus. 2011;8:53–8.
31. Kocsi S, Demeter G, Fogas J, Erces D, Kaszaki J, Molnar Z. Central venous oxygen saturation is a good indicator of altered oxygen balance in isovolemic anemia. Acta Anaesthesiol Scand. 2012;56:291–7.
32. Mikor A, Trasy D, Nemeth MF, Osztroluczki A, Kocsi S, Kovacs I, et al. Continuous central venous oxygen saturation assisted intraoperative hemodynamic management during major abdominal surgery: a randomized, controlled trial. BMC Anesthesiol. 2015;15:82.
33. Nemeth M, Tanczos K, Demeter G, Erces D, Kaszaki J, Mikor A, et al. Central venous oxygen saturation and carbon dioxide gap as resuscitation targets in a hemorrhagic shock. Acta Anaesthesiol Scand. 2014;58:611–9.
34. Cecconi M, Corredor C, Arulkumaran N, Abuella G, Ball J, Grounds RM, et al. Clinical review: goal-directed therapy-what is the evidence in surgical patients? The effect on different risk groups. Crit Care. 2013;17:209.
35. Molnar Z, Szabo Z, Nemeth M. Multimodal individualized concept of hemodynamic monitoring. Curr Opin Anaesthesiol. 2017;30:171–7.
36. Legrand M, Vallée F, Mateo J, Payen D. Influence of arterial dissolved oxygen level on venous oxygen saturation: don't forget the PaO_2! Shock. 2014;41:510–3.

The PCO_2 Gaps

Gustavo A. Ospina-Tascón

M. R. Pinsky et al. (eds.), *Hemodynamic Monitoring*, Lessons from the ICU,
https://doi.org/10.1007/978-3-319-69269-2_16

Learning Objectives

Carbon dioxide is a catabolic product generated during the Krebs cycle under normoxic condition. As a final product of cellular respiration, carbon dioxide-derived variables could be potentially used to monitor tissue perfusion and to detect the appearance of anaerobic metabolism during shock states.

In this chapter we will analyze some physiological aspects, prognostic value, clinical meaning, and possible clinical applications of the venous-to-arterial carbon dioxide difference ($Pv\text{-}aCO_2$) and the venous-arterial carbon dioxide to arterial-venous oxygen content difference ratio ($Cv\text{-}aCO_2/Ca\text{-}vO_2$) during shock states.

16.1 Introduction

Shock is a life-threatening condition in which the circulatory system is unable to deliver sufficient oxygen to maintain the metabolic demand of tissues, resulting in cellular dysfunction [1]. Thus, early recognition of tissue hypoperfusion and its reversion are pivotal factors in limiting progression to multiorgan dysfunction and death [2]. Current techniques for monitoring tissue perfusion have largely focused on systemic blood flow and the balance between oxygen demand and supply to the tissues [3, 4]. In fact, early hemodynamic optimization using resuscitation bundles targeting central venous oxygen saturation ($ScvO_2$) and macro hemodynamics were initially related with significant reduction of mortality in septic shock [5]. However, the usefulness of oxygen-derived parameters has been strongly questioned [6], and recent studies have failed to demonstrate its clinical benefits [7–9]. In fact, $ScvO_2$ is often normal or near normal at ICU admission [10], and attaining normal macro hemodynamics and global oxygen-derived parameters do not rule out the presence or persistence of tissue hypoxia. In this context, other variables such as carbon dioxide (CO_2)-derived parameters might provide valuable information about macro and micro hemodynamics during early phases of shock, even when oxygen variables seem to have been corrected [11–15]. Importantly, CO_2 variations occur faster than changes in lactate levels, which make attractive the CO_2 parameters as monitoring tool during early stages of resuscitation.

In this chapter we will analyze the physiological principles, prognostic value, clinical significance, and potential clinical applications of the venous-to-arterial carbon dioxide difference ($Pv\text{-}aCO_2$) and the venous-arterial carbon dioxide to arterial-venous oxygen content difference ratio ($Cv\text{-}aCO_2/Ca\text{-}vO_2$) during shock states.

16.2 Physiological Background

16.2.1 Aerobic Carbon Dioxide Production

Carbon dioxide (CO_2) is a terminal metabolic product generated under normoxic conditions during the Krebs cycle. Total CO_2 production (VCO_2) is directly related to the global oxygen consumption (VO_2) by the relation, $VCO_2 = RQ \times VO_2$, where RQ represents the respiratory quotient. This RQ reflects the ratio of moles of CO_2 generated per mole of oxygen consumed at the tissue level, and it will vary from 0.6 to 1.0 according to the metabolic conditions and the predominant energetic substrate consumed. Consequently, aerobic VCO_2 will increase either during increased oxidative metabolism (i.e., with simultaneous VO_2 increase) or when at constant VO_2; dietary regimen is substituted by a high carbohydrate intake [16]. Under aerobic resting conditions, RQ will never be >1.0 since CO_2 production should not surpass that amount of O_2 consumed. However, during exhaustive muscular activity or during certain pathological situations, anaerobic CO_2 generation could account for VCO_2/VO_2 ratios >1.0. However, regardless of the mechanism increasing aerobic VCO_2, Pv-aCO_2 will increase only when compensatory increase in cardiac output is not sufficient to clear the CO_2 produced by tissues.

16.2.2 Anaerobic Carbon Dioxide Production

When tissue hypoxia occurs, aerobic VCO_2 decreases, while anaerobic VCO_2 turns on. Increased anaerobic VCO_2 is the final consequence of proton [H^+] buffering by cytosolic and plasmatic bicarbonate (HCO_3^-). The "gross H^+ release" observed during hypoxia results from the sum of all cellular reactions liberating H^+ (e.g., the ATPase, hexokinase [HK], phosphofructokinase [PFK], and glyceraldehyde-3-phosphate dehydrogenase [G_3PDH] reactions), which are counterbalanced by metabolic reactions consuming H^+ (e.g., the creatine kinase [CK], AMP deaminase [AMPDase], pyruvate kinase [PK], and lactate dehydrogenase [LDH] reactions). Consequently, the difference between the "gross H^+ release" and the chemical reactions consuming H^+ (i.e., the "metabolic buffering") will result in the "net H^+ release," which ultimately will be regulated by the intra- and extracellular structural buffering (e.g., amino acids) and the bicarbonate buffering system [17]. This later is the main responsible for the anaerobic VCO_2 increase, when HCO_3^- captures the H^+ excess to become H_2CO_3 and subsequently dissociate in CO_2 and H_2O. An additional source of anaerobic VCO_2 results from anaerobic decarboxylation of some substrates such as α-ketoglutarate and oxaloacetate which occurred during intermediate metabolism, but its contribution to the total VCO_2 is quite small [18].

Despite its biochemical importance, clinical demonstration of anaerobic CO_2 increase might be very difficult because total VCO_2 decreases under hypoxic conditions and the efferent venous blood flow might be sufficient to wash out the total CO_2 produced at the tissues, thus masking the portion of increased anaerobic CO_2.

16.2.3 CO_2 Transport in Blood

Carbon dioxide excretion is a passive phenomenon in which CO_2 is transferred down an electrochemical gradient from cells to the environment. The efficiency of this transport is a function of convention (blood flow) and capacity of the carrier (blood content). Fortunately, evolution has led to transport large quantities of CO_2 in blood without large variations in blood flow. Carbon dioxide is approximately 20–30 times more soluble than oxygen, whereby dissolved CO_2 plays a key role in its total transport. As a lipophilic molecule, CO_2 rapidly diffuses through the lipid bilayer of cells and erythrocytes to be hydrated and finally converted into HCO_3^- and H^+. Thus, in general, blood carries both CO_2 and its related compounds in five forms:

1. Dissolved CO_2: $[CO_2]_{DIS}$ follows Henry's law, which establishes that, at constant temperature, any gas dissolves in a liquid phase proportionally to its partial pressure in the gas phase, adjusted by a solubility factor that differs from one gas to another. Under normal conditions, ~ 5% of the total CO_2 content is transported as $[CO_2]_{DIS}$. Despite its relatively low capacitance in blood, $[CO_2]_{DIS}$ has a critical role in gas transport since it can rapidly cross the vascular endothelium, while other forms of CO_2 must be converted into free CO_2 to enter or leave blood.

2. Carbonic acid: $[H_2CO_3]$ results from the reaction between CO_2 and H_2O. At the pH of most physiological fluids, H_2CO_3 instantly dissociates into H^+ and HCO_3^-. Hence, $[H_2CO_3]$ represents only the 1/400 part of $[CO_2]$, whereby this is not quantitatively important for total CO_2 carriage.
3. Bicarbonate: $[HCO_3^-]$ can form in three ways – by dissociation of H_2CO_3 into H^+ and HCO_3^-, by direct combination of CO_2 and OH^- (a reaction catalyzed by the carbonic anhydrase), and by combination of carbonate (CO_3^{2-}) and H^+. In arterial blood, HCO_3^- accounts for ~ 90% of the total CO_2 content. Thus, CO_2 combines with water (H_2O) to form carbonic acid (H_2CO_3), and this dissociates into HCO_3^- and hydrogen ion: $CO_2 + H_2O = H_2CO_3 = HCO_3^- + H^+$. Carbonic anhydrase catalyzes almost instantaneously this first reaction mainly in red blood cells (RBC) and pulmonary capillary endothelial cells, while the uncatalyzed second reaction occurs at a much slower rate. When H_2CO_3 dissociates within RBC into H^+ and HCO_3^-, H^+ is buffered by hemoglobin, while the excess HCO_3^- is transported out of RBC into the plasma by an electrically neutral bicarbonate-chloride exchanger (◘ Fig. 16.1).
4. Carbonate: $[CO_3^{2-}]$ is mainly formed from the dissociation of bicarbonate: $HCO_3^- \rightarrow CO_3^{2-} + H^+$. Thus, $[CO_3^{2-}]$ is ~ 1/1000 as high as HCO_3^- at pH 7.40. Consequently, CO_3^{2-} is not quantitatively important for CO_2 transport.
5. Carbamino compounds: uncharged amino groups of proteins can reversibly bind to both H^+ and CO_2. By far, the most important carbamino compound is the carbamino hemoglobin (Hb-NH-COO$^-$), which forms rapidly and reversibly as CO_2 reacts with free amino group on hemoglobin. Carbamino compounds account for ~ 5% of the total CO_2 content in arterial blood.

16

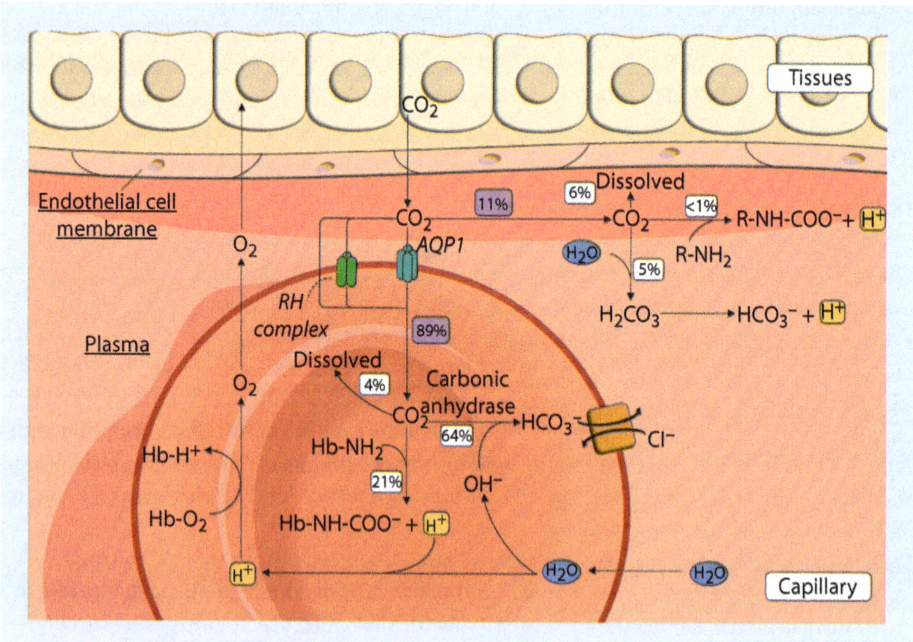

◘ **Fig. 16.1** Intracellular and extracellular events of CO_2 carriage in blood

The total CO_2 content (CCO_2) in arterial blood is ~ 48 mL of CO_2 gas/dL measured at standard temperature and pressure/dry (STPD), corresponding to a $PaCO_2$ of 40 mmHg. From that 48 mL/dL, ~ 90% corresponds to HCO_3^-, while carbamino compound contributes with ~ 5%. As blood flows along the microcirculatory bed, it picks up ~ 4 mL/dL of CO_2, so that the total CCO_2 in mixed-venous blood will rise to ~ 52 mL/dL. From that incremental CCO_2, about 10% corresponds to dissolved CO_2, ~ 69% to HCO_3^-, and ~ 21% to carbamino compounds. Accordingly, dissolved CO_2 and carbamino compounds are far more important for carrying incremental CO_2 to the lungs as a result of their contribution to the total increase in CO_2 in venous blood. In as much as oxidative metabolism occurs and Krebs cycle maintains its function, mitochondria generates CO_2, which diffuses out of the cells through the extracellular space, across the capillary endothelium, and into the blood plasma. Near 11% of incremental CO_2 remains in blood plasma throughout its way to the lungs, while ~ 89% enters red blood cells, at least initially. The aforesaid ~ 11% of plasma incremental CO_2 will in turn be transported as dissolved CO_2 (~ 6%, considering a hematocrit of 40%), as HCO_3^- (~ 6%) and small quantities as carbamino compounds. The remaining ~ 89% of incremental CO_2 enters red blood cells through two "gas channels": the aquaporin 1 and the Rh complex. This intra-RBC CO_2 will be transported as dissolved cytosolic CO_2 (~ 4%), while ~ 21% of such increment will be transported as carbamino compounds of Hb (i.e., the CO_2 linked to hemoglobin). Intra-RBC carbamino compounds are far more important than those formed in plasma because hemoglobin concentration in RBC is significantly higher (~ 33 gr/dL) than that represented by albumin, globulins, and other plasma proteins (~ 7 gr/dL total plasma proteins). Furthermore, the affinity of CO_2 for hemoglobin far surpasses that for major plasma proteins. In addition, the affinity of hemoglobin for H^+ and CO_2 will be modified as long as O_2 concentrations vary when blood enters tissue microcirculation or returns to the lungs. The remaining incremental CO_2 in RBC will be represented by HCO_3^- (~ 64%) because of the carbonic anhydrase activity accelerating the conversion of CO_2 into HCO_3^-. In absence of such enzymatic activity, HCO_3^- would hardly be synthesized inside RBCs during the short transit time of RBCs along the capillary bed. Furthermore, the Cl-HCO_3 exchanger AE1 (anion exchanger 1) carries the newly synthesized HCO_3^- out of the cell, promoting further HCO_3^- generation. ◘ Figure 16.1 resumes the combined intra-RBC and plasmatic events of CO_2 transportation.

16.2.4 The CO_2 Dissociation Curve

The carriage of total CO_2 will depend on PCO_2, plasma pH, and PO_2 [19, 20]. The CO_2 dissociation curve is characterized by a near-linear relationship within the physiological ranges of PCO_2 and PO_2 values (◘ Fig. 16.2, panel a). Moreover, at any PCO_2, the total CO_2 content rises as PO_2 falls. As a result, as blood enters the systemic microcirculation and releases O_2, the CO_2-carrying capacity increases, so that blood may remove the extra CO_2. Conversely, as blood enters the pulmonary capillaries and binds O_2, the CO_2-carrying capacity decreases, and blood loses the capacity to transport the extra CO_2. Because of the CO_2 dissociation curve slope, PCO_2 must increase from 40 mmHg in arterial blood to only 46 mmHg in mixed-venous blood to increase the total CO_2 content by ~ 4 mL/dL (i.e., from 48 to 52 mL of CO_2 gas/dL), which is required to remove the CO_2 generated by aerobic mitochondrial functioning.

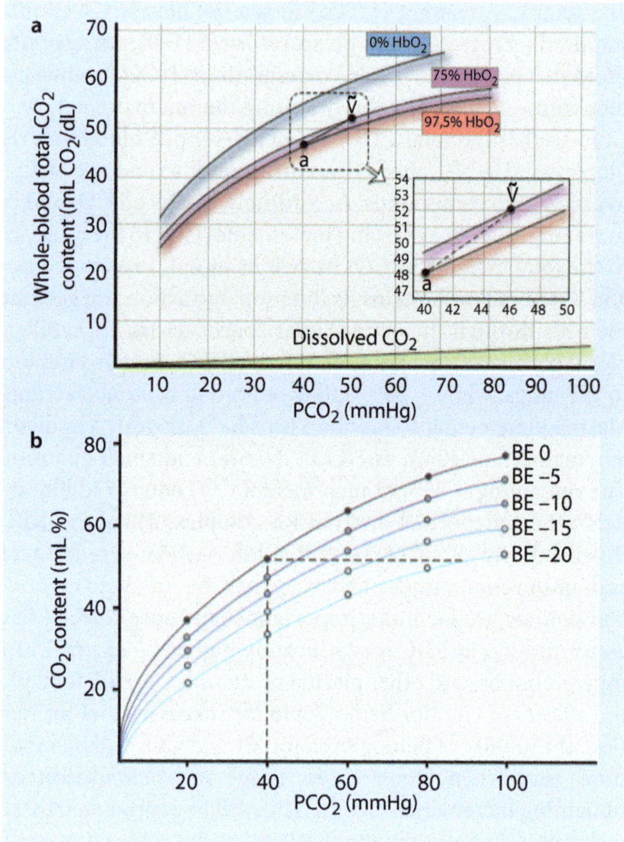

Fig. 16.2 Carbon dioxide dissociation curve. Panel **a** Relationships between whole-blood total CO_2 content (CCO_2) and blood CO_2 pressures (PCO_2) according to SpO_2 variations (Haldane effect). Panel **b** Influence of H^+ load on whole-blood total CO_2 content (CCO_2) and blood CO_2 pressures (PCO_2)

16.3 The Venous-to-Arterial Carbon Dioxide Difference (Pv-aCO_2)

16.3.1 Pv-aCO_2 and Its Relationship with Cardiac Output

The venous-to-arterial carbon dioxide difference (Pv-aCO_2) refers to the gradient of partial pressures exerted by the dissolved CO_2 on the mixed or central venous and the arterial blood. Overall, Pv-aCO_2 depends on the total carbon dioxide (CO_2) production, cardiac output, the complex relationship between CO_2 partial pressures and CO_2 blood contents, and, probably, the microcirculatory blood flow distribution.

16

The Fick equation indicates that CO_2 excretion, i.e., the equivalent to CO_2 production (VCO_2) at steady state, should equal the product of cardiac output (CO) and the venous-to-arterial CO_2 difference:

$$\dot{V}CO_2 = CO \times \left(CvCO_2 - CaCO_2\right)$$

As mentioned above, CCO_2 and PCO_2 maintain a relatively linear relationship at usual physiological ranges. Thus, PCO_2 values have been suggested as a surrogate for CCO_2 when assessing the venous-to-arterial CO_2 difference at the bedside [20–23]. As a result, a modified Fick equation can be obtained by substituting PCO_2 for CCO_2:

$$\Delta PCO_2 = k\left(\dot{V}CO_2 / CO\right)$$

where *k* is a pseudo-linear coefficient assumed to be constant during physiological conditions [22]. However, under severe hypoxic conditions, the *k* factor may rise up to sixfold as metabolic acidosis increases, causing shifts in the curvilinear relation between CCO_2 and PCO_2 (Fig. 16.2, panel b). Thus, the *k* factor increases as VCO_2 decreases, but the resultant effect on Pv-aCO_2 will depend on the cardiac output and probably on the microcirculatory blood flow distribution.

According to the modified Fick equation, Pv-aCO_2 and cardiac output keep an inverse curvilinear relationship in which rises in Pv-aCO_2 follow progressive reductions in cardiac output, especially in its lower values. As a result, under stable conditions of both VO_2 and VCO_2, the Pv-aCO_2 progressively increases in response to reductions in cardiac output due to the CO_2-stagnation phenomenon in which the delayed transit time of red blood cells leads to higher addition of CO_2 per unit of blood flowing through efferent microvessels. Early observations during cardiac arrest in both animal and human models clearly revealed a link between slowing (or stopping) blood flow and venous CO_2 accumulation [24, 25]. Similarly, experimental models of hemorrhage, hypovolemia, and obstructive shock demonstrated this inverse relationship between Pv-aCO_2 and cardiac output, thus highlighting the importance of blood flow stagnation on venous CO_2 accumulation [26–29]. Nevertheless, Pv-aCO_2 increases were originally interpreted as a reflection of tissue dysoxia since critical oxygen delivery values appeared to be consistent with the point at which venous CO_2 starts to increase [26, 27]. In a canine experimental model of cardiac tamponade using the Dill nomogram, Schlichtig and Bowles [30] suggested the appearance of anaerobic VCO_2 below critical DO_2, thus suggesting the link between dysoxia and tissue CO_2 accumulation. However, experimental models in which progressive flow decrements are used to achieve critical oxygen delivery (DO_2) with subsequent decrease in oxygen consumption (VO_2) may yield confusing results given the impossibility to distinguish tissue hypoperfusion from tissue dysoxia [31]. To solve this problem, Vallet et al. [32] designed an experiment to measure Pv-aCO_2 changes in canine hind limb preparations isolated from systemic circulation and connected to a roller pump-membrane oxygenator circuit. Comparable decreases in DO_2 were produced by two different mechanisms of tissue hypoxia: one group underwent progressive decrease in blood flow by slowing the roller pump velocity (ischemic hypoxia), while the other group underwent progressive decrease in arterial PO_2 by manipulating the inspired O_2 fraction (hypoxic hypoxia) but preserving flow velocity. Both groups experienced similar declines in DO_2 and VO_2, suggesting similar degrees of tissue dysoxia. However, the regional hind limb Pv-aCO_2 remained constant during hypoxic hypoxia, while it showed a more than twofold increase during ischemic hypoxia. Accordingly, the authors concluded that blood flow is the major determinant of Pv-aCO_2, and therefore, the absence of an increased Pv-aCO_2 does not preclude the presence of tissue dysoxia. Assessing a similar hypothesis, Nevière et al. [33] compared the effects of a reduced inspired oxygen fraction (hypoxic hypoxia) vs. decreased blood flow (ischemic hypoxia) on the gut mucosal-to-arterial CO_2 difference (Pmtis-aCO_2). Pmtis-aCO_2 increased up to 60 mmHg during ischemic hypoxia, while it remained almost constant over a wide range of DO_2 values during hypoxic hypoxia. Interestingly, Pmtis-aCO_2 slightly increased when extremely low FiO_2 values were used. The authors concluded that the increase in Pmtis-aCO_2 is mainly explained by blood flow alterations, although they admitted that an increased intramucosal PCO_2 in very severe hypoxic hypoxia conditions might indicate some local CO_2 generation. Nevertheless, the fact that DO_2/VO_2 dependency was attained earlier than increases in Pmtis-aCO_2 during hypoxic hypoxia conditions implies that Pmtis-aCO_2 should not be used as a marker of tissue dysoxia.

Similarly, in a hemorrhagic model of hypoxia without hypoperfusion in which progressive blood loss was replaced by isovolemic doses of dextran, Pv-aCO_2 showed no increases when blood flow was restituted, hence confirming the leading role of blood flow on increased venous CO_2 [34].

Thus, increases in Pv-aCO_2 are closely related to cardiac output changes during non-inflammatory conditions. Nevertheless, the concordance observed between cardiac output and Pv-aCO_2 during septic shock is weak [14, 35–37], which suggests that other mechanisms might be involved.

16.3.2 Pv-aCO_2 and Microcirculatory Blood Flow Alterations

Microcirculatory dysfunction in septic shock is a generalized phenomenon characterized by decreased functional capillary density (FCD) associated with increased heterogeneity of blood flow involving areas with well-perfused vessels in close vicinity to non-perfused capillaries [38, 39]. In normal conditions, the heterogeneity of microvascular blood flow is negligible [40], and the matching of perfusion to metabolism usually improves during hypoxic or low-flow states [41]. However, increases in heterogeneity of the microcirculatory blood flow with the subsequent reduction of FCD could be responsible for the abnormal oxygen extraction capacity occurring in sepsis [42, 43]. In fact, the heterogeneous flow cessation of individual capillaries could be an important factor determining the phenomenon of oxygen supply dependence during the most severe cases of septic shock [42, 44]. Importantly, microcirculatory alterations may occur even when global oxygen parameters appear to be adequate, and it seems to trigger the development of multiple organ dysfunction [45]. Furthermore, such microcirculatory derangements are stronger determinants of clinical outcomes than global hemodynamic parameters, with progressive increase in the risk of death in quartiles representing the most severe disturbances [46].

The link between microcirculatory alterations and tissue CO_2 accumulation in septic shock was proposed by Creteur et al. [47] by simultaneous evaluations of sublingual microcirculation, sublingual tissue CO_2, and gastric mucosal CO_2 during the infusion of a low fixed dose of dobutamine. They observed increases in cardiac output and SvO_2, while sublingual-to-arterial CO_2 difference (Psl-aCO_2) significantly decreased (from 40 ± 15 to 17 ± 8 mmHg). The proportion of well-perfused small vessels was inversely related with Psl-aCO_2 ($R^2 = 0.80$, $p < 0.01$), indicating that increases in the proportion of well-perfused capillaries paralleled inverse variations in tissue CO_2 pressure. Similarly, Nevière and colleagues [48] found that dobutamine-induced changes in gastric microvascular blood flow were well reflected by the changes in gastric mucosal-to-arterial CO_2 differences (Pgtis-aCO_2), thus supporting the leading role of microvascular blood flow on gastric-tissue CO_2 accumulation.

16

Recent observations have also suggested a close relationship between microcirculatory blood flow alterations and Pv-aCO_2 during the early stages of septic shock [11]. Particularly, the increased heterogeneity of microcirculatory blood flow and decreased functional capillary densities were well related with progressive increases of Pv-aCO_2. Interestingly, variations in cardiac output were not well correlated with changes in microcirculatory blood flow parameters, although admittedly, higher Pv-aCO_2 values were generally observed at lower cardiac output values.

During tissue hypoxia, total VCO_2 decreases despite some anaerobic CO_2 generation. However, venous CCO_2 will increase as macro blood flow decreases or microvascular blood flow turns more heterogeneous. In fact, considering a constant VCO_2, venous CO_2 will increase even at apparent "normal" cardiac output values when microcirculatory blood flow becomes heterogeneous and capillary densities fall (Fig. 16.3). In this manner, monitoring PCO_2 gaps may provide important information about microcirculatory blood flow alterations even in patients with apparently normalized cardiac output and oxygen-derived parameters.

16.3.3 The Clinical Value of Pv-aCO_2

Pv-aCO_2 changes reflect macro blood flow variations during abnormal noninflammatory conditions such as cardiac arrest, hypovolemic or hemorrhagic shock, and cardiac tamponade [24–28]. However, during septic shock, Pv-aCO_2 could be potentially influenced by microcirculatory blood flow distribution, whereby the relationship between cardiac output and Pv-aCO_2 has not been consistently observed in clinical and experimental studies.

Early observations in septic shock demonstrated that patients with Pv-aCO_2 > 6 mmHg showed lower cardiac output values than those with Pv-aCO_2 ≤ 6 mmHg [36]. Interestingly, positive responders to fluid loads exhibited simultaneous reductions in Pv-aCO_2, although the mathematical agreement between Pv-aCO_2 and cardiac output changes was actually poor ($r = 0.42$ or $R^2 = 0.18$, $p < 0.001$). Likewise, an inverse (although mathematically weak) relationship between cardiac output and Pv-aCO_2 ($r = 0.41$ or $R^2 = 0.17$, $p < 0.001$) was reported by Bakker et al. [35], and although cardiac output and DO_2 were lower in patients with Pv-aCO_2 > 6 mmHg, identical VO_2 was observed in both groups due to the adaptive ERO_2 changes.

A Pv-aCO_2 > 6.0 mmHg in patients with septic shock attaining a $ScvO_2$ > 70% after initial resuscitation has also been related with more severe multiorgan dysfunction [15]. Similarly, Ospina-Tascón et al. [14] showed that the persistence of high Pv-aCO_2 during early resuscitation of septic shock is associated with more severe multiorgan dysfunction and poorer outcomes at day 28. Increases in Pv-aCO_2 were associated with adverse clinical outcomes even when attaining $ScvO_2$ and $ScvO_2$ goals. Furthermore, higher lactate levels and slower lactate recovery were observed in those patients with persistently high Pv-aCO_2 values during the first 6 h of resuscitation. Importantly, PCO_2 gaps obtained from central venous and mixed-venous blood samples exhibited good agreement. However, as also suggested in another recent study in septic shock patients [37], no agreement was observed between Pv-aCO_2 and cardiac output.

Interestingly, although Pv-aCO_2 has been associated with adverse outcomes in septic shock [14, 15, 37, 49, 50] and high-risk surgical procedures [51], its predictive value in cardiac surgery remains controversial [52, 53].

Thus, a high Pv-aCO_2 may identify septic patients who remain inadequately resuscitated despite attaining oxygen metabolism targets, reinforcing the notion about the Pv-aCO_2 as a marker of global perfusion due to its ability to detect blood flow alterations. Nevertheless, a normal Pv-aCO_2 may not detect the presence of tissue hypoxia as elevated cardiac output values could prevent venous CO_2 increases by simple tissue washout.

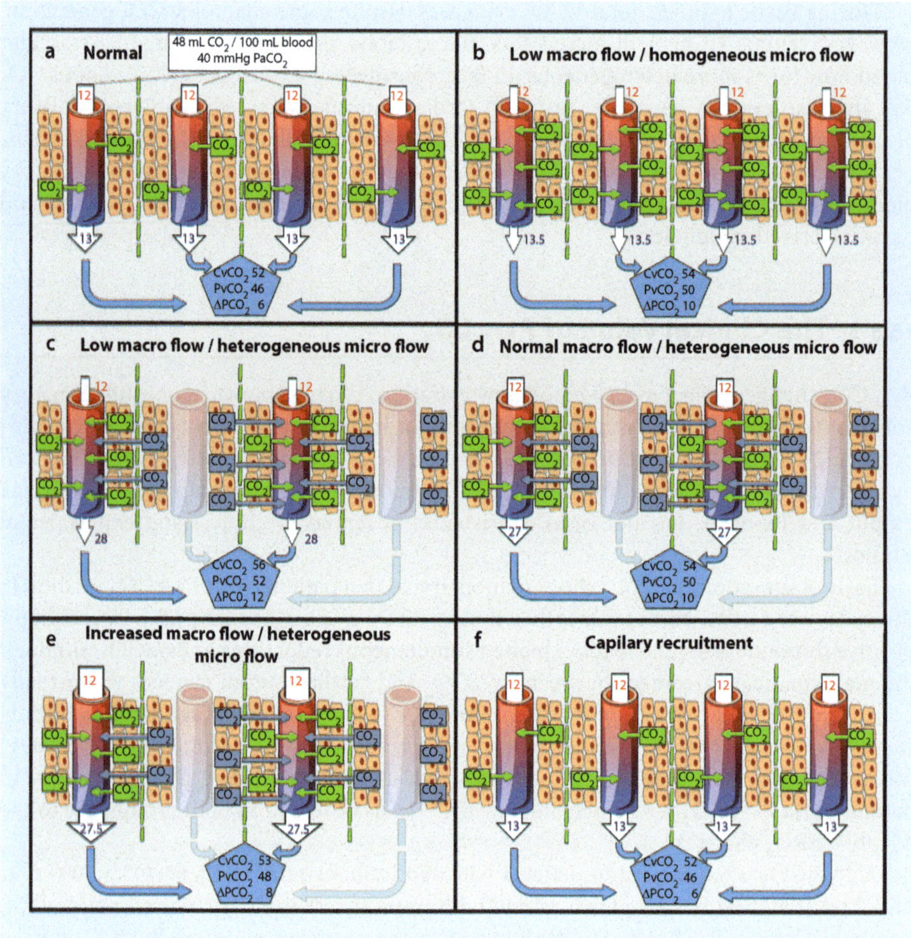

Fig. 16.3 Macro- and microcirculatory blood flow variations and its effects on Pv-aCO_2. Panel **a** Normal conditions of macro and micro blood flow: 48 mL CO_2/dL (or PCO_2 40 mmHg) are conducted throughout four capillaries with normal continuous convective flow (white arrows throughout capillaries). Venous effluent will come loaded with aerobic-produced CO_2 leading to CvCO_2 of 52 mL/dL (or PvCO_2 46 mmHg) generating a Pv-aCO_2 of 6 mmHg. Panel **b** Low cardiac output with homogeneous microvascular blood flow. Delayed transit time of capillary blood (thin white arrows throughout capillaries) will conduct to higher CO_2 loads at the venous effluent even aerobic metabolism is maintained (stagnation phenomenon). Venous effluent will be charged with extra aerobic CO_2 leading to CvCO_2 of 54 mL/dL (or PvCO_2 50 mmHg) and Pv-aCO_2 of 10 mmHg. Panel **c** Low cardiac output and heterogeneous microvascular blood flow. Patent capillaries will be loaded with higher amounts of aerobic CO_2 from adjacent cellular groups because of vascular stagnation (thin white arrows throughout open capillaries represent low convective flow). Furthermore, venous effluent will be also loaded with additional CO_2 from distant cellular groups. This additional CO_2 will be in part a product from the reduced aerobic metabolism, and most will proceed from anaerobic CO_2 generation because of the buffering of net H^+ release (see the text for details). Thus, venous effluent will be charged with extra aerobic and anaerobic CO_2 leading to CvCO_2 of 56 mL/dL (or PvCO_2 52 mmHg) and Pv-aCO_2 of 12 mmHg. Panel **d** Normal cardiac output and heterogeneous microvascular blood flow. Anaerobic CO_2 will be generated into the blood as a product of buffering of net H^+ release (increased because of O_2 limitation secondary to blood flow misdistribution – see text for details). Despite apparent normal cardiac output, this is not enough to wash out the excess of CO_2. Thus, venous effluent will be charged with extra aerobic and anaerobic CO_2 leading to CvCO_2 of 54 mL/dL (or PvCO_2 50 mmHg), and Pv-aCO_2 will remain high (10 mmHg). Panel

16.4 The Venous-Arterial CO_2 to Arterial-Venous O_2 Ratio ($Cv\text{-}aCO_2/Ca\text{-}vO_2$ Ratio)

16.4.1 Physiological Rationale

According to the Fick equation, oxygen consumption (VO_2) and CO_2 production (VCO_2) are directly proportional to the cardiac output and their respective arterial-to-venous and venous-to-arterial content differences. Under aerobic steady-state conditions, VCO_2 approaches VO_2, whereby the mixed venous-to-arterial CO_2 content difference ($Cv\text{-}aCO_2$) approximates to the arterial-to-mixed-venous CO_2 content difference ($Ca\text{-}vO_2$). Accordingly, VCO_2 should not exceed O_2 availability, and, therefore, the VCO_2/VO_2 ratio (i.e., the respiratory quotient (RQ)) should not be >1.0 during such aerobic resting conditions. $Cv\text{-}aCO_2/Ca\text{-}vO_2$ ratio could be a surrogate of the VCO_2/VO_2 ratio or RQ, and, to some extent, it should be independent of flow variations since, according to the Fick equation, the cardiac output is present in both the numerator and denominator components. A recent subanalysis from an experimental shock model of progressive hemorrhage suggested that the $Pv\text{-}aCO_2/Ca\text{-}vO_2$ ratio is a poor surrogate of anaerobic metabolism during hemodilution [54]. However, other authors have observed simultaneous increases in $Cv\text{-}aCO_2/Ca\text{-}vO_2$ ratio, the respiratory quotient (measured by indirect calorimetry), and lactate levels during circulatory failure in mechanically ventilated patients [55], thus reinforcing the idea about the link between anaerobic metabolism and increased $Cv\text{-}aCO_2/Ca\text{-}vO_2$ ratio.

Experimental blockade of mitochondrial O_2 utilization leads to nonsymmetrical reductions in VCO_2 and VO_2 with RQ increase. This asymmetric VCO_2/VO_2 fall could be explained by increased anaerobic CO_2 production derived from the buffering of excess of protons (mainly delivered during ATP hydrolysis) that are not recycled during oxidative phosphorylation as a result of the severely limited O_2 availability (Fig. 16.4). Analogously, under conditions of excessive metabolic demand (such as during exhaustive exercise), total VCO_2 may exceed adaptive increases in VO_2, once the anaerobic threshold is attained [56]. Otherwise, during circulatory shock, a global decrease in VO_2 should be accompanied by a proportional reduction in aerobic VCO_2. However, experimental shock models also demonstrated that VCO_2 could decrease slightly less than the VO_2 fall [28, 57], with the subsequent increase in the VCO_2/VO_2 ratio. Interestingly, this VCO_2/VO_2 ratio returns to normal after shock reversion. The aforementioned then suggests that $Cv\text{-}aCO_2/Ca\text{-}vO_2$ ratio could identify the presence of anaerobic metabolism.

e Increased cardiac output and heterogeneous microvascular blood flow. An increased macro flow will wash both aerobic and anaerobic CO_2 produced in tissues (thick white arrows throughout open capillaries represent increased convective flow). However, when microvascular blood flow is severely heterogeneous, anaerobic CO_2 will increase in the venous effluent despite apparent high cardiac output values. Thus, venous effluent will be charged with extra aerobic and anaerobic CO_2 leading to $CvCO_2$ of 53 mL/dL (or $PvCO_2$ 48 mmHg) and $Pv\text{-}aCO_2$ of 8 mmHg. Panel **f** Capillary recruitment. Interventions improving microvascular blood flow distribution lead to normalize $Pv\text{-}aCO_2$ that even cardiac output apparently decreases from "high" to "normal" values. Note: green vertical dotted lines represent the limits of the theoretical cylindrical areas dependent from each capillary vessel

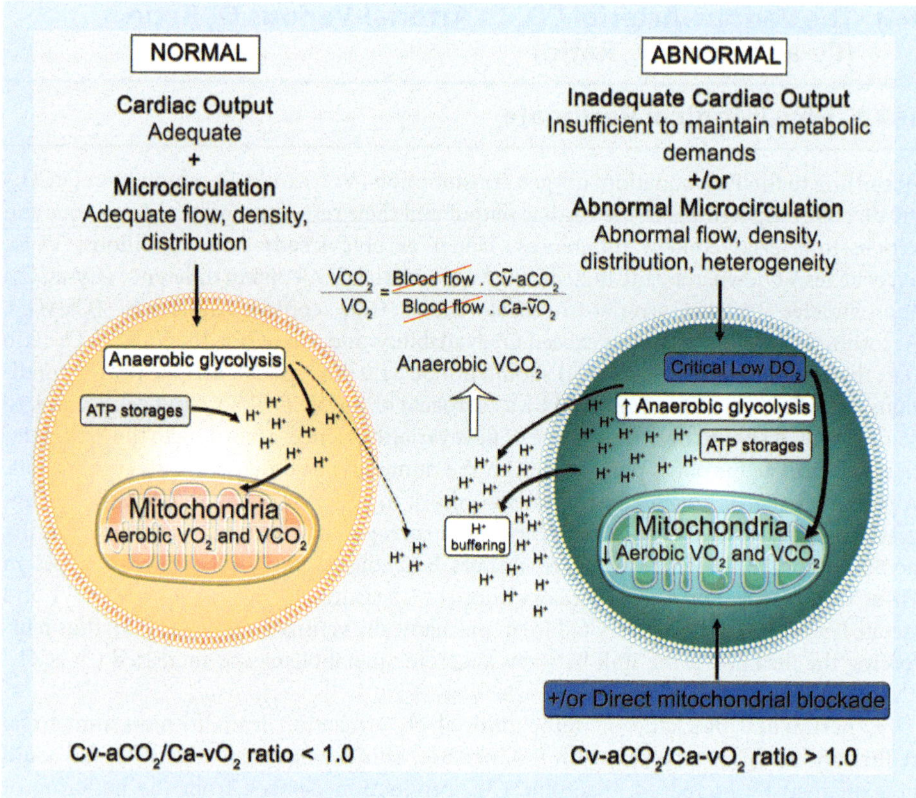

Fig. 16.4 The venous-arterial CO_2 to arterial-venous O_2 ratio (Cv-aCO_2/Ca-vO_2 ratio). Normal aerobic (left side) and anaerobic conditions (right side). Adequate cardiac output and normal microvascular blood flow distribution usually preserve cellular respiration, and Cv-aCO_2/Ca-vO_2 ratio remains ≤1.0. Conversely, inadequate cardiac output, microvascular blood flow misdistribution, and direct mitochondrial blockade decrease VO_2 with subsequent fall in aerobic VCO_2. Cellular metabolism shifts toward anaerobic glycolysis, and H^+ liberated during ATP hydrolysis is not reused in the oxidative phosphorylation. Thus, excess of non-recycled H^+ is buffered by HCO_3^- generating H_2CO_3, which dissociates into CO_2 and H_2O. This anaerobic CO_2 will increase the Cv-aCO_2/Ca-vO_2 ratio

16.4.2 The Cv-aCO_2/Ca-vO_2 Ratio and Its Clinical Implications

16

Hyperlactatemia has been traditionally recognized as a marker of anaerobic metabolism secondary to an inadequate oxygen supply to the cells. However, plasma lactate levels may increase by causes other than tissue hypoxia [58]. In fact, high lactate levels can frequently result from increased glycolytic activity, abnormal pyruvate metabolism, or altered metabolic lactate clearance [59–61], which hinder its interpretation during the resuscitation and post-resuscitation periods. Using CO_2 pressures instead of CO_2 contents, Mekontso-Dessap et al. [12] showed a good agreement between the Pv-aCO_2/Ca-vO_2 ratio (as surrogate of the Cv-aCO_2/Ca-vO_2 ratio) and lactate levels ≥2.0 mmol/L (accepting it as indicator of anaerobic metabolism). However, more important than a simple agreement, the Cv-aCO_2/Ca-vO_2 ratio can provide additional information to that provided by lactate levels. In a recent study, Ospina-Tascón et al. [13] demonstrated that persistent hyperlactatemia combined with a high $Cv\text{-}aCO_2/Ca\text{-}vO_2$ ratio was associated with more severe organ dysfunction and worse clinical outcomes in septic shock as compared to those patients with normal lactate levels and a $Cv\text{-}aCO_2/Ca\text{-}vO_2$ ratio ≤ 1.0. Intriguingly, patients attaining lactate levels <2.0 mmol/L but with persistently elevated $Cv\text{-}aCO_2/Ca\text{-}vO_2$ ratios had similar clinical outcomes than those with persistent hyperlactatemia and normal $Cv\text{-}aCO_2/Ca\text{-}vO_2$ ratios. However, whether an increased $Cv\text{-}aCO_2/Ca\text{-}vO_2$ ratio can precede increases in lactate levels during septic shock should be confirmed in the future.

Subsequent studies have corroborated the $Cv\text{-}aCO_2/Ca\text{-}vO_2$ ratio as a prognostic factor in septic shock [62, 63], while others have suggested that concomitant high $Cv\text{-}aCO_2/Ca\text{-}vO_2$ ratios and hyperlactatemia may identify an ongoing VO_2/DO_2 dependence [64, 65]. In agreement with this concept, other authors have demonstrated that VO_2 increases after a fluid load only in patients with acute circulatory failure and an increased pre-fluid $Pv\text{-}aCO_2/Ca\text{-}vO_2$ ratio [64, 65]. Furthermore, evidence from experimental septic shock models suggests that improvement of microcirculatory blood flow distribution can reverse the anaerobic metabolism reflected by proportional falls in the $Cv\text{-}aCO_2/Ca\text{-}vO_2$ ratio [41].

In conclusion, the $Cv\text{-}aCO_2/Ca\text{-}vO_2$ ratio or its equivalent, the $Pv\text{-}aCO_2/Ca\text{-}vO_2$ ratio (with the obvious limitations because the Haldane effect), might provide important prognostic information, and it could help to clarify the origin of lactate increases (from aerobic or anaerobic nature) during the early stages of shock. The $Cv\text{-}aCO_2/Ca\text{-}vO_2$ ratio reacts faster than lactate levels to short-term hemodynamic changes, which makes it an attractive variable to be monitored, and, although difficult to be calculated, its interpretation is easier, with values >1.0 suggesting probably the presence of ongoing anaerobic metabolism.

16.5 The $Pv\text{-}aCO_2$ and the Haldane Effect

The CO_2 binding to hemoglobin will vary according to the oxygenated or deoxygenated state of hemoglobin. This phenomenon known as the Haldane effect allows better loading of CO_2 from tissues to the blood when oxygen moves in the opposite direction, thereby increasing the CO_2-carrying ability of venous blood. Conversely, oxygen moving from alveoli to the capillary blood enhances unloading of CO_2 from hemoglobin, thus facilitating its pulmonary elimination. Therefore, low oxygen saturation values increase the CO_2 content (CCO_2) for a given PCO_2, whereby more CO_2 will be bound to hemoglobin. Changes in tissue oxygen extraction, pH, VCO_2, and hemoglobin concentration can influence $Pv\text{-}aCO_2$ despite a preserved or even increased tissue perfusion. For example, a combination of high blood flow and larger increases in VCO_2 compared with the respective change in oxygen consumption may lead to dissociation of the tissue-to-arterial or venous-to-arterial CO_2 gradients among different vascular beds with different baseline ERO_2 values. In fact, paradoxical increases in mucosal-to-arterial PCO_2 differences can occur during increasing splanchnic blood flow because of changes in venous oxygen saturation effluent, local VCO_2, or both [66].

Depending on baseline SvO_2, the Haldane effect may increase or decrease $Pv\text{-}aCO_2$ in response to the same changes in blood flow or metabolism [67]. Admittedly, $Pv\text{-}aCO_2/Ca\text{-}vO_2$ could be equivalent to the $Cv\text{-}aCO_2/Ca\text{-}vO_2$ ratio when PCO_2, pH, and SvO_2 approximate to normality, which occurs frequently. However, $Cv\text{-}aCO_2$ is not always represented by $Pv\text{-}aCO_2$, especially during low PCO_2 and SvO_2 conditions. In this regard, a recent study demonstrated the prognostic value of the $Cv\text{-}aCO_2/Ca\text{-}vO_2$ ratio in septic shock and the unreliability of its equivalent in terms of partial pressures, the $Pv\text{-}aCO_2/Ca\text{-}vO_2$ ratio [13]. Thus, although at low $Pv\text{-}aCO_2$ values the influence of the Haldane effect is negligible, the dispersion of $Cv\text{-}aCO_2$ vs. $Pv\text{-}aCO_2$ becomes significantly wider at higher $Pv\text{-}aCO_2$ values [13].

The simplicity of $Pv\text{-}aCO_2$ measurement makes it an attractive tool to guide resuscitation in the clinical setting. However, $Pv\text{-}aCO_2$ is a physiologically complex measurement that should be interpreted according to a number of physiological variables.

16.6 Interpreting $Pv\text{-}aCO_2$ and $Cv\text{-}aCO_2/Ca\text{-}vO_2$ Ratios in Septic Shock

Tissue-to-arterial and venous-to-arterial CO_2 differences should be considered as markers of tissue perfusion rather than indicators of tissue hypoxia. Concomitance of high $Pv\text{-}aCO_2$ (> 6.0 mmHg) and low SvO_2 levels usually reflects low cardiac output in both inflammatory and noninflammatory conditions. Likewise, normal SvO_2 accompanying persistently increased $Pv\text{-}aCO_2$ suggests the presence of a cardiac output that is insufficient to clear the CO_2 produced by tissues. Alternatively, high $Pv\text{-}aCO_2$ values with normal or even high SvO_2 values coincide with microcirculatory derangements such as decreased functional capillary densities or increased heterogeneity of microvascular blood flow, at least during the early stages of septic shock [11, 45]. In any case, an increased $Pv\text{-}aCO_2$ reflects altered macro or micro blood flow independently of the presence of anaerobic metabolism. Consequently, an elevated $Pv\text{-}aCO_2$ should encourage clinicians to optimize the cardiac output or possibly recruiting microcirculation to improve tissue perfusion, especially when lactate levels are increased and clinical signs of hypoperfusion are present. However, such decisions should take into account the clinical context and information provided by "multimodal" monitoring [68]. Under aerobic conditions, a high $Pv\text{-}aCO_2$ would mean that blood flow is not sufficient even when the cardiac output is in "normal" ranges. In this context, further efforts to increase the cardiac output aimed to prevent the possible onset of tissue hypoxia remain controversial and need to be evaluated in the future.

Under conditions of oxygen supply dependency, increases in cardiac output should be accompanied by rises in VO_2 and, consequently, by increases in aerobic VCO_2, so that $Pv\text{-}aCO_2$ may decrease by a lesser extent after such positive intervention. Thus, minor decreases in $Pv\text{-}aCO_2$ not always mean an ineffective therapeutic intervention. Consequently, in cases of probable oxygen supply dependency, interventions optimizing the cardiac output should probably be maintained until a decrease in $Pv\text{-}aCO_2$ values is obtained. Remarkably, most interventions aimed to increase the cardiac output will increase VCO_2 since vasoactive amines and inotropes positively increase the thermogenic effect [69]. In this regard, $Pv\text{-}aCO_2$ could be used as an index reflecting the VCO_2/cardiac output relationship [29], and consequently, it could help titrate drug therapy [70]. Conversely, a normal $Pv\text{-}aCO_2$ (<6.0 mmHg) suggests that the cardiac output is sufficient to clear the CO_2 produced by tissues and also suggests that the microcirculatory blood flow is adequately distributed. However, whether cardiac output or microcirculation should be manipulated during apparent hypoxic conditions with a $Pv\text{-}aCO_2$ < 6.0 mmHg remains also debatable.

A $Cv\text{-}aCO_2/Ca\text{-}vO_2$ ratio > 1.0 could suggest the presence of anaerobic metabolism. Thus, combining lactate levels and $Cv\text{-}aCO_2/Ca\text{-}vO_2$ ratios might provide relevant information during the early stages of resuscitation. An increased lactate level accompanied by $Cv\text{-}aCO_2/Ca\text{-}vO_2$ ratios >1.0 could suggest "ongoing" anaerobic metabolism; thus clinicians should be encouraged to optimize both macro and micro blood flow parameters. Conversely, increased lactate levels accompanied by $Cv\text{-}aCO_2/Ca\text{-}vO_2$ ratios ≤ 1.0 may could suggest lactate accumulation as a result of cell dysfunction in the presence of aerobic metabolism. In such cases, additional resuscitation maneuvers aimed to increase blood flow should probably be discouraged, although this should be confirmed in clinical trials. Given the faster response in CO_2 variables, a $Cv\text{-}aCO_2/Ca\text{-}vO_2$ ratio > 1.0 with normal lactate levels could eventually suggest the onset of anaerobic metabolism, even anticipating the increase in lactate levels. Nevertheless, the complexity of the $Cv\text{-}aCO_2/Ca\text{-}vO_2$ ratio merits further research and confirmation in the clinical setting.

Conclusion

Physiology determining venous CO_2 increases is complex. However, $Pv\text{-}aCO_2$ globally reflects blood flow alterations at both macro- and microvascular levels, more than tissue dysoxia. Meanwhile, an elevated $Cv\text{-}aCO_2/Ca\text{-}vO_2$ ratio could reflect anaerobic metabolism, and it could add important prognostic information in patients with shock. Despite the physiological bases of such monitoring CO_2-derived variables, its clinical utility during resuscitation in shock remains to be proved in future experimental and clinical studies.

Take-Home Messages

- $Pv\text{-}aCO_2$ is determined by the conjunction of macro- and/or microvascular blood flow, the total CO_2 production (both aerobic and anaerobic), and the complex relationship between CO_2 partial pressures and CO_2 blood contents (Haldane effect).
- $Pv\text{-}aCO_2$ should be considered as a marker of tissue perfusion but not of tissue hypoxia.
- An increased $Pv\text{-}aCO_2$ usually suggest a "low" or "insufficient" cardiac output. However, during severe inflammatory conditions, alterations in functional capillary density and heterogeneity of microvascular blood flow could also account for venous CO_2 accumulation.
- An elevated $Pv\text{-}aCO_2$ should encourage clinicians to optimize the cardiac output, especially when lactate levels are increased and clinical signs of hypoperfusion are present.
- Under aerobic conditions, further efforts to increase the cardiac output in order to prevent the possible onset of tissue hypoxia in the presence of a high $Pv\text{-}aCO_2$ remain controversial.
- An increased venous-arterial carbon dioxide to arterial-venous oxygen content difference ratio ($Cv\text{-}aCO_2/Ca\text{-}vO_2$) could reflect the presence of anaerobic metabolism. There is some experimental evidence that high $Cv\text{-}aCO_2/Ca\text{-}vO_2$ ratio can be reversed by resuscitation maneuvers, at least during early stages of shock.
- A high $Cv\text{-}aCO_2/Ca\text{-}vO_2$ ratio could offer additional prognostic information in septic shock. Whether $Cv\text{-}aCO_2/Ca\text{-}vO_2$ ratio could anticipate lactate increase during early stages of shock remains to be elucidated.

References

1. Cecconi M, De Backer D, Antonelli M, Beale R, Bakker J, Hofer C, et al. Consensus on circulatory shock and hemodynamic monitoring. Task force of the European Society of Intensive Care Medicine. Intensive Care Med. 2014;40(12):1795–815.
2. Vincent JL, De Backer D. Circulatory shock. N Engl J Med. 2013;369(18):1726–34.
3. Shoemaker WC, Appel PL, Kram HB. Tissue oxygen debt as a determinant of lethal and nonlethal postoperative organ failure. Crit Care Med. 1988;16(11):1117–20.
4. Vallet B. Vascular reactivity and tissue oxygenation. Intensive Care Med. 1998;24(1):3–11.
5. Rivers E, Nguyen B, Havstad S, Ressler J, Muzzin A, Knoblich B, et al. Early goal-directed therapy in the treatment of severe sepsis and septic shock. N Engl J Med. 2001;345(19):1368–77.
6. Bellomo R, Reade MC, Warrillow SJ. The pursuit of a high central venous oxygen saturation in sepsis: growing concerns. Crit Care. 2008;12(2):130.
7. Peake SL, Delaney A, Bailey M, Bellomo R, Cameron PA, Cooper DJ, et al. Goal-directed resuscitation for patients with early septic shock. N Engl J Med. 2014;371(16):1496–506.
8. Mouncey PR, Osborn TM, Power GS, Harrison DA, Sadique MZ, Grieve RD, et al. Trial of early, goal-directed resuscitation for septic shock. N Engl J Med. 2015;372(14):1301–11.
9. Yealy DM, Kellum JA, Huang DT, Barnato AE, Weissfeld LA, Pike F, et al. A randomized trial of protocol-based care for early septic shock. N Engl J Med. 2014;370(18):1683–93.
10. van Beest PA, Hofstra JJ, Schultz MJ, Boerma EC, Spronk PE, Kuiper MA. The incidence of low venous oxygen saturation on admission to the intensive care unit: a multi-center observational study in The Netherlands. Crit Care. 2008;12(2):R33.
11. Ospina-Tascón GA, Umaña M, Bermúdez WF, Bautista-Rincón DF, Valencia JD, Madriñán HJ, et al. Can venous-to-arterial carbon dioxide differences reflect microcirculatory alterations in patients with septic shock? Intensive Care Med. 2016;42(2):211–21.
12. Mekontso-Dessap A, Castelain V, Anguel N, Bahloul M, Schauvliege F, Richard C, et al. Combination of venoarterial PCO_2 difference with arteriovenous O_2 content difference to detect anaerobic metabolism in patients. Intensive Care Med. 2002;28(3):272–7.
13. Ospina-Tascón GA, Umaña M, Bermúdez W, Bautista-Rincón DF, Hernandez G, Bruhn A, et al. Combination of arterial lactate levels and venous-arterial CO_2 to arterial-venous O 2 content difference ratio as markers of resuscitation in patients with septic shock. Intensive Care Med. 2015;41(5):796–805.
14. Ospina-Tascón GA, Bautista-Rincón DF, Umaña M, Tafur JD, Gutiérrez A, García AF, et al. Persistently high venous-to-arterial carbon dioxide differences during early resuscitation are associated with poor outcomes in septic shock. Crit Care. 2013;17(6):R294.
15. Vallée F, Vallet B, Mathe O, Parraguette J, Mari A, Silva S, et al. Central venous-to-arterial carbon dioxide difference: an additional target for goal-directed therapy in septic shock? Intensive Care Med. 2008;34(12):2218–25.
16. Herve P, Simonneau G, Girard P, Cerrina J, Mathieu M, Duroux P. Hypercapnic acidosis induced by nutrition in mechanically ventilated patients: glucose versus fat. Crit Care Med. 1985;13(7):537–40.
17. Marcinek DJ, Kushmerick MJ, Conley KE. Lactic acidosis in vivo: testing the link between lactate generation and H+ accumulation in ischemic mouse muscle. J Appl Physiol (1985). 2010;108(6):1479–86.
18. Randall HM, Cohen JJ. Anaerobic CO_2 production by dog kidney in vitro. Am J Phys. 1966;211(2):493–505.
19. Jensen FB. Comparative analysis of autoxidation of haemoglobin. J Exp Biol. 2001;204(Pt 11):2029–33.
20. McHardy GJ. The relationship between the differences in pressure and content of carbon dioxide in arterial and venous blood. Clin Sci. 1967;32(2):299–309.
21. Cavaliere F, Giovannini I, Chiarla C, Conti G, Pennisi MA, Montini L, et al. Comparison of two methods to assess blood CO_2 equilibration curve in mechanically ventilated patients. Respir Physiol Neurobiol. 2005;146(1):77–83.
22. Lamia B, Monnet X, Teboul JL. Meaning of arterio-venous PCO_2 difference in circulatory shock. Minerva Anestesiol. 2006;72(6):597–604.
23. Giovannini I, Chiarla C, Boldrini G, Castagneto M. Calculation of venoarterial CO_2 concentration difference. J Appl Physiol (1985). 1993;74(2):959–64.
24. Grundler W, Weil MH, Rackow EC. Arteriovenous carbon dioxide and pH gradients during cardiac arrest. Circulation. 1986;74(5):1071–4.
25. Weil MH, Rackow EC, Trevino R, Grundler W, Falk JL, Griffel MI. Difference in acid-base state between venous and arterial blood during cardiopulmonary resuscitation. N Engl J Med. 1986;315(3):153–6.

26. Zhang H, Vincent JL. Arteriovenous differences in PCO_2 and pH are good indicators of critical hypoperfusion. Am Rev Respir Dis. 1993;148(4 Pt 1):867–71.
27. Van der Linden P, Rausin I, Deltell A, Bekrar Y, Gilbart E, Bakker J, et al. Detection of tissue hypoxia by arteriovenous gradient for PCO_2 and pH in anesthetized dogs during progressive hemorrhage. Anesth Analg. 1995;80(2):269–75.
28. Groeneveld AB, Vermeij CG, Thijs LG. Arterial and mixed venous blood acid-base balance during hypoperfusion with incremental positive end-expiratory pressure in the pig. Anesth Analg. 1991;73(5):576–82.
29. Teboul JL, Mercat A, Lenique F, Berton C, Richard C. Value of the venous-arterial PCO_2 gradient to reflect the oxygen supply to demand in humans: effects of dobutamine. Crit Care Med. 1998;26(6):1007–10.
30. Schlichtig R, Bowles SA. Distinguishing between aerobic and anaerobic appearance of dissolved CO_2 in intestine during low flow. J Appl Physiol (1985). 1994;76(6):2443–51.
31. Vallet B, Tavernier B, Lund N. Assessment of tissue oxygenation in the critically Ill. In: Vincent J-L, editor. Yearbook of intensive care and emergency medicine. Berlin/Heidelberg: Springer Berlin Heidelberg; 2000. p. 715–25.
32. Vallet B, Teboul JL, Cain S, Curtis S. Venoarterial CO(2) difference during regional ischemic or hypoxic hypoxia. J Appl Physiol (1985). 2000;89(4):1317–21.
33. Nevière R, Chagnon JL, Teboul JL, Vallet B, Wattel F. Small intestine intramucosal PCO(2) and microvascular blood flow during hypoxic and ischemic hypoxia. Crit Care Med. 2002;30(2):379–84.
34. Dubin A, Estenssoro E, Murias G, Pozo MO, Sottile JP, Barán M, et al. Intramucosal-arterial Pco2 gradient does not reflect intestinal dysoxia in anemic hypoxia. J Trauma. 2004;57(6):1211–7.
35. Bakker J, Vincent JL, Gris P, Leon M, Coffernils M, Kahn RJ. Veno-arterial carbon dioxide gradient in human septic shock. Chest. 1992;101(2):509–15.
36. Mecher CE, Rackow EC, Astiz ME, Weil MH. Venous hypercarbia associated with severe sepsis and systemic hypoperfusion. Crit Care Med. 1990;18(6):585–9.
37. van Beest PA, Lont MC, Holman ND, Loef B, Kuiper MA, Boerma EC. Central venous-arterial pCO_2 difference as a tool in resuscitation of septic patients. Intensive Care Med. 2013;39(6):1034–9.
38. De Backer D, Creteur J, Preiser JC, Dubois MJ, Vincent JL. Microvascular blood flow is altered in patients with sepsis. Am J Respir Crit Care Med. 2002;166(1):98–104.
39. De Backer D, Ospina-Tascon G, Salgado D, Favory R, Creteur J, Vincent JL. Monitoring the microcirculation in the critically ill patient: current methods and future approaches. Intensive Care Med. 2010;36(11):1813–25.
40. Zuurbier CJ, van Iterson M, Ince C. Functional heterogeneity of oxygen supply-consumption ratio in the heart. Cardiovasc Res. 1999;44(3):488–97.
41. Stein JC, Ellis CG, Ellsworth ML. Relationship between capillary and systemic venous PO2 during nonhypoxic and hypoxic ventilation. Am J Phys. 1993;265(2 Pt 2):H537–42.
42. Goldman D, Bateman RM, Ellis CG. Effect of decreased O2 supply on skeletal muscle oxygenation and O2 consumption during sepsis: role of heterogeneous capillary spacing and blood flow. Am J Physiol Heart Circ Physiol. 2006;290(6):H2277–85.
43. Ospina-Tascón GA, García Marin AF, Echeverri GJ, Bermudez WF, Madriñán-Navia H, Valencia JD, et al. Effects of dobutamine on intestinal microvascular blood flow heterogeneity and O2 extraction during septic shock. J Appl Physiol (1985). 2017;122(6):1406–17.
44. Humer MF, Phang PT, Friesen BP, Allard MF, Goddard CM, Walley KR. Heterogeneity of gut capillary transit times and impaired gut oxygen extraction in endotoxemic pigs. J Appl Physiol (1985). 1996;81(2):895–904.
45. Sakr Y, Dubois MJ, De Backer D, Creteur J, Vincent JL. Persistent microcirculatory alterations are associated with organ failure and death in patients with septic shock. Crit Care Med. 2004;32(9):1825–31.
46. De Backer D, Donadello K, Sakr Y, Ospina-Tascon G, Salgado D, Scolletta S, et al. Microcirculatory alterations in patients with severe sepsis: impact of time of assessment and relationship with outcome. Crit Care Med. 2013;41(3):791–9.
47. Creteur J, De Backer D, Sakr Y, Koch M, Vincent JL. Sublingual capnometry tracks microcirculatory changes in septic patients. Intensive Care Med. 2006;32(4):516–23.
48. Nevière R, Mathieu D, Chagnon JL, Lebleu N, Wattel F. The contrasting effects of dobutamine and dopamine on gastric mucosal perfusion in septic patients. Am J Respir Crit Care Med. 1996;154(6 Pt 1):1684–8.
49. Mallat J, Pepy F, Lemyze M, Gasan G, Vangrunderbeeck N, Tronchon L, et al. Central venous-to-arterial carbon dioxide partial pressure difference in early resuscitation from septic shock: a prospective observational study. Eur J Anaesthesiol. 2014;31(7):371–80.

50. Du W, Liu DW, Wang XT, Long Y, Chai WZ, Zhou X, et al. Combining central venous-to-arterial partial pressure of carbon dioxide difference and central venous oxygen saturation to guide resuscitation in septic shock. J Crit Care. 2013;28(6):1110.e1–5.
51. Robin E, Futier E, Pires O, Fleyfel M, Tavernier B, Lebuffe G, et al. Central venous-to-arterial carbon dioxide difference as a prognostic tool in high-risk surgical patients. Crit Care. 2015;19:227.
52. Guinot PG, Badoux L, Bernard E, Abou-Arab O, Lorne E, Dupont H. Central venous-to-arterial carbon dioxide partial pressure difference in patients undergoing cardiac surgery is not related to postoperative outcomes. J Cardiothorac Vasc Anesth. 2017;31(4):1190–6.
53. Morel J, Grand N, Axiotis G, Bouchet JB, Faure M, Auboyer C, et al. High veno-arterial carbon dioxide gradient is not predictive of worst outcome after an elective cardiac surgery: a retrospective cohort study. J Clin Monit Comput. 2016;30(6):783–9.
54. Dubin A, Ferrara G, Kanoore Edul VS, Martins E, Canales HS, Canullán C, et al. Venoarterial PCO_2-to-arteriovenous oxygen content difference ratio is a poor surrogate for anaerobic metabolism in hemodilution: an experimental study. Ann Intensive Care. 2017;7(1):65.
55. Danin PE, Bendjelid K. The venous-arterial CO_2 to arterial-venous O_2 content difference ratio: easy to monitor? J Crit Care. 2016;35:217–8.
56. Wasserman K, Beaver WL, Whipp BJ. Gas exchange theory and the lactic acidosis (anaerobic) threshold. Circulation. 1990;81(1 Suppl):II14–30.
57. Cohen IL, Sheikh FM, Perkins RJ, Feustel PJ, Foster ED. Effect of hemorrhagic shock and reperfusion on the respiratory quotient in swine. Crit Care Med. 1995;23(3):545–52.
58. Rimachi R, Bruzzi de Carvahlo F, Orellano-Jimenez C, Cotton F, Vincent JL, De Backer D. Lactate/pyruvate ratio as a marker of tissue hypoxia in circulatory and septic shock. Anaesth Intensive Care. 2012;40(3):427–32.
59. Gore DC, Jahoor F, Hibbert JM, DeMaria EJ. Lactic acidosis during sepsis is related to increased pyruvate production, not deficits in tissue oxygen availability. Ann Surg. 1996;224(1):97–102.
60. Levraut J, Ciebiera JP, Chave S, Rabary O, Jambou P, Carles M, et al. Mild hyperlactatemia in stable septic patients is due to impaired lactate clearance rather than overproduction. Am J Respir Crit Care Med. 1998;157(4 Pt 1):1021–6.
61. Tapia P, Soto D, Bruhn A, Alegría L, Jarufe N, Luengo C, et al. Impairment of exogenous lactate clearance in experimental hyperdynamic septic shock is not related to total liver hypoperfusion. Crit Care. 2015;19:188.
62. He HW, Liu DW, Long Y, Wang XT. High central venous-to-arterial CO_2 difference/arterial-central venous O2 difference ratio is associated with poor lactate clearance in septic patients after resuscitation. J Crit Care. 2016;31(1):76–81.
63. Mesquida J, Saludes P, Gruartmoner G, Espinal C, Torrents E, Baigorri F, et al. Central venous-to-arterial carbon dioxide difference combined with arterial-to-venous oxygen content difference is associated with lactate evolution in the hemodynamic resuscitation process in early septic shock. Crit Care. 2015;19:126.
64. Monnet X, Julien F, Ait-Hamou N, Lequoy M, Gosset C, Jozwiak M, et al. Lactate and venoarterial carbon dioxide difference/arterial-venous oxygen difference ratio, but not central venous oxygen saturation, predict increase in oxygen consumption in fluid responders. Crit Care Med. 2013;41(6):1412–20.
65. Mallat J, Lemyze M, Meddour M, Pepy F, Gasan G, Barrailler S, et al. Ratios of central venous-to-arterial carbon dioxide content or tension to arteriovenous oxygen content are better markers of global anaerobic metabolism than lactate in septic shock patients. Ann Intensive Care. 2016;6(1):10.
66. Jakob SM, Kosonen P, Ruokonen E, Parviainen I, Takala J. The Haldane effect – an alternative explanation for increasing gastric mucosal PCO_2 gradients? Br J Anaesth. 1999;83(5):740–6.
67. Hurley R, Mythen MG. The Haldane effect – an explanation for increasing gastric mucosal PCO_2 gradients? Br J Anaesth. 2000;85(1):167–9.
68. Alegría L, Vera M, Dreyse J, Castro R, Carpio D, Henriquez C, et al. A hypoperfusion context may aid to interpret hyperlactatemia in sepsis-3 septic shock patients: a proof-of-concept study. Ann Intensive Care. 2017;7(1):29.
69. Chioléro R, Flatt JP, Revelly JP, Jéquier E. Effects of catecholamines on oxygen consumption and oxygen delivery in critically ill patients. Chest. 1991;100(6):1676–84.
70. Teboul JL, Graini L, Boujdaria R, Berton C, Richard C. Cardiac index vs oxygen-derived parameters for rational use of dobutamine in patients with congestive heart failure. Chest. 1993;103(1):81–5.

Lactate

Ricardo Castro, David Carpio, and Glenn Hernández

M. R. Pinsky et al. (eds.), *Hemodynamic Monitoring*, Lessons from the ICU,
https://doi.org/10.1007/978-3-319-69269-2_17

Learning Objectives

The purpose of this chapter is to review the physiological basis of lactate production and clearance, its major determinants during shock states, and to provide some clues to aid in the interpretation of lactate levels in the intensive care unit (ICU) setting.

17.1 Introduction

Lactate is a key metabolic parameter that has traditionally been related to hypoperfusion and hypoxia during acute circulatory dysfunction [1–4]. In fact, persistent hyperlactatemia is a strong adverse prognostic factor during shock states, and on the contrary, a decrease in lactate levels during resuscitation is associated with enhanced change of recovery and has been considered as a marker of reperfusion [5–9]. For these reasons, lactate assessment is recommended as a fundamental part of the monitoring of the critically ill patient. Moreover, hyperlactatemia was incorporated into the latest septic shock definition [10] and proposed as a resuscitation goal by the Surviving Sepsis Campaign (SSC) [11].

In this chapter, we will review the physiological basis of lactate generation and clearance, its major determinants during shock states, and provide some clues to aid in the interpretation of lactate levels in the critically ill patient.

17.2 Anaerobic Lactate Generation

Lactate is produced in all human cells as part of intracellular handling of glucose [12–14]. The metabolism of glucose into two molecules of pyruvate generates two net adenosine triphosphate (ATP) molecules and does not require oxygen (O_2), thus being called anaerobic glycolysis. Pyruvate can be metabolized through different pathways, being the most relevant its conversion to lactate by the lactate dehydrogenase (LDH) or the mitochondrial Krebs cycle depending on the activity of the pyruvate dehydrogenase complex (PDH) and O_2 availability. The conversion of pyruvate into lactate regenerates nicotinamide adenine dinucleotide (NAD), a key cofactor to maintain glycolysis [12].

Anaerobic glycolysis is the mechanism by which hypoperfused cells can produce ATP, and its rate can increase several times compensating up to some point the actual decrease in mitochondrial function (▫ Fig. 17.1). During overt or occult hypoperfusion, increased anaerobically generated lactate is released into the circulation and can alert physicians on the presence of under-resuscitated tissues. Classical experimental data suggested that anaerobic lactate production increases when O_2 delivery falls below a critical threshold upon which O_2 consumption becomes supply dependent [3, 15]. In this context, when systemic and regional flow and tissue oxygenation are restored, lactate can be removed through specific monocarboxylate transporters (MCT) by the same cells where it was released and reconverted into pyruvate and enters the Krebs cycle, signaling a successful resuscitation [12]. However, severe microcirculatory abnormalities might preclude restoration of tissue oxygenation, and several studies have found a good correlation between these abnormalities and progressive hyperlactatemia [16, 17, 18].

Two clinically measurable variables that have been proposed as closely representing tissue hypoxia are the venous-arterial CO_2 to arterial-venous O_2 content difference ratio ($Cv\text{-}aCO_2/Da\text{-}vO_2$) [19] and the lactate/pyruvate (L/P) ratio [20]. Both ratios might constitute an expression of anaerobic metabolism at the cellular level and thus can be linked to hypoxia. Thus, they might aid in suggesting a hypoxic source of lactate.

17

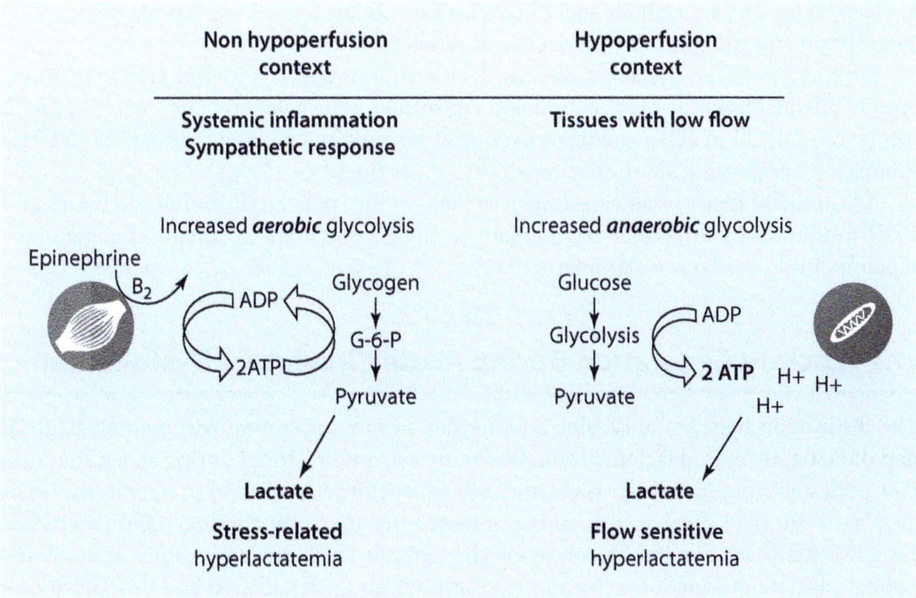

Fig. 17.1 The figure shows the two main mechanisms involved in lactate generation: anaerobic glycolysis in hypoperfused tissues and adrenergic-driven aerobic glycolysis at the muscle level

This Cv-aCO_2/Da-vO_2 ratio might be useful as a surrogate of the respiratory quotient [19, 21, 22]. A ratio ≥1.4 could identify anaerobic CO_2 generation [19, 21, 22]. A high Cv-aCO_2/Da-vO_2 ratio in the setting of hyperlactatemia may favor anaerobic metabolism as the possible source of lactate, while a normal Cv-aCO_2/Da-vO_2 ratio may suggest that lactate accumulation is due to non- hypoperfusion-related causes [19, 21, 22]. In a recent study, we observed that persistent hyperlactatemia combined with a high Cv-aCO_2/Da-vO_2 ratio was associated with severe organ dysfunctions and mortality, while simultaneous normalization of lactate and Cv-aCO_2/Da-vO_2 ratio was associated with the best outcome [19].

Several authors have suggested that pyruvate should be measured together with lactate to discriminate hypoxic from non-hypoxic sources of lactate [20, 23]. In anaerobic conditions, pyruvate is transformed to lactate, and thus the L/P ratio increases to ≥18 [23]. The L/P ratio might be one of the most reliable indexes of hypoxia in critically ill patients, but it has never been extensively used because of technical difficulties with measuring pyruvate.

17.3 Aerobic Lactate Generation

During systemic inflammation, sepsis, and shock states, activation of the compensatory adrenergic neurohormonal complex leads to an increase in epinephrine levels which is proportional to the magnitude of the injury. Epinephrine stimulates skeletal muscle beta-2 adrenergic receptors increasing cyclic AMP activity, thus promoting glycogenolysis and aerobic glycolysis with concomitant activation of the Na+/K+-ATPase pump [12, 14] (Fig. 17.1). Generated pyruvate eventually overwhelms PDH capacity during severe stress and inflammation, therefore increasing conversion to lactate. Lactate is exported and can be used as a metabolic fuel by other groups of muscle cells or remote organs such as the brain and the heart during stress and shock conditions [12].

Adrenergic-driven lactate production is an aerobic process, since it occurs in the presence of adequate muscle oxygenation and constitutes a fundamental metabolic shuttle. It can be modulated in experimental and clinical settings by blocking the Na+/K+-ATPase pump or by decreasing adrenergic tone [24, 25] (◘ Fig. 17.1).

Additionally, many other causes such as the presence of necrotic or infected tissue, and PDH inhibition by inflammatory mediators, might contribute to enhanced lactate production during systemic inflammation [12].

17.4 Lactate Generation During Acute Circulatory Dysfunction

The distinction between anaerobic and aerobic lactate generation is somehow artificial and didactic. Increased lactate production is always multifactorial during shock states. In fact, as tissue hypoperfusion evolves, the cells shift ATP generation to anaerobic glycolysis as a basic survival mechanism, and simultaneously the compensatory neurohormonal response activates aerobic glycolysis at the muscle level. In successfully resuscitated patients, lactate production decreases in relation both to reperfusion and deactivation of the adrenergic response [1]. On the contrary, persistent and progressive hyperlactatemia is a hallmark of refractory shock probably representing the sum of hypoxia, toxic hyperadrenergia, and other mechanisms [1].

17.5 Lactate Clearance and Kinetics

Approximately 1500 mmol of lactate is produced daily under physiological conditions, and the most relevant metabolizing organs are the liver and the kidneys. Together these organs account for more than 90% of systemic clearance, either by oxidation or neoglucogenesis through the Cori cycle [12–14].

Lactate clearance has been defined by a change of lactate levels between two time points and expressed as a 10–20% hourly lactate reduction or a decrease of at least 10% in 6 h during early resuscitation [12–14]. However, clearance is more strictly a pharmacokinetic term used to describe drug or endogenous substance elimination from the organism. In this sense, the term "lactate clearance" has been incorrectly used in the medical literature since a decrease in lactate levels could be induced either by a decreased aerobic or anaerobic generation or increased lactate clearance [1, 26]. Therefore, it is better to use the term "lactate kinetics" or "time course" [26].

17

A recent systematic review on lactate kinetics found a heterogeneous pattern of evolution of lactate levels in critically ill patients, where some patients decrease, others increase, and others exhibit a stable course over time in response to therapy [26]. Based on these observations, it appears that reassessing lactate every 1 or 2 h is sufficient in most clinical conditions.

The liver which is responsible for 60% of systemic lactate clearance is a vulnerable organ during sepsis-related acute circulatory dysfunction. Liver dysfunction in the context of uncontrolled sepsis or hepatosplanchnic hypoperfusion in septic shock could affect lactate handling by the liver [12, 27–29]. However, it is noteworthy that persistent hyperlactatemia has only been related to a liver dysfunction in the setting of severe shock with clear ischemia as expressed by an increase in liver enzymes or hypoglycemia or in advanced cirrhosis [27, 28]. Indeed, there is a relative lack of comprehensive physiological studies addressing the role of the liver in persistent hyperlactatemia, and experimental and clinical studies so far have provided conflicting results.

In a recent physiological study, we addressed the role of hepatosplanchnic perfusion in lactate kinetics during resuscitation [27]. A cohort of 15 hyperdynamic septic shock patients under active resuscitation were subjected to a special monitoring including serial lactate assessments, together with gastric tonometry and plasma disappearance rate of indocyanine green (ICG-PDR (LiMON, Pulsion Medical Systems, Munich, Germany)). ICG-PDR depends on liver flow and function, but since function does not change in short periods of time, a decrease in PDR from a normal range of 20–30%/min is assumed to reflect hypoperfusion. Patients with versus without an impaired lactate decrease at 6 h exhibited hepatosplanchnic hypoperfusion as revealed by both techniques (ICG-PDR (9.7 vs 19.6%/min, $p < 0.05$) and pCO_2 gap (33 vs 7.7 mmHg, $p < 0.05$)). Systemic hemodynamics was comparable between groups, once again highlighting the fact that normal macrohemodynamics does not rule out the presence of hepatosplanchnic hypoperfusion. However, the most interesting aspect is that liver enzymes including transaminases did not differentiate patients that decreased or not lactate [27]. This could mean that a potential role for liver dysfunction in abnormal lactate kinetics cannot be ruled out just by looking at systemic parameters of any kind.

A moderate impairment of whole body lactate clearance was demonstrated by Levraut et al. in a cohort of stable septic patients with mildly elevated lactate levels but without vasopressors [30]. For real clearance assessment, a bolus of 1 mmol/kg of sodium lactate was infused via a central venous catheter over 15 min. Serial arterial blood samples for lactate assessment were taken at baseline, during the infusion, and, then, sequentially for 40 min after the lactate bolus. Clearance was later analyzed using the least squares method with semi-logarithmic coordinates [30]. This study demonstrated that lactate clearance can be impaired in septic patients in a subclinical way even without evident circulatory dysfunction, suggesting a metabolic dysfunction.

To explore this subject more profoundly, we performed a series of experimental studies [31, 32]. Our objectives were to establish the kinetics and severity of exogenous lactate clearance impairment during endotoxic (LPS) shock and to explore a potential role for liver hypoperfusion in the early phase of shock [31]. After anesthesia, 12 sheep were subjected to hemodynamic/perfusion monitoring including hepatic vein and portal catheterization, and a hepatic ultrasound flow probe, and then randomized to LPS or sham. After 60 min of shock, the LPS animals were resuscitated with fluid and vasopressors. Serial assessments of all parameters including repeated exogenous lactate and sorbitol clearances were performed up to 2 h after shock resuscitation. Progressive hyperlactatemia was observed in LPS animals reaching 10.2 mmol/L at 2 h. In parallel, exogenous lactate clearance decreased to 10% of the value of sham animals at the end of the experiment. This severe impairment was not related to liver hypoperfusion since hepatic oxygen transport, consumption and extraction, total hepatic blood flow, ex vivo mitochondrial respiration, transaminases, and sorbitol clearance (a flow-related parameter) were comparable between LPS and sham animals [31]. In a subsequent study using the same model, we demonstrated that abnormalities in exogenous whole body and hepatic lactate clearance could be attenuated with the use of adrenergic modulators such as dexmedetomidine and esmolol [32]. In this later study, parallel samples of hepatic vein and portal and arterial catheters were taken for serial lactate assessment after the sodium lactate bolus, finding that there was no gradient between hepatic vein and portal lactate levels, suggesting a negligible liver extraction (non-published observations on study [31]).

In summary, it appears that the contribution of the liver to persistent hyperlactatemia might be much higher than previously thought, and the mechanisms are probably multifactorial. Doubtlessly, hepatosplanchnic ischemia could contribute in some cases especially in, but not limited to, severe septic shock and with or without alterations in classic liver enzymes.

On the other hand, a severe impairment of exogenous lactate clearance not related to liver hypoperfusion has been shown in experimental conditions. If this is adaptive or maladaptive, a metabolic dysfunction or eventually is caused by liver microcirculatory abnormalities is a matter for further research.

17.6 Transition to Hyperlactatemia

The balance between production and clearance maintains normal lactate levels even under conditions of increased lactate generation as in systemic inflammation or mild circulatory dysfunction. The transition from normal lactate levels to hyperlactatemia reflects the transition from a physiological equilibrium to a pathophysiological decompensated state affecting one or more of the mechanisms involved in normal lactate metabolism [1].

Therefore, and not surprisingly, progressive hyperlactatemia is associated to a bad prognosis in different clinical settings [2, 4, 6, 7, 33]. Indeed, since the report by Scherer in 1843, a significant amount of evidence accumulated in the literature demonstrates that progressive hyperlactatemia is associated with significant morbidity and mortality [33–35]. Many studies have emphasized the prognostic relevance of either a single elevated lactate level or impaired lactate decrease during resuscitation. Remarkably, the prognostic value of lactate levels seems to be independent from the underlying critical illness and the presence of shock and is superior to macrohemodynamic parameters in predicting outcome in different critical patients' populations, including sepsis. More recently, an analysis of a large SSC dataset confirmed that persistent hyperlactatemia is a useful predictor of outcome in severe sepsis and septic shock patients [33].

Practical Implications

1. Both the recent Sepsis-3 consensus [10] and the fourth hemodynamic recommendations of the SSC [11] fail to address a key issue: the heterogeneity of the mechanisms that can lead to progressive hyperlactatemia in patients with sepsis-related acute circulatory dysfunction [36, 37]. The apparently homogeneous risk of death among septic shock patients brought by the Sepsis-3 definition and the proposal of lactate normalization as the main resuscitation goal by SSC guidelines are highly controversial issues that lack strong physiologic foundations [35–37].

   In fact, persistent hyperlactatemia is particularly difficult to interpret in the clinical setting. As stated above, at least three possible pathogenic mechanisms might be involved: anaerobic glycolysis in hypoperfused territories especially in the presence of severe microcirculatory abnormalities [1, 17, 18, 38], stress-related adrenergic-induced aerobic glycolysis [12], and impaired hepatic lactate clearance [30–32]. The most crucial challenge is to try to identify the predominant mechanism for each patient. This is a key aspect since only some of these mechanisms such as persistent hypoperfusion might respond to systemic flow optimization, a condition that we call flow sensitivity, and others will clearly not.

To recognize a clinical pattern of hypoperfusion-related hyperlactatemia is highly relevant since optimizing systemic blood flow in this setting could revert ongoing hypoperfusion and improve prognosis. In contrast, pursuing additional resuscitation in non-hypoperfusion-related cases might lead to the toxicity of fluid overload and excessive vasoactive drugs, eventually increasing morbidity or mortality [1].

2. The rate of lactate decrease or normalization has been related to survival and tested as a goal in two important studies with conflicting results [9, 39]. More recently, Shapiro et al. reported that lactate normalization was the strongest predictor of survival (adjusted OR, 5.2; 95% CI, 1.7–15.8), followed by lactate decrease >50% in 6 h (OR, 4.0; 95% CI, 1.6–10.0) in a cohort of 187 septic shock patients subjected to early resuscitation [40].

   However, there are several unresolved aspects and concerns about the role of lactate as an appropriate resuscitation target. First, it is not clear if selecting lactate decrease versus lactate normalization as resuscitation goals is equivalent but, more importantly, if this decision leads to similar timely resolution of tissue hypoperfusion or hypoxia. Eventually, only lactate normalization may assure the absence of hypoxia, although this is controversial [40]. Second, since non-hypoperfusion-related causes of hyperlactatemia might predominate in an unknown number of patients, this could lead to over-resuscitation in at least some of them as stated above. Third, the kinetics of recovery of lactate might exhibit a biphasic pattern, and therefore, the real-time response of lactate to fluid challenges could be not straightforward depending on the hypoperfusion context [41]. Some survivors might even normalize lactate only after 24 h of evolution [41].

3. We recently proposed that a simultaneous analysis of central venous O_2 saturation ($ScvO_2$), central venous-arterial pCO_2 gradient ($P(cv\text{-}a)CO_2$), and peripheral perfusion assessed by the capillary refill time (CRT) might be helpful in suggesting a hypoperfusion context for patients with or without hyperlactatemia [1] (◘ Fig. 17.2). The presence of a low $ScvO_2$ clearly indicates an imbalance in the O_2 transport/O_2 consumption relationship [1]. In the case of $P(cv\text{-}a)CO_2$, an inverse curvilinear relationship between $Pcv\text{-}aCO_2$ and cardiac output exists, highlighting the importance of blood flow on venous CO_2 accumulation [1, 42]. Even more, high $Pcv\text{-}aCO_2$ could potentially identify septic patients who remain inadequately resuscitated despite achieving oxygen metabolism targets, reinforcing the notion of $P(cv\text{-}a)CO_2$ as a better marker of global perfusion [42]. The assessment of peripheral perfusion may provide additional physiological information. An abnormal peripheral perfusion may be caused by adrenergic-induced skin vasoconstriction secondary to a low systemic blood flow and should prompt at least a reassessment of preload status [43].

   In a retrospective proof-of-concept study in 90 hyperlactatemic septic shock patients, we tested if these criteria could effectively identify a subgroup with higher risk [44]. Patients exhibiting either a $ScvO_2 < 70\%$, a $P(cv\text{-}a)CO_2 \geq 6$ mmHg, or a CRT ≥ 4 sec at ICU admission were categorized as patients with a hypoperfusion context. Seventy patients met this category and required more vasopressors and inodilators. They also tended to have higher ICU and hospital length of stay, mechanical ventilation days, positive fluid balance, and rescue therapy requirements. Only 1 of 20 hyperlactatemic patients without a hypoperfusion context died (5%) compared to 11 of the 70 with hypoperfusion-related hyperlactatemia (16%), although this difference fell short of significance [44].

4. From a theoretical point of view, these three easily assessable perfusion-related variables offer an important advantage over lactate as potential targets for fluid resuscitation in septic shock patients: they are clearly flow-sensitive and exhibit a faster recovery rate after systemic blood flow optimization. In other words, these parameters might clear in minutes in fluid-responsive patients as compared to lactate which sometimes takes hours to recover. We demonstrated this point by analyzing the kinetics of recovery of these parameters in a cohort of ultimately surviving septic shock patients. $ScvO_2$, $P(cv\text{-}a)CO_2$, and CRT were already normal in almost 70% of the patients after 2 h of fluid resuscitation, as compared with only 15% in the case of lactate [41].

   However, there are also a couple of drawbacks for some of these perfusion-related flow-sensitive parameters. $ScvO_2$ is a complex physiological variable. It was widely used until recently as the resuscitation goal in critically ill patients [1], although several limitations may preclude a straightforward interpretation of its changes [1]. For instance, normal or even supranormal $ScvO_2$ values do not rule out global or regional tissue hypoxia for several reasons that have been highlighted elsewhere, but that include severe microcirculatory derangements impairing tissue O_2 extraction capabilities [1]. Vallee et al. found persistent abnormal $P(cv\text{-}a)CO_2$ values in 50% of septic shock patients who had already achieved normal $ScvO_2$ values after initial resuscitation [42]. Nevertheless, in some hyperdynamic states, a high efferent venous blood flow could be sufficient to wash out the global CO_2 generation from hypoperfused tissues, and thus, $Pcv\text{-}aCO_2$ could be normal despite the presence of tissue hypoxia [1]. Another problem for these two variables is that they necessarily require a central venous catheterization to be assessed, a task that might be complex to perform in limited-resource settings or emergency departments (ED).

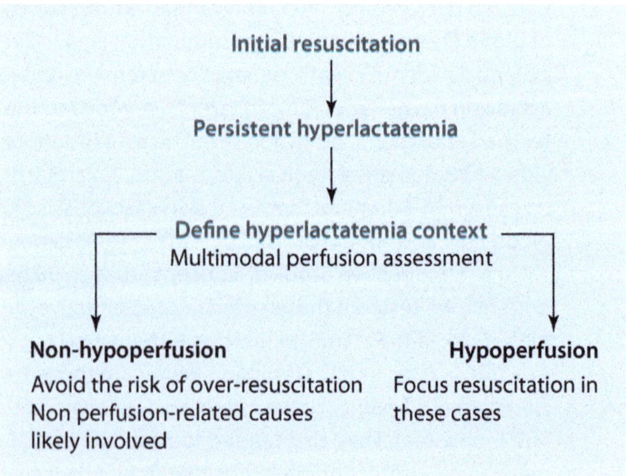

Fig. 17.2 A simple algorithm to approach persistent hyperlactatemia based on the presence of a hypoperfusion context

17

Conclusions

Persistent hyperlactatemia after shock resuscitation is associated to increased morbidity and mortality but is particularly difficult to interpret in the clinical setting. At least three possible pathogenic mechanisms might be involved: anaerobic glycolysis in hypoperfused territories, stress-related aerobic glycolysis, and impaired hepatic lactate clearance. A multimodal perfusion assessment might aid in suggesting a hypoperfusion context in patients with hyperlactatemia to focus resuscitation in these cases and avoid the risk of over-resuscitation when other non-perfusion-related causes are likely involved.

Take-Home Messages

- Lactate is a key metabolic parameter that has traditionally been related to hypoperfusion and hypoxia during acute circulatory dysfunction.
- Lactate assessment is recommended as a fundamental part of the monitoring of the critically ill patient.
- Persistent hyperlactatemia after shock resuscitation is associated to increased morbidity and mortality.
- Persistent hyperlactatemia is particularly difficult to interpret in the clinical setting. At least three possible pathogenic mechanisms might be involved: anaerobic glycolysis in hypoperfused territories, stress-related adrenergic-induced aerobic glycolysis, and impaired hepatic lactate clearance.
- A multimodal perfusion assessment might aid in suggesting a hypoperfusion context in patients with persistent hyperlactatemia.

References

1. Hernandez G, Bruhn A, Castro R, Regueira T. The holistic view on perfusion monitoring in septic shock. Curr Opin Crit Care. 2012;18:280–6.
2. Bakker J, Nijsten MW, Jansen TC. Clinical use of lactate monitoring in critically ill patients. Ann Intensive Care. 2013;3:12.
3. Bakker J, Vincent JL. The oxygen-supply dependency phenomenon is associated with increased blood lactate levels. J Crit Care. 1991;6:152–9.
4. Bakker J, Coffernils M, Leon M, Gris P, Vincent JL. Blood lactate levels are superior to oxygen-derived variables in predicting outcome in human septic shock. Chest. 1991;99:956–62.
5. Nguyen HB, Rivers EP, Knoblich BP, Jacobsen G, Muzzin A, Ressler JA, et al. Early lactate clearance is associated with improved outcome in severe sepsis and septic shock. Crit Care Med. 2004;32:1637–42.
6. Arnold RC, Shapiro NI, Jones AE, Schorr C, Pope J, Casner E, et al. Multicenter study of early lactate clearance as a determinant of survival in patients with presumed sepsis. Shock. 2009;32:35–9.
7. Mikkelsen ME, Miltiades AN, Gaieski DF, Goyal M, Fuchs BD, Shah CV, et al. Serum lactate is associated with mortality in severe sepsis independent of organ failure and shock. Crit Care Med. 2009;37:1670–7.
8. Gu WJ, Wang F, Bakker J, Tang L, Liu JC. The effect of goal-directed therapy on mortality in patients with sepsis - earlier is better: a meta-analysis of randomized controlled trials. Crit Care. 2014;18:570.
9. Jansen TC, van Bommel J, Schoonderbeek FJ, Visser SJS, van der Klooster JM, Lima AP, et al. Early lactate-guided therapy in intensive care unit patients: a multicenter, open-label, randomized controlled trial. Am J Respir Crit Care Med. 2010;182:752–61.
10. Singer M, Deutschman CS, Seymour CW, Shankar-Hari M, Annane D, Bauer M, et al. The third international consensus definitions for sepsis and septic shock (Sepsis-3). JAMA. 2016;315:801–10.

11. Rhodes A, Evans LE, Alhazzani W, Levy MM, Antonelli M, Ferrer R, et al. Surviving Sepsis Campaign: international guidelines for management of sepsis and septic shock: 2016. Intensive Care Med. 2017;43:304–77.
12. Garcia-Alvarez M, Marik P, Bellomo R. Sepsis-associated hyperlactatemia. Crit Care. 2014;18:503.
13. Cori CF. Mammalian carbohydrate metabolism. Physiol Rev. 1931;11:143–275.
14. Levy B. Lactate and shock state: the metabolic view. Curr Opin Crit Care. 2006;12:315–21.
15. Friedman G, De Backer D, Shahla M, Vincent JL. Oxygen supply dependency can characterize septic shock. Intensive Care Med. 1998;24:118–23.
16. De Backer D, Donadello K, Sakr Y, Ospina-Tascon G, Salgado D, Scolletta S, et al. Microcirculatory alterations in patients with severe sepsis: impact of time of assessment and relationship with outcome. Crit Care Med. 2013;41:791–9.
17. Hernandez G, Boerma EC, Dubin A, Bruhn A, Koopmans M, Edul VK, et al. Severe abnormalities in microvascular perfused vessel density are associated to organ dysfunctions and mortality and can be predicted by hyperlactatemia and norepinephrine requirements in septic shock patients. J Crit Care. 2013;28:538.e9–14.
18. Hernandez G, Bruhn A, Ince C. Microcirculation in sepsis: new perspectives. Curr Vasc Pharmacol. 2013;11:161–9.
19. Ospina-Tascón GA, Umaña M, Bermúdez W, Bautista-Rincón DF, Hernandez G, Bruhn A, et al. Combination of arterial lactate levels and venous-arterial CO_2 to arterial-venous O_2 content difference ratio as markers of resuscitation in patients with septic shock. Intensive Care Med. 2015;41:796–805.
20. Rimachi R, Bruzzi de Carvahlo F, Orellano-Jimenez C, Cotton F, Vincent JL, De Backer D. Lactate/pyruvate ratio as a marker of tissue hypoxia in circulatory and septic shock. Anaesth Intensive Care. 2012;40:427–32.
21. Ospina-Tascón GA, Hernández G, Cecconi M. Understanding the venous-arterial CO_2 to arterial-venous O_2 content difference ratio. Intensive Care Med. 2016;42:1801–4.
22. Monnet X, Julien F, Ait-Hamou N, Lequoy M, Gosset C, Jozwiak M, et al. Lactate and venoarterial carbon dioxide difference/arterial-venous oxygen difference ratio, but not central venous oxygen saturation, predict increase in oxygen consumption in fluid responders. Crit Care Med. 2013;41:1412–20.
23. Minton J, Sidebotham DA. Hyperlactatemia and cardiac surgery. J Extra Corpor Technol. 2017;49:7–15.
24. Levy B, Desebbe O, Montemont C, Gibot S. Increased aerobic glycolysis through beta2 stimulation is a common mechanism involved in lactate formation during shock states. Shock. 2008;30:417–21.
25. Levy B, Gibot S, Franck P, Cravoisy A, Bollaert PE. Relation between muscle Na+K+ ATPase activity and raised lactate concentrations in septic shock: a prospective study. Lancet. 2005;365:871–5.
26. Vincent JL, Quintairos E, Silva A, Couto L Jr, Taccone FS. The value of blood lactate kinetics in critically ill patients: a systematic review. Crit Care. 2016;20:257.
27. Hernandez G, Regueira T, Bruhn A, Castro R, Rovegno M, Fuentealba A, et al. Relationship of systemic, hepatosplanchnic, and microcirculatory perfusion parameters with 6-hour lactate clearance in hyperdynamic septic shock patients: an acute, clinical-physiological, pilot study. Ann Intensive Care. 2012;2:44.
28. Mizock B. The hepatosplanchnic area and hyperlactatemia: a tale of two lactates. Crit Care Med. 2001;29:447–9.
29. De Backer D, Creteur J, Silva E, Vincent JL. The hepatosplanchnic area is not a common source of lactate in patients with severe sepsis. Crit Care Med. 2001;29:256–61.
30. Levraut J, Ciebiera JP, Chave S, Rabary O, Jambou P, Carles M, et al. Mild hyperlactatemia in stable septic patients is due to impaired lactate clearance rather than overproduction. Am J Respir Crit Care Med. 1998;157:1021–6.
31. Tapia P, Soto D, Bruhn A, Alegría L, Jarufe N, Luengo C, et al. Impairment of exogenous lactate clearance in experimental hyperdynamic septic shock is not related to total liver hypoperfusion. Crit Care. 2015;19:188.
32. Hernández G, Tapia P, Alegría L, Soto D, Luengo C, Gomez J, et al. Effects of dexmedetomidine and esmolol on systemic hemodynamics and exogenous lactate clearance in early experimental septic shock. Crit Care. 2016;20:234.
33. Casserly B, Phillips GS, Schorr C, Dellinger RP, Townsend SR, Osborn TM, et al. Lactate measurements in sepsis-induced tissue hypoperfusion: results from the Surviving Sepsis Campaign database. Crit Care Med. 2015;43:567–73.

34. Kompanje EJO, Jansen TC, van der Hoven B, Bakker J. The first demonstration of lactic acid in human blood in shock by Johann Joseph Scherer (1814–1869) in January 1843. Intensive Care Med. 2007;33:1967–71.
35. Bakker J. Lost in translation: on lactate, hypotension, sepsis-induced tissue hypoperfusion, quantitative resuscitation and Surviving Sepsis Campaign bundles. Crit Care Med. 2015;43:705–6.
36. Bakker J, de Backer D, Hernandez G. Lactate-guided resuscitation saves lives: we are not sure. Intensive Care Med. 2016;42:472–4.
37. Hernández G, Teboul JL. Fourth Surviving Sepsis Campaign's hemodynamic recommendations: a step forward or a return to chaos? Crit Care. 2017;21:133.
38. Vellinga NAR, Boerma EC, Koopmans M, Donati A, Dubin A, Shapiro NI, et al. Mildly elevated lactate levels are associated with microcirculatory flow abnormalities and increased mortality: a microSOAP post hoc analysis. Crit Care. 2017;21:255.
39. Jones AE, Shapiro NI, Trzeciak S, Arnold RC, Claremont HA, Kline JA, et al. Lactate clearance vs central venous oxygen saturation as goals of early sepsis therapy: a randomized clinical trial. JAMA. 2010;303:739–46.
40. Puskarich MA, Trzeciak S, Shapiro NI, Albers AB, Heffner AC, Kline JA, et al. Whole blood lactate kinetics in patients undergoing quantitative resuscitation for severe sepsis and septic shock. Chest. 2013;143:1548–53.
41. Hernandez G, Luengo C, Bruhn A, Kattan E, Friedman G, Ospina-Tascon GA, et al. When to stop septic shock resuscitation: clues from a dynamic perfusion monitoring. Ann Intensive Care. 2014;4:30.
42. Vallée F, Vallet B, Mathe O, Parraguette J, Mari A, Silva S, et al. Central venous-to-arterial carbon dioxide difference: an additional target for goal-directed therapy in septic shock? Intensive Care Med. 2008;34:2218–25.
43. Lara B, Enberg L, Ortega M, Leon P, Kripper C, Aguilera P, et al. Capillary refill time during fluid resuscitation in patients with sepsis-related hyperlactatemia at the emergency department is related to mortality. PLoS One. 2017;12:e0188548.
44. Alegría L, Vera M, Dreyse J, Castro R, Carpio D, Henriquez C. A hypoperfusion context may aid to interpret hyperlactatemia in sepsis-3 septic shock patients: a proof-of-concept study. Ann Intensive Care. 2017;7:29.

The Techniques

Contents

Cardiac Ultrasound Examination in Shock

Guillaume Geri and Antoine Vieillard-Baron

M. R. Pinsky et al. (eds.), *Hemodynamic Monitoring*, Lessons from the ICU,
https://doi.org/10.1007/978-3-319-69269-2_18

Learning Objectives

Critical care echocardiography (CCE) is very suitable to manage patients with circulatory failure, especially when associated with respiratory failure.

Transesophageal echocardiography (TEE) is more suitable than transthoracic echocardiography (TTE) for hemodynamic monitoring when performed in intubated patients, allowing reproducible and sequential hemodynamic assessments. TEE allows an easy evaluation of four important parameters: the respiratory variation of the superior vena cava (SVC), the LV systolic function, the RV size, and the existence of a paradoxical septal motion. Since echocardiography only allows a discontinuous hemodynamic monitoring, it has to be associated with a more continuous device as invasive blood pressure monitoring.

In this chapter, we will describe different ICU situations where TEE is useful to evaluate hemodynamic instability in ICU mechanically ventilated patients treated for respiratory and circulatory failures.

18.1 Introduction

Echocardiography is increasingly being used in the critically ill patients. Papolos et al. recently reported a 3.4% increase per year of hospital use of echocardiography in the USA between 2001 and 2011 and a global volume of more than 7,000,000 echocardiographic (echo) examinations performed in the Nationwide Inpatient Sample (NIS) population [1]. Interestingly, critical care echocardiography (CCE) was more frequently used than the pulmonary artery catheter in patients with sepsis or congestive heart failure [1]. Similar results were obtained from French data in ARDS patients with a significant increase over time [2]. CCE is very suitable to manage patients with respiratory or circulatory failure [3]. It may have a direct diagnostic and therapeutic impact. In a mini review, including 2508 patients, on the use and safety of transesophageal echocardiography (TEE) in general ICU, TEE was mostly performed in the case of hemodynamic instability and had a diagnostic impact in 88.4% of cases [4]. TEE diagnosed left ventricular (LV) dysfunction in 27% and right ventricular (RV) dysfunction and hypovolemia in 11% and 16%, respectively. In 68.5% of patients, the findings had therapeutic implications, either surgical interventions or changes in medical therapy. A surgical intervention without additional investigations was performed in 5.6% [4].

In 2011, a consensus of 16 experts in the field of hemodynamic monitoring has recognized CCE as a true hemodynamic monitoring device, although discontinuous [5]. An echo study has to be done very quickly in case of hemodynamic instability after having evaluated whether the patient is obviously fluid responsive with a low central venous pressure [5]. While echocardiography is operator-dependent, TEE is expected to be less operator-dependent than transthoracic echocardiography (TTE) because the windows for visualization, movement artifact, and anatomical landmark are more precise and regular. Thus, TEE is more suitable than TTE for hemodynamic monitoring when performed in intubated patients, allowing reproducible and sequential hemodynamic assessments [6]. Rather than performing many measurements, it has also been reported that TEE may allow the intensivist to obtain a qualitative and accurate hemodynamic evaluation based on four main parameters to know the respiratory variation of the superior vena cava (SVC), the LV systolic function, the RV size, and the existence of a paradoxical septal motion [7].

Since echocardiography only allows a discontinuous hemodynamic monitoring, it has to be associated with a more continuous device. Then, combining invasive blood pressure monitoring and CCE is mandatory, especially in mechanically ventilated ARDS patients [8]. While the former may be used as a "warning" signal, the latter helps intensivists to understand the reason of a low blood pressure or pulse pressure variations (PPV). Furthermore, CCE is not blindly performed because of abnormal vital signs suggesting poor organ perfusion, as skin mottling, elevated lactate, oliguria, etc. Thus, CCE really led to a paradigm shift from an invasive, quantitative, and continuous hemodynamic monitoring to a less invasive, qualitative, discontinuous, and functional one [9, 10]. This is why single measurement of cardiac output is probably less informative than longitudinal evaluation (before/after fluids, before/after dobutamine) for hemodynamic monitoring using CCE. In a systematic review, Wetterslev et al. reported that cardiac output measurements using either echocardiography or thermodilution were not interchangeable while trends were [11].

In this chapter, rather than writing another review on the use of CCE in patients with shock, we prefer to illustrate and briefly discuss four typical frequently encountered ICU situations, where CCE is very useful for treatment adjustment: (i) detection of fluid responsiveness (ii and iii), detection of RV failure in ARDS patients and its consequence, and (iv) septic cardiomyopathy involving the left ventricle. While these cases are illustrated with TEE, similar information may be obtained using TTE except for SVC but with a greater operator dependency.

Clinical Vignette 1: Detection of Fluid Responsiveness (Fig. 18.1)

A 35-year-old man was admitted to the ICU after drug poisoning and aspiration. He was initially intubated and ventilated in zero PEEP without hemodynamic instability. The systolic arterial pressure was 90 mmHg and the serum lactate level non-elevated. The initial evaluation reported a PPV of 9% with mild decrease in RV stroke volume during tidal ventilation and respiratory variation of the SVC. After applying a PEEP (required by severe hypoxemia), the cardiac index (CI) dropped, as well as the blood pressure, and the PPV increased. TEE evaluation demonstrated a complete collapse of SVC at inspiration with a huge decrease in RV stroke volume. After fluid expansion, CI increased, and SVC collapse disappeared, as well as the respiratory variation of RV stroke volume leading to hemodynamic improvement.

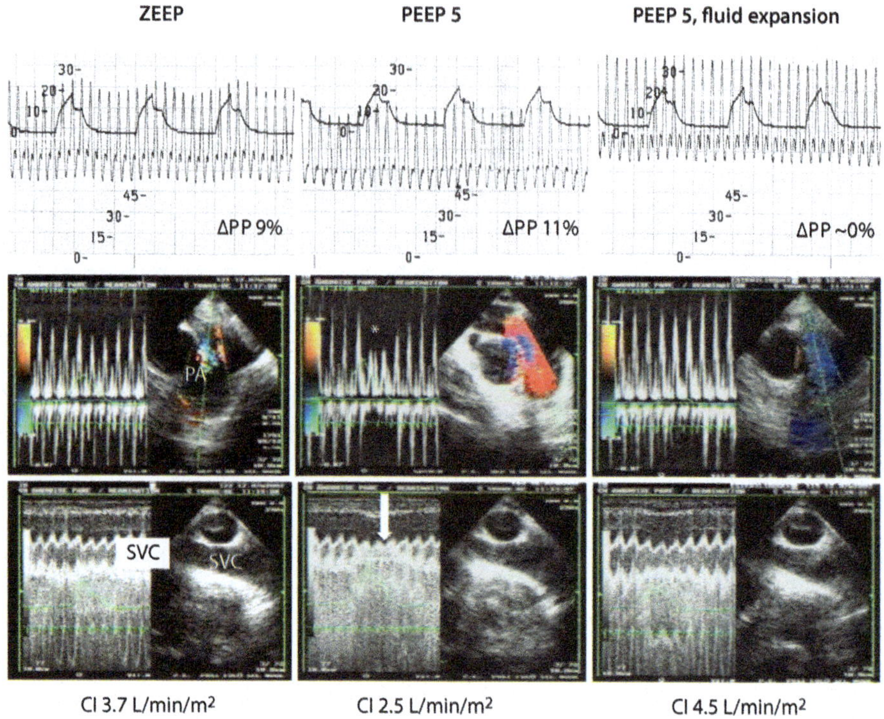

Fig. 18.1 SVC collapses (arrow) and decreases in RV stroke (asterisk) during tidal ventilation using PEEP 5 cmH_2O compared to zero PEEP (ZEEP). These findings disappeared after fluid expansion. CI cardiac index, PEEP positive expiratory pressure, ΔPP respiratory variations of pulse pressure, SVC superior vena cava, PA pulmonary artery

Take-Home Messages

This case illustrates different important points for hemodynamic management with echo.

- The need for fluids may change according to the respiratory settings. Echo evaluation has then to be done with regard to the mechanical ventilation settings, and a reassessment is required as soon as these settings are modified.
- Pulsed-wave Doppler into the main pulmonary artery allows recording the respiratory changes of RV stroke volume. When significant, it gives the intensivist the hemodynamic information that there is some "bad" interaction between the right ventricle and the ventilator, which is mediated either by a lack of enough fluid content into the thorax (preload effect) or by a RV systolic overload (afterload effect; see also Vignette 2) [8]. Such a cyclic decrease in RV stroke volume is the cause of the observed PPV and may be corrected by fluid expansion in this clinical case.
- TEE may be used before and after fluid expansion, when decided, to look for respiratory variations of SVC and RV stroke volume, as well as the efficacy of such a fluid challenge (increased CI).
- SVC respiratory variations are the most specific parameter of fluid responsiveness as recently reported in a multicenter study prospectively including 540 unselected patients with shock [12]. This parameter requires a TEE approach.

Clinical Vignette 2: Detection of RV Failure I (Fig. 18.2)

A 55-year-old man was admitted to the ICU for septic shock related to severe pneumonia. He rapidly required to be intubated and ventilated with a lung protective approach. At the time of TEE evaluation, PaO_2/FiO_2 was 110 mmHg and $PaCO_2$ 55 mmHg. The patient was in shock with a low blood pressure and a high lactate level (5 mmol/L). Significant PPV were observed. TEE study was performed and reported RV failure with a pattern of severe acute cor pulmonale (ACP) with a huge RV dilatation. Fluid expansion was inefficient and even deteriorated the patient with an increase in PPV and an enlargement of the RV. Norepinephrine was then started, allowing to increase blood pressure, to correct PPV, and to slightly decrease the RV size.

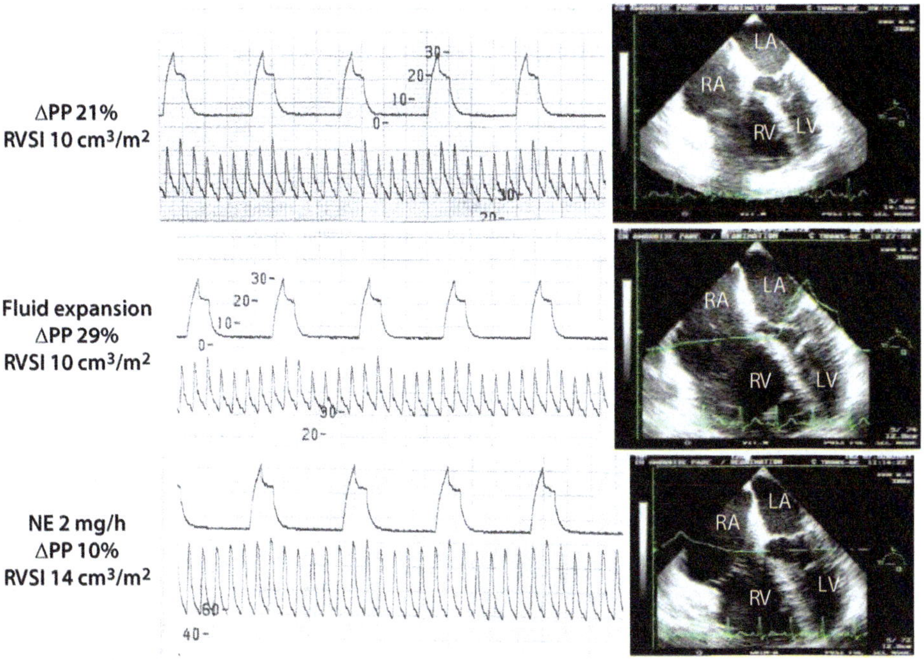

Fig. 18.2 Significant respiratory variations of pulse pressure (ΔPP) are observed in the first panel (top) as well as an acute cor pulmonale pattern with right ventricle dilatation. After fluid expansion (second panel, medium), hemodynamic worsened with regard to an increase of ΔPP and an enlargement of the right ventricle. After norepinephrine infusion (third panel, bottom), ΔPP was corrected and the right ventricle size decreased. RVSI right ventricle stroke index, NE norepinephrine, LA left atrium, LV left ventricle, RA right atrium, RV right ventricle

Take-Home Messages

This case illustrates different important points for hemodynamic management with echo.

- In this patient, PPV was due to RV failure and the related respiratory variations in RV stroke volume (not reported here). TEE allowed the intensivist to understand the cause of such shock with significant PPV.
- Fluid expansion does not permit in this situation any hemodynamic improvement and even may induce deterioration. Based on TEE evaluation, it is useless. It is usually recommended not to infuse fluids when the right ventricle is

severely dilated [13]. A clinical study done in patients with massive pulmonary embolism has reported that the higher the RV size the lower the increase in CO induced after fluid expansion [14].

- Norepinephrine is a powerful therapy to improve RV function. It increases blood pressure and then RV coronary blood flow by stopping the vicious circle of functional RV ischemia. At small or moderate dose, its potential vasoconstriction of the pulmonary circulation is very limited.

Clinical Vignette 3: Detection of RV Failure II (Fig. 18.3)

A 41-year-old man was admitted to the ICU for acute respiratory failure due to pneumonia. He was quickly intubated and ventilated. He developed an ARDS. Few hours after intubation, he developed a circulatory failure with a systolic arterial pressure (SAP) of 90 mmHg, a heart rate of 128 bpm, and an elevated serum lactate level. At the time of TEE examination, the plateau pressure and driving pressure were 33 cmH_2O and 28 cmH_2O, respectively. Blood gas analysis revealed a PaO_2/FiO_2 ratio of 100 and a $PaCO_2$ of 67 mmHg. TEE showed an enlargement of the right ventricle associated with a paradoxical septal motion, named *acute cor pulmonale* (ACP). Based on the echo findings, tidal volume was slightly decreased to limit plateau and driving pressures. In the same time, instrumental dead space was removed in order to control hypercapnia. Hemodynamics very rapidly improved (SAP 123 mmHg, heart rate 90 bmp) as the RV size decreased. The paradoxical septal motion did not completely disappear but was less pronounced.

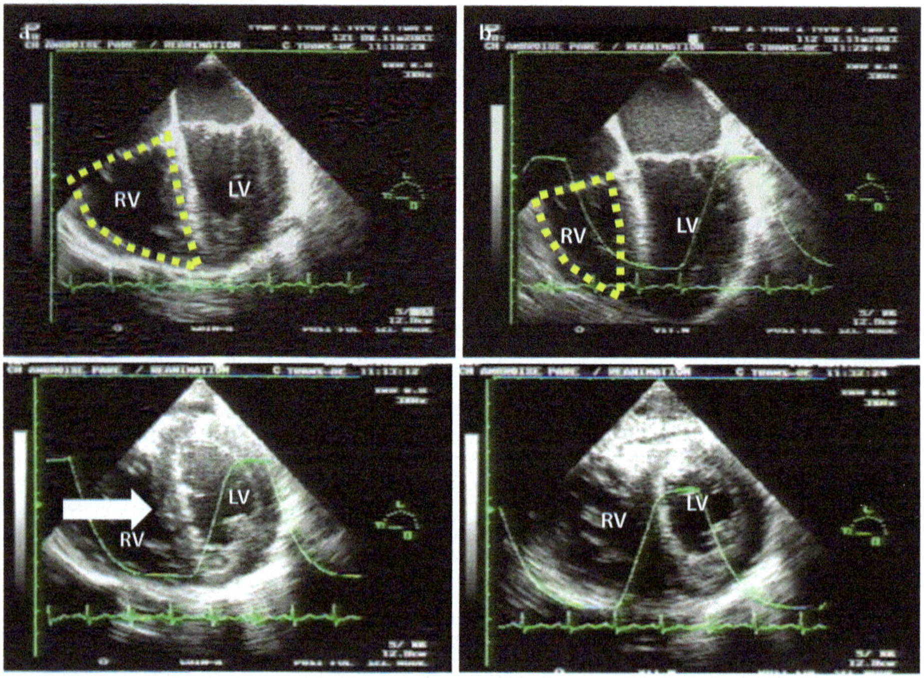

Fig. 18.3 Panel **a**: Enlargement of the right ventricle on a transverse mid-esophageal view (top) with paradoxical septal motion on a transgastric short-axis view (arrow, bottom). Panel **b**: After adaptation of respiratory settings (see the manuscript), the right ventricular size decreased, and paradoxical septal motion was less pronounced. LV left ventricle, RV right ventricle

Take-Home Messages

This case illustrates different important points for hemodynamic management with echo.

- RV failure, named ACP, is frequently encountered in ARDS treated with protective ventilation. A 22% incidence has been reported in 752 patients [15]. This means that a systematic detection has to be done by echocardiography, at least during the first 3 days following mechanical ventilation, especially in the case of circulatory failure. TEE has been reported to be more sensitive than TTE for detection [16]. This is generally true that TEE is more efficient than TTE in patients with high PEEP, fluid overload, and chest tubes [17].
- ACP may lead to hemodynamic compromise [18] and then must be corrected.
- We have reported that four risk factors are associated with RV failure, pneumonia as the cause of ARDS, driving pressure ≥ 18 cmH$_2$O, PaO$_2$/FiO$_2$ < 150, and PaCO$_2$ ≥ 48 mmHg [15]. The incidence of ACP increases with the number of risk factors. Thus, managing hemodynamics using CCE in such patients also means to adapt the respiratory strategy to the RV function.

Clinical Vignette 4: Septic Cardiomyopathy (Fig. 18.4)

A 66-year-old woman was admitted to the ICU for a septic shock related to urinary tract infection. She was intubated and mechanically ventilated. After fluid optimization, she was still in shock with a low blood pressure (SAP 75 mmHg, base deficit 19 mmol/L). Despite the absence of ARDS, TEE demonstrated RV failure with an ACP pattern. RV function as well as hemodynamics was corrected by infusion of high-dose norepinephrine and continuous veno-venous hemofiltration (see also Vignette 3). A few hours later, a worsening of hemodynamics occurred with new lactic acidosis. TEE now demonstrated severe LV systolic dysfunction. Dobutamine was then infused at small dose, allowing increase in LV ejection fraction, correction of acidosis, and hemodynamic stabilization.

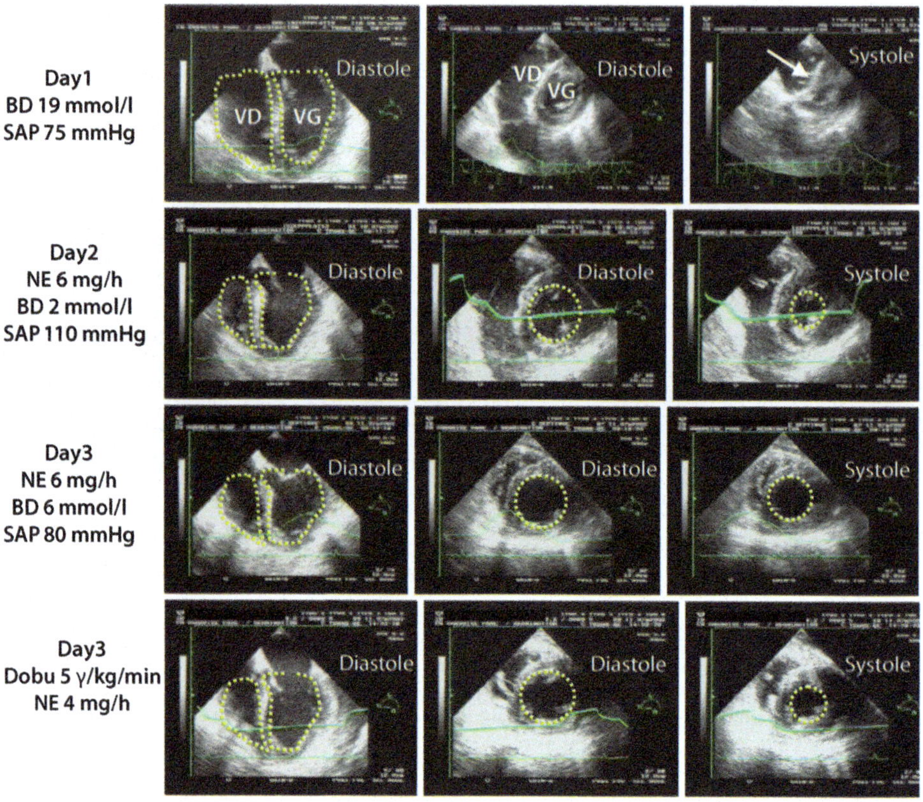

Fig. 18.4 Left column: Transverse mid-esophageal view; middle column, transgastric short-axis view in diastole; right column, transgastric short-axis view in systole. Right ventricular failure and acute cor pulmonale pattern were present at day 1 (top). After norepinephrine infusion, RV function normalized at day 2 but was followed by secondary worsening related to LV systolic dysfunction (day 3). Dobutamine infusion restored LV systolic function (bottom). BD base deficit, SAP systolic arterial pressure, RV right ventricle, LV left ventricle, NE norepinephrine, Dobu dobutamine. Arrow marks the paradoxical septal motion. Dotted yellow lines mark RV and LV endocardial border

Take-Home Messages

This case illustrates different important points for hemodynamic management with echo.

- Septic cardiomyopathy may injure the right and the left side.
- The most efficient way to detect such a complication is to use CCE. In particular, S_cVO_2 has been reported to be normal in the case of severe LV systolic dysfunction with low cardiac index in septic shock patients [19].
- ACP pattern may be observed in the absence of ARDS, especially when sepsis and profound acidosis, which impair RV systolic function, are associated with positive pressure ventilation which increases RV afterload.
- Different hemodynamic profiles may occur at different time during the evolution of a septic shock. This requires frequent reassessment of cardiac function by CCE.
- Infusion of small dose of dobutamine, when appropriate (poor organ perfusion, low LV ejection fraction, optimization of fluid resuscitation), is useful to improve hemodynamics despite no evidence of decreased ICU mortality in this setting has been published so far.

Conclusion

CCE is an amazing device for monitoring hemodynamics in the most complicated situations as septic shock and ARDS. It may allow to independently diagnose the need for more fluids, for norepinephrine or dobutamine infusion, or for adjustment of the mechanical ventilation settings. Since CCE is never blindly performed, intensivists must remind that CCE is a help to improve patients' management and not a goal for itself. In other words, intensivists should not treat an "abnormal" echo picture but have to interpret echo studies in the light of the clinical situation. Since CCE is a discontinuous hemodynamic monitoring device, it always has to be associated with a continuous monitoring of invasive blood pressure, as well as serial dosage of serum lactate or base deficit, at least in the most severe patients. In the future, development of cheap esophageal echo probe that could be left in place into the patient is desirable [20].

Take-Home Messages

- CCE is key to manage patients with circulatory failure.
- TEE is probably more suitable than TTE in ventilated patients for hemodynamic monitoring, as it is less operator dependent.
- Echo evaluation may be very simply based on four parameters: SVC respiratory variation, RV size, LV systolic function, and movement of the interventricular septum.

References

1. Papolos A, Narula J, Bavishi C, Chaudry F, Sengupta P. U.S. Hospital use of echocardiography. Insights from the nationwide inpatient sample. J Am Coll Cardiol. 2016;67(5):502–11.
2. Dres M, Austin P, Pham T, Aegerter P, Guidet B, Demoule A, Vieillard-Baron A, Brochard L, Geri G. Acute respiratory distress syndrome cases volume and intensive care unit mortality in medical patients. Crit Care Med. 2018; 46(1): e33–e40 [Epub ahead of print].
3. De Backer D, Cholley B, Slama M, Vieillard-Baron A, Vignon P, editors. Hemodynamic monitoring using echocardiography in the critically ill. Berlin/Heidelberg: Springer-Verlag; 2011.
4. Hüttemann E, Schelenz C, Kara F, Chatzinikolaou K, Reinhart K. The use and safety of transesophageal echocardiography in the general ICU – a mini review. Acta Anaesthesiol Scand. 2004;48(7):827–36.
5. Vincent JL, Rhodes A, Perel A, Martin GS, Della Rocca G, Vallet B, Pinsky MR, Hofer CK, Teboul JL, de Boode WP, Scolletta S, Vieillard-Baron A, De Backer D, Walley KR, Maggiorini M, Singer M. Clinical review: update on hemodynamic monitoring – a consensus of 16. Crit Care. 2011;15(4):229.
6. Vignon P, Merz TM, Vieillard-Baron A. Ten reasons for performing hemodynamic monitoring using transesophageal echocardiography. Intensive Care Med. 2017;43(7):1048–51.
7. Vieillard-Baron A, Charron C, Chergui K, Peyrouset O, Jardin F. Bedside echocardiographic evaluation of hemodynamics in sepsis: is a qualitative evaluation sufficient? Intensive Care Med. 2006;32(10):1547–52.
8. Vieillard-Baron A, Matthay M, Teboul JL, Bein T, Schultz M, Magder S, Marini JJ. Experts' opinion on management of hemodynamics in ARDS patients: focus on the effects of mechanical ventilation. Intensive Care Med. 2016;42:739–49.
9. Jardin F. Ventricular interdependence: how does it impact on hemodynamic evaluation in clinical practice? Intensive Care Med. 2003;29(3):361–3.
10. Pinsky MR, Payen D. Functional hemodynamic monitoring. Crit Care. 2005;9(6):566–72.
11. Wetterslev M, Moller-Sorensen H, Johansen RR, Perner A. Systematic review of cardiac output measurements by echocardiography vs. thermodilution: the techniques are not interchangeable. Intensive Care Med. 2016;42(8):1223–33.
12. Vignon P, Repesse X, Bégot E, Léger J, jacob C, Bouferrache K, Slama M, Prat G, Vieillard-Baron A. Comparison of echocardiographic indices used to predict fluid responsiveness in ventilated patients. Am J Respir Crit Care Med. 2017;195(8):1022–32.

13. Teboul JL. SRLF experts recommendations; indications of volume resuscitation during circulatory failure. Reanimation. 2004;13:255–63.
14. Mercat A, Diehl JL, Meyer G, Teboul JL, Sors H. Hemodynamic effects of fluid loading in acute massive pulmonary embolism. Crit Care Med. 1999;27(3):540–4.
15. Mekontso-Dessap A, Boissier F, Charron C, Bégot E, Repessé X, Legras Y, Brun-Buisson C, Vignon P, Vieillard-Baron A. Acute cor pulmonale during protective ventilation for acute respiratory distress syndrome: prevalence, predictors, and clinical impact. Intensive Care Med. 2016;42:862–70.
16. Lhéritier G, Legras A, Caille A, Lherm T, Mathonnet A, Frat JP, Courte A, Martin-Lefèvre L, Gouëllo JP, Amiel JB, Garot D, Vignon P. Prevalence and prognostic value of acute cor pulmonale and patent foramen ovale in ventilated patients with early acute respiratory distress syndrome: a multicenter study. Intensive Care Med. 2013;39(10):1734–42.
17. Cook CH, Praba AC, Beery PR, Martin LC. Transthoracic echocardiography is not cost-effective in critically ill surgical patients. J Trauma. 2002;52(2):280–4.
18. Vieillard-Baron A, Prin S, Chergui K, Dubourg O, Jardin F. Echo-Doppler demonstration of acute cor pulmonale at the bedside in the medical intensive care unit. Am J Respir Crit Care Med. 2002;166:1310–9.
19. Bouferrache K, Amiel JB, Chimot L, Caille V, Charron C, Vignon P, Vieillard-Baron A. Initial resuscitation guided by the Surviving Sepsis Campaign recommendations and early echocardiographic assessment of hemodynamics in intensive care unit septic patients: a pilot study. Crit Care Med. 2012;40:2821-7.
20. Vieillard-Baron A, Slama M, Mayo P, Charron C, Amiel JB, Esterez C, Leleu F, Repesse X, Vignon P. A pilot study on safety and clinical utility of a single-use 72-hour indwelling transesophageal echocardiography probe. Intensive Care Med. 2013;39:629–35.

Non-cardiac Ultrasound Signs in Shock

Becky X. Lou and Paul H. Mayo

Electronic Supplementary Material The online version of this chapter (https://doi.org/10.1007/978-3-319-69269-2_19) contains supplementary material, which is available to authorized users.

M. R. Pinsky et al. (eds.), *Hemodynamic Monitoring*, Lessons from the ICU,
https://doi.org/10.1007/978-3-319-69269-2_19

Learning Objectives

- Review the utility of ultrasonography for detection of bleeding in the trauma and non-trauma patient.
- Review the utility of ultrasonography for identification of source of infection in septic shock.

19.1 Introduction

The intensivist uses echocardiography at the bedside of the patient to identify imminently life-threatening causes of shock, to categorize its cause, and to guide management. While echocardiography is preeminent for the evaluation of hemodynamic failure, other aspects of critical care ultrasonography are productively combined with it using a whole-body ultrasonography (WBU) approach [1]. The WBU consists of thoracic (lung and pleura) and screening abdominal examinations as well as a vascular diagnostic ultrasonography for the detection of deep venous thrombosis. This combined approach is useful for rendering the cause of the shock state with early and accurate diagnosis leading to therapeutic interventions [2–4]. While recognizing the importance of echocardiography, this chapter will focus on the utility of other aspects of ultrasonography as they pertain to the diagnosis and management of shock. The authors will use a case-based approach that includes narrated video material that can be accessed from the online library.

Severe reduction in intravascular volume results in shock. The history and physical examination are key aspects of the evaluation. In some cases, the diagnosis is obvious. Massive gastrointestinal hemorrhage with hematemesis and/or melenic stool does not require ultrasonography nor does a patient presenting with obvious whole-body hypovolemia due to major body fluid loss from cholera or an environmental exposure without access to fluid repletion. Ultrasonography becomes helpful in situations where there is clinical suspicion for hypovolemic shock without apparent explanation for the critical loss of effective circulation volume, such as in the patient who has major internal bleeding that is not evident by history or physical examination.

Clinical Case 1

This 39-year-old male patient presents to the emergency department following a motor vehicle accident that involved a high-speed deceleration event. He is hypotensive with cutaneous abdominal and chest wall injury suggestive of a steering column impact. The critical care team performs an immediate extended FAST (focused assessment with sonography in trauma) exam, while the trauma team manages other key aspects of resuscitation.

Rapid evaluation for life-threatening internal bleeding with ultrasonography is widely used by trauma teams. The FAST exam was originally described as a limited examination of the abdominal compartment in the trauma victim [5]. If fluid is present on FAST exam within the abdominal compartment, it is taken as evidence that the fluid is blood. This indicates that there is a high probability of significant injury to an intraabdominal organ. This technique has replaced peritoneal lavage for the detection of intraabdominal bleeding. It is safe, rapid and has similar predictive value to detect blood accumulation within the peritoneal compartment when compared to peritoneal lavage [6, 7]. When free fluid is identified in a normotensive blunt trauma patient on FAST exam, this method has a sensitivity and specificity of 75.8% and 97.4%, respectively [8]. Larger amounts of blood accumulate in the prehepatic, perisplenic, subphrenic, and pelvic spaces. But even a small fluid collection within the hepatorenal or splenorenal space is considered a positive result, and as little as 120–150 cc of fluid can be detected by ultrasonography [9].

A commonly applied algorithm holds that if the FAST exam for intraabdominal fluid is positive in a patient who is hemodynamically unstable, the patient is taken to the operating theater without the need for additional imaging. Delay in operating on patients with positive FAST exams is associated with both early and late in-hospital mortality [10, 11]. If the initial examination is negative for fluid, it can be performed in a serial fashion, and further imaging such as computerized tomography or serial FAST examinations may be indicated.

To perform a FAST exam, the operator, using a low-frequency (2.0–5.0 MHz) phased array or curvilinear probe, images the hepatorenal and splenorenal spaces in the coronal axis. Ascites appears as a hypoechoic collection within the space. Blood accumulates in these spaces as they are dependent in position when the patient is supine. The operator then images the pelvic area by placing the probe above the pubic bone in transverse scanning axis. The tomographic plane is angled into the pelvis to check for pelvic fluid collection.

Case 1 ◘ Video 19.1 shows fluid collection in the hepatorenal recess of the Case 1 patient. There was no detectable pelvic fluid.

◘ Video 19.2 shows an example of absence of fluid in the hepatorenal space.

◘ Video 19.3 shows an example of pelvic fluid collection.

◘ Video 19.4 shows an example of prehepatic fluid collection.

◘ Video 19.5 shows an example of fluid collection in splenorenal and presplenic spaces.

In the trauma patient, all of these examples except for ◘ Video 19.2 would be considered a positive FAST exam.

As a standard approach to thoracic trauma, the critical care team extended the ultrasonography examination to include the thorax. The extended FAST (eFAST) exam includes evaluation for pneumothorax, intrapleural blood, and hemopericardium. It can be performed rapidly with the patient in supine position [12]. If any component of the examination is positive, the team may need to take immediate action (e.g., chest tube insertion, emergency thoracotomy). If the initial examination is negative, further imaging, such as computerized tomography or serial FAST examinations, may be indicated.

In the supine trauma patient, ultrasonography evaluation for pneumothorax can be performed rapidly and is superior to standard chest radiography when chest computerized tomography (CT) scan is used as the "gold standard" [13]. Ultrasonography has similar operating characteristics as chest CT for this application with the added advantage of speed and bedside utility with no need to transport the critically ill patient to the CT scanner. In the context of thoracic trauma, this finding of absent lung sliding is an indication for insertion of a pleural drainage device, particularly if there is clinical concern for a tension pneumothorax.

There are several characteristics of a pneumothorax that can be identified via US. The presence of lung sliding indicates that there is no pneumothorax with 100% negative predictive value at the site of the probe at the chest wall. The presence of B lines, lung consolidation, or pleural effusion rules out the pneumothorax at the site of the probe at the chest wall. The absence of lung sliding is consistent but not diagnostic for a pneumothorax [14]. With ultrasonography, multiple interspaces can be examined in a short period of time. In the case of thoracic trauma, absence of lung sliding, barring alterative explanation is strong evidence for a pneumothorax. The presence of a lung point is diagnostic of a pneumothorax. This finding may be difficult to detect; so, while 100% specific for pneumothorax, its absence does not rule out pneumothorax [15].

Following evaluation for pneumothorax, the operator then examines the posterolateral thorax for blood. The presence of a pleural effusion in a patient with thoracic trauma is assumed to be a hemothorax. Intervention is predicated on the clinical condition of the patient. A large pleural effusion with internal echogenicity is consistent with acute hemorrhage and may warrant urgent thoracotomy for source control.

The extended FAST exam concludes with a subcostal long axis view of the heart to rule out hemopericardium. This comes under the definition of echocardiographic evaluation of shock and will not be reviewed in this chapter.

Case 1 ◘ Video 19.6 shows the presence of lung sliding which was present bilaterally thereby ruling out pneumothorax in this Case 1 patient.

◘ Videos 19.7 and 19.8 show an example of absent lung sliding and the presence of lung point, respectively, the former being consistent with pneumothorax and the latter being diagnostic of pneumothorax.

Case 1 ◼ Video 19.9 shows a large left-sided pleural effusion which has a swirling echogenic pattern ("hematocrit sign") characteristic of an acute hemothorax in the Case 1 patient. The descending aorta has a dissection and perforation which explains the acute hemothorax.

In this Case 1 patient, based upon the results of the ultrasonography examination, the trauma team performed an immediate left-sided thoracotomy and was able to cross-clamp the aorta with immediate source control followed by successful repair of the aortic injury. Based upon the identification of intraabdominal fluid, the patient also underwent exploratory laparotomy, which identified bowel injury with successful repair.

Case 1 provides an example of the utility of ultrasonography to detect an imminently life-threatening cause for shock in the form of internal bleeding that was not readily detected by physical examination.

Clinical Case 2

This is a 54-year-old male patient, who presents with massive recurrent ascites due to hepatic cirrhosis complicated by portal hypertension. Several hours following a routine high-volume paracentesis, he develops hypotension. The critical care team performs immediate abdominal ultrasonography.

Severe bleeding from injury due to an aberrantly positioned vascular structure or inadvertent injury of a normally positioned vessel is an occasional complication of paracentesis.

Case 2 ◼ Video 19.10 shows ascites with a sedimentation effect in the Case 2 patient. Typical of peritoneal bleeding is that the red cells by gravitational effect sediment in dependent fashion. If the patient remains inactive, the sedimentation effect yields a linear interface between the echoic red cell collection and the anechoic plasma component of blood. This has operational consequence. A diagnostic paracentesis will show a paucity of red cells if the fluid is sampled from the anechoic area (i.e., plasma), thereby confusing the clinical team. To avoid a false-negative result, the paracentesis is performed when the patient has been moved sufficiently to assure uniform distribution of red cells within the fluid.

Sekiguchi et al. [16] described a case of lethal peritoneal bleeding following laceration of an inferior gastric vein after a paracentesis in which ultrasonography was not used to guide the procedure. They propose a measure to improve the safety of paracentesis. Ultrasonography, using a low-frequency phased-array or curvilinear probe, identifies a safe site, angle, and depth for needle insertion. The site is then scanned with a high-frequency linear vascular probe with doppler to detect any blood vessels that would contraindicate needle insertion. The color doppler examination is straightforward and adds little time to the procedure.

In the Case 2 patient, an urgent interventional radiology procedure was able to stop the bleeding with embolization of an aberrant peritoneal vessel.

Clinical Case 3

A 45-year-old female patient presents with a recurrent pleural effusion due to breast cancer. Several hours following a routine therapeutic thoracentesis, the patient develops dyspnea and hypotension. The critical care team performs immediate thoracic ultrasonography exam.

As with paracenteses, thoracenteses can be complicated by severe bleeding from an aberrantly positioned vascular structure or inadvertent injury of a normally positioned vessel. This can be detected with characteristic findings on ultrasonography. Unlike trauma, where blood loss can be rapid, bleeding from a peritoneal or intercostal vessel presents in a delayed fashion – often hours after the procedure. Ultrasonography allows for immediate identification of this form of internal blood loss.

Severe bleeding from injury to an intercostal vessel is an occasional complication of thoracentesis. The intercostal vessels are usually located along the inferior aspect of the ribs. However, these vessels may be tortuous, and collaterals can cross the proposed thoracentesis site especially in elderly patients. Several studies have examined the position of intercostal vessels with patients and human cadavers. There is significant variability of vessel position in the posterior medial thorax, so the operator avoids needle insertion within 10 cm of the posterior midline [17–19].

Kanai and Sekiguchi [20] described severe pleural bleeding after injury to an intercostal artery during a seemingly uncomplicated thoracentesis. As with paracentesis, they proposed the use of color doppler to identify aberrantly positioned intercostal vessels. Ultrasonography is used to identify a safe site, angle, and depth for needle insertion. The site is then scanned with a high-frequency linear vascular probe using color doppler to detect any vascular structure that would contraindicate needle insertion. If an aberrant vessel is identified, then the insertion site can be adjusted accordingly.

Case 3 ▣ Video 19.11 shows a discrete, mobile, homogeneous, and hypoechoic structure that has the typical appearance of an intrapleural thrombus. Because of the delayed presentation, the blood had sufficient time to clot with the resultant thrombus. The examination included evaluation for pneumothorax in order to rule out delayed presentation of a tension pneumothorax. In the Case 3 patient, lung sliding was present at multiple sites on the thorax, thereby ruling out pneumothorax. An urgent interventional radiology procedure was able to stop the bleeding with embolism of an intercostal vessel.

In Case 3, the cause of the shock state was from blood loss into the pleural space. Without bleeding, large pleural effusions have been implicated as a cause for shock, the presumed mechanism being due to cardiac chamber compression with tamponade physiology [21, 22].

Clinical Case 4

This 57-year-old male patient presents with hypotension and an acute reduction in hemoglobin level following initiation of low molecular weight heparin for pulmonary embolism. In association with treatment, the critical care team performed an immediate ultrasonography exam.

When the cause for bleeding is not readily apparent from history and physical examination, the operator uses ultrasonography to examine for cryptic sources. Potential sites include retroperitoneal, gastric, or bladder bleeding.

To examine for retroperitoneal bleeding, the operator examines the posterior flank area bilaterally using the low-frequency phased-array or curvilinear probe with the tomographic plane oriented in longitudinal scanning axis. The tomographic plane is adjusted to achieve a coronal axis view of the retroperitoneum, which is posterior to the peritoneal compartment, containing the intestinal structures. Patient-specific factors such as body habitus, dressings, and difficulty with positioning the probe may degrade image quality. In these cases, abdominal CT is superior to ultrasonography for detection of a retroperitoneal bleed.

Case 4 ▣ Video 19.12 shows a fluid collection within the retroperitoneum with a sedimentation effect that is characteristic of blood collection.

In the Case 4 patient, an urgent interventional radiologic procedure was able to stop the bleeding with embolism of a culprit vessel.

The following videos show other situations of unexplained hemorrhagic shock. ▣ Video 19.13 shows an example of gastric blood collection. ▣ Video 19.14 shows an example of blood collection in the bladder.

Clinical Case 5

This 82-year-old female patient presents with hypotension and abdominal pain. Six months before admission, the patient had an aortic abdominal repair with insertion of a graft.

Vascular injury with internal bleeding may occur acutely from an aortic aneurysm leak or as a late complication of vascular surgery. Aorto-duodenal fistula is a well-described though rare delayed complication of aortic aneurysm repair [23]. Graft failure with bleeding from the site is also a possibility.

Case 5 ◘ Video 19.15, taken with a phased-array probe placed in the abdominal midline using a transverse scanning plane, shows an aortic aneurysm with a double-lumen graft within it. Case 5 ◘ Video 19.16 using color doppler shows blood flow within the graft and through the wall of the graft into a periaortic collection.

In Case 5, the patient required emergent surgical repair of the leaking graft. There was a large aortic pseudoaneurysm.

Ultrasonography has utility for identification of the source of infection in the patient with septic shock. As with standard chest radiographs and CT scans, ultrasonography findings are integrated into the results of the history, physical examination, and laboratory values thereby allowing the clinician to establish a diagnosis.

Clinical Case 6

This 29-year-old male patient presented with hypotension, fever, and tachycardia. The presentation was consistent with septic shock. Following the early use of appropriate antibiotics and hemodynamic management, the critical care team performed a whole-body ultrasonography examination.

Thoracic (pleural and lung), abdominal, and soft tissue ultrasonography may identify the source for sepsis. This information may be used to refine antibiotic selection, obtain diagnostic material, and achieve source control.

Ultrasonography is superior to standard chest radiography for identification of lung consolidation and parapneumonic effusion and is similar to chest CT scan for these applications [24, 25]. It is also useful for identification of a variety of intraabdominal infections such as liver abscess, cholecystitis, ascending cholangitis, complex ascitic collections, and pyelonephritis. Soft tissue abscess is readily found with ultrasonography as are fluid collections within joint spaces. In addition to identification of the source, ultrasonography is used to guide aspiration of diagnostic material and intervention for source control.

Case 6 ◘ Video 19.17 shows a liver abscess in the Case 6 patient. The study was performed using a phased-array probe to examine the right upper quadrant. The abscess is identified as a round structure in the liver with heterogeneous echogenicity pattern including hyperechoic foci representing air within the abscess cavity.

In the Case 6 patient, the patient had a drainage catheter inserted, which guided final antibiotic selection based upon culture results and was a key component of successful resolution of the sepsis.

◘ Videos 19.18, 19.19, 19.20, and 19.21 are examples of lung consolidation, infected septated pleural effusion, emphysematous pyelonephritis, and a soft tissue abscess, respectively. These findings had impact on the management of septic shock in terms of antibiotic choice, diagnostic material, and source control.

Practical Implications

While echocardiography is a key component for the diagnosis and management of shock, other aspects of ultrasonography have utility for identification of the cause of hemodynamic failure. By utilizing a methodical ultrasonography exam (e.g., WBU and FAST exams), the examiner can evaluate for source of hemorrhage or source of septic shock.

Clinical Protocol

When the critical care clinician evaluates the patient with shock, ultrasonography may be useful in identifying a source for shock that is independent of the echocardiography evaluation. The components of WBU approach include a search for occult blood loss within intraabdominal, intrathoracic, bladder, retroperitoneal, intraperitoneal spaces and for site of infection as the source of septic shock.

Conclusions

Echocardiography is the primary method for evaluating the patient with shock. It is useful to supplement echocardiography assessment with other aspects of ultrasonography. These include detection of occult hemorrhage and source of sepsis.

Take-Home Messages

- Ultrasonography examination is useful in assessing the trauma patient for bleeding into the abdomen or pleural space. The use of ultrasonography in trauma has been codified into the FAST and extended FAST exam that is in widespread use by trauma teams.
- Ultrasonography examination is useful in assessing for internal bleeding that results in hemorrhagic shock in the non-trauma patient. Blood can be detected in the peritoneal and pleural spaces as a complication of paracentesis or thoracentesis. Blood loss into the retroperitoneum, bladder, and stomach and as a result of vascular injury can be detected with ultrasonography. Identification of bleeding source may lead to lifesaving interventions.
- Ultrasonography is useful in the detection of a source of infection in the patient with septic shock. Identification of the source for infection allows for appropriate antibiotic selection, sampling for accurate bacteriologic analysis, and intervention for source control.

Conflicts of Interest Becky Lou MD and Paul H. Mayo MD have no conflicts of interest regarding the content of this chapter.

References

1. Narasimhan M, Koenig SJ, Mayo PH. A whole-body approach to point of care ultrasound. Chest. 2016;150(4):772–6.
2. Volpicelli G, Lamorte A, Tullio M, Cardinale L, Giraudo M, Stefanone V, Boero E, Nazerian P, Pozzi R, Frascisco MF. Point-of-care multiorgan ultrasonography for the evaluation of undifferentiated hypotension in the emergency department. Intensive Care Med. 2013;39(7):1290–8.
3. Laursen CB, Sloth E, Lambrechtsen J, Lassen AT, Madsen PH, Henriksen DP, Davidsen JR, Rasmussen F. Focused sonography of the heart, lungs, and deep veins identifies missed life-threatening conditions in admitted patients with acute respiratory symptoms. Chest. 2013;144(6):1868–75.
4. Lichtenstein D, Axler O. Intensive use of general ultrasound in the intensive care unit. Intensive Care Med. 1993;19(6):353–5.

5. Scalea TM, Rodriguez A, Chiu WC, Brenneman FD, Fallon WF, Kato K, McKenney MG, Nerlich ML, Ochsner MG, Yoshii H. Focused assessment with sonography for trauma (FAST): results from an international consensus conference. J Trauma. 1999;46(3):466–72.
6. Moylan M, Newgard CD, Ma OJ, Sabbaj A, Rogers T, Douglass R. Association between a positive ED FAST examination and therapeutic laparotomy in normotensive blunt trauma patients. J Emerg Med. 2007;33(3):265–71.
7. Ollerton JE, Sugrue M, Balogh Z, D'Amours SK, Giles A, Wyllie P. Prospective study to evaluate the influence of FAST on trauma patient management. J Trauma. 2006;60(4):785–91.
8. Savatmongkorngul S, Wongwaisayawan S, Kaewlai R. Focused assessment with sonography for trauma: current perspectives. Open Access Emerg Med. 2017;9:57.
9. Jehle DV, Stiller G, Wagner D. Sensitivity in detecting free intraperitoneal fluid with the pelvic views of the FAST exam. Am J Emerg Med. 2003;21(6):476–8.
10. Barbosa RR, Rowell SE, Fox EE, Holcomb JB, Bulger EM, Phelan HA, Alarcon LH, Myers JG, Brasel KJ, Muskat PC, Del Junco DJ. Increasing time to operation is associated with decreased survival in patients with a positive FAST exam requiring emergent laparotomy. J Trauma. 2013;75(101):S48.
11. Richards JR, McGahan JP. Focused assessment with sonography in trauma (FAST) in 2017: what radiologists can learn. Radiology. 2017;283(1):30–48.
12. Reardon R, Moscati R. Beyond the FAST Exam: additional applications of sonography in trauma. In: Jehle D, Heller M, editors. Ultrasonography in trauma: the FAST exam. Dallas, TX: American College of Emergency Physicians; 2003. p. 107–26.
13. Rowan KR, Kirkpatrick AW, Liu D, Forkheim KE, Mayo JR, Nicolaou S. Traumatic pneumothorax detection with thoracic US: correlation with chest radiography and CT—initial experience. Radiology. 2002;225(1):210–4.
14. Lichtenstein D. Lung ultrasound in the critically ill. Curr Opin Crit Care. 2014;20:315–22.
15. Volpicelli G. Sonographic diagnosis of pneumothorax. Intensive Care Med. 2011;37(2):224–32.
16. Sekiguchi H, Suzuki J, Daniels CE. Making paracentesis safer: a proposal for the use of bedside abdominal and vascular ultrasonography to prevent a fatal complication. Chest. 2013;143(4):1136–9.
17. Choi S, Trieu J, Ridley L. Radiological review of intercostal artery: anatomical considerations when performing procedures via intercostal space. J Med Imaging Radiat Oncol. 2010;54(4):302–6.
18. Helm EJ, Rahman NM, Talakoub O, Fox DL, Gleeson FV. Course and variation of the intercostal artery by CT scan. Chest. 2013;143(3):634–9.
19. Shurtleff E, Olinger A. Posterior intercostal artery tortuosity and collateral branch points: a cadaveric study. Folia Morphol (Warsz). 2012;71(4):254–1.
20. Kanai M, Sekiguchi H. Avoiding vessel laceration in thoracentesis: a role of vascular ultrasound with color doppler. Chest. 2015;147(1):e5–7.
21. Kopterides P, Lignos M, Papanikolaou S, Papadomichelakis E, Mentzelopoulos S, Armaganidis A, Panou F. Pleural effusion causing cardiac tamponade: report of two cases and review of the literature. Heart Lung. 2006;35(1):66–7.
22. Traylor JJ, Chan K, Wong I, Roxas JN, Chandraratna PA. Large pleural effusions producing signs of cardiac tamponade resolved by thoracentesis. Am J Cardiol. 2002;89(1):106–8.
23. Antoniou GA, Koutsias S, Antoniou SA, Georgiakakis A, Lazarides MK, Giannoukas AD. Outcome after endovascular stent graft repair of aortoenteric fistula: a systematic review. J Vasc Surg. 2009;49(3):782–9.
24. Xirouchaki N, Magkanas E, Vaporidi K, Kondili E, Plataki M, Patrianakos A, Akoumianaki E, Georgopoulos D. Lung ultrasound in critically ill patients: comparison with bedside chest radiography. Intensive Care Med. 2011;37(9):1488.
25. Lichtenstein D, Goldstein I, Mourgeon E, Cluzel P, Grenier P, Rouby JJ. Comparative diagnostic performances of auscultation, chest radiography, and lung ultrasonography in acute respiratory distress syndrome. Anesthesiology. 2004;100(1):9–15.

Central Venous Pressure

Sheldon Magder

M. R. Pinsky et al. (eds.), *Hemodynamic Monitoring*, Lessons from the ICU,
https://doi.org/10.1007/978-3-319-69269-2_20

Learning Objectives

- CVP represents the equilibrium of cardiac and return functions.
- CVP is altered by changes in cardiac function or changes in return functions.
- The physiological range of CVP is small so that precise measurements are crucial.
- Patterns of CVP and indices of blood flow can be used to diagnose changes in haemodynamic status and help assess the response to fluid infusions.
- CVP gives diagnostic information beyond just the preload of the heart.

20.1 Introduction

Central venous pressure (CVP) is an easily accessible value that is readily available in any patient who has a central venous line. In many patients it even can be estimated by simple clinical exam. However, it often is argued that CVP is of little clinical use. A large part of these criticisms comes from a lack of appreciation of what CVP means and its determinants [1]. Failure to appreciate these leads to errors in its use and unfairly discredits its value.

20.2 Determinants of CVP

Ernest Starling was one of the first to indicate that output from the heart is dependent upon the return of blood back to it [2]. Arthur Guyton more fully developed this concept by describing how cardiac output is determined by a function that describes the return of blood to the heart (venous return function) and a function that describes the output from the heart (cardiac function) [3–5]. In the intact circulation, CVP is the equilibrium value of these two functions. When the heart is isolated from the venous return, CVP indicates the pressure on the walls of the heart in diastole that sets the initial length of cardiac sarcomeres based on the compliance of the ventricular walls. Sarcomere length determines the force of cardiac contraction as expressed by the Frank-Starling relationship [6]. When venous return is isolated from the heart, CVP determines the pressure difference for the return of blood to the heart. When the circulation is intact, the heart controls the return of blood by lowering right atrial pressure, and there is little change in the upstream venous reservoir during the cardiac cycle [7]. A change in CVP should not be considered simply as a change in preload but rather as a change in the equilibrium of the cardiac and return functions (◘ Fig. 20.1).

An important consideration for the interaction of the cardiac and return functions is that these two functions have limits (◘ Fig. 20.1). The ventricles have a limit to filling which is created by the pericardium when it is present or by the cardiac cytoskeleton when the pericardium is absent. At the limit of cardiac filling, sarcomeres cannot be stretched further, and diastolic filling pressure rises without a change in stroke volume. The break in the cardiac function curve is sharp [8] and creates an almost flat cardiac function curve (◘ Fig. 20.1). When cardiac function is limited, increasing the return function by giving volume, or by decreasing venous resistance, does not increase cardiac output. This can be considered 'wasted preload' because ventricular diastolic pressure rises without a change in stroke volume. The return function is limited when CVP is less than zero in a spontaneously breathing person or less than pleural pressure in someone on a ventilator. This occurs because veins have soft walls and collapse when the pressure inside the vein is less

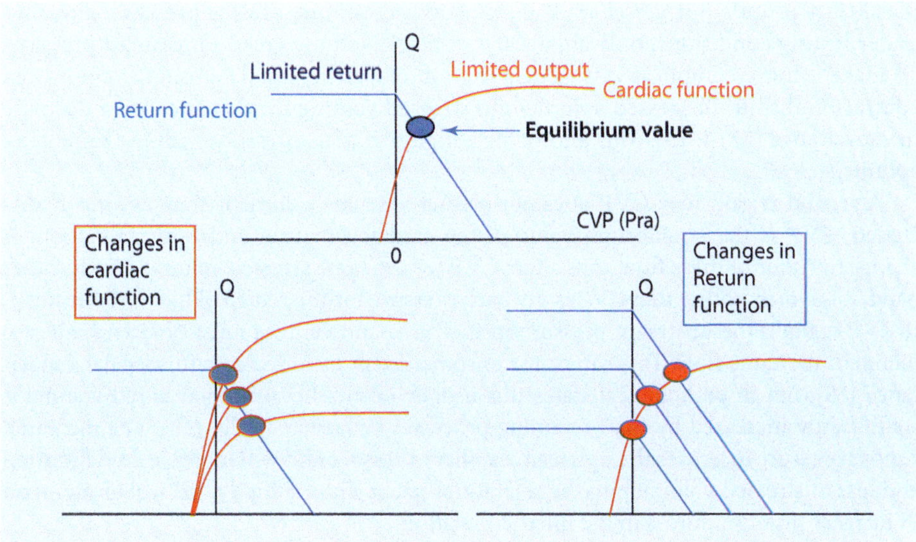

Fig. 20.1 Interactions of the cardiac and return functions. The upper figure shows the cardiac function and return function and the intersection at an equilibrium value. When breathing is spontaneous, the return function is limited (flatline) when CVP is <0. The cardiac function is limited when it reaches a plateau (the value is variable). The bottom left shows changes only in cardiac function; changes in cardiac output and CVP move in opposite directions. The bottom left shows changes in return function; changes in cardiac output and CVP move in the same direction

than the pressure surrounding the vein in what is called a vascular waterfall [9]. Under waterfall conditions, lowering the pressure in a vein below the collapse point does not increase flow, and flow is determined by the pressure difference from the upstream source to the collapse pressure. Accordingly, when return function is limited, lowering CVP further, either by increasing cardiac function or with the use of a mechanical device, does not increase the return of blood to the heart and thus cannot increase cardiac output.

An understanding of the significance of the interaction of the cardiac and return functions is helped by considering what happens during exercise. Cardiac output in a young male can go from 5 to 25 L/min with little change in CVP after an initial small increase [10]. For this to happen, cardiac function must increase at the same rate as the return function increases. If cardiac output increases faster than the return function, CVP would fall, and if cardiac function increases more slowly than the return function, CVP would increase. Furthermore, because the slope of the cardiac function curve is so steep at peak exercise, the effect of a change in CVP on cardiac output is five times greater than in the resting state, and the heart appears to be more preload sensitive. This is because the more rapid heart rate, increased contractility and lower peripheral resistance allow larger stroke volume for the same preload.

20.3 What Does CVP Not Tell You?

A common error is to think that CVP indicates blood volume [11]. In a 70 kg male, total blood volume is about 5.5 L, but only about 1.3–1.4 L is stressed, which is the volume that stretches vessel walls [12, 13]. The rest of the blood volume is unstressed in that it just rounds out vessel walls. Only stressed volume creates pressure, and thus under resting conditions, only about 30% of blood volume creates measured pressure. To make it more complicated, vascular smooth muscle in small veins and venules can contract and shift unstressed volume into stressed volume in what is called a decrease in capacitance [7, 14, 15]. This allows for a higher venous pressure with the same total volume.

A second reason why CVP does not predict vascular volume is that, as already discussed, CVP is the equilibrium value of the cardiac function and return function. A change in either of these functions alters CVP for the same stressed volume. On the other hand, it is worth noting that CVP is the back pressure for the return of blood to the heart. If CVP is high, the upstream pressure in the veins and venules must be even higher to maintain the same flow. This can occur to some extent by a decrease in vascular capacitance [15], but in pathological states this usually occurs because total blood volume is significantly increased by fluid retaining processes or iatrogenically [16]. The increased venous pressure increases the upstream capillary pressure and will increase fluid filtration and loss of stressed volume into the interstitial space. Thus, a high CVP will always tend to increase filtration forces in the microcirculation.

CVP also does not predict volume responsiveness. When the right heart is functioning close to the maximum possible end-diastolic volume, increasing the return function by increasing stressed volume only increases end-diastolic pressure but not sarcomere length. This produces the plateau of the cardiac function curve. The plateau value is very variable among individuals because it depends upon the heart rate, the right ventricular afterload, the slope of the end-systolic pressure-flow relationship and the compliance of the right heart. The volume of the left ventricle can affect it, too, because when left heart volume is increased, it takes up a greater proportion of the limited pericardial space. However, despite some arguments to the contrary [17], high values of CVP make it less likely that volume will increase cardiac output, and low values make it more likely [18, 19]. An important selection bias in almost all the studies in this area is that boluses are given based on clinicians' belief that volume will be helpful, and thus patients with higher CVP values, and who are less likely to respond, are not included [18].

20.4 Proper Measurement

Pressures measured with fluid-filled systems are always made relative to a reference level. This is because the fluid in the measuring device creates an additional force which is due to the force of gravity acting on the mass of the fluid in the line used for the measurement. On physical exam, the recommended reference level is 5 cm below the sternal angle, which is where the second rib is attached to the sternum [20] and can be identified as a bump on the sternum. This landmark is approximately 5 cm above the midpoint of the right atrium. The right atrium is a round and anterior structure [21], and thus the centre of the right atrium remains in the same position relative to the sternal angle even with the person sitting with the head at 60° from the horizontal. In my unit we reference our transducers to 5 cm below the sternal angle with a carpenter's levelling device, and the transducer is re-levelled if the head of the bed is moved up or down. Far more frequently, the reference level is set at the mid-thoracic (also called mid-axillary) position. This produces a pressure approximately 3 mmHg higher than the sternal angle-based measurement [19]. The mid-thoracic position is used more often as the reference level because it is easier to identify and does not require a carpenter's level, but that also is the problem. Because the assessment is easier, the measurement often is done with a casual estimation, which reduces reproducibility among members of the treating team, whereas repeated measures with the sternal angle-based measurement give very reproducible values [22].

Not only is the level of the transducer important but so is the reference pressure for the transducer. When initially set up, the pressure transducer is exposed to atmospheric pressure, which becomes the zero value for the measurements, although it is not really zero, but rather atmospheric pressure, which is 760 mmHg at sea level on a calm day. The pressure across the wall of vascular structures is called transmural pressure. When the outside pressure is atmospheric pressure, and it is used as the zero reference, transmural pressure simply is the inside pressure minus the outside pressure, which is zero. However, when the pressure surrounding intrathoracic vascular structures is not atmospheric pressure, and it varies during the respiratory cycle, this surrounding pressure is needed to know the transmural pressure rather than atmospheric pressure. To minimize the consequent error in measurement of transmural pressure when pleural pressure is not known, CVP is measured at end-expiration because this is when pleural pressure is closest to the atmospheric pressure. However, if the physiological question is what the downstream pressure is in the right heart for venous drainage, the CVP value relative to atmospheric pressure is the value to use.

When the reference level is standardized, and the proper timing in the respiratory cycle is chosen, the next question is where in the cardiac cycle should CVP be measured. CVP varies during the cardiac cycle. There usually is a prominent 'a' wave after atrial systole, a 'c' wave with closure of the tricuspid valve and a 'v' wave at the end of systole (◘ Fig. 20.2). The recommended place to measure CVP is at the base of the 'c' wave because that is the final pressure in the ventricle before the onset of systole. This is called the 'z' point, and it is the best estimate of the preload of the heart, which is the most frequent reason for measuring CVP. If the 'c' wave cannot be seen, the base of the 'a' wave usually is a reasonable substitute. The position of the 'c' wave also can be identified by drawing a vertical line from the 'S' wave of the QRS wave if the ECG is synchronized with the haemodynamic pressure tracing (◘ Fig. 20.2). The 'S' wave is used instead of the 'Q' wave because transmission of the fluid haemodynamic pressure is slower than the electrical ECG signal.

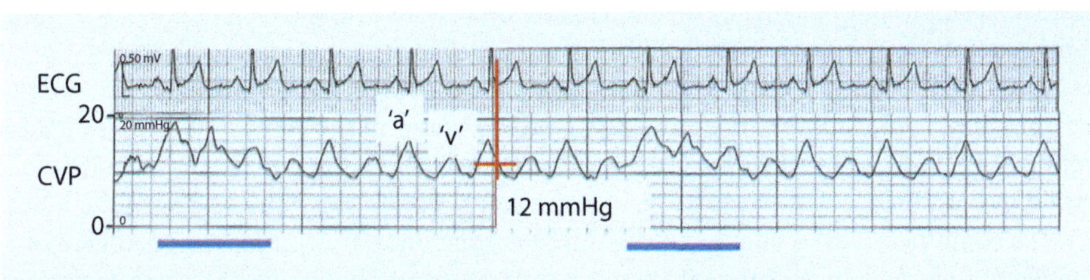

◘ **Fig. 20.2** Example of CVP tracing and ECG with controlled mechanical breaths. The lines at the bottom indicate inspiration. CVP rises during this phase. In this subject the expiratory phase is flat, and the pressure is measured close to the end of expiration. The 'a' and 'v' waves are marked. There is no obvious 'c' wave, and the appropriate place to measure the CVP is determined by drawing a vertical line down from the S wave of the ECG. The value in this example is 12 mmHg

20.5 Proper Use of the CVP

In the upright posture at rest, CVP is below atmospheric pressure (i.e. below zero) in most people. Thus, a CVP above 4 mmHg relative to the mid-right atrium is an abnormal value. This does not mean that it needs to be treated, but it should make the clinician think of why the CVP is elevated.

If the patient is awake and alert, urinating and appears well perfused, a low CVP offers little useful information. However, a low CVP does not mean that everything is okay. The CVP could be low because of inadequate venous return due to depletion of vascular volume or because of increased venous resistance. This even can occur in someone with decreased cardiac function. CVP also can be low because the heart is hyperdynamic and lowered the cardiac function-return function equilibrium value.

On the other hand, CVP can be high in a normal heart because there is excess vascular volume, either because of failure of renal excretion or because of excessive administration of intravenous fluid. CVP can be high because cardiac function is decreased or because of an obstructive process in the heart, while the return function remains normal. It also can be high because the return function is increased because of decreased venous resistance. The latter likely is an important factor in septic patients [23] with high cardiac outputs or in patients with large arterial-venous shunts such as an aortocaval fistula.

The key message is that when examining the CVP, the order of events should be to first identify a clinical problem and only then look at the CVP to help with the interpretation of the clinical problem, rather than look first at the CVP and then consider giving volume outside of a clinical context [1]. If a patient is in shock, and the diagnosis of a massive pulmonary embolism is considered, a CVP close to zero makes this diagnosis very unlikely unless there is another process at the same time, such as a major volume loss. This is because a pulmonary embolism causes shock by being an obstructive process, and increased CVP inhibits the normal return of blood to the right heart. On the other side, if shock is considered to be due to a major volume loss, and the CVP is markedly elevated, this makes the diagnosis of hypovolemia very unlikely unless there is another pathological process going on at the same time, for example, cardiac tamponade which is contributing an obstructive component.

It is important to differentiate a high CVP based on a deviation from normal values [19], which indicates an abnormal process, from a value of CVP that may predict volume responsiveness [17]. Patients can sometimes respond to fluids at high CVP values, but there is a price to pay because of the high upstream venous pressure [1]. On the other side, some patients do not respond to volume infusions, even at low values of CVP [19].

CVP often is called a 'static' measure, but it is no more static than any other physiological measures, which all vary over time. CVP is only 'static' in the context of an investigator taking a single value for a study. CVP is most useful in the dynamic state when it is followed over time and compared to changing clinical conditions. This is best done when CVP is combined with a change in measured cardiac output or at least a surrogate of a change in flow such as a change in central venous saturation, change in serum lactate or change in skin perfusion. A rise in CVP and a fall in cardiac output indicate a primary decrease in cardiac function; this is best addressed by improving cardiac function. A fall in CVP and a rise in cardiac output indicate that there has been a primary increase in cardiac function (◘ Figs. 20.1 and 20.3). A fall in CVP with a fall in cardiac output indicates a primary decrease in the return function. This most often is due to a decrease in

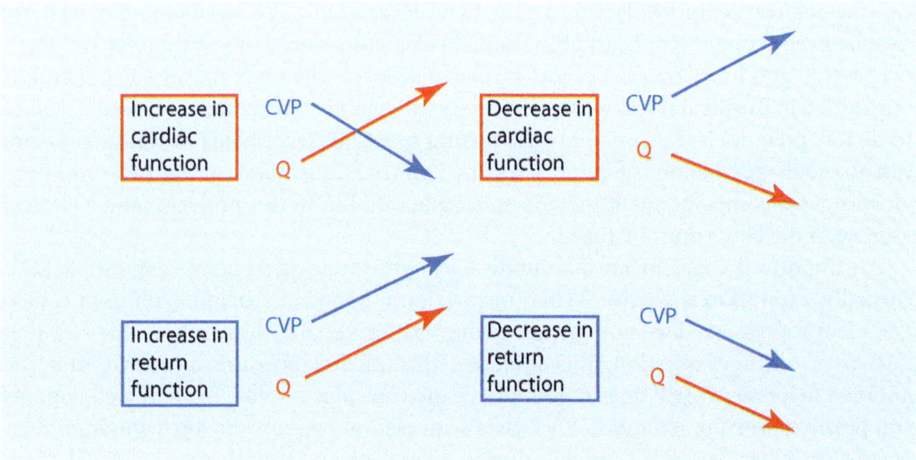

Fig. 20.3 Use of CVP and cardiac output (Q) to indicate changes in cardiac function versus changes in return function. With changes in cardiac function (upper part of figure), changes in Q and CVP are in opposite directions. With changes in the return function (bottom of the figure), changes in Q and CVP are in the same direction. These patterns can be used to distinguish a primary cardiac function change from a primary return change

stressed volume so that giving volume is a reasonable choice if clinically indicated. A rise in CVP with a rise in cardiac output indicates a primary increase in the return function, which most often is due to an increase in stressed volume.

CVP also has a useful role in assessing the response to a fluid bolus. The logic is the same as the diagnostic reasoning in the previous section. A fluid bolus corrects perceived inadequate tissue perfusion by increasing cardiac filling pressures which increases cardiac output. If the identified clinical problem is not corrected by a volume bolus, this could be because the patient's right heart is operating on the flat part of the cardiac function curve and is not volume responsive or because insufficient volume was given to increase the cardiac filling pressure enough to observe a response in cardiac output. In the first case, more volume is not useful. In the second, more volume needs to be given to test the hypothesis. These two possibilities can be distinguished by observing what happened to the CVP with the volume bolus. If CVP went up without a correction in indices of perfusion or without correcting the clinical problem, giving more volume is not the answer. If the CVP did not increase, and I arbitrarily define this as an increase of 2 mmHg because this is a value that can be detected with confidence on a monitor, more volume can be tried.

20.6 Pitfalls

The pressure difference that determines venous return normally only is in the range of 4–6 mmHg. Thus, small changes in CVP are significant, and errors in measurement can have significant impact on clinical decisions. Besides the technical issues discussed above, the breathing pattern can have important effects. Pleural pressure at end-expiration during spontaneous respiratory efforts normally is subatmospheric, but with positive-pressure mechanical breaths, pleural pressure is positive during inspiration and increases further with the application of PEEP. This results in an increase in CVP relative to atmospheric pressure even though right heart filling actually decreases during inspiration (Fig. 20.2). If chest wall and lung compliance are normal, a little less than half the airway pressure is transmitted to the pleural space [24]. However, when lung compliance is decreased, less of the airway pressure is transmitted to the pleural space. Measurements of pleural pressure with an esophageal balloon allow an assessment of true transmural cardiac pressures [24], but without this measurement there is no simple solution to this problem, and a clinical estimate of the effect must be made.

An important cause of an inaccurate CVP measurement is active expiration [22]. Normally, expiration is passive. When inspiration is spontaneous and expiration is passive, pleural pressure does not change during expiration and thus neither does CVP. If CVP rises during expiration, this indicates that pleural pressure increased, and the observed increase in CVP does not represent the transmural value. In ventilated patients with positive-pressure inflations, CVP rises with pleural pressure during inspiration relative to atmospheric pressure and falls during expiration, but if all the air is exhaled, there should be a plateau in the CVP and pleural pressure before the next inspiration. If CVP does not reach a plateau, the transmural pressure is overestimated because functional reserve capacity was not reached and pleural pressure is a positive value. The greatest error occurs when there is a progressive rise in CVP during expiration. This only can occur if there is significant recruitment of expiratory muscles and the CVP value at end-expiration greatly exaggerates true CVP transmural pressure [22, 25].

20.7 Other Uses of CVP

There is much information that can be gleamed from the CVP waveform beyond just assessing cardiac filling pressure [26, 27]. A large 'y' descent in the CVP indicates that the right heart has restrictive physiology and it is unlikely that cardiac output will increase with a volume bolus [28]. The presence of 'a' waves indicates that there is atrial activity. Prominent 'a' waves indicate decreased compliance of the right atrium. Cannon 'a' waves indicate that there is atrial-ventricular dissociation. During spontaneous breaths the magnitude of the fall in CVP gives an indication of the inspiratory effort. During positive-pressure breaths, the rise in CVP during inspiration gives an indication of chest wall compliance [26].

Take-Home Message

The CVP gives an indication of the function of the heart and of the return of blood to the heart and, accordingly, must be interpreted considering these two functions. The pressure driving blood back to the heart from the veins is small, and thus the measurement must be carefully done. A low CVP can be normal but also occurs with hypovolemia. An elevated CVP is always abnormal, but the problem can be due to decreased heart function, increased total vascular volume or both. CVP is most useful when changes over time are compared to haemodynamic changes. The most important haemodynamic measure for interpretation of CVP is the corresponding change in cardiac output either measured directly or through surrogates. Finally, the CVP waveform itself gives an indication of cardiac as well as respiratory function, which the careful clinician can use to follow patient's conditions.

References

1. De Backer D, Vincent JL. Should we measure the central venous pressure to guide fluid management? Ten answers to 10 questions. Crit Care. 2018;22(1):43.
2. Patterson SW, Starling EH. On the mechanical factors which determine the output of the ventricles. J Physiol. 1914;48(5):357–79.
3. Magder S. An approach to hemodynamic monitoring: Guyton at the beside. Crit Care. 2012;16:236–43.
4. Guyton AC, Lindsey AW, Kaufman BN. Effect of mean circulatory filling pressure and other peripheral circulatory factors on cardiac output. Am J Physiol. 1955;180:463–8.
5. Guyton AC. Determination of cardiac output by equating venous return curves with cardiac response curves. Physiol Rev. 1955;35:123–9.
6. Katz AM. Ernest Henry Starling, his predecessors, and the "Law of the Heart". Circulation. 2002;106(23):2986–92.
7. Magder S. Volume and its relationship to cardiac output and venous return. Crit Care. 2016;20:271.
8. Bishop VS, Stone HL, Guyton AC. Cardiac function curves in conscious dogs. Am J Physiol. 1964;207(3):677–82.
9. Permutt S, Riley S. Hemodynamics of collapsible vessels with tone: the vascular waterfall. J Appl Physiol. 1963;18(5):924–32.
10. Notarius CF, Levy RD, Tully A, Fitchett D, Magder S. Cardiac vs. non-cardiac limits to exercise following heart transplantation. Am Heart J. 1998;135:339–48.
11. Marik PE, Baram M, Vahid B. Does central venous pressure predict fluid responsiveness? A systematic review of the literature and the tale of seven mares. Chest. 2008;134(1):172–8.
12. Magder S, De Varennes B. Clinical death and the measurement of stressed vascular volume. Crit Care Med. 1998;26:1061–4.
13. West JB. Physiology of the body fluids. Physiological basis of medical practice. 11th ed. Baltimore/London: Williams & Wilkins; 1985. p. 438–50.
14. Rothe C. Venous system: physiology of the capacitance vessels. In: Shepherd JT, Abboud FM, editors. Handbook of physiology. The cardiovascular system. Section 2. III. Bethesda: American Physiological Society; 1983. p. 397–452.
15. Rothe CF. Reflex control of veins and vascular capacitance. Physiol Rev. 1983;63(4):1281–95.
16. Marik PE. Iatrogenic salt water drowning and the hazards of a high central venous pressure. Ann Intensive Care. 2014;4:21.
17. Eskesen TG, Wetterslev M, Perner A. Reanalysis of central venous pressure as an indicator of fluid responsiveness. Intensive Care Med. 2015;42:324–32.
18. Magder S. Value of CVP: an epidemiological or physiological question? Intensive Care Med. 2016;42(3):458–9.
19. Magder S, Bafaqeeh F. The clinical role of central venous pressure measurements. J Intensive Care Med. 2007;22(1):44–51.
20. Bickley LS, Hoekelman RA, editors. Bates guide to physical examination and history taking. Philadelphia: Lippincott; 1999. p. 299–303.
21. Magder S. Is all on the level? Hemodynamics during supine versus prone ventilation. Am J Respir Crit Care Med. 2013;188(12):1390–1.
22. Magder S, Serri K, Verscheure S, Chauvin R, Goldberg P. Active expiration and the measurement of central venous pressure. J Intensive Care Med. 2018;33(7):430–5.
23. Magder S. Heart-lung interactions in sepsis. In: Scharf SM, Pinsky M, Magder S, editors. Respiratory-circulatory interactions in health and disease. 2nd ed. New York: Marcel Dekker, Inc.; 2001. p. 739–62.
24. Akoumianaki E, Maggiore SM, Valenza F, Bellani G, Jubran A, Loring SH, et al. The application of esophageal pressure measurement in patients with respiratory failure. Am J Respir Crit Care Med. 2014;189(5):520–31.
25. Verscheure S, Massion PB, Gottfried S, Goldberg P, Samy L, Damas P, et al. Measurement of pleural pressure swings with a fluid-filled esophageal catheter vs pulmonary artery occlusion pressure. J Crit Care. 2017;37:65–71.
26. Magder S. Right atrial pressure in the critically ill: how to measure, what is the value, what are the limitations? Chest. 2017;151(4):908–16.
27. Magder S. Diagnostic information from the respiratory variations in central hemodynamics pressures. In: Scharf SM, Pinsky MR, Magder S, editors. Respiratory-circulatory interactions in health and disease. New York: Marcel Dekker, Inc.; 2001. p. 861–82.
28. Magder S, Erice F, Lagonidis D. Determinants of the 'y' descent and its usefulness as a predictor of ventricular filling. J Intensive Care Med. 2000;15:262–9.

Arterial Blood Pressure

Bernd Saugel, Thomas W. L. Scheeren, and Jean-Louis Teboul

M. R. Pinsky et al. (eds.), *Hemodynamic Monitoring*, Lessons from the ICU,
https://doi.org/10.1007/978-3-319-69269-2_21

Learning Objectives

The measurement of blood pressure (BP) is a key component of hemodynamic monitoring in various fields of medicine, including intensive care medicine, emergency medicine, and anesthesiology. Thus, it is crucial to understand the different technologies available for BP monitoring. This includes understanding the underlying measurement principles of invasive and noninvasive techniques and knowing their advantages and limitations in different clinical settings. In this chapter, we give a brief overview of the history of technologies for BP measurement, and we describe the available technologies for BP monitoring used in intensive care medicine with regard to their measurement principles, advantages, limitations, and clinical applicability.

21.1 Introduction

The serial or continuous measurement of arterial BP is a cornerstone of hemodynamic monitoring in intensive care medicine. The measurement of BP is crucial for the timely detection of hemodynamic instability and hypotension (BP monitoring to ensure patient safety) and for individually targeting BP values (BP management). Today, various technologies are available to assess BP either invasively (via an arterial catheter) or noninvasively (Fig. 21.1). Noninvasive BP measurements are usually performed in an intermittent manner with an inflatable occluding (upper arm) cuff using the auscultatory method, palpatory method, or automated techniques such as oscillometry. Recently, however, noninvasive BP monitoring technologies that enable the arterial BP waveform to be recorded and displayed continuously have become available for clinical practice. A profound under-

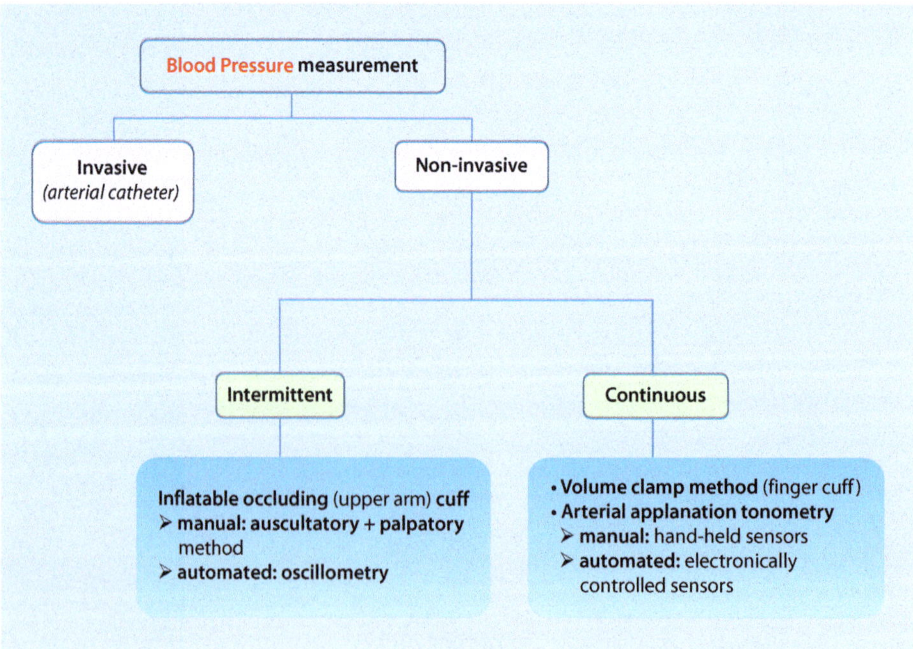

Fig. 21.1 Arterial blood pressure measurement: the different techniques

standing of the principles of BP measurement and of the indications and contraindications of each technique in intensive care medicine is important to choose the optimal way to measure BP in the individual patient.

21.2 History of Blood Pressure Measurement

BP was first measured directly (i.e., invasively) in the middle of the eighteenth century when Reverend Stephen Hales performed physiologic experiments and aimed to quantify the pressure in the cardiovascular circulation of different animals by measuring the height of the blood column in a long glass tube directly inserted into the animals' arteries [1–3].

In 1828, the French physician Jean Léonard Marie Poiseuille invasively measured BP in animals using a cannula inserted into an artery and a mercury manometer (he called it "hemodynamometer") and coined the unit "centimeters of mercury" to quantify BP readings [1, 3].

In 1847, the German physiologist Carl Ludwig, for the first time, continuously recorded and graphically displayed BP by attaching a floating pen to Poiseuille's mercury manometer and called his invention the "kymograph" [1, 3].

In 1856, the French surgeon Jean Faivre performed the first invasive direct systolic BP measurements in humans using a mercury manometer connected to a cannula inserted in an artery (femoral or brachial) during surgery [1, 3].

Beginning in the middle of the nineteenth century, different physiologists and physicians developed methods to assess BP noninvasively based on the idea to quantify an external counterpressure required to intermittently stop the intra-arterial blood flow.

A noninvasive simple transducer recording the BP waveform at the radial artery using external weights to determine the closing pressure of the artery was developed in 1855 by the German physiologist Karl von Vierordt [1, 3, 4]. This "sphygmograph" was improved by the French physiologist Étienne-Jules Marey in 1860 who invented a brilliant – but very complicated – system combining a water-filled glass chamber enclosing the arm, a sphygmograph, and a kymograph [1, 5].

The British physician Frederick Akbar Mahomed explored the physiology of the radial artery BP waveform and laid the foundation for the science of pulse contour analysis (from 1872 to 1884) [6, 7].

The first modern "sphygmomanometer" was developed in 1881 by the Austrian physician Samuel Siegfried Karl von Basch who placed a water-filled rubber bag surrounding a bulb that was connected to a mercury column over the radial artery [1, 3]. By increasing the amount of water in the bag and thus the pressure on the radial artery, the arterial pulsation was impaired and eventually stopped so that systolic BP could be determined by observing the corresponding height of the mercury column [1]. Interestingly, the *British Medical Journal* back then stated that by the use of a sphygmomanometer to assess BP "we pauperize our senses and weaken clinical acuity" [1].

The French cardiologist Pierre Potain improved von Basch's sphygmomanometer by using air instead of water to compress the artery and a portable aneroid manometer [1].

In 1896, BP assessment using sphygmomanometry with an inflatable non-expanding occluding upper arm cuff (developed by Dunlop) and a mercury manometer was described by the Italian physician Scipione Riva-Rocci [1, 3, 8]. This approach still forms the basis of present-day BP measurement techniques. However, Riva-Rocci used a too narrow cuff with a width of only 5 cm. In 1901, Heinrich von Recklinghausen suggested using a wider cuff (12 cm) [1, 3]. In addition, the palpatory method suggested by Riva-Rocci allowed the assessment of systolic BP but not of diastolic BP.

Due to the advances made by Riva-Rocci and the physicians who came after, the portability and usefulness of the sphygmomanometer became apparent to surgeons and anesthesiologists. In 1897, Leonard Hill and Harold Barnard described a decline in systolic BP after induction of anesthesia with chloroform [9].

The determination of diastolic BP became possible with the discovery of the auscultatory method for BP determination by the Russian army physician Nikolai Sergejewitsch Korotkow [1, 3]. He famously proposed to obtain the "Korotkoff sounds" with the help of a stethoscope placed distally from the cuff over the brachial artery during slow deflation of the upper arm cuff.

Another crucial step toward the routine measurement of both systolic and diastolic BP was the development of oscillometric methods that allowed recording the oscillations within the cuff. In the early twentieth century, the oscillometric method, which had been described by Marey as early as 1876, was further developed and refined by Joseph Erlanger and Victor Pachon who eventually provided a portable "sphygmo-oscillometer" [3, 10].

Since the first description of oscillometry, the technique was further refined and improved and was used for BP measurement in research and clinical routine [3].

However, as late as in 1969, it was demonstrated that the point of maximum oscillation actually corresponds to the mean BP [11–13]. Later, a more detailed understanding of the oscillations observed during cuff deflation allowed defining certain points corresponding to systolic and diastolic BP [12, 14]. In the 1970s, electronic pressure sensors and microprocessors allowed the development of automated oscillometry [12]. The algorithms used to analyze the oscillometric waveforms and the hardware/software of the oscillometric BP monitors were constantly refined since then [12]. Today, automated sphygmomanometers using oscillometry are widely used in all fields of medicine, including medical care sites and home BP monitoring.

21.3 Invasive Arterial Blood Pressure Measurement (Arterial Catheter)

The invasive and continuous recording of the BP waveform and assessment of BP values with a catheter placed in an artery, a fluid-filled tubing system, and an electronic system are also called "direct" measurement and are considered the clinical "gold standard" method for measuring BP.

Arterial cannulation for BP monitoring is routinely performed in critically ill patients. Arteries used for direct BP measurements are the radial, femoral, brachial, and dorsalis pedis artery. The placement of an arterial catheter is usually straightforward when performed by a well-trained operator, but it can be challenging in certain clinical situations, e.g., in pediatric patients or in patients with arteriosclerosis or circulatory shock with peripheral vasoconstriction. Ultrasound guidance has been suggested to improve the success rate and quality of arterial catheter placement [15]. The overall complication rate associated with arterial catheter placement is relatively low, but complications related to the placement or presence of an arterial catheter can be major (embolism, ischemic damage, bleeding, pseudoaneurysm, infection) [16]. In addition, it has been shown that arterial cannulation can decrease blood flow distal to the catheter [17].

It is important to understand the underlying principle of direct BP measurement, which requires an intra-arterial catheter connected to a fluid-filled tubing system and a pressure transducer containing an impermeable diaphragm [18]. The intra-arterial catheter connects the system to the vascular system, picks up BP, and transmits it to the fluid-filled tubing system. The fluid column in the tubing system, in turn, transmits the pressure signal to the diaphragm of the pressure transducer and deforms it physically leading to changes in the electrical resistance of strain gauges attached to the diaphragm and the other side if the diaphragm is open to atmospheric pressure [18]. The pressure-induced changes in electrical resistance show a linear relationship with the intra-arterial pressure and can thus be mathematically translated in a waveform. Thus, the pressure transducer converts the mechanical signal into an electrical signal, which is processed by the monitor and translated into a BP waveform and numeric BP values.

To avoid erroneous BP readings, the tubing system and pressure transducer must be correctly set up and maintained. This includes meticulously priming the tubing system with fluid, referencing (or leveling) the transducer to the level of the patient's right atrium, and zeroing the transducer to atmospheric pressure [18, 19]. Although the correct point for leveling the transducer is a matter of discussion, in clinical practice the phlebostatic axis (located at the fourth intercostal space, halfway between the anterior and posterior chest wall) approximates the location of the right atrium and can be used for referencing the transducer.

For zeroing, the zeroing button of the monitor is pressed after the transducer has been opened to atmospheric pressure. This defines the transducer level as the hydrostatic zero reference point and ensures that the monitor uses atmospheric pressure as the atmospheric zero reference point [18, 19].

In addition, testing the dynamic response of the catheter/tubing system is key for reliable BP readings. The dynamic response is determined by its natural frequency and the damping coefficient. BP readings can be falsely low when the damping properties of the arterial catheter/tubing system are too high (and vice versa) [20].

A fast flush test needs to be performed to verify the natural frequency and damping of the direct BP monitoring system [7, 18, 19, 21]. The flush test consists of inspecting the arterial waveform after flushing the system with 300 mmHg and abruptly terminating the flushing manoeuver.

When deciding whether arterial cannulation is necessary, one should balance the risks (complications associated with catheter placement and maintenance) and the benefits (direct "gold standard" BP readings, blood sampling) of an arterial catheter for each individual patient.

21.4 Intermittent Noninvasive Arterial Blood Pressure Measurement

Inflatable air-filled cuffs that occlude the artery at the measurement site are used for intermittent noninvasive (manually or automated) BP measurements. An appropriately sized cuff is a prerequisite for valid measurements [22].

Manual intermittent noninvasive BP measurements obtained during gradual deflation of the occluding cuff (with a manometer indicating the applied pressure) can be performed by the palpatory or auscultatory method [14]. The palpatory method, i.e., palpating the pulse distal to the occluding cuff during slow cuff deflation, only allows assessing systolic BP. The auscultatory method (auscultation of Korotkoff sounds distal to the cuff with a stethoscope) yields systolic (onset of the sounds) and diastolic pressures (disappearance of sounds).

Different technologies for automated intermittent noninvasive assessment of BP with an occluding cuff are available, with "oscillometry," a technique detecting oscillations of the arterial wall, being the most widely used [13]. Small oscillations occur when the cuff pressure is higher than the systolic BP. During cuff deflation, the oscillations increase until they reach a maximum at mean BP [23] and then again decrease toward the diastolic BP. From the pressure with maximal oscillations (mean BP), algorithms help deriving systolic and diastolic pressures. The cuff pressure at the time of the initial occurrence of oscillations corresponds to the maximum systolic BP, and the lowest cuff pressure just prior to the time that oscillations stop decreasing in amplitude corresponds to the diastolic BP [4, 7]. Today, automatic oscillometry is widely used in intensive care medicine and anesthesiology but also in physician offices, on hospital wards, for 24-h ambulatory BP monitoring, and for home BP monitoring. It needs to be stressed, however, that oscillometry is not a standardized technique. There are numerous different proprietary algorithms to derive BP that are not made publicly available by the manufacturers [12, 24, 25]. Although oscillometry can basically be applied easily and rapidly and provides BP readings in an automated way without the need for trained personnel, the choice of the appropriate cuff size is key in order to avoid erroneously low (too large cuff size) or high (too small cuff size) BP measurements [26]. In addition, oscillometric BP measurements are prone to artifacts (potentially resulting in false BP values) caused by active or passive movement at the measurement site [12]. Oscillometry tends to underestimate the systolic BP and overestimate the diastolic BP compared with invasively measured BP [27]. Data on the measurement performance of oscillometry in critically ill patients are – in part – conflicting. On the one hand, it has been proposed that oscillometry can be used in intensive care unit patients with hypotension or vasopressor infusion [28]. In addition, it has been shown that oscillometry provides accurate BP measurements compared with invasive reference measurements in critically ill patients with cardiac arrhythmia [29, 30]. On the other hand, Lehman et al. [31] analyzed a database of intensive care unit patients and compared oscillometric BP values with direct BP measurements (arterial catheter) and observed marked and clinically relevant discrepancies between the methods. In noncardiac surgery patients, Wax et al. [32] demonstrated that oscillometric BP measurements were generally higher compared with invasive BP measurements during hypotension and lower during hypertension.

21.5 Continuous Noninvasive Arterial Blood Pressure Measurement

Two different technologies for automated continuous noninvasive assessment and analysis of the BP waveform are now available, namely, the volume clamp method (also called vascular unloading technology or "finger cuff technology") and radial artery applanation tonometry [7]. Although these technologies are often referred to as "new and innovative" technologies, the basic principles of both measurement techniques have been described many years ago [33, 34].

The volume clamp method uses an inflatable single- or double-finger cuff (with an integrated infrared light and an infrared transmission plethysmograph) that adjusts its pressure multiple times per second to keep the volume in the finger artery constant. From this pressure a BP curve can be derived. This method was described by the Czech physiologist Peňáz in 1973 [33]. Further technical developments and refinements of this method [35–38] led to monitoring systems that are now commercially available for bedside use. The ClearSight system (Edwards Lifesciences, Irvine, California, USA) uses a transfer function, an algorithm called "Physiocal" that adjusts for finger BP changes related to changes in the vasomotor tone, and a "heart reference system" that automatically adjusts for the hydrostatic difference between the level of the finger sensor and the level of the heart [35, 39–41]. In contrast, the CNAP system (CNSystems Medizintechnik AG, Graz, Austria) calibrates the systolic and diastolic BP values obtained with the finger cuff to oscillometric BP measurements assessed with an integrated upper arm cuff using a proprietary algorithm. To adjust and correct for long-term tracking of the finger BP, the CNAP system uses concentrically interlocking control loops [38].

The volume clamp method has some limitations due to the distal BP measurement site. In clinical circumstances with altered or impaired finger perfusion, such as finger edema, peripheral vasoconstriction, peripheral vascular disease, or marked hypothermia, the quality of the BP signal recorded with the finger cuff might be not good enough. Moreover, BP measurements with a finger cuff technology can be influenced and disturbed by excessive active or passive movement of the patient (especially of the arm or hand used for the measurements). When used in awake patients, the finger cuff technologies can cause discomfort or pain because the cuff impairs venous return from the finger and causes venous congestion. In addition to these general limitations of the vascular unloading technology, a specific limitation of the CNAP system might be the calibration of the BP values to brachial BP values assessed with oscillometry because, as discussed above, oscillometry also has some limitations with regard to the measurement performance and the clinical applicability.

A different technology for continuous noninvasive BP monitoring is the radial artery applanation tonometry that uses a pressure sensor applied over the radial artery based on the principle first described by Pressman and Newgard in the 1960s [34] and further developed by other researchers [42, 43]. The basic principle of arterial tonometry is that external flattening (applanation) of the arterial wall causes the pulse pressure amplitude (that is assessed with a sensor over this artery) to be maximal. To be able to flatten an artery with an external sensor, the artery must be superficial and supported by a bony structure (e.g., radial artery supported by styloid bone). The technology enables the mean arterial BP to be measured directly and the systolic and diastolic BP values to be calculated (e.g., using population-based algorithms) [44]. Nonautomatic systems using handheld sensors have been used for many years by cardiologists to estimate central vascular pressures [45]. Automatic radial artery applanation tonometry systems using a sensor attached to the patient's wrist have been developed for BP monitoring in the intensive care unit or the operating room [46]. Automatic artery applanation tonometry systems need to constantly adjust the pressure of the sensor flattening the underlying artery to obtain the optimal contact pressure and thus the optimal BP signal. One device for automatic radial artery applanation tonometry is the T-Line system (Tensys Medical, San Diego, CA, USA) that uses a disposable wrist splint for optimal positioning (slight extension) of the hand

and a "bracelet" housing the sensor and two motors that electromechanically drive the sensor over the artery to achieve the optimal sensor position and applanation pressure [7, 47]. The mean BP can be obtained from the maximal pulse pressure; systolic and diastolic BP is derived after scaling of the BP waveform using a proprietary algorithm that considers biometric data and a large invasive radial artery reference database [47, 48].

The main limitation of radial artery applanation tonometry is its high sensitivity to motion artifacts caused by movement of the measurement site. The system has been evaluated in a variety of clinical settings [44, 47, 49–52].

Numerous validation studies have been carried out to evaluate the measurement performance of these innovative noninvasive technologies for continuous BP monitoring in comparison with invasive reference measurements [53–55]. For all the technologies and devices described above, the validation studies revealed contradicting results. Some studies showed good agreement between the test and the reference method and recommended the use of noninvasive technologies as an alternative to invasive BP monitoring. Other studies reported a poor agreement with reference methods and concluded that these technologies should not be used in clinical routine to guide BP management. A meta-analysis on the accuracy and precision of different continuous noninvasive BP monitoring technologies including 28 studies revealed an overall random effect pooled mean of the differences of 3.2 mmHg, with a standard deviation of ±8.4 mmHg and 95% limits of agreement −13.4 to 19.7 mmHg for mean BP [54]. The authors stratified the results according to the different devices and reported a mean of the differences ± standard deviation of 3.5 ± 6.8 mmHg, 5.5 ± 9.3 mmHg, and 1.3 ± 5.7 mmHg, for the ClearSight (volume clamp method), CNAP (volume clamp method), and T-Line system (radial artery applanation tonometry), respectively [54].

However, how to define clinically acceptable agreement between noninvasive test methods and reference methods remains a matter of debate [56]. In addition, innovative noninvasive technologies should probably not only be tested against an invasive reference method but also against intermittent noninvasive BP monitoring techniques (such as oscillometry). Vos et al. [57] recently concluded that noninvasive continuous BP monitoring with the ClearSight system was interchangeable with monitoring by an oscillometric technique.

21.6 The Future of Arterial Blood Pressure Measurement

In the future, innovative, sophisticated, tiny sensors able to record biosignals such as BP and heart rate might change the way we perform clinical, ambulatory, and home BP monitoring.

For instance, it has been shown that flexible pressure-sensitive organic thin film transistors can be used for noninvasive continuous recording of the radial artery BP waveform [58]. In addition, thin conformable piezoelectric pressure sensors placed on the skin enable BP signals to be registered and analyzed [59]. Recently, it was demonstrated that nanocomposites (graphene added to polysilicon) can be used as highly sensitive electromechanical sensors that can measure pulse and BP [60].

These innovative materials might be used to develop flexible and wearable sensors that allow noninvasive transcutaneous recording of BP signals. Wireless and wearable sensors might offer intriguing possibilities for long-time continuous monitoring of BP, other vital signs, and the cardiovascular status ("mobile health monitoring," "mobile biomonitoring") [61–64]. Innovative sensor technologies might thus improve ambulatory and clinic BP monitoring and might be used in a variety of clinical applications in critical care, anesthesiology, emergency medicine, and cardiology [62–64].

Practical Implications

In clinical practice, the choice of the type of BP monitoring device is based on a variety of factors, with patient-specific factors being the most important ones. Considering the specific advantages and limitations of each technology and the clinical circumstances, the optimal BP monitoring device needs to be selected for the individual patient.

For critically ill patients with circulatory shock, invasive direct BP monitoring with an arterial catheter is required and recommended [65]. Besides the direct measurement of BP, an arterial catheter allows regular blood sampling for laboratory testing and blood gas analysis.

Patients undergoing high-risk surgery (e.g., cardiothoracic surgery, major abdominal surgery) and high-risk patients undergoing low- or intermediate-risk surgery also require invasive BP monitoring with an arterial catheter.

In the perioperative setting, the majority of the remaining patients will be monitored using noninvasive BP monitoring techniques. In certain groups of surgical patients, the continuous noninvasive BP monitoring allows a better stability of BP compared with intermittent BP measurements [66–68]. Future research needs to identify specific clinical settings in which continuous noninvasive BP monitoring can improve the quality of care or patient safety compared with intermittent noninvasive BP measurements. Because even short periods of intraoperative hypotension are associated with postoperative organ failure [69], continuous BP monitoring or the use of closed-loop systems might in the future help to avoid hypotension-related postoperative complications.

In acutely ill patients treated in the emergency department or patients undergoing complex diagnostic or therapeutic interventions [70–72], continuous noninvasive BP monitoring might enable BP instability to be detected earlier compared with serial intermittent BP measurements.

Conclusion

BP is a crucial hemodynamic variable in critically ill patients. The understanding of BP monitoring technologies is key to choose the optimal BP monitoring method for the individual patient and to avoid erroneous BP measurements. In critically ill patients, the direct invasive continuous BP measurement with an arterial catheter remains the reference method. In hemodynamically stable patients, BP monitoring can be performed in an intermittent manner using oscillometry. Noninvasive technologies that enable BP to be monitored continuously are now available for routine clinical use. Current research aims to evaluate whether these technologies for continuous noninvasive BP monitoring can improve patient outcome or the quality of care in certain clinical settings (perioperative medicine, emergency medicine).

Take-Home Messages

- BP monitoring is a mainstay of hemodynamic monitoring in various fields of medicine, including intensive care medicine, anesthesiology, and emergency medicine.
- Different technologies for invasive and noninvasive BP monitoring are available.
- An arterial catheter connected to a fluid-filled tubing system and a pressure transducer is the clinical reference method for invasive continuous BP monitoring.
- Noninvasive BP measurements are usually performed in an intermittent manner with an inflatable occluding cuff using the auscultatory method, palpatory method, or automated techniques such as oscillometry.
- Noninvasive BP monitoring technologies that enable the arterial BP waveform to be recorded and displayed continuously are now available for clinical practice.
- It is important to know the principles, the advantages, and the limitations of each BP measurement technique to be able to choose the optimal method to measure BP in the individual patient.

Conflict of Interest BS collaborates with Pulsion Medical Systems SE (Feldkirchen, Germany) as a member of the medical advisory board and received honoraria for giving lectures and refunds of travel expenses from Pulsion Medical Systems SE. BS received research support from Edwards Lifesciences (Irvine, CA, USA). BS received institutional research grants, unrestricted research grants, and refunds of travel expenses from Tensys Medical Inc. (San Diego, CA, USA). BS received honoraria for giving lectures and refunds of travel expenses from CNSystems Medizintechnik AG (Graz, Austria).

TWLS received honoraria from Edwards Lifesciences (Irvine, CA, USA) and Masimo Inc. (Irvine, CA, USA) for consulting and lecturing.

JLT is a member of the medical advisory board of Pulsion Medical systems and received honoraria from Edwards Lifesciences and Masimo Inc. for consulting.

References

1. Booth J. A short history of blood pressure measurement. Proc R Soc Med. 1977;70:793–9.
2. Lewis O. Stephen Hales and the measurement of blood pressure. J Hum Hypertens. 1994;8:865–71.
3. O'Brien E, Fitzgerald D. The history of blood pressure measurement. J Hum Hypertens. 1994;8:73–84.
4. Nichols WW, Nichols WW, McDonald DA. McDonald's blood flow in arteries: theoretic, experimental, and clinical principles. 6th ed. London: CRC Press; 2011.
5. Marey E-J. Recherches sur le pouls au moyen d'un nouvel appareil enregistreur le sphygmographe. Paris: Thunot; 1860.
6. Mahomed F. The physiology and clinical use of the sphygmograph. Med Times Gazette. 1872;1:62.
7. Saugel B, Dueck R, Wagner JY. Measurement of blood pressure. Best Pract Res Clin Anaesthesiol. 2014;28:309–22.
8. Perloff D, Grim C, Flack J, Frohlich ED, Hill M, McDonald M, et al. Human blood pressure determination by sphygmomanometry. Circulation. 1993;88:2460–70.
9. Hill L, Barnard H. A simple and accurate form of sphygmometer or arterial pressure gauge contrived for clinical use. Br Med J. 1897;2:904.
10. Erlanger J, Hooker DR. An experimental study of blood-pressure and of pulse-pressure in man. John Hopkins Hosp Rep. 1904;XII:145–378.
11. Posey JA, Geddes LA, Williams H, Moore AG. The meaning of the point of maximum oscillations in cuff pressure in the indirect measurement of blood pressure. 1. Cardiovasc Res Cent Bull. 1969;8:15–25.

12. Alpert BS, Quinn D, Gallick D. Oscillometric blood pressure: a review for clinicians. J Am Soc Hypertens. 2014;8:930–8.
13. Ogedegbe G, Pickering T. Principles and techniques of blood pressure measurement. Cardiol Clin. 2010;28:571–86.
14. Geddes LA, Voelz M, Combs C, Reiner D, Babbs CF. Characterization of the oscillometric method for measuring indirect blood pressure. Ann Biomed Eng. 1982;10:271–80.
15. Gu WJ, Tie HT, Liu JC, Zeng XT. Efficacy of ultrasound-guided radial artery catheterization: a systematic review and meta-analysis of randomized controlled trials. Crit Care. 2014;18:R93.
16. Scheer B, Perel A, Pfeiffer UJ. Clinical review: complications and risk factors of peripheral arterial catheters used for haemodynamic monitoring in anaesthesia and intensive care medicine. Crit Care. 2002;6:199–204.
17. Numaguchi A, Adachi YU, Aoki Y, Ishii Y, Suzuki K, Obata Y, et al. Radial artery cannulation decreases the distal arterial blood flow measured by power Doppler ultrasound. J Clin Monit Comput. 2015;29:653–7.
18. Ortega R, Connor C, Kotova F, Deng W, Lacerra C. Use of pressure transducers. N Engl J Med. 2017;376:e26.
19. McGhee BH, Bridges EJ. Monitoring arterial blood pressure: what you may not know. Crit Care Nurse. 2002;22:60–4, 66–70, 3 passim.
20. Gardner RM. Direct blood pressure measurement–dynamic response requirements. Anesthesiology. 1981;54:227–36.
21. Kleinman B, Powell S, Kumar P, Gardner RM. The fast flush test measures the dynamic response of the entire blood pressure monitoring system. Anesthesiology. 1992;77:1215–20.
22. Petrie JC, O'Brien ET, Littler WA, de Swiet M. Recommendations on blood pressure measurement. Br Med J (Clin Res Ed). 1986;293:611–5.
23. Ramsey M 3rd. Noninvasive automatic determination of mean arterial pressure. Med Biol Eng Comput. 1979;17:11–8.
24. Smulyan H, Safar ME. Blood pressure measurement: retrospective and prospective views. Am J Hypertens. 2011;24:628–34.
25. van Montfrans GA. Oscillometric blood pressure measurement: progress and problems. Blood Press Monit. 2001;6:287–90.
26. Pickering TG, Hall JE, Appel LJ, Falkner BE, Graves J, Hill MN, et al. Recommendations for blood pressure measurement in humans and experimental animals: part 1: blood pressure measurement in humans: a statement for professionals from the Subcommittee of Professional and Public Education of the American Heart Association Council on High Blood Pressure Research. Circulation. 2005;111:697–716.
27. Picone DS, Schultz MG, Otahal P, Aakhus S, Al-Jumaily AM, Black JA, et al. Accuracy of cuff-measured blood pressure: systematic reviews and meta-analyses. J Am Coll Cardiol. 2017;70:572–86.
28. Lakhal K, Ehrmann S, Boulain T. Non-invasive blood pressure monitoring in the critically ill: time to abandon the intra-arterial catheter? Chest. 2018;153:1023–39.
29. Lakhal K, Ehrmann S, Martin M, Faiz S, Reminiac F, Cinotti R, et al. Blood pressure monitoring during arrhythmia: agreement between automated brachial cuff and intra-arterial measurements. Br J Anaesth. 2015;115:540–9.
30. Lakhal K, Martin M, Ehrmann S, Faiz S, Rozec B, Boulain T. Non-invasive blood pressure monitoring with an oscillometric brachial cuff: impact of arrhythmia. J Clin Monit Comput. 2018;32:707–15.
31. Lehman LW, Saeed M, Talmor D, Mark R, Malhotra A. Methods of blood pressure measurement in the ICU. Crit Care Med. 2013;41:34–40.
32. Wax DB, Lin HM, Leibowitz AB. Invasive and concomitant noninvasive intraoperative blood pressure monitoring: observed differences in measurements and associated therapeutic interventions. Anesthesiology. 2011;115:973–8.
33. Penaz J, Voigt A, Teichmann W. Contribution to the continuous indirect blood pressure measurement. Z Gesamte Inn Med. 1976;31:1030–3.
34. Pressman GL, Newgard PM. A transducer for the continuous external measurement of arterial blood pressure. IEEE Trans Biomed Eng. 1963;10:73–81.
35. Wesseling KH, Settels JJ, van der Hoeven GM, Nijboer JA, Butijn MW, Dorlas JC. Effects of peripheral vasoconstriction on the measurement of blood pressure in a finger. Cardiovasc Res. 1985;19:139–45.
36. Takazawa K, O'Rourke MF, Fujita M, Tanaka N, Takeda K, Kurosu F, et al. Estimation of ascending aortic pressure from radial arterial pressure using a generalised transfer function. Z Kardiol. 1996;85(Suppl 3):137–9.

37. Imholz BP, Parati G, Mancia G, Wesseling KH. Effects of graded vasoconstriction upon the measurement of finger arterial pressure. J Hypertens. 1992;10:979–84.
38. Fortin J, Marte W, Grullenberger R, Hacker A, Habenbacher W, Heller A, et al. Continuous non-invasive blood pressure monitoring using concentrically interlocking control loops. Comput Biol Med. 2006;36:941–57.
39. Wesseling KH. Finger arterial pressure measurement with Finapres. Z Kardiol. 1996;85(Suppl 3):38–44.
40. Martina JR, Westerhof BE, van Goudoever J, de Beaumont EM, Truijen J, Kim YS, et al. Noninvasive continuous arterial blood pressure monitoring with Nexfin(R). Anesthesiology. 2012;116:1092–103.
41. Gizdulich P, Prentza A, Wesseling KH. Models of brachial to finger pulse wave distortion and pressure decrement. Cardiovasc Res. 1997;33:698–705.
42. Stein PD, Blick EF. Arterial tonometry for the atraumatic measurement of arterial blood pressure. J Appl Physiol. 1971;30:593–6.
43. Drzewiecki GM, Melbin J, Noordergraaf A. Arterial tonometry: review and analysis. J Biomech. 1983;16:141–52.
44. Meidert AS, Huber W, Hapfelmeier A, Schofthaler M, Muller JN, Langwieser N, et al. Evaluation of the radial artery applanation tonometry technology for continuous noninvasive blood pressure monitoring compared with central aortic blood pressure measurements in patients with multiple organ dysfunction syndrome. J Crit Care. 2013;28:908–12.
45. Nelson MR, Stepanek J, Cevette M, Covalciuc M, Hurst RT, Tajik AJ. Noninvasive measurement of central vascular pressures with arterial tonometry: clinical revival of the pulse pressure waveform. Mayo Clin Proc. 2010;85:460–72.
46. Kemmotsu O, Ueda M, Otsuka H, Yamamura T, Okamura A, Ishikawa T, et al. Blood pressure measurement by arterial tonometry in controlled hypotension. Anesth Analg. 1991;73:54–8.
47. Dueck R, Goedje O, Clopton P. Noninvasive continuous beat-to-beat radial artery pressure via TL-200 applanation tonometry. J Clin Monit Comput. 2012;26:75–83.
48. Drzewiecki G, Hood R, Apple H. Theory of the oscillometric maximum and the systolic and diastolic detection ratios. Ann Biomed Eng. 1994;22:88–96.
49. Saugel B, Fassio F, Hapfelmeier A, Meidert AS, Schmid RM, Huber W. The T-Line TL-200 system for continuous non-invasive blood pressure measurement in medical intensive care unit patients. Intensive Care Med. 2012;38:1471–7.
50. Saugel B, Meidert AS, Hapfelmeier A, Eyer F, Schmid RM, Huber W. Non-invasive continuous arterial pressure measurement based on radial artery tonometry in the intensive care unit: a method comparison study using the T-Line TL-200pro device. Br J Anaesth. 2013;111:185–90.
51. Meidert AS, Huber W, Muller JN, Schofthaler M, Hapfelmeier A, Langwieser N, et al. Radial artery applanation tonometry for continuous non-invasive arterial pressure monitoring in intensive care unit patients: comparison with invasively assessed radial arterial pressure. Br J Anaesth. 2014;112:521–8.
52. Szmuk P, Pivalizza E, Warters RD, Ezri T, Gebhard R. An evaluation of the T-Line Tensymeter continuous noninvasive blood pressure device during induced hypotension. Anaesthesia. 2008;63:307–12.
53. Bartels K, Esper SA, Thiele RH. Blood pressure monitoring for the anesthesiologist: a practical review. Anesth Analg. 2016;122:1866–79.
54. Kim SH, Lilot M, Sidhu KS, Rinehart J, Yu Z, Canales C, et al. Accuracy and precision of continuous noninvasive arterial pressure monitoring compared with invasive arterial pressure: a systematic review and meta-analysis. Anesthesiology. 2014;120:1080–97.
55. Ameloot K, Palmers PJ, Malbrain ML. The accuracy of noninvasive cardiac output and pressure measurements with finger cuff: a concise review. Curr Opin Crit Care. 2015;21:232–9.
56. Saugel B, Reuter DA. Are we ready for the age of non-invasive haemodynamic monitoring? Br J Anaesth. 2014;113:340–3.
57. Vos JJ, Poterman M, Mooyaart EA, Weening M, Struys MM, Scheeren TW, et al. Comparison of continuous non-invasive finger arterial pressure monitoring with conventional intermittent automated arm arterial pressure measurement in patients under general anaesthesia. Br J Anaesth. 2014;113:67–74.
58. Schwartz G, Tee BC, Mei J, Appleton AL, Kim do H, Wang H, et al. Flexible polymer transistors with high pressure sensitivity for application in electronic skin and health monitoring. Nat Commun. 2013;4:1859.
59. Dagdeviren C, Su Y, Joe P, Yona R, Liu Y, Kim YS, et al. Conformable amplified lead zirconate titanate sensors with enhanced piezoelectric response for cutaneous pressure monitoring. Nat Commun. 2014;5:4496.

60. Boland CS, Khan U, Ryan G, Barwich S, Charifou R, Harvey A, et al. Sensitive electromechanical sensors using viscoelastic graphene-polymer nanocomposites. Science. 2016;354:1257–60.
61. Michard F. Hemodynamic monitoring in the era of digital health. Ann Intensive Care. 2016;6:15.
62. Michard F. A sneak peek into digital innovations and wearable sensors for cardiac monitoring. J Clin Monit Comput. 2017;31:253–9.
63. Michard F, Pinsky MR, Vincent JL. Intensive care medicine in 2050: NEWS for hemodynamic monitoring. Intensive Care Med. 2017;43:440–2.
64. Michard F, Gan TJ, Kehlet H. Digital innovations and emerging technologies for enhanced recovery programmes. Br J Anaesth. 2017;119:31.
65. Teboul JL, Saugel B, Cecconi M, De Backer D, Hofer CK, Monnet X, et al. Less invasive hemodynamic monitoring in critically ill patients. Intensive Care Med. 2016;42:1350–9.
66. Benes J, Simanova A, Tovarnicka T, Sevcikova S, Kletecka J, Zatloukal J, et al. Continuous non-invasive monitoring improves blood pressure stability in upright position: randomized controlled trial. J Clin Monit Comput. 2015;29:11–7.
67. Meidert AS, Nold JS, Hornung R, Paulus AC, Zwissler B, Czerner S. The impact of continuous non-invasive arterial blood pressure monitoring on blood pressure stability during general anaesthesia in orthopaedic patients: a randomised trial. Eur J Anaesthesiol. 2017;34:716.
68. Ilies C, Kiskalt H, Siedenhans D, Meybohm P, Steinfath M, Bein B, et al. Detection of hypotension during Caesarean section with continuous non-invasive arterial pressure device or intermittent oscillometric arterial pressure measurement. Br J Anaesth. 2012;109:413–9.
69. Walsh M, Devereaux PJ, Garg AX, Kurz A, Turan A, Rodseth RN, et al. Relationship between intraoperative mean arterial pressure and clinical outcomes after noncardiac surgery: toward an empirical definition of hypotension. Anesthesiology. 2013;119:507–15.
70. Nowak RM, Sen A, Garcia AJ, Wilkie H, Yang JJ, Nowak MR, et al. Noninvasive continuous or intermittent blood pressure and heart rate patient monitoring in the ED. Am J Emerg Med. 2011;29:782–9.
71. Wagner JY, Prantner JS, Meidert AS, Hapfelmeier A, Schmid RM, Saugel B. Noninvasive continuous versus intermittent arterial pressure monitoring: evaluation of the vascular unloading technique (CNAP device) in the emergency department. Scand J Trauma Resusc Emerg Med. 2014;22:8.
72. Siebig S, Rockmann F, Sabel K, Zuber-Jerger I, Dierkes C, Brunnler T, et al. Continuous non-invasive arterial pressure technique improves patient monitoring during interventional endoscopy. Int J Med Sci. 2009;6:37–42.

Cardiac Output Monitors

Daniel A. Reuter and Sebastian A. Haas

M. R. Pinsky et al. (eds.), *Hemodynamic Monitoring*, Lessons from the ICU,
https://doi.org/10.1007/978-3-319-69269-2_22

22

Learning Objectives

Understanding of the historical evolution of cardiac output monitoring in intensive care medicine; understanding the (historical) reasons, why cardiac output monitoring is still not used as routine monitoring in critically ill patients; overview of currently used technological concepts for bedside cardiac output monitoring.

22.1 Introduction

Cardiac output, i.e., the quantification of the blood flow that is generated by the heart, is by far the most important macrohemodynamic variable in the assessment of hemodynamic instable, critically ill patient. Although of course, also cardiac output can only be of significant help, if its values (and much more importantly its changes under therapy) are interpreted within the context of other hemodynamic and metabolic parameters, its assessment frequently determines and changes the direction of therapeutic interventions. This chapter will try to give an overview of the methodological and technical principles of cardiac output monitors (please see ◘ Table 22.1) and the impact of each of them on their clinical usability. It therefore tries to function as a bracket around the following chapters, where each of the methods that are presently available is separately described and discussed in depth.

22.2 Historical View Back

Historically, cardiac output monitors have not been used routinely in critically ill patients. And also, when looking at recent data from European ICU's, cardiac output monitoring is performed only in a small minority of our patients [1]. The reason for that – and the

◘ **Table 22.1** Clinically available technologies for cardiac output monitoring

Measurement technique	Description
Indicator dilution	Application as pulmonary artery thermodilution or transpulmonary thermodilution Serve as clinical gold standard for CO measurement Additional parameters provided: right ventricular ejection fraction, right ventricular end-diastolic volume (both for pulmonary artery thermodilution), global end-diastolic volume, extravascular lung water (both for transpulmonary thermodilution)
Doppler-derived blood flow measurement	Low invasiveness High user dependency Not suitable for long-term use
Pulse wave analysis	Low-intermediate invasiveness Not suitable for patients with arrhythmias Prone to artifacts Limited exactness; focus is in trending
Bioimpedance and bioreactance	Noninvasiveness Limited validity compared to clinical gold standard

overwhelming interest in blood pressures – is easy to explain; for many decades, the assessment of blood flow was technically simply too difficult and cumbersome for a routine use. Methods derived in the nineteenth century were based on the principle of indicator dilution. Salt solutions or dyes, injected into the venous system and then detected in arterial blood samples, served as indicators [2]. Not only the fact that handling these indicators properly was not really user-friendly, but also the detection of downslope concentrations was not possible at the bedside, but needed additional technical and human resources. Similarly, the CO2 rebreathing method based on the Fick principle did not reach the clinical routine use due to inhomogeneity of measurement results and technical complexity.

Thus, "monitoring" by its principle meaning was simply not possible with these methods. Other technical principles, such as the arterial pulse contour analysis (or pulse wave analysis), which were also described already more than 100 years ago, had theoretically already overcome those problems of "discontinuity" and "time delay"; however, also their practical usability remained theory, until the evolution of computerization within the 1980s and 1990s of the last century, making the automated use of calculation algorithms at the bedside possible [3, 4]. However, the "historical breakthrough" for clinical cardiac output monitoring was made by the technical modification of an indicator dilution principle: Thermodilution within the pulmonary artery, using the pulmonary artery catheter (PAC), or named after their pioneers William Ganz and Jeremy Swan the "Swan-Ganz catheter," became a technique, which allowed quantifying cardiac output in clinical routine at the bedside [5]. However, also the PA catheter remained an exotic monitoring tool within the ICUs with its use restricted to a small group of highly complex critically ill patients. This is because as a highly invasive method, its use is of course associated with a certain risk profile, but it is even more problematic that, for its implementation and its proper use, this method is still dependent on the presence of highly skilled personnel – it is simply not an easy "plug and play device" [6, 7]. Amelioration of these method immanent drawbacks and at least a small increase in the use of thermodilution cardiac output monitoring outside the small community of PAC enthusiasts came with the availability of transpulmonary thermodilution devices in the mid-1990s [2]. However, the limitation of discontinuity and non-automatization remained also here.

The next big milestone and opportunity for cardiac output monitoring to become much more integral part of bedside monitoring as a continuous variable were the clinical implementation of ultrasound and in particular echocardiography. Besides manifold other highly important diagnostic opportunities, which make this technology indispensable from the ICU, echocardiography-based cardiac output determination seemed to fulfill the criteria such as "real-time," easy-to-use," and "noninvasive" [8]. However, its drawbacks of being user-dependent, noncontinuous, and time- (and personnel-) consuming have prevented this technology to become a real "cardiac output monitor." This is different with the application of Doppler by miniaturized transnasal esophageal probes, which has found its place as cardiac output monitoring for short-term use in perioperative medicine [9].

In parallel to this evolution of ultrasound, the historical technique of pulse wave or pulse contour analysis has become available within the 1990s of the last century. The principle, as Otto Frank, physiologist, and one part of the well-known "Frank-Starling mechanism" have described already in 1899, has remained the same until today: "Under certain circumstances, it might be possible to generate information of blood flow from the shape of the blood pressure curve." However, now analysis has become automated and available at the bedside, and the principle has been transformed from central arteries and invasively deducted signals to peripheral pulse signals, which are assessed completely noninvasive, using even not only the arterial pressure signal but also other signals, such as the photoplesmythographic pulse signal [10].

22.3 What Do We Need from a Cardiac Output Monitor?

Clinical utility of cardiac output monitors is defined by the following modalities: (a) Measurements need to be reliable, i.e., exactness of measurements should be high in terms of bias and precision; (b) the method should be noninvasive in order not to place additional risks to the patient because of the measurements; (c) the method should provide continuous and real-time measurements; (d) it should be automated in order to save human resources; (e) if not automated, it should be as user-independent as possible in order to minimize inter-user discrepancies in results; and (f) it should be easy to implement and use in order to reach a high degree of acceptance in daily clinical practice.

22.4 Methods of Measurement

So up today, the following principle methods are available for cardiac output monitoring.

22.4.1 Indicator Dilution

This comprises pulmonary artery thermodilution using a sensor-tipped PAC; transpulmonary thermodilution with a femoral, axillary, or brachial sensor-tipped arterial catheter; and lithium dilution, again with a peripheral sensor-tipped arterial catheter. The common basic principle is that a known amount of indicator is brought as a bolus within the circulation, and further downstream, its concentration over time is measured. The faster the blood flow is, the faster is the rise, as well as the decline of the indicator concentration downslope. All these technologies, and for historical reasons in particular the pulmonary artery thermodilution are seen as the "clinical gold standard" [2]. So determination of absolute values of cardiac output, also repetitive over time, is most reliable using one of those techniques. However, bolus application already implies the most prominent disadvantage; all indicator dilution techniques, also when bolus application is automated, remain intermittent, discontinuous measurement techniques.

22.4.2 Doppler-Derived Blood Flow Measurement

Doppler-based cardiac output measurements can be achieved by transthoracic, transesophageal echocardiography or using miniaturized esophageal Doppler probes [8, 9]. The principle is as follows: With the use of the Doppler effect, the flow profile of the ultrasound-reflecting erythrocytes through a vascular structure is continuously assessed and quantified as a velocity-time integral. If now the vascular diameter (right/left ventricular outflow tract, descending aorta) is known (or estimated), stroke volume and thus cardiac output can be continuously assessed. The striking advantages are the noninvasiveness and the real-time/beat-to-beat assessment. However, all these techniques remain user-dependent and (with the exemption of esophageal Doppler) are only temporary snapshots – echocardiography is by nature not a monitoring modality.

22.4.3 Pulse Wave Analysis

If the elastic properties of the arterial wall remain constant, then the integral of the systolic portion of the arterial pressure curve is directly correlated to the left ventricular stroke volume. This is the basic assumption of most arterial pulse contour algorithms currently in use [11]. Its use, which was initially just assumed to be "clinically valid enough" in central arteries, i.e., the aorta, has been extended to pressure tracings derived from peripheral arteries, both measured invasively and noninvasively, as, for example, with volume clamp technology [12]. The advantage of all of those variants of pulse contour analysis is that it is an automated, beat-by-beat, continuous, and user-independent measurement technique. However, on the other side, the exactness of arterial pulse contour analysis, compared to the clinical gold standards of thermodilution, in particular in terms of absolute values, is limited. Further, this technique is quite sensible for measurement errors produced by artifacts within the raw signal (pressure curve).

22.4.4 Bioimpedance and Bioreactance

Recently, two other noninvasive cardiac monitoring technologies were clinically introduced, which both use the assessment of changes in electrical conductivity within the thorax to quantify stroke volume and cardiac output [13]. The principle idea behind it is that if intrathoracic blood volume is changing due to blood ejection into the circulation, accordingly, electrical conductivity of a high-frequency but low-magnitude current, which is applied to the thorax via a skin electrode, is changing accordingly. Literally, stroke volume serves as an electrical contrast medium, which is continuously assessed. The advantages of those methods are noninvasive, real-time, continuous, and automated monitoring. However, the most important drawback so far is the limited exactness of these technologies in comparison to the clinical gold standards of cardiac output monitors [10].

Take-Home Messages

Availability and applicability of cardiac output monitors have tremendously increased during the last two decades, making assessment and monitoring of this very central hemodynamic variable feasible theoretically in all patients on the ICU, which show signs of hemodynamic instability. Each method has its own profile of advantages and disadvantages in particular in terms of invasiveness versus exactness of results. However, the needs for the individual patients in intensive care differ: In patients where cardiac output monitoring is performed in order to preemptively avoid phases of hemodynamic instability and to routinely guide standard therapies, as in elective perioperative patients, automatization and low invasiveness dominate over exactness, whereas in the highly complex, hemodynamically instable, critically ill patient in shock, precision of measurement and the availability of other associated hemodynamic parameters have much higher importance.

References

1. Funcke S, Sander M, Goepfert MS, et al. Practice of hemodynamic monitoring and management in German, Austrian, and Swiss intensive care units: the multicenter cross-sectional ICU-CardioMan Study. Ann Intensive Care. 2016;6:49.
2. Reuter DA, Huang C, Edrich T, et al. Cardiac output monitoring using indicator-dilution techniques: basics, limits, and perspectives. Anesth Analg. 2010;110:799–811.
3. Sagawa K, Lie RK, Schaefer J. Translation of Otto Frank's paper "Die Grundform des arteriellen Pulses" Zeitschrift für Biologie 37: 483–526 (1899). J Mol Cell Cardiol. 1990;22:253–4.
4. Frank O. The basic shape of the arterial pulse. First treatise: mathematical analysis. J Mol Cell Cardiol. 1990;22:255–77.
5. Swan HJ, Ganz W, Forrester J. Catheterization of the heart in man with use of a flow-directed balloon-tipped catheter. N Engl J Med. 1970;283:447–51.
6. Ramsay J. Pro: is the pulmonary artery catheter dead? J Cardiothorac Vasc Anesth. 2007;21:144–6.
7. Murphy GS, Vender JS. Con: is the pulmonary artery catheter dead? J Cardiothorac Vasc Anesth. 2007;21:147–9.
8. Wetterslev M, Møller-Sørensen H, Johansen RR, Perner A. Systematic review of cardiac output measurements by echocardiography vs. thermodilution: the techniques are not interchangeable. Intensive Care Med. 2016;42:1223–33.
9. Singer M. Oesophageal Doppler. Curr Opin Crit Care. 2009;15:244–8.
10. Teboul JL, Saugel B, Cecconi M, et al. Less invasive hemodynamic monitoring in critically ill patients. Intensive Care Med. 2016;42:1350–9.
11. Thiele RH, Durieux ME. Arterial waveform analysis for the anesthesiologist: past, present, and future concepts. Anesth Analg. 2011;113:766–76.
12. Saugel B, Cecconi M, Wagner JY, Reuter DA. Noninvasive continuous cardiac output monitoring in perioperative and intensive care medicine. Br J Anaesth. 2015;114(4):562–75.
13. Fellahi JL, Fischer MO. Electrical bioimpedance cardiography: an old technology with new hopes for the future. J Cardiothorac Vasc Anesth. 2014;28:755–60.

Volumetric Monitoring in Critically Ill Patients

Manu L. N. G. Malbrain

M. R. Pinsky et al. (eds.), *Hemodynamic Monitoring*, Lessons from the ICU,
https://doi.org/10.1007/978-3-319-69269-2_23

Learning Objectives

In this chapter we will discuss the different available volumetric monitoring techniques. After finishing this chapter, the reader will understand the differences between pulmonary thermodilution and transpulmonary thermodilution and single and double dye dilution techniques. Each technique has indications and contraindications and pros and cons, and the user must understand the different pitfalls that may affect the results and when one technique is preferred over another. Echocardiography should be seen as an additional tool or the modern stethoscope to assess cardiac function and to obtain a "volumetric" idea of preload in combination with cardiac function and afterload. It is not a real continuous monitoring tool; however, the aforementioned indicator dilution techniques will only provide "static" volumetric data intermittently at each calibration with thermo- or dye dilution. The user will also understand the basic principles of volumetric monitoring with bioelectrical impedance analysis.

23.1 Introduction

Correct assessment of preload is important in critically ill patients with shock. This chapter will focus on the different volumetric monitoring techniques currently available for the critically ill patient and not on pressure monitoring. Both play independent and linked roles in defining health, disease, and response to treatment. In the past barometric preload parameters like central venous pressure (CVP) and pulmonary artery occlusion pressure (PAOP) have been suggested as the gold standard. The reader must be aware that filling pressures and even absolute static volumetric parameters are both relative estimates of preload and can be used to assess ventricular pump function, but not fluid responsiveness. Fluid responsiveness and functional hemodynamic monitoring will be discussed elsewhere. Clearly CVP and PAOP are more sensitive to peripheral and pulmonary edema etiologies. However, in situations where intrathoracic pressure (ITP) is increased as seen with positive-pressure ventilation, the addition of positive end-expiratory pressure (PEEP), the presence of auto-PEEP, or increased intra-abdominal pressure (IAP), the traditional barometric preload parameters may be erroneously increased because in fact they are zeroed against atmospheric pressure instead of ITP. Intra-abdominal hypertension (IAH) is defined as a sustained increase in IAP above 12 mmHg. In those conditions and in general, volumetric monitoring may provide more meaningful results.

Volumetric monitoring includes right ventricular end-diastolic volume (RVEDV), global end-diastolic volume (GEDV), and intrathoracic blood volume (ITBV) that can be obtained with thermodilution techniques. Furthermore, left ventricle end-diastolic area (LVEDA) can be evaluated with transthoracic (TTE) or transesophageal echocardiography (TEE). All the above listed parameters can also be indexed according to body surface area (BSA). Extravascular lung water (EVLW) is another volumetric parameter that can be obtained with transpulmonary thermodilution. Traditionally EVLW is indexed to predicted body weight (PBW). Finally, in order to be concise, we will briefly mention volumetric monitoring that can be obtained with bioelectrical impedance analysis (BIA).

23.2 Limitations of Barometric Preload

According to Frank-Starling mechanism, preload of the left ventricle is defined as the fiber length of the myocardial muscles at end-diastole (Fig. 23.1). The clinical parameter that correlates best with this is the left ventricular end-diastolic volume (LVEDV), but this parameter cannot be easily measured, let alone that it can be estimated repeatedly to assess the effect of treatment [1, 2]. Assuming that left ventricular compliance remains constant or stable, changes in volume should be accompanied by changes in pressure:

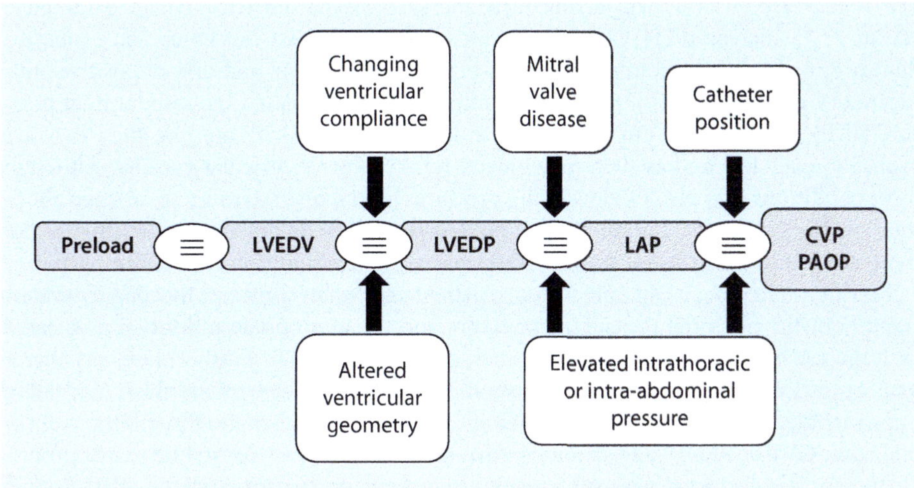

Fig. 23.1 "The PAOP assumption": Why intracardiac filling pressures like pulmonary artery occlusion pressure do not accurately estimate preload status. First, ventricular compliance is constantly changing in the critically ill, resulting in a variable relationship between pressure and volume. As a result, changes in intracardiac pressure no longer directly reflect changes in intravascular volume. The presence of increased ITP will decrease LV compliance by rightward shift and flattening of the Frank-Starling curve. Second, elevated ITP (as in intra-abdominal hypertension) has been demonstrated to increase PAOP and CVP measurements by an amount that is difficult to predict, further confounding their validity. This apparent deviation from Starling's law of the heart is due to the fact that both PAOP and CVP are measured relative to atmospheric pressure but are actually the sum of both intravascular pressure and ITP. Third, mitral valve disease can confound the use of PAOP as an estimate of intravascular volume status. Patients with IAH-induced pulmonary hypertension or acute lung injury demonstrate increased PVR and are at significant risk for mitral valve regurgitation. Fourth, accurate PAOP measurements are dependent upon proper placement of the PAC. Compression of the pulmonary parenchyma as a result of elevated IAP can markedly alter the normal progression of alveolar distention and pulmonary capillary pressures defined in West's lung zones 1, 2, and 3. IAH-induced cardiac and pulmonary dysfunction can further alter the normal pulmonary artery waveforms making proper placement of the PAC tip in West's lung zone 2 difficult. Inadvertent placement of the tip in apical zone 1 commonly results in PAOP measurements that more appropriately reflect alveolar pressure. (Adapted from Cheatham et al. [1]). CVP central venous pressure, LAP left atrial pressure, LVEDV left ventricular end-diastolic volume, LVEDP left ventricular end-diastolic pressure, PAOP pulmonary artery occlusion pressure

$$\text{Compliance} = \Delta\text{Volume} / \Delta\text{Pressure}$$

and

$$\Delta\text{Volume} \cong \Delta\text{Pressure}$$

Following this assumption, pressure-based (barometric) preload parameters like CVP, PAOP, left atrial pressure (LAP), and left ventricular end-diastolic pressure have traditionally been used at the bedside as intravascular volume surrogate estimates. Although they may likely be valid in healthy normal individuals, the multiple assumptions that need to be made in order to use CVP and PAOP as correct estimates of right and left preload, respectively, do not necessarily hold true in the critically ill unstable patient, especially if ITP is increased as this will erroneously increase the barometric preload parameters (◘ Fig. 23.1). Increased ITP can be related to diminished chest wall compliance (obesity, fluid overload, post sternotomy), positive-pressure ventilation, addition of positive end-expiratory pressure (PEEP), presence of auto-PEEP, or increased intra-abdominal pressure (IAP) and IAH [3]. On the other hand, if CVP and PAOP are low, then they are probably really low and as such may indeed reflect a low ventricular preload. Although some conditions may result in low filling pressures like an open sternum or an open abdomen (with a temporary abdominal closure). However, they do not indicate whether or not the patient may or may not be fluid responsive [4]. Hemodynamic monitoring per se cannot alter outcome; it can only improve patient care when clinicians thoroughly understand both the potential measurement errors and the appropriate utilization associated with the use of barometric parameters such as CVP and PAOP. Furthermore, any therapeutic protocol or treatment algorithm should follow physiology; otherwise, it may fail to improve outcome [5]. Due to the physiologic complexity, resuscitation to arbitrary, absolute, static CVP or PAOP values should be avoided as such a practice can lead to inappropriate therapeutic decisions, with subsequent under- or over-resuscitation and related organ dysfunction or failure. Volumetric (as opposed to barometric) preload monitoring may therefore provide more meaningful information as it more closely reflects the true filling status of the patient even in conditions of increased ITP that may be present in more than 30% of critically ill patients [6]. However, as stated above and similar to barometric preload parameters, "static" volumetric preload parameters also do not reflect fluid responsiveness.

23.3 Pulmonary Thermodilution

Pulmonary thermodilution (TD) can only be performed with a pulmonary artery catheter (PAC) and consists of injecting a bolus of iced fluid (usually normal saline) via the proximal lumen (with the opening in the right atrium) [7]. ◘ Figure 23.2 shows a classic pulmonary TD curve. A thermistor on the tip of the PAC, located in the pulmonary artery, records the resulting thermodilution curve. Cardiac output (CO) can then be calculated and is inversely related to the area under the dilution curve (time integral), according to the Stewart-Hamilton equation. Several variations of the PAC have been developed, also allowing the measurement of right ventricular ejection fraction (RVEF) and assessment of a "volumetric" parameter, namely, RVEDV. The RVEF provides information on right ventricular contractility, while the right ventricular preload is reflected by RVEDV. The RVEF can be determined through a beat-to-beat analysis of the thermodilution curve via estimation of the exponential decay time constant (τ) of the thermodilution curve and heart rate:

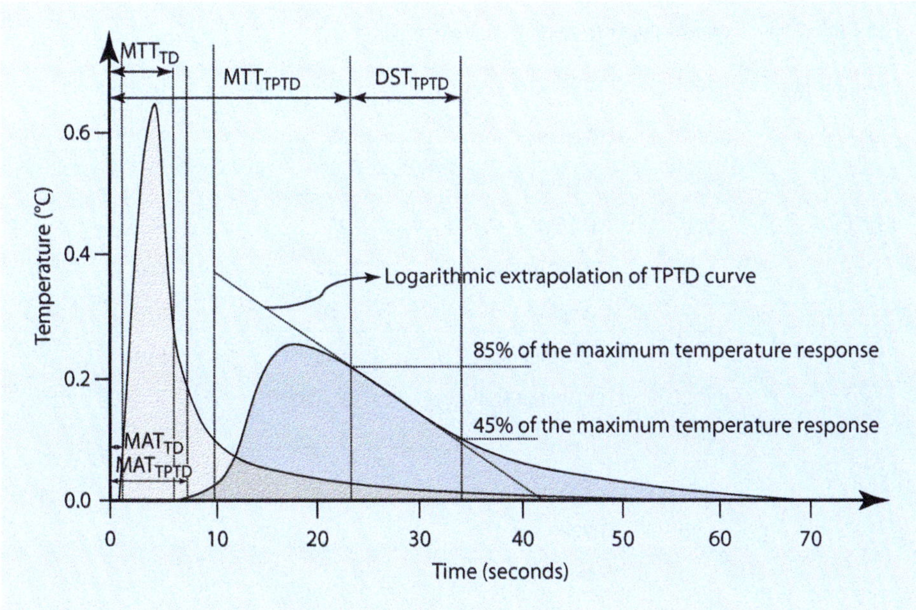

Fig. 23.2 Sample of a pulmonary and transpulmonary thermodilution curve. DST downslope time, MAT mean appearance time, MTT mean transit time, TD thermodilution, TPTD transpulmonary thermodilution

$$\text{RVEF} = 1 - \exp\left[-60/\left(\text{heart rate} \times \tau\right)\right]$$

The RVEDV can be calculated using the following equation [8]:

$$\text{RVEDV} = \text{CO}/\left(\text{heart rate} \times \text{RVEF}\right)$$

The RVEDV is a true volumetric, as opposed to barometric, estimate of intravascular volume. Initially, this technology still depended upon the traditional method of intermittent TD, but it provided valuable hemodynamic data not previously available [9]. In the late 1990s, the current generation of volumetric PACs was introduced, allowing continuous cardiac output (CCO), continuous RVEF (cRVEF), and continuous RVEDV (cRVEDV)(Edwards Lifesciences, Irvine, CA, USA). These catheters differ significantly from the original PAC in several important respects. Measurement of CCO was achieved by adding a "heating coil" so that TD curves could be obtained automatically by heating a certain volume of blood instead of the traditional cooling after injection of an iced bolus. The new cRVEF algorithm generates a waveform resembling the bolus TD curves. These "volumetric" PACs have a rapid (between 50 and 70 ms) response thermistor. In order to calculate the RVEF, the R-R interval needs to be monitored. This can be done by connecting the "Vigilance" monitor (Edwards Lifesciences, Irvine, USA) to the ECG tracing although some PACs also have intracardiac electrodes (but these are mainly used for cardiac pacing and not for R-R interval estimation). As a consequence, RVEF and RVEDV cannot be reliably assessed in patients with atrial fibrillation. Theoretically, the continuous assessment of cRVEDV and cRVEF could be used for better guidance of fluid treatment (as static resuscitation target). It should be noted that one should take RVEF (influenced by contractility and afterload) into consideration when interpreting RVEDV [10, 11]. Table 23.1 lists the normal values and ranges for RVEF and

Table 23.1 Normal values of volumetric parameters

Monitoring technique	Parameter	Lower limit	Upper limit
TD	RVEF (%)	35	45
	RVEDVI (ml/m^2)	80	120
TPTD	GEF (%)	25	35
	GEDVI (ml/m^2)	680	800
	Sepsis	760	820
	Postoperative	680	810
	EVLWI (ml/kg PBW)	3	7
	Sepsis	7	8
	Postoperative	9	13
	PVPI	1	2
	MAT (sec)	5	10
	MTT (sec)	10	15
	DST (sec)	15	20
TPDD	ITBVI (ml/m^2)	850	1000
Echo	LVEDAI (cm^2/m^2)	6	12
	LA volume (cm^2/m^2)	20	29
	FAC (%)	35	45
BIA	TBW men (%)	50	60
	TBW women (%)	45	50
	ECW/ICW ratio	0.8	0.9
	VE (ml)	−1000	1000

DST downslope time, ECW extracellular water, EVLWI extravascular lung water index, FAC fractional area contraction, GEF global ejection fraction, GEDVI global end-diastolic volume index, ICW intracellular water, ITBVI intrathoracic blood volume index, LA left atrium, LVEDAI left ventricular end-diastolic area index, MAT mean appearance time, MTT mean transit time, RVEF right ventricular ejection fraction, RVEDVI right ventricular end-diastolic volume index, TBW total body water, TD thermodilution, TPDD transpulmonary double dye dilution, TPTD transpulmonary thermodilution, VE volume excess

RVEDV. Indications for PAC are right ventricular failure, pulmonary hypertension, and monitoring of pulmonary artery pressure during the use of inhalation therapy (e.g., ilomedine or nitric oxide (NO)) in acute respiratory distress syndrome (ARDS). The PAC is still the most widely used CO monitoring catheter. With the modern PACs, continuous measurement of CCO, cRVEF, cRVEDV, and SvO2 is possible; there is no need for extra fluid administration and calibration is automatic. The obtained values are operator independent with low intra- and interobserver variability. Table 23.2 lists the indications and contraindications and advantages and disadvantages of the different volumetric monitoring techniques.

Table 23.2 Comparison of different volumetric monitoring techniques

	Technique	Indications	Contraindications	Advantages	Disadvantages
PAC	Pulmonary thermodilution, gold standard	Right heart failure Pulmonary hypertension ARDS Assessment of effect of inhalation therapy (e.g., NO)	Volumetric monitoring not possible in AF	No added fluid No need for manual calibration Information on right heart function (RVEF) Continuous RVEDV Continuous SvO2	Invasive Expensive and difficult catheter No beat-to-beat data (average 5 min) Cannot be used for fluid responsiveness Complications (PA rupture, arrhythmia) Slow response time to changes in preload or afterload Poor signal-to-noise ratio
PiCCO	Transpulmonary thermodilution, new surrogate gold standard	Well validated against PAC Critically ill with shock, new-onset organ failure, respiratory failure Increased ITP	Recent vascular surgery femoral artery Presence of (pseudo) aneurysm Brachial position not trustworthy for volumetric monitoring	Less invasive Beat-to-beat data Can be used for FR Additional parameters (GEDV, EVLW, PVPI) Identification of *R/L* shunt (no loss of indicator) Less dependent on respiratory variations	Effect of valvulopathy on TPTD Volumetric monitoring not continuous Need for recalibration after changes in preload, afterload, contractility
EV1000	Transpulmonary thermodilution, PiCCO clone	Not well validated Same as PiCCO	Same as PiCCO	Less invasive Same as PiCCO	Continuous CVP tracing needed for calculations Effect of valvulopathy on TPTD Volumetric monitoring not continuous Need for recalibration after changes in preload, afterload, contractility

(continued)

23

Table 23.2 (continued)

	Technique	Indications	Contraindications	Advantages	Disadvantages
LiDCO	TP lithium dilution	Less validated	Treatment with lithium salts Neuromuscular blockers Small children Pregnancy	Less invasive Uses existing access No central venous line needed Only measures ITBV	Less additional parameters Need for recalibration after changes in preload, afterload, contractility
TEE	Ultrasound obtained LVEDA and FAC	Minimal invasive Well validated	Coagulopathy Esophageal varices Upper gastrointestinal bleeding Esophageal diverticle (Zencker) Hernia hiatale (relative)	Provides additional anatomical and functional information	Learning curve Not really continuous Contraindications
hTEE	Ultrasound obtained LVEDA and FAC	Minimal invasive Not well validated	Same as TEE	Direct cardiac visualization	Expensive only monoplane Not really continuous No Doppler No color or tissue doppler imaging Contraindications
TTE	Ultrasound obtained LVEDA and FAC	Well validated	Virtually none Thoracic wound or burns	Noninvasive Modern stethoscope for the intensivist, no contraindications	Learning curve, not really continuous
BIA	Bioelectrical impedance analysis	Not well validated in critically ill	Pacemaker AICD	Noninvasive Provides information on TBW, ECW, ICW, and volume excess	Less reproducible in peripheral edema

Adapted from Huygh et al. with permission [12]. See text for explanation. AF atrial fibrillation, AICD automated implantable cardioverter defibrillator, ARDS acute respiratory distress syndrome, BIA bioelectrical impedance analysis, CVP central venous pressure, ECW extracellular water, EVLW extravascular lung water, FAC fractional area contraction, GEF global ejection fraction, GEDV global end-diastolic volume, ICW intracellular water, ITBV intrathoracic blood volume, ITP intrathoracic pressure, LA left atrium, LVEDA left ventricular end-diastolic area, NO nitric oxide, PA(C) pulmonary artery (catheter), PVPI pulmonary vascular permeability index, RVEF right ventricular ejection fraction, RVEDV right ventricular end-diastolic volume, TBW total body water, TD thermodilution, TEE transesophageal echocardiography, TP transpulmonary, TPTD transpulmonary thermodilution, TTE transthoracic echocardiography

23.4 Transpulmonary Double Indicator Dilution

Following the intensive discussions after negative results of some major trails about the use of PAC in critically ill patients [13], especially also regarding its invasiveness, there has been an increasing interest in recent years in less invasive hemodynamic monitoring tools, also allowing volumetric preload assessment [7, 14]. Initially, the COLD device (PULSION Medical Systems, Munich, Germany) used a double (thermo-dye) indicator dilution technique. The combination of an indicator (indocyanine green dye) that does not diffuse into the extravascular compartment with an indicator (cold saline) that does allows simultaneous assessment of volume (ITBV and EVLW) and flow (CO), respectively. ◘ Figure 23.2 also shows a classic transpulmonary TD (TPTD) curve. The mean appearance time (MAT) is defined as the time between injection for the cold (or dye) bolus and start of cooling (or dye dilution). A normal MAT is around 5–10 s. The concentration of the indicator is distributed over time because of the intravascular volume, i.e., there is a given time for each indicator particle to travel between the point of injection and the point of detection. This time is called the transit time and each particle has its own transit time. The MTT is the mean value of all these transit times. The MTT is defined as the time between injection and the short period after the maximal cooling. A normal MTT is around 10–15 s. The downslope time (DST) is detected by plotting the thermodilution curve with the temperature change (indicator concentration) on a logarithmic scale and time change on a linear scale. When you plot the thermodilution curve as a linear-ln graph, the indicator decay approximates a linear function. Two points, the starting point located at 85% of the maximum temperature response and an endpoint defined as 45% of the maximum temperature response, are identified. This time difference is determined and labeled as DST and reflects passage of the indicator through the largest mixing chamber, usually the pulmonary blood volume (PBV). The normal DST is around 15–20 s. The calculation of EVLW with the double indicator technique is explained below:

$$\text{ITBVdye} = \text{CO} \times \text{MTTdye}$$

$$\text{PBVdye} = \text{CO} \times \text{DSTdye}$$

$$\text{GEDVdye} = \text{ITBVdye} - \text{PBVdye}$$

$$\text{ITTVice} = \text{CO} \times \text{MTTice}$$

$$\text{PTVice} = \text{CO} \times \text{DSTice}$$

$$\text{GEDVice} = \text{ITTVice} - \text{PTVice}$$

$$\text{EVLW} = \text{ITTVice} - \text{ITBVdye}$$

with ITTV, the intrathoracic thermal volume, and PTV, the pulmonary thermal volume. The COLD technique has been used in different patient populations: mechanically ventilated [15], coronary artery bypass grafting [16], sepsis and septic shock [17], postoperative [18], and neonates and infants [19]. Although effective at the bedside, due to the preparation (and the cost) of the indocyanine green (ICG) solution, the transpulmonary double indicator dilution technique is relatively time-consuming, cumbersome, and expensive [20]. This technique has been abandoned in the early 2000s and replaced by the less expensive and easier single transpulmonary thermodilution technique as will be discussed further.

23.5 Transpulmonary Thermodilution

23

To simplify and reduce the manipulations for monitoring, research led to the development of a device based on the transpulmonary thermodilution technique (TPTD) with one single thermal indicator [20]. The intermittent CO is measured using a transpulmonary thermodilution technique also based on the Stewart-Hamilton equation:

$$\mathrm{CO} = \frac{(T_\mathrm{b} - T_\mathrm{i}) \times V_\mathrm{inj} \times K}{\int \Delta T_\mathrm{b} \times \mathrm{dt}}$$

where T_b is blood temperature, T_i is injectate temperature, V_inj is injectate volume, K is the correction constant, and $\int \Delta T_\mathrm{b} \times \mathrm{dt}$ (area under the thermodilution curve) [7]. The first commercially available device using transpulmonary thermodilution was the PiCCO system (PULSION Medical Systems, Feldkirchen, Germany, later integrated in Maquet, Rastatt, Germany, and now in Getinge, Gothenburg, Sweden). The PiCCO device allows the measurement of GEDV and intrathoracic blood volume (ITBV), with ITBV = 1.25 × GEDV as surrogate preload markers together with extravascular lung water (EVLW) and pulmonary vascular permeability index (PVPI) [9, 21]. Determination of EVLW by single transpulmonary thermodilution depends on the measurement of the intrathoracic thermal volume (ITTV), and the pulmonary thermal volume (PTV), which is the largest accessible volume transversed by the thermal indicator [7]. The ITTV and PTV are calculated from the mean transit time (MTT) and the exponential downslope time (DST) of the thermodilution curve of the cold injectate [7]:

$$\mathrm{ITTV} = \mathrm{CO} \times \mathrm{MTT}$$

$$\mathrm{PTV} = \mathrm{CO} \times \mathrm{DST}$$

The ITTV consists of the PTV and the sum of the end-diastolic volumes of all cardiac chambers. Accordingly, the global end-diastolic volume (GEDV) can be calculated as [7]:

$$\mathrm{GEDV} = \mathrm{ITTV} - \mathrm{PTV}$$

Based on the before-mentioned linear relation between GEDV and ITBV, the EVLW can be calculated as follows [7]:

$$\mathrm{ITBV} = 1.25 \times \mathrm{GEDV}$$

$$\mathrm{EVLW} = \mathrm{ITTV} - \mathrm{ITBV}$$

Figure 23.3 shows schematically the different volumetric indices and how they are connected/correlated to each other. Recently, an alternative system for transpulmonary thermodilution has been developed by Edwards Lifesciences (Irvine, California, USA), consisting of the VolumeView thermistor-tipped arterial catheter and EV1000 monitoring platform/software [7]. The concept is very similar to the TPTD technique employed by the PiCCO system as discussed above; both use the Stewart-Hamilton equation in order to calculate the thermodilution-derived CO [7]. However, in order to calculate GEDV, the VolumeView/EV1000 system uses a formula implementing the maximum upstroke (*S*1) and downslope (*S*2) time of the thermodilution curve, whereas the PiCCO system employs time constants derived from the mean appearance, mean transit, and downslope of the thermodilution curve:

$$\mathrm{GEDV\ VolumeView} = \mathrm{CO} \times \mathrm{MTT} \times f\left(S1/S2\right)$$

where MTT is the mean transit time, *S*1 is maximum upstroke, and *S*2 is maximum downslope. The EVLW is calculated using the same formula as the PiCCO.

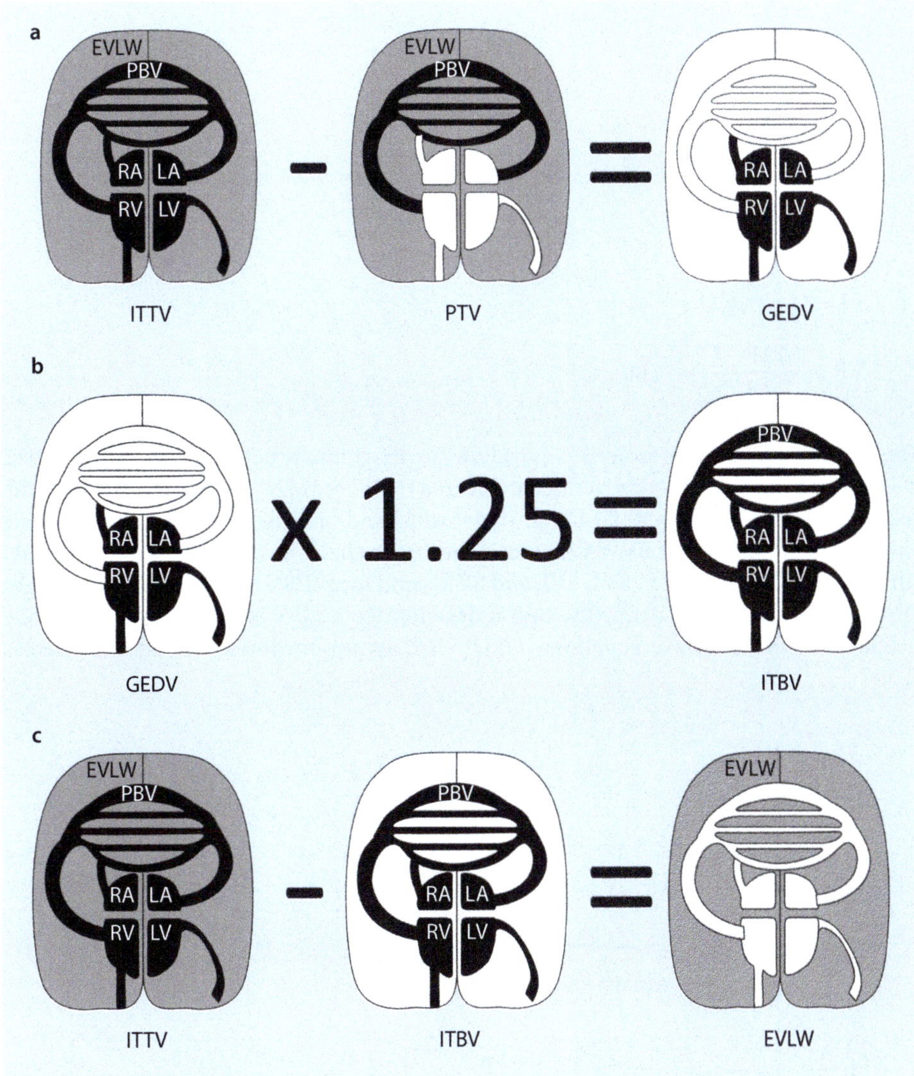

Fig. 23.3 Schematic presentation of the calculation of volumetric parameters with transpulmonary thermodilution. Panel **a** Calculation of global end-diastolic volume, Panel **b** Estimation of intrathoracic blood volume, Panel **c** Calculation of extravascular lung water. water. EVLW extravascular lung water, GEDV global end-diastolic volume, ITBV intrathoracic blood volume, ITTV intrathoracic thermal volume, LA left atrium, LV left ventricle, PBV pulmonary blood volume, PTV pulmonary thermal volume, RA right atrium, RV right ventricle,

Both the PiCCO and VolumeView also calculate pulmonary blood volume (PBV), PVPI, SV, global ejection fraction (GEF), cardiac function index (CFI), cardiac power index (CPI), and systemic vascular resistance (SVR). These parameters are derived from the values obtained with TPTD:

$$PBV = ITBV - GEDV$$

$$PVPI = \frac{EVLW}{PBV}$$

$$SV = \frac{CO}{\text{heart rate}}$$

$$GEF = \frac{4 \times SV}{GEDV}$$

23

$$CFI = \frac{CO}{GEDV}$$

$$CPI = MAP \times CO$$

$$SVR = \frac{MAP - CVP}{CO} \times 80$$

The PVPI (normal values around 1–1.5) allows to discriminate between hydrostatic (PVPI 2–2.5) and hyperpermeability pulmonary edema (PVPI > 3) [22]. ◘ Figure 23.4 shows the relation between EVLW and GEDV during normal and increased permeability. Absolute values for CO, GEDV, ITBV, SV, and SVR are normalized as indexed by BSA or body surface area (CI, GEDVI, ITBVI, SVI, and SVRI) and for EVLW by predicted body weight (EVLWI) [7], although ideally the best indexation for EVLW seems according to body height [23]. In the above equations, GEDV is correctly measured/calculated, whereas

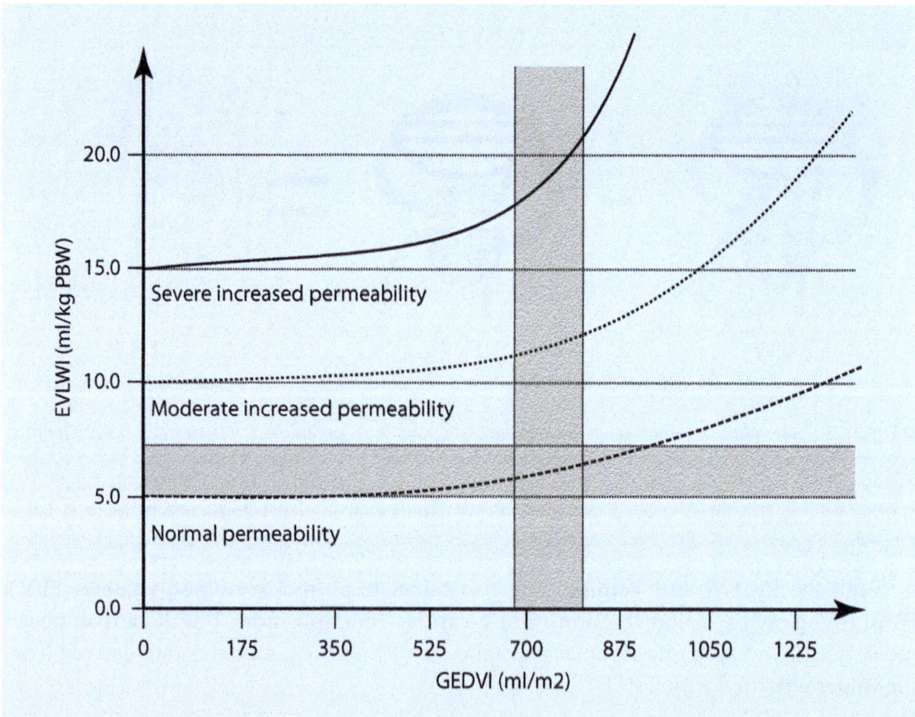

◘ **Fig. 23.4** Relation between extravascular lung water and global end-diastolic volume. Relation between extravascular lung water index (EVLWI) and global end-diastolic volume index (GEDVI) at different levels of permeability (normal vs moderately increased vs severely increased permeability). The shaded gray zones indicate the normal range of EVLWI (5–7 ml/kg predicted body weight) and GEDVI (680–800 ml/m²)

ITBV is estimated based on the correlation obtained between the single transpulmonary and the double indicator technique, namely, ITBV = 1.25 × GEDV [24]. It is assumable that this linear relationship is not constant but could depend upon patient characteristics and underlying pathology and comorbidities.

The TPTD technique has been extensively validated in different patent populations: lung transplantation [25], sepsis and septic shock [26], and cardiac surgery [27], among others [7, 20]. ◘ Table 23.1 lists the normal values for GEF, GEDVI, EVLWI, and ITBVI. Indications for transpulmonary thermodilution are shock states with unclear fluid status, new-onset organ failure (e.g., kidney failure), or respiratory insufficiency (ARDS, pulmonary edema, capillary leak). Transpulmonary thermodilution is less invasive than PAC; the TPTD CO measurement is less dependent on the respiratory cycle. The parameters are rapidly available and directly clinically applicable. The volumetric quantification is independent of ITP, PEEP, or IAP and can be used in a broad range of patients (from adults to small children). In the situation of a right-to-left shunt (as can be the case in ARDS with pulmonary hypertension and open foramen ovale), there is no loss of indicator (◘ Table 23.2). Moreover, after calibration with TPTD, the pulse contour analysis gives real-time beat-to-beat CO, functional hemodynamics, and afterload (as will be discussed elsewhere). Head-to-head comparison between RVEDVI, obtained with PAC, and GEDVI, obtained with PiCCO, showed that GEDVI better reflects echocardiographic changes in left ventricular preload in response to fluid administration in 20 patients undergoing elective cardiac surgery [27]. As the TPTD technique is less invasive, it has evolved as the new gold standard for validation of other less invasive and uncalibrated CO monitoring techniques [14].

23.6 Transpulmonary Single Dye Dilution

The original technique used ICG as indicator. However, as this technique initially required frequent blood sampling and manual analysis of the dye dilution curve and was cumbersome and time-consuming, it has been abandoned in the clinical setting. Using the Stewart-Hamilton equation, CO can be calculated by the use of any intravascular indicator. In another dye dilution technique, lithium is injected via a central or peripheral vein, and lithium concentrations are measured in a peripheral artery using a specialized sensor probe attached to the pressure line in order to construct a lithium decay curve [28]. Correct application of this equation requires three conditions to be present: a homogenous mixing of blood and indicator, a constant blood flow, and the absence of loss of indicator between injection and detection site. The CO is then calculated as follows:

$$\mathrm{CO} = \frac{\mathrm{LiCl} \times 60}{A \times 1(1 - \mathrm{PCV})}$$

where LiCl is the dose of lithium chloride in mmol, A is the area under the lithium dilution curve, and PCV is the packed cell volume (that can be derived from hemoglobin concentration). Currently, only one commercially available device exists, using lithium dilution (LiDCO; LiDCO Ltd., London, UK). Lithium, like ICG is a nondiffusible indicator. The method of using bolus indicator dilution to measure volume is similar as for other dilution techniques. The method of ITBV calculation is as follows (with MTT representing the mean transit time of the lithium indicator from injection to detection):

$$\mathrm{ITBV} = \mathrm{CO} \times \mathrm{MTT}$$

The normal values for ITBVI are listed in ◘ Table 23.1. The lithium dilution technique is less invasive than the PAC, and the data are rapidly available. It uses existing access and does not require central circulation catheterization. In contrast to the PiCCO and EV1000, extravascular lung water quantification is not possible, and the technique must be used with caution in small children and patients under muscle relaxants or lithium treatment (manic depression). The technique has not been validated as extensively as compared to other TPTD techniques. The ion-selective lithium electrode needs to be replaced every 3 days, but this technique is not more expensive than other TPTD techniques (◘ Table 23.2).

23.7 Volumetric Integration

In patients in whom the measurement of pulmonary artery pressure (PAP) and the management of RV function are crucial such as in ARDS patients with IAH, the combination of a pulmonary and transpulmonary TD (e.g., via PAC and PiCCO/VolumeView) could be very interesting from a theoretical point of view [29–31]. The combined (trans)pulmonary TD curves allow calculation of right heart end-diastolic volume (RHEDV) and RVEDV after obtaining the MTT and DST, respectively, of the cold injectate within the right heart and pulmonary circulation (◘ Fig. 23.2):

$$\mathrm{RHEDV} = \mathrm{CO} \times \mathrm{MTT}$$

$$\mathrm{RVEDV} = \mathrm{CO} \times \mathrm{DST}$$

$$\mathrm{RVEF} = \mathrm{SV} / \mathrm{RVEDV}$$

$$\mathrm{LHEDV} = \mathrm{GEDV} - \mathrm{RHEDV}$$

$$R / L\,\mathrm{ratio} = \mathrm{RHEDV} / \mathrm{LHEDV}$$

The integration of all these parameters in the clinical setting and especially in patients with IAH needs further evaluation; however, they may be useful in the optimization of pulmonary circulation and oxygenation or the adjustment of vasoactive and inhalation agents (NO, ilomedin, or prostacyclin). ◘ Figure 23.5 schematically shows the right and left heart volumes. Where the GEDV provides information on the total amount of cardiac preload, the cardiac sub-volumes offer the possibility to differentiate between left or right heart failure and heart-lung interactions. Continuous monitoring of these parameters as with cRVEDV could provide additional benefits. However, in a study in 20 patients undergoing cardiac surgery, Hofer et al. found that both left ventricular end-diastolic area index (LVEDAI) and GEDVI significantly increased after fluid administration while this correlation was not present for LHEDVI [31].

23.8 Echocardiography

Ultrasound machines generate a vibration within the transducer that, when put next to tissue surfaces, vibrates the surrounding tissue, and this allows to noninvasively visualize structures inside the body [7]. During vibration, particles within the tissue compress (compression) and then spread apart (rarefaction). The sequence of compression and rarefaction is described by sinusoidal waves and is characterized in terms of wavelength,

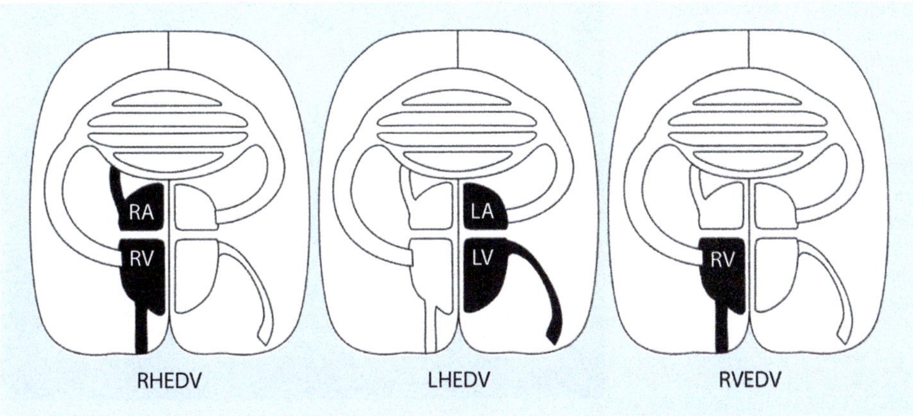

Fig. 23.5 Volumetric integration. LA left atrium, LHEDV left heart end-diastolic volume, LV left ventricle, RA right atrium, RHEDV right heart end-diastolic volume, RV right ventricle, RVEDV right ventricular end-diastolic volume

frequency, amplitude, and propagation velocity [32]. Wavelength is the distance (in millimeters) between two peaks of the sinusoidal wave. Frequency is the number of cycles that occur in 1 s. One cycle per second is defined as 1 hertz (abbreviated Hz). Ultrasound uses frequencies higher than the audible range for humans (greater than 20,000 cycles per second or 20 kHz). Frequencies typically used for ultrasound imaging are 2–10 megahertz (MHz). The wavelength is inversely related to the frequency. The amplitude is a measure of tissue compression and represents the loudness of an ultrasound wave and is described by decibels (dB). Decibels are a logarithmic transformation that allows large amplitudes to be presented next to small amplitudes (i.e., 1000 and 0.001) on the same display. The propagation velocity describes the speed of an ultrasound wave traveling through tissue (e.g., for blood this is 1540 m/s). The relationship between propagation velocity, frequency, and wavelength is described as follows:

$$\text{Propagation velocity} = \text{Frequency} \times \text{Wavelength}$$

Assuming that propagation velocity is constant, the wavelength for any frequency can hence be calculated. To generate 2D images, ultrasound machines were configured to sequentially redirect the beam over an area (sector) of interest. Transducers contain a row of piezoelectric crystals (a linear array). By introducing a small delay in the firing of adjacent crystals in the array (a phased array), the ultrasound machine is able to guide the resultant ultrasound beam through a sector of interest. The heart can be examined with transthoracic (TTE) and transesophageal echocardiography (TEE). Since TEE is not without risk, its use is restricted to selected indications as much of the information gathered by TEE can also be obtained by less invasive TTE. Guidelines published by ACA reflect this in saying that TEE should be used for critical care patients with persistent hypotension or hypoxia when diagnostic information expected to alter management cannot be obtained by TTE or other modalities in a timely manner [32].

The left ventricular end-diastolic area (LVEDA) is a “volumetric” method to assess preload status. The LVEDA is measured at the level of the papillary muscles in the para-

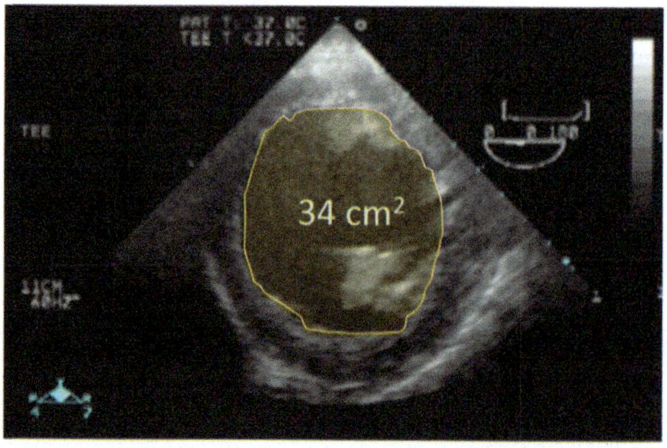

Fig. 23.6 Left ventricular end-diastolic area. Large left ventricular end-diastolic area obtained with transesophageal echocardiography in a patient with dilated cardiomyopathy. Note that the papillary muscles are included within the surface area. The LVEDA can also be assessed on the parasternal short axis with transthoracic echocardiography

sternal short-axis view obtained with TTE by tracing the endocardial border [33] or in a mid-esophageal long-axis view with TEE (Fig. 23.6). A LVEDA of less than 10 cm^2 or a LVEDAI of less than 5.5 cm^2/m^2 indicates significant hypovolemia (normal range of LVEDAI is between 8 and 12 cm^2/m^2, Table 23.1) [34]. However, in critically ill patients, the identification of a low threshold seems more cumbersome [35]. On the other hand, a LVEDA of more than 24 cm^2 suggests volume overload. It should be mentioned that severe concentric hypertrophy can reduce LVEDA without the presence of hypovolemia [36]. Previous studies showed no correlation between PAOP and LVEDAI [35, 37, 38]. In cardiac surgical patients, LVEDAI is a sensitive marker to detect changes in blood volume, even if regional wall motion is abnormal.

Fluid administration will increase LVEDAI up to a certain level, when it will remain constant, concordant with CO [39, 40], whereas PAOP, on the contrary, will continue to rise. Therefore, LVEDAI is superior to barometric static preload parameters in cardiac surgery [41]. Left ventricular end-diastolic diameter [42], taken, can also be utilized as a static variable. When assessing LVEDA it is important to also look at the fractional area contraction as a surrogate marker for left ventricular EF. The fractional area contraction (FAC) can be derived by calculating the linear shortening of the following measurements, with LVEDA as the left ventricular end-diastolic area and LVESA as the left ventricular end-systolic area:

$$\mathrm{FAC} = \left[(\mathrm{LVEDA} - \mathrm{LVESA}) / \mathrm{LVEDA}\right] \times 100$$

The assessment of the left atrium (LA) and the presence of LA dilation are usually the consequence of long-standing LA pressure and/or volume overload [36]. Thus, LA enlargement indicates a likelihood of elevated LA pressure (LAP). A normal LA_{vol}/BSA is below 29 ml/m^2 (Table 23.1).

23.9 Bioelectrical Impedance Analysis

The last method, BIA, is a promising noninvasive tool to assess not only total body water (TBW) but also extra- (ECW) and intracellular water (ICW), ECW/ICW ratio, and volume excess (VE) [43]. Classic whole-body BIA can be performed with many different commercially available devices. However, three devices are currently available for use in (critically ill) patients: the Fresenius Medical Care (BCM) body composition monitor

(Fresenius Medical Care, Bad Homburg, Germany), the SECA medical body composition analyzer mBCA 525 (SECA, Chino, CA, USA), and the Maltron BioScan 920 or the new touch i8 bioScan (Maltron International Ltd., Rayleigh, Essex, UK) [44]. However, so far, no large study with head-to-head comparison has been performed in critically ill patients. In the future other parameters like intravascular and extravascular fluid volume may become readily available.

In the future, two devices may supply BIA-defined estimates of total thoracic fluid content, Bio-Z (Sonosite, Seattle, WA, USA) and NICOM (Cheetah Medical, Tel Aviv, Israel).

We will briefly discuss the electrical parameters measured by BIA [43]. A conductor is a tissue that allows electricity to flow easily. Examples are muscles or tissue that consists of mainly water with low resistance and low impedance. An insulator is a tissue that consists of cells that are not conducting electrical signals. Examples are fat cells with high resistance and high impedance. In electrical terms, the capacitance (C) is the storage of an electrical charge by a condenser for a short moment in time. The capacitance measurement in a human being is related to the amount and health status of cell membranes (the more and the healthier the cells, the higher the capacitance value). The resistance (R) of an electrical conductor is the opposition to the passage of an electric current through that conductor and is inversely related to the water content. The opposition of an electrical circuit element (due to that element's capacitance) to a change of electric current is called reactance (X) and is related to the cell mass. The impedance (Z) represents the ratio between insulation tissue over the conductive tissue or, thus, the resistance divided by the conductance. BIA allows calculation of body composition and volumes using an electric current going through the body at different frequencies. Some assumptions are made to obtain a reproducible measurement: the human body is considered as a cylinder; this cylinder consists of five smaller cylinders (one central, two for the arms, and two for the legs); body composition is homogenous without individual variations; and finally, there is no impact from the environment (temperature, stress, fluid infusions, etc.). It is obvious that in critically ill patients, those assumptions may not hold true [43]. When electric current goes through a cylinder-shaped body, the impedance (Z) is related to the length (L) and specific resistivity (ρ) of the tissue and inversely related to the cross-sectional area (A) of the cylinder. The volume of a cylinder (V) can be calculated as L multiplied with A. Bioelectrical impedance analysis calculates volumes as follows:

$$Z = \rho \times \frac{L}{A}$$

$$Z = \rho \times \frac{L}{A} \times \frac{L}{L}$$

$$Z = \rho \times \frac{L^2}{V}$$

Extrapolated to a critically ill patient, L stands for the patient's height (in cm) so that the body composition and the specific volume (V) can be calculated as follows:

$$V = \rho \times \frac{L^2}{Z}$$

where $\frac{L^2}{Z}$ corresponds to the impedance index that can be calculated with bioelectrical impedance analysis.

23

The use of tetrapolar electrodes is preferred with two current electrodes to drive electricity into the human body and two electrodes to detect impedance placed on hands and feet to obtain reproducible measurements [43]. Modern devices also use multiple frequencies that may further improve the accuracy and reproducibility of the measurement. The frequency is the number of repetitions per second of a complete electric waveform (one repetition per second is 1 Hz) [45]. A current with a frequency below 100 Hz will not pass the cell membranes and will only measure extracellular water (ECW). Currents with frequencies above 100 Hz will go through cells and measure total body water (TBW) [44]. The intracellular water (ICW) can then be calculated as follows:

$$\text{ICW} = \text{TBW} - \text{ECW}$$

The *phase angle* is the time delay that occurs when electric current passes the cell membrane and reflects the relationship between resistance and reactance. A phase angle of 0° is an indicator of the absence of cell membranes,whereas 90° represents a capacitive circuit which consists of only membranes without fluid [44]. The presence of cell membranes causes time delays caused by the time current takes when passing through extracellular water. Hence, the more cells, the greater the phase angle and the greater the proportion of ICW compared to ECW [46].

For the ICU clinician, it is important to be aware that the normal ECW/ICW ratio is usually less than 1 (around 0.8). Increase in ICW is seen in patients with heart failure and liver cirrhosis and in patients with chronic kidney disease (especially in early stage). A decrease in ICW is related to osmotic factors. Increases in ECW are mostly due to shift from the intra- to extracellular space as seen with second- and third-space edema and in the late stages of heart, liver, or kidney failure. Increase ECW is also seen in patients with septic shock with capillary leak and fluid overload. Peripheral edema (anasarca) is the most common sign of increased ECW. Monitoring ECW and ICW changes over time can be helpful to guide fluid therapy. In addition to TBW, ECW, and ICW, the assessment of volume excess (VE) can help to identify patients that may be eligible for deresuscitation [47].

Critically ill patients, especially those with sepsis or septic shock, easily develop changes in the distribution of body fluids with the migration of fluid from the intravascular to the extravascular space. As suspected, Plank showed that although changes in TBW were similar, patients with peritonitis and sepsis (n = 12) had higher ECW values compared to those with blunt trauma (n = 18) [48]. A retrospective study comparing BIA data in critically ill patients (n = 101) with healthy volunteers (n = 101) showed significant differences in body water composition [49]. Patients had higher values for TBW, ECW, and ECW/ICW ratio, while ICW remained unchanged. Patients had an average VE of 6.2 L vs −0.2 L in healthy volunteers. Non-survivors (n = 40) had similar values of ECW and TBW, but significantly lower values for ICW, resulting in an increased ECW/ICW ratio (1.1 ± 0.2 vs 1 ± 0.2, P = 0,002). Non-survivors had a mean VE of 7.5 L vs 4.6 L in survivors (P = 0.029). More recently, Samoni and colleagues found similar results in a large dual-center study (n = 125). The presence of fluid overload was the only variable found to be significantly associated with ICU mortality [50]. However, in critically ill patients, many conditions may coexist like the presence of ascites, anasarca, severe peripheral edema, pleural effusions, and massive fluid overload that in combination with other clinical conditions may alter fluid and electrolyte distribution. In these situations, conventional BIA may be a poor measure of TBW [43].

The body of evidence regarding the usefulness of BIA-derived parameters in critically ill patients is steadily increasing; however, more data is needed before general acceptance [49–52]. The newer devices (e.g., Maltron, touch i8) will not only be able to obtain an idea of VE but also further separate this into intravascular vs extravascular fluid volume.

23.10 Normal Volumetric Values and Tips and Tricks

In this paragraph we will discuss in depth some tips and tricks regarding the TPTD method (regardless of the indicator used, either iced saline, indocyanine green, or lithium), as this is the most widely used technique for volumetric preload assessment. However, it must be noted that more research has been performed using iced saline as indicator (valid for PICCO or VolumeView). As discussed above, the hemodynamic parameters such as the ITBVI, GEDVI, and EVLWI, derived by transpulmonary thermodilution, have gained increasing interest for guiding fluid therapy in critically ill patients. However, the proposed normal values of 680–800 ml/m^2 for GEDVI and 3–7 ml/kg predicted body weight for EVLWI are based on measurements in healthy individuals and expert opinion and are assumed to be suitable for all patients [53]. The published data for GEDVI and EVLWI has been recently analyzed [53]. The authors investigated the differences between a cohort of septic patients and patients undergoing major surgery, respectively. Data from 1925 patients corresponding to 64 studies were included [53]. In the group of septic patients, GEDVI and EVLWI were significantly higher than in the group of patients undergoing major surgery. On comparison of both groups, mean GEDVI was 94 ml/m^2 higher in septic (788 ml/m^2) compared to surgical patients (694 ml/m^2). Mean EVLWI was 3.3 ml/kg higher in septic (11.0 ml/kg) compared to surgical patients (7.2 ml/kg). The published data for GEDVI and EVLWI are heterogeneous, particularly in critically ill patients, and often exceed the proposed normal values derived from healthy individuals. This points to the need for defining different therapeutic targets for different patient populations. The normal ranges for the available volumetric parameters are listed in ◘ Table 23.1.

Within this respect it is also important that the ICU physician is aware of the underlying conditions that may interfere with the volumetric indices obtained with TPTD. Moreover, any measurement stands or falls with its accuracy and reproducibility, and correct measurement is of paramount importance. A recent review listed some common pitfalls and tips and tricks in relation to transpulmonary thermodilution [54].

These can be summarized in 10 steps for the nurse or the one performing the TPTD calibration [54]:

1. *Assessment of arterial pressure curve and rapid flush test.* Visual inspection of the arterial waveform should be done before performing a TPTD measurement with PiCCO, VolumeView, or LidCO. The square waveform and oscillations generated by a rapid flush are suitable to assess the dynamic response properties of the monitoring system and to identify and treat over- or underdamping.
2. *Zeroing the pressure system.* As a general rule, the pressure transducer needs to be zeroed at the level of the phlebostatic axis (right atrium) against atmospheric pressure. This should be done at least once every nursing shift.

3. *Importance of demographic data.* Most of the human mistakes are probably made before performing the actual TPTD measurement. As mentioned previously, entering appropriate and accurate patient data is important for calculation of the indexed volumes. This pertains to biometric data such as height, weight and gender, injectate volume, as well as the relative positions of the arterial and central venous catheters.
4. *Entering the CVP.* It is a misconception among nurses that entering the CVP is necessary for the calculation of the TPTD parameters; however, the sole purpose is for the calculation of the systemic vascular resistance.
5. *Impact of indicator bolus volume.* It is important to adjust the indicator volume according to the patient's body weight. A volume of 0.2 ml/kg is recommended. It is important to inject the exact amount that was preset on the TPTD monitor. An injected volume that is smaller than the one set or expected by the device will falsely increase CO, ITBV, GEDV, and EVLW. For PiCCO and VolumeView, the bolus temperature should be lower than 8 °C. Theoretically room temperature can be used, but this will lead to a systematic overestimation of CO, GEDV, and EVLW [55, 56]. Therefore, the colder the bolus for TPTD, the better.
6. *Effect of injection site.* The most distal lumen of the central venous catheter is preferred, and the injection should be as close to the patient as possible.
7. *Effect of injection speed.* A fast and steady injection is recommended at a speed above 2.5 ml/s; the whole bolus hence should be injected within 8 s (for a 20 ml bolus). A slow or interrupted bolus will cause a deformed TPTD curve and may alter the volumetric data.
8. *Observation of the TPTD curve.* The morphology and timing of the TPTD curve are important. A typical TPTD curve has a flat portion which reflects the transit time of the cold injectate from injection site to thermistor (MAT), followed by a rise and fall in $\Delta T°$ with an exponential decrease, ending in a plateau due to physiological recirculation of the indicator (DST). If the mean transit and downslope times are increased, the value of CO can be expected to be low, while the volumes are usually increased.
9. *Checking the numbers.* At least three ice boluses or one indocyanine green or lithium bolus is necessary to obtain an acceptable precision, and any measured CO, ITBV, GEDV, and EVLW should not deviate more than 15% from the mean value.
10. *Obtaining maximal cooling or $\Delta T°$ (only for thermal TPTD with PiCCO and VolumeView).* The minimum $\Delta T°$ (cooling) to ascertain correct volumetric measurement is 0.2 °C, and if necessary, a colder or higher volume bolus can be tried in order to obtain a $\Delta T°$ above 0.2 °C.

Assuming that a correct TPTD calibration has been obtained, the ICU physician further needs to take into account 10 more steps [54]:

1. *Observation of the TPTD curve.* An interrupted injection can cause a distortion of the TPTD curve with a premature hump leading to over- or underestimation of the volumetric indices. The specific shape of the TPTD curve can point toward specific diagnoses as will be discussed further.
2. *Checking for shunts.* A right-to-left shunt (via patent foramen ovale) typically gives a TPTD curve with premature hump caused by right-to-left passage of a portion of

the indicator, reaching the thermistor at the tip of the femoral arterial line more rapidly. This has also been named "camel curve" [57].

3. *Effect of catheter position (thermal TPTD).* The TPTD values obtained after bolus injection via a femoral central venous catheter will result in increased values for CO, ITBV, GEDV, and EVLW. If the venous and arterial lines are both femoral and inserted on the same side with the same length, a premature hump, similar to one seen in right-to-left shunt, can occur due to changes in venous temperature sensed by the thermistor on the arterial catheter tip. This phenomenon has been named "cross talk" and may also falsely increase the volumetric parameters [58].
4. *Effect of extracorporeal circuit.* Continuous renal replacement therapy (CRRT) seems to have no major clinical impact albeit a small statistically significant decrease in CI and GEDV and a small increase in EVLW have been observed [54]. This effect will be more pronounced when the central venous and dialysis catheter are in the femoral and subclavian/internal jugular position, respectively. In extracorporeal heart and lung assist systems, due to indicator loss in the extracorporeal circuit, the above-described changes may become clinically important, especially when high extracorporeal blood flows are applied (high-flow ECMO). However, some reports suggest that volumetric measurements are reliable, if extracorporeal blood flow does not exceed 20% of cardiac output [54].
5. *Effect of valvulopathy and heart function.* Regurgitation of the thermodilution injectate can prolong the MTT and DST of the indicator or can interfere with the TPTD curve. The long and flat running of the TD curve may result in an overestimation in the GEDV and EVLW. Usually in aortic stenosis, one can observe increased volumes that may differ at each TPTD, whereas mitral valve regurgitation gives a consistent increase in the volumetric preload parameters. In case of right ventricular failure, GEF may underestimate left ventricular function, as it represents global myocardial contraction; on the other hand, if GEF is normal, left ventricular function is usually normal [54].
6. *Effect of pleural effusions.* The etiology of pulmonary opacities, especially when bilateral, can be heterogeneous. EVLW has shown a good correlation with the degree of pulmonary edema either hydrostatic (cardiogenic) or hyperpermeability (septic). As already mentioned, the PVPI may help to differentiate between hyperpermeability versus hydrostatic edema in patients with increased EVLW. Pleural effusions do not contribute to the dilution of the thermal indicator and consequently do not increase TPTD-derived EVLW [59, 60]. Therefore, if EVLWI is normal (< = 10 ml/kg PBW), the presence of opacities on chest X-ray suggests the clinician to perform a lung ultrasound to check for pleural effusion.
7. *Normal values and indexation.* Initially, actual body weight and derived BSA were used for indexing CO and volumetric parameters. Later predicted rather than actual body weight and the derived predicted BSA were used for indexing. This improved accuracy in obese patients and correlates better with severity of illness and survival in acute lung injury patients. Recent data for EVLW show that indexation related to height is better [23]. A problem is that so far, there are no real normal ranges in different types of patients.
8. *Effect of pneumonectomy.* The available data suggests that correct calculation of GEDV is still possible while EVLW is underestimated. TPTD can be useful to detect

postpneumonectomy pulmonary edema by examining the trend of CO and EVLW. The EVLW underestimation is dependent on the amount of lung resected.

9. *Effect of other conditions.* Situations like pulmonary embolism, aortic or left ventricular aneurysm (hidden volumes), or cardiac tamponade may also affect TPTD values. If the patient is known with an aortic aneurysm and a femoral arterial catheter is used, GEDV is increased. In this case a brachial, long radial, or axillary catheter is recommended. In case of pulmonary embolism or acute respiratory distress syndrome (ARDS) due to microthrombi and/or high PEEP levels, GEDV will be overestimated, while EVLW will be underestimated. EVLW values are influenced by the amount of EVLW, permeability, tidal volume, PaO2/FiO2 ratio, and level of PEEP. Although it may seem controversial, recruitment of edematous lung areas or thoracocentesis can relieve the compression of pulmonary vessels and resolve hypoxic pulmonary vasoconstriction, so that the resulting increase in PBV may lead to a paradoxal increase in EVLW.
10. *Influence of mode of ventilation.* Body positioning (proning) can increase EVLW and GEDV, although the effects are clinically insignificant. In case of one-lung ventilation, the area under the thermodilution curve will not change; however, the MTT and DST and associated volumetric variables are affected and may not be correct. As discussed above, the effect of PEEP on EVLW measurement is controversial. On one hand, the use of high levels of PEEP may be responsible for pulmonary vascular defects resulting in a decrease in EVLW. On the other hand, by recruiting the lungs, PEEP may induce a redistribution of pulmonary blood flow toward previously excluded areas hence artificially "increasing" EVLW. Importantly, PEEP may have an effect not only on the TPTD measurement of EVLW but also on the actual amount. Indeed, PEEP may decrease EVLW by concomitant decrease in CO and pulmonary capillary pressure. On the other hand, PEEP may also increase EVLW by reducing lymph flow and pulmonary interstitial pressure (increasing lung volume).

▫ Table 23.3 lists some common conditions and problems that may either increase (overestimate) or decrease (underestimate) the EVLW and GEDV values obtained with TPTD.

23.11 Mathematical Coupling

Mathematical coupling, or the interdependence of two variables when one is used to calculate the other, may account for the significant correlation between CO and ITBV and GEDV or RVEDV measurements [61]. The relationship between two such variables is due, in part, to their common derivation, calculation, and shared measurement error [62]. Since RVEDV is calculated using SV, and CO is calculated as heart rate multiplied by SV, by definition CO and RVEDV are mathematically coupled variables. This is also the case for ITBV and GEDV since they are calculated using CO. In the past, Durham, Chang, and Nelson have separately addressed the potential impact of mathematical coupling on the reliability of RVEDV as an adequate preload measurement. Durham used mathematical modeling to correct for the shared measurement error introduced by mathematical coupling and found CI to remain significantly correlated with RVEDV [63]. Chang measured CO via indirect calorimetry and demonstrated a significant correlation between mathematically uncoupled CO and

Table 23.3 Common conditions and problem that may either increase or decrease the values obtained for extravascular lung water (EVLW) and global end-diastolic volume (GEDV). ARDS acute respiratory distress syndrome, CRRT continuous renal replacement therapy, ECCO2R extracorporeal CO2 removal, ECMO extracorporeal membrane oxygenation, PEEP positive end-expiratory pressure, TPTD transpulmonary thermodilution

	EVLW	GEDV
Increase (overestimation)	Wrong demographic data Too low injectate volume Femoral venous access Long radial arterial access Presence of shunt Cross talk phenomenon Aortic stenosis Mitral regurgitation Tricuspid regurgitation CRRT ECCO2R ECMO After thoracocentesis (paradoxal) After recruitment (paradoxal) High PEEP application (paradoxal) Prone positioning	Wrong demographic data Too low injectate volume Femoral venous access Long radial arterial access Presence of shunt Cross talk phenomenon Aortic stenosis Mitral regurgitation Tricuspid regurgitation Aortic aneurysm Pulmonary embolism Cardiac tamponade ARDS (microthrombi) Prone positioning
Decrease (underestimation)	Wrong demographic data Too high injectate volume Cross talk phenomenon (rapid TPTD interruption) Pleural effusions Edematous lungs Atelectasis High tidal volume PEEP application Low P/F ratio Postpneumonectomy ARDS (microthrombi)	Wrong demographic data Too high injectate volume Cross talk phenomenon (rapid TPTD interruption) CRRT ECCO2R ECMO

thermodilution RVEDV [64]. Nelson compared CO with RVEDV measurements determined using two different thermodilution technologies and confirmed the significant correlation between mathematically uncoupled CO and RVEDV [65]. Buhre investigated whether a variation in CO induced by high-dose beta-blockade influences thermodilution measurements of ITBV and GEDV in the absence of changes in intravascular volume in 16 patients undergoing minimally invasive direct coronary artery bypass surgery [66]. They found that the administration of a beta-blocker decreased CO significantly while volumetric parameters remained unchanged suggesting the absence of mathematical coupling. The same was found in an interesting study in 36 septic patients by Michard and colleagues, demonstrating that, in contrast to CVP, the transpulmonary thermodilution GEDV behaves as an indicator of cardiac preload [26]. Volume loading induced a significant increase in CVP, GEDV, SV, and CO. Changes in GEDV were correlated with changes in SV, while changes in CVP were not. The preinfusion GEDV was lower in the cases of positive response and was negatively correlated with the percentage increase in GEDV. Dobutamine infusion induced an increase in SV and in CO, but no significant change in CVP and in GEDV occurred. Mathematical coupling does not negate the validity of RVEDV and GEDV as predictors of intravascular volume status.

23.12 How to Improve Volumetric Monitoring

Static monitoring of the volumetric parameters (GEDV) has not consistently been shown to be able to predict changes in CO. For any patient admitted to the ICU that becomes hemodynamically unstable, it is important to know what his/her Frank-Starling curve looks like and where the patient is situated on the curve (Fig. 23.7).

The initial studies describing the use of volumetric PAC and PiCCO/VolumeView technologies described "optimal" RVEDVI values of approximately 130–140 mL/m^2 and optimal GEDVI values of 680–800 mL/m^2 above which patients felt to no longer respond to further volume administration with increases in CI [26, 63, 67]. As clinical experience with volumetric technology has increased, these "optimal" values have been disputed and found to oversimplify what is actually a complex and dynamic relationship between preload, contractility, and afterload [54]. New insights have learned that the patient's RVEF

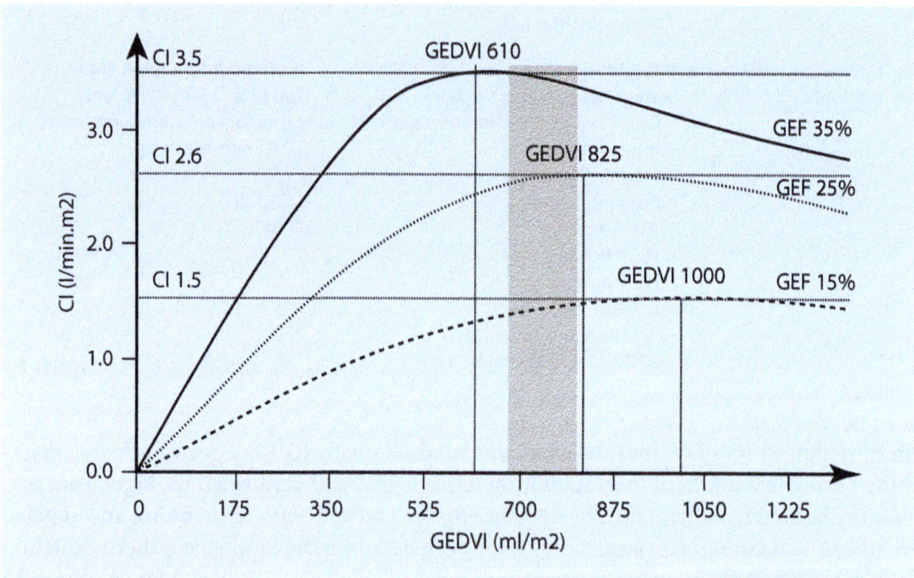

Fig. 23.7 Relation between global end-diastolic volume and ventricular function. Cardiac contractility in the critically ill can be described as a series of "ventricular function curves." Each curve has an associated global ejection fraction (GEF), describing the ventricle's contractility, and an optimal global end-diastolic volume index (GEDVI), identifying the plateau of the ventricular function curve [1]. Resuscitation to this plateau end-diastolic volume is widely believed to optimize a patient's intravascular volume, cardiac function, and end-organ perfusion. For a GEF of 35%, this plateau is at a GEDVI of 610 ml/m^2 and 825 and 1000, respectively, for a GEF of 25% and 15% [1]. As ventricular function changes, the patient "shifts" from one Frank-Starling curve to another with identification of both a new, optimal plateau GEDVI as a resuscitation endpoint and a new GEF. Therefore, the patient's GEDVI must be interpreted in conjunction with the patient's GEF. Shaded area indicates normal range of GEDVI (680–800 ml/m^2). (Adapted from Malbrain et al. [3])

and GEF must be taken into consideration when assessing the adequacy of RVEDVI or GEDVI as a resuscitation endpoint [30].

Cardiac contractility can be described as a series of "ventricular function curves" [1]. Each of these curves is associated with both an ejection fraction, which describes the ventricle's contractility, and an end-diastolic volume, which identifies the plateau of the patient's ventricular function curve [1]. Resuscitation to this plateau end-diastolic volume is widely believed to optimize a patient's intravascular volume, cardiac function, and end-organ perfusion [63].

Ventricular function (contractility), preload, afterload, and compliance are constantly changing in the critically ill. As ventricular function changes, the patient "shifts" from one GEF-defined Starling curve to another with identification of a new, optimal plateau GEDVI as a resuscitation endpoint (◘ Fig. 23.7)[1]. Thus, each GEDVI and RVEDVI must be considered in the context of the simultaneous GEF and RVEF measurement to determine whether the patient's left or right ventricular function is increasing, decreasing, or stable [1]. In the presence of unchanging ventricular contractility and afterload (as evidenced by a stable EF), EDVI assessment is relatively straightforward, as the target EDVI remains unchanged. In the critically ill patient with deteriorating ventricular contractility or increasing ventricular afterload, however, EDVI assessment becomes more complex. Thus, since ventricular compliance (and therefore RVEF and GEF) is subject to change in the critically ill, there cannot be a single value of RVEDVI or GEDVI that can be considered the ultimate goal of resuscitation for all patients. Each patient must be resuscitated to restore end-organ perfusion and function rather than to a single, arbitrary value [1].

Therefore, a reasonable resuscitation protocol is to initially fluid resuscitate patients to a "RVEF-corrected" RVEDVI of 100 mL/m^2, assuming that normal RVEF is approximately 40%. In analogy, one might postulate to resuscitate patients to a "GEF-corrected" GEDVI of 625 mL/m^2, assuming normal GEF in the critically ill is approximately 30% [1]. Patients with lower RVEF or GEF measurements are resuscitated to proportionally higher RVEDVI or GEDVI values. ◘ Figure 23.8 shows EF-nomogram for GEDVI resuscitation target values related to GEF values. A patient with a GEF of 25% might have a target GEDVI value of 775 mL/m^2, whereas a patient with a GEF of 15% might have a target GEDVI value of 950 mL/m^2. The EF measurement is also useful in determining the need for and choice of vasoactive infusion as it represents the relationship between ventricular contractility and afterload. Patients with a high EF will usually respond to fluid administration alone, while those with a low EF almost invariably benefit from early administration of inotropic support. It is important to recognize that patients should be volume resuscitated to the EDVI that restores end-organ perfusion and function and normalizes the patient's markers of resuscitation adequacy [1]. Patients may achieve these endpoints at EDVI values below their EF-corrected target values. Unnecessary over-resuscitation past these values will not benefit the patient and may induce possible harm.

Conclusions

Correct assessment of preload is important in critically ill patients with shock. In situations where intrathoracic pressure is increased as seen with positive-pressure ventilation, the addition of positive end-expiratory pressure, presence of auto-PEEP, or increased intra-abdominal pressure traditional barometric preload parameters like central venous pressure and pulmonary artery occlusion pressure may be erroneously increased because in fact they are zeroed against atmospheric pressure. In those conditions and in general, volumetric monitoring

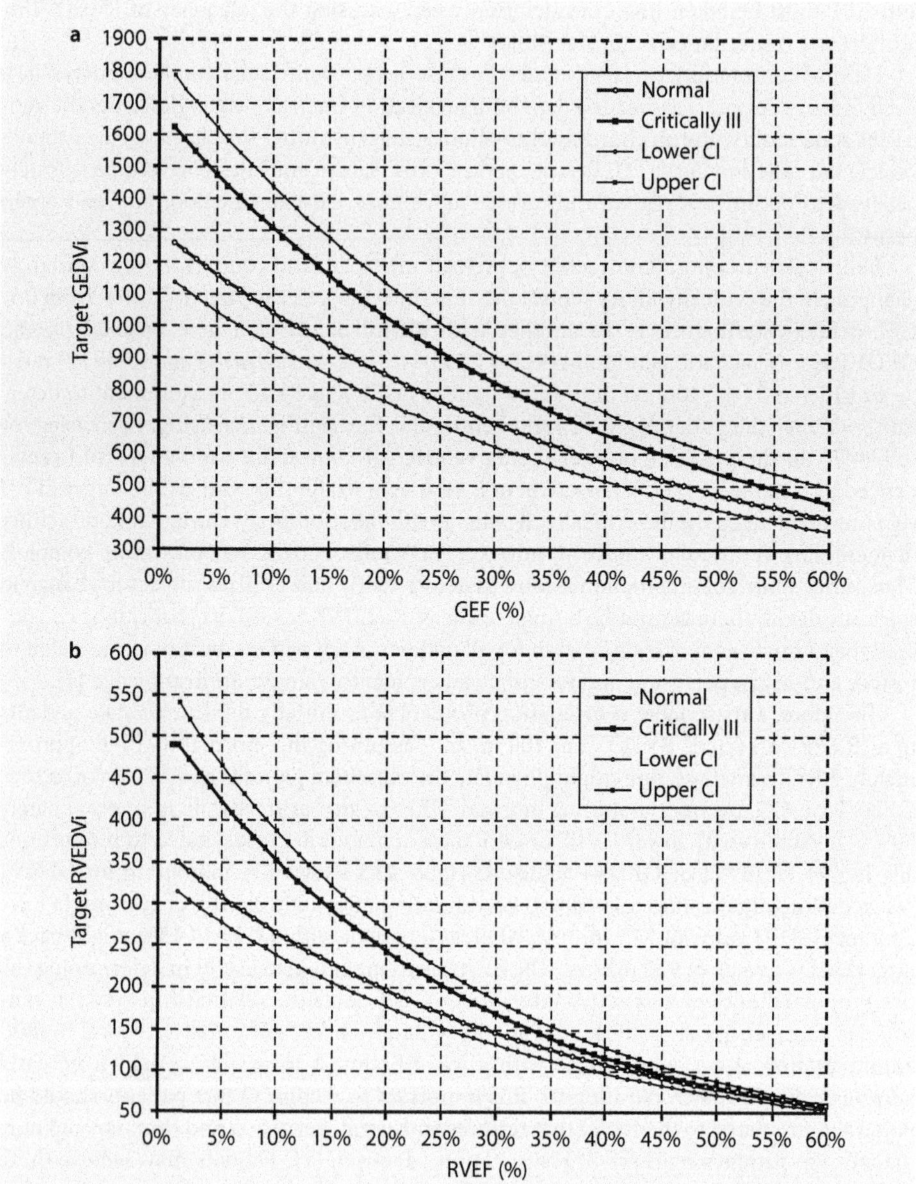

Fig. 23.8 Ejection fraction nomograms. Ejection fraction (EF) nomograms for global end-diastolic volume index (GEDVI) and right ventricular end-diastolic volume index (RVEDVI) resuscitation target values related to global ejection fraction (GEF) (panel **a**) and right ventricular ejection fraction (RVEF) (panel **b**) values. (Adapted from Malbrain et al. [30])

may provide more meaningful results. There are different volumetric monitoring techniques available at the moment. Each technique is different, needs to be assessed on its merits, and has a learning curve, indications and contraindications, and pros and cons, and the ICU physician must understand the different pitfalls that may affect the interpretation of the results and when one technique is preferred over another.

Take-Home Messages

- Assessment of the volumetric status (and especially intravascular hypo- or hypervolemia) is very important in hemodynamically unstable critically ill patients.
- Correct assessment of volumetric status is difficult at the bedside.
- Volumetric preload assessment in combination with functional hemodynamics and tests to evaluate fluid responsiveness (like passive leg raising) are superior over barometric preload indices.
- Barometric preload parameters are erroneously increased in conditions with increased intrathoracic pressure (mechanical ventilation, positive end-expiratory pressure (PEEP) or presence of auto-PEEP, diminished chest wall compliance, increased intra-abdominal pressure).
- There are different ways to assess volumetric preload and the most widely used are the volumetric pulmonary artery catheter (with measurement of right ventricular end-diastolic volume – RVEDV) and transpulmonary thermodilution techniques (with measurement of global end-diastolic volume – GEDV and extravascular lung water – EVLW).
- Each technique has its pitfalls and has a learning curve.

Conflict of Interest Manu Malbrain is professor at the Faculty of Medicine and Pharmacy at the Vrije Universiteit Brussel (VUB) and the founding president and the current treasurer of WSACS, the Abdominal Compartment Society (▶ www.wsacs.org); he is a member of the Medical Advisory Board of Getinge (formerly Pulsion Medical Systems) and consults for ConvaTec, Acelity, Maltron, Spiegelberg, Serenno Medical, Cytosorbents and Holtech Medical. He is the co-founder of the IFA, the International Fluid Academy (▶ www.fluidacademy.org).

References

1. Cheatham ML, Malbrain ML. Cardiovascular implications of abdominal compartment syndrome. Acta Clin Belg Suppl. 2007;62(1):98–112.
2. Malbrain ML, Ameloot K, Gillebert C, Cheatham ML. Cardiopulmonary monitoring in intra-abdominal hypertension. Am Surg. 2011;77(Suppl 1):S23–30.
3. Malbrain ML, De Waele JJ, De Keulenaer BL. What every ICU clinician needs to know about the cardiovascular effects caused by abdominal hypertension. Anaesthesiol Intensive Ther. 2015;47(4):388–99.

4. Marik PE, Cavallazzi R. Does the central venous pressure predict fluid responsiveness? An updated meta-analysis and a plea for some common sense. Crit Care Med. 2013;41(7):1774–81.
5. Malbrain MLNG, Reuter D. Hemodynamic treatment algorithms should follow physiology or they fail to improve outcome. Crit Care Med. 2012;40(10):2923–4.
6. Malbrain ML, Chiumello D, Cesana BM, Reintam Blaser A, Starkopf J, Sugrue M, et al. A systematic review and individual patient data meta-analysis on intra-abdominal hypertension in critically ill patients: the wake-up project. World initiative on abdominal hypertension epidemiology, a unifying project (WAKE-Up!). Minerva Anestesiol. 2014;80(3):293–306.
7. Peeters Y, Bernards J, Mekeirele M, Hoffmann B, De Raes M, Malbrain ML. Hemodynamic monitoring: to calibrate or not to calibrate? Part 1 - Calibrated techniques. Anaesthesiol Intensive Ther. 2015;47(5):487–500.
8. Robin E, Costecalde M, Lebuffe G, Vallet B. Clinical relevance of data from the pulmonary artery catheter. Crit Care. 2006;10(Suppl 3):S3.
9. Malbrain ML, De Potter T, Deeren D. Cost-effectiveness of minimally invasive hemodynamic monitoring. In: Vincent J-L, editor. Yearbook of intensive care and emergency medicine. Berlin: Springer; 2005. p. 603–31.
10. Cheatham ML, Safcsak K, Block EF, Nelson LD. Preload assessment in patients with an open abdomen. J Trauma. 1999;46(1):16–22.
11. Cheatham ML, Nelson LD, Chang MC, Safcsak K. Right ventricular end-diastolic volume index as a predictor of preload status in patients on positive end-expiratory pressure. Crit Care Med. 1998;26(11):1801–6.
12. Huygh J, Peeters Y, Bernards J, Malbrain ML. Hemodynamic monitoring in the critically ill: an overview of current cardiac output monitoring methods. F1000Res. 2016;5 https://doi.org/10.12688/f1000research.8991.1.
13. Harvey S, Harrison DA, Singer M, Ashcroft J, Jones CM, Elbourne D, et al. Assessment of the clinical effectiveness of pulmonary artery catheters in management of patients in intensive care (PAC-Man): a randomised controlled trial. Lancet. 2005;366(9484):472–7.
14. Bernards J, Mekeirele M, Hoffmann B, Peeters Y, De Raes M, Malbrain ML. Hemodynamic monitoring: to calibrate or not to calibrate? Part 2 - Non-calibrated techniques. Anaesthesiol Intensive Ther. 2015;47(5):501–16.
15. Lichtwarck-Aschoff M, Zeravik J, Pfeiffer UJ. Intrathoracic blood volume accurately reflects circulatory volume status in critically ill patients with mechanical ventilation. Intensive Care Med. 1992;18(3):142–7.
16. Godje O, Peyerl M, Seebauer T, Lamm P, Mair H, Reichart B. Central venous pressure, pulmonary capillary wedge pressure and intrathoracic blood volumes as preload indicators in cardiac surgery patients. Eur J Cardiothorac Surg. 1998;13(5):533–9; discussion 9–40.
17. Sakka SG, Bredle DL, Reinhart K, Meier-Hellmann A. Comparison between intrathoracic blood volume and cardiac filling pressures in the early phase of hemodynamic instability of patients with sepsis or septic shock. J Crit Care. 1999;14(2):78–83.
18. Brock H, Gabriel C, Bibl D, Necek S. Monitoring intravascular volumes for postoperative volume therapy. Eur J Anaesthesiol. 2002;19(4):288–94.
19. Schiffmann H, Singer M, Harms K, Buhre W, Hoeft A. Transpulmonary Indicator-Dilution (TPID): a new method for cardiovascular monitoring in critically ill neonates and infants. Appl Cardiopulm Pathophysiol. 1995;5:237–44.
20. Della Rocca G, Costa MG, Pietropaoli P. How to measure and interpret volumetric measures of preload. Curr Opin Crit Care. 2007;13(3):297–302.
21. Godje O, Peyerl M, Seebauer T, Dewald O, Reichart B. Reproducibility of double indicator dilution measurements of intrathoracic blood volume compartments, extravascular lung water, and liver function. Chest. 1998;113(4):1070–7.
22. Monnet X, Anguel N, Osman D, Hamzaoui O, Richard C, Teboul JL. Assessing pulmonary permeability by transpulmonary thermodilution allows differentiation of hydrostatic pulmonary edema from ALI/ARDS. Intensive Care Med. 2007;33(3):448–53.
23. Huber W, Hollthaler J, Schuster T, Umgelter A, Franzen M, Saugel B, et al. Association between different indexations of extravascular lung water (EVLW) and PaO2/FiO2: a two-center study in 231 patients. PLoS One. 2014;9(8):e103854.
24. Sakka SG, Ruhl CC, Pfeiffer UJ, Beale R, McLuckie A, Reinhart K, et al. Assessment of cardiac preload and extravascular lung water by single transpulmonary thermodilution. Intensive Care Med. 2000;26(2):180–7.
25. Della Rocca G, Costa GM, Coccia C, Pompei L, Di Marco P, Pietropaoli P. Preload index: pulmonary artery occlusion pressure versus intrathoracic blood volume monitoring during lung transplantation. Anesth Analg. 2002;95(4):835–43, table of contents.

26. Michard F, Alaya S, Zarka V, Bahloul M, Richard C, Teboul JL. Global end-diastolic volume as an indicator of cardiac preload in patients with septic shock. Chest. 2003;124(5):1900–8.
27. Hofer CK, Furrer L, Matter-Ensner S, Maloigne M, Klaghofer R, Genoni M, et al. Volumetric preload measurement by thermodilution: a comparison with transoesophageal echocardiography. Br J Anaesth. 2005;94(6):748–55.
28. Jonas MM, Tanser SJ. Lithium dilution measurement of cardiac output and arterial pulse waveform analysis: an indicator dilution calibrated beat-by-beat system for continuous estimation of cardiac output. Curr Opin Crit Care. 2002;8(3):257–61.
29. Malbrain ML, De Potter P, Deeren D. Cost-effectiveness of minimally invasive hemodynamic monitoring. In: Vincent J-L, editor. Yearbook of intensive care and emergency medicine. Berlin: Springer; 2005. p. 603–31.
30. Malbrain ML, De Potter TJ, Dits H, Reuter DA. Global and right ventricular end-diastolic volumes correlate better with preload after correction for ejection fraction. Acta Anaesthesiol Scand. 2010;54(5):622–31.
31. Hofer CK, Ganter MT, Matter-Ensner S, Furrer L, Klaghofer R, Genoni M, et al. Volumetric assessment of left heart preload by thermodilution: comparing the PiCCO-VoLEF system with transoesophageal echocardiography. Anaesthesia. 2006;61(4):316–21.
32. American Society of A, Society of Cardiovascular Anesthesiologists Task Force on Transesophageal E. Practice guidelines for perioperative transesophageal echocardiography. An updated report by the American Society of Anesthesiologists and the Society of Cardiovascular Anesthesiologists Task Force on Transesophageal Echocardiography. Anesthesiology. 2010;112(5):1084–96.
33. Mullany D. Benefits of using ultrasound and non-invasive haemodynamic monitoring for critically ill and cardiac surgical patients. Anaesth Intensive Care. 2013;41(6):706–9.
34. Skarvan K, Lambert A, Filipovic M, Seeberger M. Reference values for left ventricular function in subjects under general anaesthesia and controlled ventilation assessed by two-dimensional transoesophageal echocardiography. Eur J Anaesthesiol. 2001;18:713–22.
35. Tousignant C, Walsh F, Mazer C. The use of transesophageal echocardiography for preload assessment in critically ill patients. Anesthesia Analgesia. 2000;90:351–5.
36. Vermeiren GL, Malbrain ML, Walpot JM. Cardiac ultrasonography in the critical care setting: a practical approach to assess cardiac function and preload for the "non-cardiologist". Anaesthesiol Intensive Ther. 2015;47 Spec No:s89–104.
37. Thys D, Hillel Z, Goldman M, Mindich B, Kaplan J. A comparison of hemodynamic indices derived by invasive monitoring and two-dimensional echocardiography. Anesthesiology. 1987;67:630–4.
38. Cheung MM, Smallhorn JF, Redington AN, Vogel M. The effects of changes in loading conditions and modulation of inotropic state on the myocardial performance index: comparison with conductance catheter measurements. Eur Heart J. 2004;25(24):2238–42.
39. van Daele ME, Trouwborst A, van Woerkens LC, Tenbrinck R, Fraser AG, Roelandt JR. Transesophageal echocardiographic monitoring of preoperative acute hypervolemic hemodilution. Anesthesiology. 1994;81(3):602–9.
40. Swenson JD, Harkin C, Pace NL, Astle K, Bailey P. Transesophageal echocardiography: An objective tool in determining maximum ventricular response to intravenous fluid therapy. Anesthesia Analgesia. 1996;83:1149–53.
41. Wiesenack C, Prasser C, Rodig G, Keyl C. Stroke volume variation as an indicator of fluid responsiveness using pulse contour analysis in mechanically ventilated patients. Anesth Analg. 2003;96(5):1254–7.
42. Slama M, Masson H, Teboul JL, Arnout ML, Susic D, Frohlich E, et al. Respiratory variations of aortic VTI: a new index of hypovolemia and fluid responsiveness. Am J Physiol Heart Circ Physiol. 2002;283(4):H1729–33.
43. Malbrain MLNG, Huygh J, Dabrowski W, De Waele J, Wauters J. The use of bio-electrical impedance analysis (BIA) to guide fluid management, resuscitation and deresuscitation in critically ill patients: a bench-to-bedside review. Anaesthesiol Intensive Ther. 2014;46(5):381–91.
44. Bioelectrical impedance analysis in body composition measurement: National Institutes of Health Technology Assessment Conference Statement. Am J Clin Nutr. 1996;64(3):524S–532S. https://doi: 10.1093/ajcn/64.3.524S.
45. Streat SJ, Plank LD, Hill GL. Overview of modern management of patients with critical injury and severe sepsis. World J Surg. 2000;24(6):655–63.
46. Foster KR, Lukaski HC. Whole-body impedance--what does it measure? Am J Clin Nutr. 1996;64(3 Suppl):388S–96S.
47. Malbrain ML, Marik PE, Witters I, Cordemans C, Kirkpatrick AW, Roberts DJ, et al. Fluid overload, de-resuscitation, and outcomes in critically ill or injured patients: a systematic review with suggestions for clinical practice. Anaesthesiol Intensive Ther. 2014;46(5):361–80.

48. Plank LD, Hill GL. Similarity of changes in body composition in intensive care patients following severe sepsis or major blunt injury. Ann N Y Acad Sci. 2000;904:592–602.
49. Vandervelden S, Teering S, Hoffman B, Peeters Y, Bernards J, Mekeirele M, et al. Prognostic value of bioelectrical impedance analysis (BIA) derived parameters in critically ill patients. Anaesth Intensive Therapy. 2015;47(Supplem 2):14–6.
50. Samoni S, Vigo V, Resendiz LI, Villa G, De Rosa S, Nalesso F, et al. Impact of hyperhydration on the mortality risk in critically ill patients admitted in intensive care units: comparison between bioelectrical impedance vector analysis and cumulative fluid balance recording. Crit Care. 2016;20:95.
51. Basso F, Berdin G, Virzi GM, Mason G, Piccinni P, Day S, et al. Fluid management in the intensive care unit: bioelectrical impedance vector analysis as a tool to assess hydration status and optimal fluid balance in critically ill patients. Blood Purif. 2013;36(3–4):192–9.
52. House AA, Haapio M, Lentini P, Bobek I, de Cal M, Cruz DN, et al. Volume assessment in mechanically ventilated critical care patients using bioimpedance vectorial analysis, brain natriuretic Peptide, and central venous pressure. Int J Nephrol. 2011;2011:413760.
53. Eichhorn V, Goepfert MS, Eulenburg C, Malbrain ML, Reuter DA. Comparison of values in critically ill patients for global end-diastolic volume and extravascular lung water measured by transcardiopulmonary thermodilution: a metaanalysis of the literature. Med Intensiva. 2012;36:467.
54. Hofkens PJ, Verrijcken A, Merveille K, Neirynck S, Van Regenmortel N, De Laet I, et al. Common pitfalls and tips and tricks to get the most out of your transpulmonary thermodilution device: results of a survey and state-of-the-art review. Anaesthesiol Intensive Ther. 2015;47(2):89–116.
55. Faybik P, Hetz H, Baker A, Yankovskaya E, Krenn CG, Steltzer H. Iced versus room temperature injectate for assessment of cardiac output, intrathoracic blood volume, and extravascular lung water by single transpulmonary thermodilution. J Crit Care. 2004;19(2):103–7.
56. Huber W, Kraski T, Haller B, Mair S, Saugel B, Beitz A, et al. Room-temperature vs. iced saline indicator injection for transpulmonary thermodilution. J Crit Care. 2014;29(6):1133.e7–1133.e14.
57. Michard F, Phillips C. The camel curve: the icing on the transpulmonary thermodilution cake. Crit Care Med. 2011;39(3):611–2; author reply 2.
58. Michard F. Looking at transpulmonary thermodilution curves: the cross-talk phenomenon. Chest. 2004;126(2):656–7.
59. Deeren DH, Dits H, Daelemans R, Malbrain ML. Effect of pleural fluid on the measurement of extravascular lung water by single transpulmonary thermodilution. Clin Intensive Care. 2004;15:119–22.
60. Saugel B, Phillip V, Ernesti C, Messer M, Meidert AS, Schmid RM, et al. Impact of large-volume thoracentesis on transpulmonary thermodilution-derived extravascular lung water in medical intensive care unit patients. J Crit Care. 2013;28(2):196–201.
61. McNamee JE, Abel FL. Mathematical coupling and Starling's law of the heart. Shock. 1996;6(5):330.
62. Stratton HH, Feustel PJ, Newell JC. Regression of calculated variables in the presence of shared measurement error. J Appl Physiol (1985). 1987;62(5):2083–93.
63. Durham R, Neunaber K, Vogler G, Shapiro M, Mazuski J. Right ventricular end-diastolic volume as a measure of preload. J Trauma. 1995;39(2):218–23; discussion 23–4.
64. Chang MC, Black CS, Meredith JW. Volumetric assessment of preload in trauma patients: addressing the problem of mathematical coupling. Shock. 1996;6(5):326–9.
65. Nelson LD, Safcsak K, Cheatham ML, Block EF. Mathematical coupling does not explain the relationship between right ventricular end-diastolic volume and cardiac output. Crit Care Med. 2001;29(5):940–3.
66. Buhre W, Kazmaier S, Sonntag H, Weyland A. Changes in cardiac output and intrathoracic blood volume: a mathematical coupling of data? Acta Anaesthesiol Scand. 2001;45(7):863–7.
67. Diebel LN, Wilson RF, Tagett MG, Kline RA. End-diastolic volume. A better indicator of preload in the critically ill. Arch Surg. 1992;127(7):817–21; discussion 21–2.

Assessment of Fluid Responsiveness

Xavier Monnet and Jean-Louis Teboul

M. R. Pinsky et al. (eds.), *Hemodynamic Monitoring*, Lessons from the ICU,
https://doi.org/10.1007/978-3-319-69269-2_24

Learning Objectives

In this chapter, students will learn the physiology of preload responsiveness and its consequences in clinical practice. They will also learn the different tests that can be used to predict fluid responsiveness at the bedside, their principle, the way to perform them in practice and their limitations.

24.1 Introduction

Volume expansion is the treatment that is most often undertaken as first-line therapy during shock. It creates a crucial therapeutic dilemma. On the one hand, it is likely to increase stroke volume and cardiac output and ultimately oxygen delivery. On the other hand, it may cause deleterious effects that have been well demonstrated: aggravation of tissue oedema, including lung oedema, worsening of organ dysfunction and haemodilution. It has been clearly established that fluid overload is a poor prognostic factor in critically ill patients, particularly in the case of acute respiratory distress syndrome (ARDS) [1–3], acute kidney injury [4, 5], sepsis [6–8] and/or intra-abdominal hypertension [9]. The problem is compounded by the fact that the beneficial haemodynamic effect of volume expansion is inconsistent. The Frank-Starling's relationship between cardiac preload and stroke volume has a variable slope, which depends on ventricular systolic function (◘ Fig. 24.1). Depending on the slope of the curve on which the patient's heart is working, the preload increase induced by volume expansion may induce a negligible or significant response in terms of stroke volume and cardiac output [10].

The first way to solve the therapeutic conflict created by volume expansion is to perform it only if it is certain that it will result in haemodynamic improvement. This is the

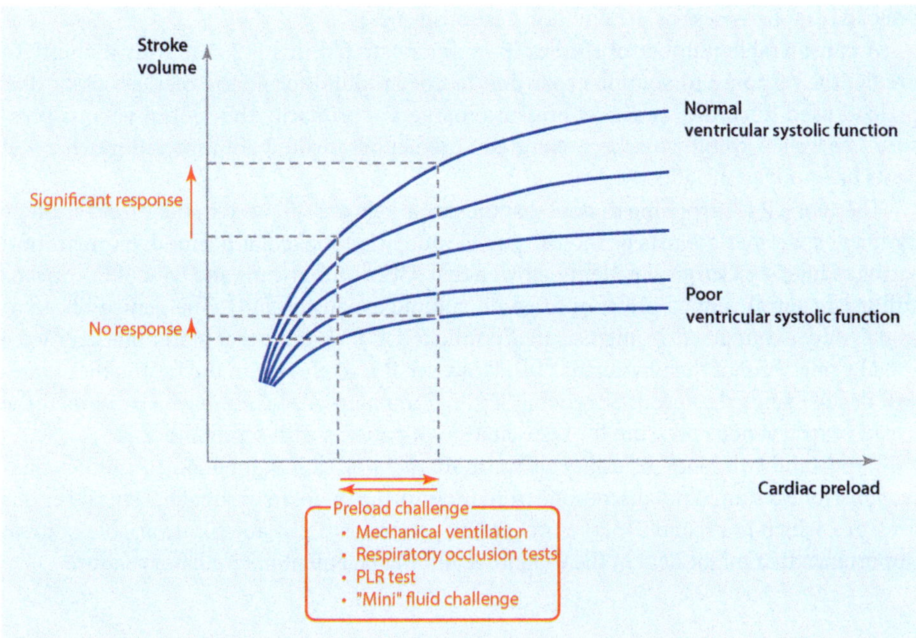

◘ **Fig. 24.1** Frank-Starling relationship. PLR passive leg raising

case when the fluid loss is obvious, during haemorrhagic or hypovolemic shock, or at the initial phase of septic shock. In the other cases, it is less easy to a priori predict the haemodynamic response to volume expansion. Numerous studies have shown that, in these cases, only half of the patients (usually called fluid responders) respond to fluid administration by the expected increase in cardiac output [11].

24

It is for this purpose that several methods have been developed to predict fluid responsiveness. In addition to "static" markers of cardiac preload, the futility of which has been clearly established, many "dynamic" tests have been developed. In this chapter, we will review them, indicating in particular their validity conditions, their advantages and their limitations.

When Should We Test Fluid Responsiveness?

1. Only in patients with haemodynamic instability and/or signs of peripheral hypoperfusion (mottling, increased capillary refill time, low urine output, elevated lactate, etc)
2. Not if hypovolemia is clinically obvious: hypovolemic shock, initial phase of septic shock when no treatment has been administered yet

24.2 Static Markers of Cardiac Preload: The Wrong Solution

For decades, the decision to administer or not fluid has been guided by the simple estimation of cardiac preload. The principle was that when cardiac preload is low, the response to volume expansion is likely and vice versa. However, this method is inefficient. Above all, the reason is physiological. By observing the family of Frank-Starling curves (◘ Fig. 24.1), it is obvious that a given "static" level of cardiac preload may correspond to preload responsiveness or preload non-responsiveness.

A considerable number of studies have demonstrated this [12, 13]. This inability to predict the response to volume expansion has been found for all the markers of cardiac preload used in clinical practice: pressure markers – primarily the central venous pressure – as well as volume markers. None can predict before fluid administration what will be its haemodynamic effectiveness.

Therefore, it is surprising to note that these markers are still used in their fluid strategy by many anaesthesiologists or intensivists. A study that looked at haemodynamic monitoring of high-risk surgical patients showed that 73% of Americans and 84% of Europeans still used central venous pressure to guide volume expansion [14]. The Fenice observational study, conducted in intensive care units (ICU), showed that static markers were used by one-third of the physicians [14]. However, it is likely that in the future, these rates will decline since the recent Surviving Sepsis Campaign guidelines have abandoned the use of central venous pressure for resuscitation of patients with septic shock [15]

Importantly, the lack of utility of static markers of cardiac preload to predict fluid responsiveness should not discourage from monitoring them. In particular, central venous pressure, which is a reliable marker of cardiac preload, is a physiological variable of great importance that might help in the diagnosis and management of circulatory failure.

24.3 Respiratory Variations in Arterial Pulse Pressure and Stroke Volume

The respiratory variations of the arterial pulse pressure (PPV) and of stroke volume (SVV) are the first dynamic indices that have been developed to predict fluid responsiveness and the ones whose reliability has been best demonstrated.

24.3.1 Physiological Principle

During positive pressure ventilation, insufflation increases the intrathoracic pressure. This increase is transmitted to the right atrium. The resulting decrease in the pressure gradient of venous return leads to a decrease in the preload of the right ventricle. If the latter is preload-dependent, its stroke volume is lowered. After the time required for the transit through the pulmonary circulation, that is to say at expiration, the left ventricular preload is lowered in turn. If this ventricle is also preload-dependent, stroke volume decreases. Other haemodynamic phenomena occur during positive pressure inspiration. It stretches the pulmonary arterial vessels and increases their resistance, so that the right ventricular afterload increases. This contributes to the decrease in the right ventricular stroke volume. Also, the inspiratory increase in intrathoracic pressure decreases the transmural pressure of the left ventricle, which tends to increase its stroke volume. Thus, all the phenomena concur so that stroke volume decreases at the end of expiration and increases at the end of inspiration [16].

24.3.2 Reliability and Practical Use

Arterial pulse pressure is the first estimate of stroke volume whose respiratory variation has been demonstrated to predict fluid responsiveness [17]. This predictive ability has been confirmed by a considerable number of studies and several meta-analyses [13, 18, 19]. The diagnostic threshold is 12% [18] (▫ Table 24.1).

PPV is calculated as the difference between the maximum pulse pressure and minimum during a respiratory cycle divided by the average of the two values. The measurement is today automatically performed by the majority of bedside monitors.

Following that of invasive arterial pressure, the respiratory variation of many other substitutes for stroke volume was studied: the arterial pulse pressure estimated noninvasively from the volume-clamp technique [20]; the stroke volume estimated by pulse contour analysis; the maximum velocity of the flow in the left ventricular outflow tract, measured by echocardiography; the descending aortic flow measured by oesophageal Doppler [21]; or even the amplitude of the carotid or arterial femoral flow measured with vascular Doppler. The amplitude of the plethysmography signal was used for the same purpose [22]. While studies have led to positive results, others have been less affirmative, especially in patients receiving vasopressors, which could alter the relationship between stroke volume and plethysmography signal [23, 24].

24

Table 24.1 Summary of methods predicting preload responsiveness with diagnostic threshold and limitations

Method	Threshold	Main limitations
Pulse pressure/stroke volume variations	12%	Cannot be used in case of spontaneous breathing, cardiac arrhythmias, low tidal volume/lung compliance
Tidal volume challenge	3.5% (PPV)	Cannot be used in case of spontaneous breathing, cardiac arrhythmias
	2.5% (SVV)	
Inferior vena cava diameter variations	12%	Cannot be used in case of spontaneous breathing, low tidal volume/lung compliance
Superior vena cava diameter variations	36%[a]	Requires performing transoesophageal Doppler
		Cannot be used in case of spontaneous breathing, low tidal volume/lung compliance
Passive leg raising	10%	Requires a direct measurement of cardiac output
End-expiratory occlusion test	5%	Cannot be used in non-intubated patients
		Cannot be used in patients who interrupt a 15-sec respiratory hold
End-inspiratory + end-expiratory occlusion test	15%	Cannot be used in non-intubated patients
		Cannot be used in patients who interrupt a 15-sec respiratory
"Mini"-fluid challenge (100 mL)	6%[b]	Requires a precise technique for measuring cardiac output
"Standard" fluid challenge (300–500 mL)	15%	Requires a direct measurement of cardiac output
		Induces fluid overload if repeated

Citations indicate the most important reference regarding the test
[a]Thresholds from 12% to 40% have been reported
[b]10% is more compatible with echography precision

24.3.3 Limitations

Although the reliability of PPV and SVV is well established, there are some conditions in which they are no longer reliable. The main ones are listed in Table 24.1. These include spontaneous breathing (even in an intubated patient) and cardiac arrhythmias, two conditions that lead to false positives. ARDS leads to false-negative results. In this case, the low tidal volume that is used for ventilation reduces the magnitude of the change in intrathoracic pressure that causes PPV and SVV. If the compliance of the respiratory system is low, the transmission of alveolar pressures to intravascular and cardiac pressures are reduced, and the reliability of PPV and SVV is reduced [25].

A recent study showed that in patients with ARDS ventilated with a tidal volume at 6 mL/kg, this limitation of PPV could be circumvented by a "tidal volume challenge". It consists in transiently increasing the tidal volume to 8 mL/kg. If this causes an increase in the absolute value of PPV ≥ 3.5% or SVV ≥ 2.5%, the presence of fluid responsiveness at 6 mL/kg is very likely [26].

Intra-abdominal hypertension is also recognised as another condition that limits the accuracy of PPV and SVV [27] (◘ Table 24.1). In this case, the respiratory variations of stroke volume are not exclusively related to the volume status [28], and the threshold values identifying fluid responders and non-responders could be higher than in case of normal intra-abdominal pressure.

Finally, it has been suggested that in cases of right heart failure, the increase in right ventricular afterload during mechanical insufflation may be the cause of some false positives to PPV and SVV. Nevertheless, this has been poorly documented. A study suggesting this limitation has reported an incidence of false positives that has never been reported in any of the numerous studies of PPV or SVV, even in patients with ARDS [29].

In ICU practice, the conditions under which the reliability of PPV and SVV is decreased are quite common. This is especially true today as patients are less sedated and low tidal volume ventilation is more common than before. By contrast, in the operating room, PPV and SVV (obtained invasively or noninvasively) retain their predictive value since the conditions of applicability are generally fulfilled. The limitations of PPV and SVV should always be taken into account by intensivists or anaesthesiologists, as ignoring them may lead to serious misinterpretations. However, a recent survey showed that a large proportion of intensivists did not know all the factors confusing the PPV and SVV interpretation [30].

Summary

PPV and SVV are the predictors of fluid responsiveness that are the most established and of which measurement is automatic. They suffer from restrictive conditions of use, especially in the ICU, which must be kept in mind at the bedside.

24.4 Respiratory Variability of the Diameter of the Venae Cavae

24.4.1 Principle

Two factors underlie the variability of the diameter of the venae cavae during mechanical ventilation in case of preload responsiveness [31]. Firstly, changes in intrathoracic pressure lead to greater compression of the intrathoracic veins if they are more compliant, that is to say, if the central blood volume is lower, than if they are not. Secondly, the respiratory variation in central venous pressure and, therefore, in the pressure gradient of systemic venous return is greater if both ventricles are preload-responsive than if they are not. These two factors mean that, in the case of preload responsiveness, the vena cava expands upon insufflation compared to expiration. Reported diagnostic thresholds range from 12% to 40% (◘ Table 24.1).

24.4.2 Reliability and Practical Use

The respiratory variation of the inferior vena cava diameter is easily measured with transthoracic echocardiography, while the measurement of the respiratory change in the superior vena cava diameter is performed only transoesophageally.

24

Compared with PPV and SVV, the respiratory variation of the venae cavae diameters has been less studied. In addition, the results of the validation studies are generally less convincing. In a meta-analysis that included eight studies, sensitivity was only 76% and specificity was 86% [32]. In a recent study of a large population of 540 ICU mechanically ventilated patients most of them with low tidal volume, the area under the receiver operating characteristic curve was only 0.755 for the respiratory variation diameter of the superior vena cava and 0.635 for that of the inferior vena cava [33]. Nevertheless, it must be admitted that, in this pragmatic study, PPV also had a poor diagnostic performance, even in the subgroup of patients ventilated with normal tidal volume. This latter result goes against results of many publications as well as against the principles of physiology mentioned above, which must call into question the methodological value of the pragmatic study [33].

24.4.3 Limitations

It is important to emphasise that the respiratory variability of the venae cavae shares with PPV and SVV several restrictive conditions of use (▫ Table 24.1). In case of spontaneous ventilation, the irregularity of the inspiratory efforts prevents the determination of a diagnostic threshold. This has been confirmed by several studies [13, 34]. One study showed that in case of spontaneous breathing, only the very high values of the inferior vena cava diameter variation were of diagnostic value [35].

Although this has not been formally investigated, it is logical that the use of a small tidal volume leads to false negatives for the respiratory variation of the venae cavae dimensions as for PPV and SVV. The decrease in pulmonary compliance logically has the same effect. Nonetheless, cardiac arrhythmias do not influence the diagnostic performance of the method, the variation of the venae cavae not depending on the cardiac rhythm.

Summary
The respiratory variation of the inferior vena cava dimensions has the advantage of being measured quite easily by transthoracic echocardiography. It is therefore interesting when no haemodynamic monitoring technique is in place and the patient is not equipped with an arterial catheter. Nevertheless, in this case, it must be kept in mind that PPV and SVV have a higher diagnostic value and almost identical applicability conditions. The variability of the superior vena cava may have a slightly higher diagnostic value than that of the inferior vena cava, but its measurement requires a transoesophageal echocardiography.

24.5 Passive Leg Raising Test

24.5.1 Principle

The transition from the semi-recumbent position to a position in which the lower limbs are raised to 45° and the trunk is horizontal induces the transfer of venous blood from the lower limbs but also from the splanchnic territory, towards the cardiac cavities. This results in a significant increase in mean systemic pressure [36] and in the right and left cardiac preload [37]. Therefore, the passive leg raising (PLR) can be used as a preload responsiveness test. If cardiac output increases in response to the PLR manoeuvres, both ventricles are most likely preload-responsive. It has been shown that a PLR test was equivalent to about 300 mL of fluid challenge [38], but this is only an average value, this volume being highly variable depending on the circumstances and on the patient.

24.5.2 Reliability

As a matter of fact, many studies have shown that the PLR test can reliably detect preload responsiveness. The diagnostic threshold that was the most frequently found was a 10% increase in cardiac output [39] (◘ Table 24.1). A great advantage of the test is that it remains valid even in clinical circumstances where PPV and SVV cannot be used [40]. In particular, the PLR test keeps all its diagnostic value in case of spontaneous breathing, cardiac arrhythmia, low tidal volume ventilation and low lung compliance [25] (◘ Fig. 24.2).

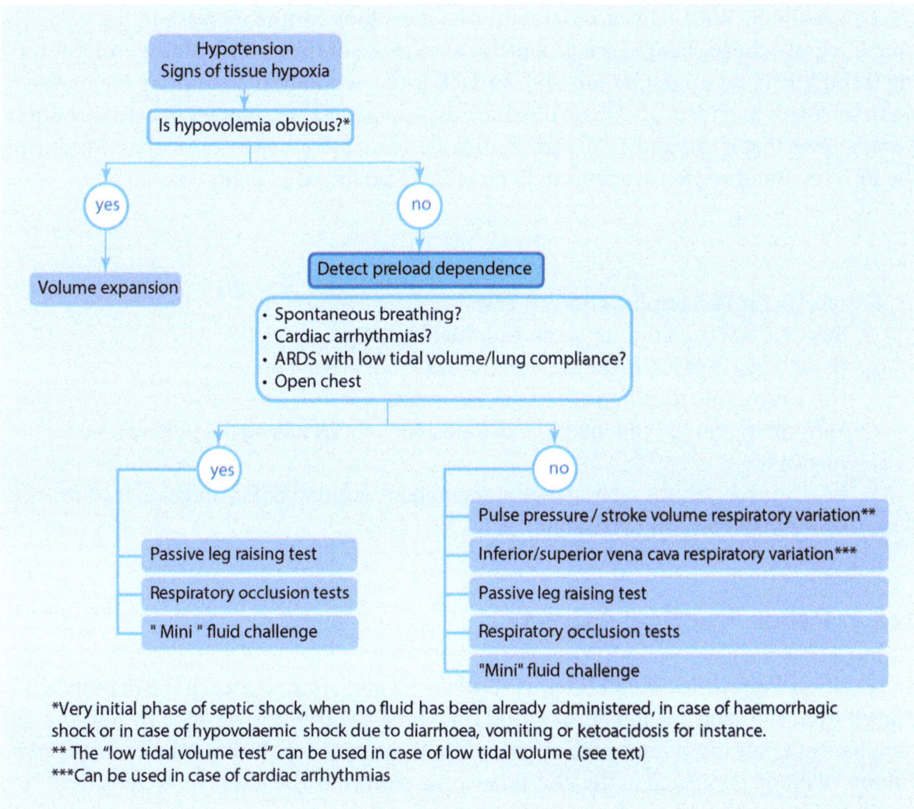

◘ **Fig. 24.2** Decisional algorithm for detecting preload responsiveness. ARDS acute respiratory distress syndrome

Two meta-analyses confirmed the diagnostic value of the PLR test [39, 41]. It has been included in the most recent version of the Surviving Sepsis Campaign Guidelines [15] and in a consensus conference of the European Society of Intensive Care Medicine [42].

24.5.3 Cardiac Output Measurement Technique

The effects of the PLR test should be measured directly on cardiac output [43]. Indeed, if these effects are assessed on arterial pressure, even pulse pressure, the sensitivity of the test is lower and the number of false negatives is greater [39, 41] (◘ Table 24.1). From this point of view, the PLR test is similar to the fluid challenge, the effects of which are poorly estimated by the only arterial pressure [44, 45].

Several cardiac output measurement techniques can be used to perform the PLR test. They must meet the requirement to measure flow continuously and in real time, in order to capture the maximum effect of the test. In fact, when the PLR test is positive, the increase in cardiac output occurs during the first minute [40]. Nevertheless, it may occur that cardiac output decreases after reaching this maximum. This effect is particularly observed in patients with severe septic shock, whose vasodilatation is marked. This is, for example, not possible with thermodilution, neither classic pulmonary nor transpulmonary.

Oesophageal Doppler and calibrated or non-calibrated pulse wave contour analysis can be used [40]. With echocardiography, one must look for the increase in the velocity-time integral, whose changes are proportional to those of the stroke volume. An interesting technique is capnography [46–48]. In fact, if the ventilation conditions are perfectly stable, changes in end-tidal carbon dioxide are proportional to changes in cardiac output. It was shown that if this end-tidal carbon dioxide value increased by more than 5% during the PLR test, fluid responsiveness could be reliably predicted [47, 48].

Five Rules for Performing the PLR Test

1. Start the test from the 45°-semi-recumbent position.
2. Use a direct measurement of cardiac output (not arterial pressure).
3. Use a real-time measurement of cardiac output.
4. Perform the test by changing the bed position, not by raising the patient's legs manually.
5. Reassess cardiac output in the semi-recumbent position before infusing fluid to check that it returns to baseline.

24.5.4 Other Practical Aspects

The position from which the PLR test is started is of great importance. Indeed, if the test is started from the semi-recumbent position, in which the trunk is elevated by 45°, the test mobilises not only the volume of the venous blood contained in the lower limbs but also the volume of blood contained in the vast splanchnic reservoir. The test is more sensitive [38].

The PLR test should ideally be performed using the automatic movements of the bed. Indeed, the "manual" embodiment, which involves holding the patient's heels, can cause discomfort, or even pain, which could distort the analysis of changes in cardiac output [43].

Finally, it is important to measure cardiac output after performing the test, when the patient has been returned to the semi-recumbent position, in order to verify that it has returned to its baseline value and that the changes observed during PLR were only attributable to the test [43].

24.5.5 Limitations

As stated above, the essential limit of the PLR test is that it requires a direct measurement of cardiac output. Also, the test is difficult or impossible to use during a surgical procedure. It is probably less sensitive in patients with venous compression stocking.

In case of intra-abdominal hypertension, it has been suspected that the venous blood mobilisation of the lower limbs through the vena cava could be observed and that this condition is responsible for false negatives [49] (◘ Table 24.1).

Summary

The PLR test is a way of predicting fluid responsiveness which reliability is well established. It has the advantage of supplying PPV and SVV under the conditions where these heart-lung interaction indices cannot be used. Its major disadvantage is that it requires to directly measuring cardiac output, even if several noninvasive means can be used to do this. Finally, one must pay attention to the technique of performing the test because it determines its reliability.

24.6 Respiratory Occlusion Tests

24.6.1 Principle

Like PPV and SVV, these tests use heart-lung interactions to induce a change in cardiac preload which effects on cardiac output are used to detect preload responsiveness (◘ Fig. 24.1). During mechanical ventilation, each insufflation increases the intrathoracic pressure and, consequently, the pressure in the right atrium, which opposes the systemic venous return. When mechanical ventilation is interrupted at end-expiration for a few seconds, the cyclical decrease in cardiac preload is interrupted. Cardiac preload increases transiently. If, in response, cardiac output increases, this means that both ventricles are preload responsive. Conversely, an end-inspiratory occlusion should decrease cardiac output in case of preload responsiveness.

24.6.2 End-Expiratory Occlusion Test

It has been shown that if cardiac output measured by the pulse contour analysis increased by more than 5% at the end of a 15-sec end-expiratory occlusion (EEO), the cardiac output response to a subsequent volume expansion is very likely [50]. An important point is that the EEO must be extended enough to allow the increase in cardiac preload to cross the pulmonary circulation and pass on the left side. Duration of 5 sec is insufficient.

Changes in cardiac output must be measured continuously and in real time. But also, the technique must be precise enough to detect changes of a few percent only. From this point of view, pulse contour analysis is perfectly adapted. Nevertheless, it requires an arterial catheter or, alternatively, a noninvasive system that estimates blood pressure in a continuous and noninvasive way.

24.6.3 Combination of End-Expiratory and End-Inspiratory Occlusions

For assessing the effects of the EEO test, echocardiography may raise the problem of its accuracy. Indeed, even though it allows a continuous and real-time measurement of cardiac output, only changes of more than 10% of the velocity-time integral can be reliably detected. In a recent study, increasing the velocity-time integral during a 15-sec EEO predicted fluid responsiveness, but the diagnostic threshold was 4%. Interestingly, the effects of an end-inspiratory occlusion were also tested [51]. A decrease of more than 5% in the velocity-time integral during such a 15-sec end-inspiratory occlusion also predicted fluid responsiveness, with a diagnostic threshold of 5%. Thus, when the effects of the two respiratory occlusions were added (in absolute value), the response to the volume expansion could be predicted with a diagnostic threshold of 15%, which is compatible with the precision of cardiac ultrasound [51].

The method is somewhat restrictive, since it imposes a careful measurement of the velocity-time integral during two successive respiratory breaks, but it could be an alternative when no other techniques than echocardiography is available for measuring cardiac output. When cardiac output is measured by a technique that cannot reliably detect changes in cardiac output less than 5%, it seems interesting to associate the end-expiratory and end-inspiratory occlusions.

24.6.4 Limitations

Of course, the first limitation of the method of respiratory occlusions is that it requires the patient to be ventilated invasively (Table 24.1). In addition, the method requires that the patient can tolerate a 15-sec ventilatory pause without interrupting it. This is of course not always possible. As far as we can conclude from a single clinical study, the level of positive expiratory pressure does not seem to influence the haemodynamic effects of the end-expiratory occlusion test and does not disturb its diagnostic value, at least between 5 and 11 cmH_2O [52].

Summary
Several studies converge today to establish the reliability of the expiratory occlusion test. If cardiac output is measured continuously, as for example with the analysis of the contour of the pulse wave, the test has the advantage of being very simple to achieve.

24.7 Other Tests Using Heart-Lung Interactions

An increase in the level of positive expiratory pressure from 5 to 10 cmH_2O induces a decrease in cardiac preload that can be used to detect a preload responsiveness. This was shown in a study where the effects of the manoeuvre were measured on end-tidal carbon dioxide, used as an estimate of cardiac output in patients who were stably ventilated [53].

Recruitment manoeuvres induce an increase in intrathoracic pressure with similar haemodynamic effects. Concomitant cardiac output changes can predict the response to volume expansion. The respiratory systolic variation test (RSVT) consists of measuring the changes in systolic arterial pressure induced by a series of three respiratory cycles performed with increasing airway pressure [54]. The essential advantage of the test is that it does not depend on the tidal volume. It can be automatically performed by some ventilators of anaesthesia.

24.8 Fluid Challenge

24.8.1 The Standard Fluid Challenge

The most direct way to assess the response to volume expansion is to administer fluid. Nevertheless, the conventional 300–500 mL fluid challenge suffers from two major disadvantages. The first is that its effects should be measured directly on cardiac output. As with the PLR test, changes in systemic blood pressure alone do not reliably detect the effects of the fluid challenge on cardiac output [44, 45]. The second drawback is that the fluid challenge is more a treatment than a diagnostic test itself. Unlike the PLR test, once preload responsiveness has been challenged, it is not reversible. Repetitive fluid challenges are inherently associated with fluid overload, especially when they do not result in any haemodynamic improvement. For example, in a patient with haemodynamic instability, in whom five hypotensive episodes occur during the day, guiding fluid therapy with 300-mL fluid challenges would result in infusing 1500 mL which would not increase cardiac output but only contribute to fluid overload and haemodilution.

24.8.2 "Mini"-Fluid Challenge

The idea has emerged to perform the fluid challenge with a smaller volume than the conventional 300 or 500 mL. In a study where a "mini"-fluid challenge was performed with 100 mL of colloid, an increase in the velocity-time integral, measured by transthoracic echocardiography, by more than 6% predicted fluid responsiveness reliably [55]. However, since this threshold is below the accuracy of echocardiography, the authors suggested using a diagnostic threshold of 10% despite a lower diagnostic value [55].

The mini-fluid challenge poses two problems. On the one hand, the volume used to change cardiac preload must be sufficient to stress the system. Recently, it has been suggested that a bolus of 4 mL/kg administered over 5 min was the minimum volume that increases the mean systemic pressure and can make the fluid challenge interpretable [56].

In keeping with this, it has been shown that a fluid challenge performed with only 50 mL of fluid does not predict the response to volume expansion [57]. On the other hand, the mini-fluid challenge requires a very accurate measurement of cardiac output. As we have seen, this may not be the case with echocardiography. Pulse contour analysis, the accuracy of which is very high [58], could be more appropriate.

24

Summary
The standard fluid challenge with 300–500 mL fluid is inherently associated with the risk of fluid overload. It may be less problematic in patients with no lung impairment or in the operating room. The 100-mL mini-fluid challenge requires a very precise measurement of cardiac output.

Conclusion

Volume expansion must be considered as a treatment in its own right, which side effects are dose-dependent and which efficacy is often uncertain. It is reasonable to try to predict its haemodynamic effects before undertaking it. About 20 years after the development of PPV and SVV, several tests are now available to evaluate preload responsiveness. The advantage is that their conditions of use and their limitations are different. It is up to the clinician to select the appropriate tests depending on the clinical situation and the haemodynamic monitoring techniques in place.

Take-Home Messages

- After the initial phase of septic shock and in the absence of obvious fluid losses, fluid responsiveness should be predicted before performing volume expansion in order to avoid unnecessary fluid infusion and fluid overload.
- Static markers of cardiac preload, such as central venous pressure, do not reliably predict fluid responsiveness.
- Pulse pressure and stroke volume variations are reliable but can be used only under strict conditions, in particular in the absence of ARDS, spontaneous breathing activity and cardiac arrhythmias.
- The variations of the superior and inferior venae cavae diameters cannot be used in case of ARDS and spontaneous breathing activity.
- Passive leg raising is reliable to predict fluid responsiveness. It requires a direct measurement of cardiac output, which can be invasive or noninvasive.
- The end-expiratory occlusion test can be used in ventilated patients with no strong spontaneous breathing activity. The combination of end-expiratory and end-inspiratory tests induces larger changes in cardiac output in fluid responders and makes the test assessable by echocardiography.
- The traditional fluid challenge with 300 to 500 mL of fluid requires a direct measurement of cardiac output. It is more a treatment than a test and it inherently contributes to fluid overload.
- The "mini"-fluid challenge might advantageously replace the traditional one, but it requires a precise technique for measuring cardiac output.

Conflicts of Interest Prof. Xavier MONNET and Prof. Jean-Louis TEBOUL are members of the Medical Advisory Board of Pulsion Medical Systems and have received honoraria for lectures from Masimo and Cheetah.

References

1. Murphy CV, Schramm GE, Doherty JA, Reichley RM, Gajic O, Afessa B, Micek ST, Kollef MH. The importance of fluid management in acute lung injury secondary to septic shock. Chest. 2009;136:102–9.
2. Rosenberg AL, Dechert RE, Park PK, Bartlett RH, Network NNA. Review of a large clinical series: association of cumulative fluid balance on outcome in acute lung injury: a retrospective review of the ARDSnet tidal volume study cohort. J Intensive Care Med. 2009;24:35–46.
3. Jozwiak M, Silva S, Persichini R, Anguel N, Osman D, Richard C, Teboul JL, Monnet X. Extravascular lung water is an independent prognostic factor in patients with acute respiratory distress syndrome. Crit Care Med. 2013;41:472–80.
4. Bouchard J, Soroko SB, Chertow GM, Himmelfarb J, Ikizler TA, Paganini EP, Mehta RL, Program to Improve Care in Acute Renal Disease Study G. Fluid accumulation, survival and recovery of kidney function in critically ill patients with acute kidney injury. Kidney Int. 2009;76:422–7.
5. Payen D, de Pont AC, Sakr Y, Spies C, Reinhart K, Vincent JL, Sepsis Occurrence in Acutely Ill Patients I. A positive fluid balance is associated with a worse outcome in patients with acute renal failure. Crit Care. 2008;12:R74.
6. Boyd JH, Forbes J, Nakada TA, Walley KR, Russell JA. Fluid resuscitation in septic shock: a positive fluid balance and elevated central venous pressure are associated with increased mortality. Crit Care Med. 2011;39:259–65.
7. Vincent JL, Sakr Y, Sprung CL, Ranieri VM, Reinhart K, Gerlach H, Moreno R, Carlet J, Le Gall JR, Payen D. Sepsis in European intensive care units: results of the SOAP study. Crit Care Med. 2006;34:344–53.
8. Micek ST, McEvoy C, McKenzie M, Hampton N, Doherty JA, Kollef MH. Fluid balance and cardiac function in septic shock as predictors of hospital mortality. Crit Care. 2013;17:R246.
9. Kirkpatrick AW, Roberts DJ, De Waele J, Jaeschke R, Malbrain ML, De Keulenaer B, Duchesne J, Bjorck M, Leppaniemi A, Ejike JC, Sugrue M, Cheatham M, Ivatury R, Ball CG, Reintam Blaser A, Regli A, Balogh ZJ, D'Amours S, Debergh D, Kaplan M, Kimball E, Olvera C, Pediatric Guidelines Sub-Committee for the World Society of the Abdominal Compartment S. Intra-abdominal hypertension and the abdominal compartment syndrome: updated consensus definitions and clinical practice guidelines from the World Society of the Abdominal Compartment Syndrome. Intensive Care Med. 2013;39:1190–206.
10. Monnet X, Marik PE, Teboul JL. Prediction of fluid responsiveness: an update. Ann Intensive Care. 2016;6:111.
11. Michard F, Teboul JL. Predicting fluid responsiveness in ICU patients: a critical analysis of the evidence. Chest. 2002;121:2000–8.
12. Marik PE, Cavallazzi R. Does the central venous pressure predict fluid responsiveness? An updated meta-analysis and a plea for some common sense. Crit Care Med. 2013;41:1774–81.
13. Bentzer P, Griesdale DE, Boyd J, MacLean K, Sirounis D, Ayas NT. Will this hemodynamically unstable patient respond to a bolus of intravenous fluids. JAMA. 2016;316:1298–309.
14. Cannesson M, Pestel G, Ricks C, Hoeft A, Perel A. Hemodynamic monitoring and management in patients undergoing high risk surgery: a survey among North American and European anesthesiologists. Crit Care. 2011;15:R197.
15. Rhodes A, Evans LE, Alhazzani W, Levy MM, Antonelli M, Ferrer R, Kumar A, Sevransky JE, Sprung CL, Nunnally ME, Rochwerg B, Rubenfeld GD, Angus DC, Annane D, Beale RJ, Bellinghan GJ, Bernard GR, Chiche JD, Coopersmith C, De Backer DP, French CJ, Fujishima S, Gerlach H, Hidalgo JL, Hollenberg SM, Jones AE, Karnad DR, Kleinpell RM, Koh Y, Lisboa TC, Machado FR, Marini JJ, Marshall JC, Mazuski JE, McIntyre LA, McLean AS, Mehta S, Moreno RP, Myburgh J, Navalesi P, Nishida O, Osborn TM, Perner A, Plunkett CM, Ranieri M, Schorr CA, Seckel MA, Seymour CW, Shieh L, Shukri KA, Simpson SQ, Singer M, Thompson BT, Townsend SR, Van der Poll T, Vincent JL, Wiersinga WJ, Zimmerman JL, Dellinger RP. Surviving sepsis campaign: international guidelines for management of sepsis and septic shock: 2016. Intensive Care Med. 2017;43:304–77.
16. Marik PE, Monnet X, Teboul JL. Hemodynamic parameters to guide fluid therapy. Ann Intensive Care. 2011;1:1.

17. Michard F, Boussat S, Chemla D, Anguel N, Mercat A, Lecarpentier Y, Richard C, Pinsky MR, Teboul JL. Relation between respiratory changes in arterial pulse pressure and fluid responsiveness in septic patients with acute circulatory failure. Am J Respir Crit Care Med. 2000;162:134–8.
18. Yang X, Du B. Does pulse pressure variation predict fluid responsiveness in critically ill patients? A systematic review and meta-analysis. Crit Care. 2014;18:650.
19. Marik PE, Cavallazzi R, Vasu T, Hirani A. Dynamic changes in arterial waveform derived variables and fluid responsiveness in mechanically ventilated patients: a systematic review of the literature. Crit Care Med. 2009;37:2642–7.
20. Monnet X, Dres M, Ferre A, Le Teuff G, Jozwiak M, Bleibtreu A, Le Deley MC, Chemla D, Richard C, Teboul JL. Prediction of fluid responsiveness by a continuous non-invasive assessment of arterial pressure in critically ill patients: comparison with four other dynamic indices. Br J Anaesth. 2012;109:330–8.
21. Monnet X, Rienzo M, Osman D, Anguel N, Richard C, Pinsky MR, Teboul JL. Esophageal Doppler monitoring predicts fluid responsiveness in critically ill ventilated patients. Intensive Care Med. 2005;31:1195–201.
22. Sandroni C, Cavallaro F, Marano C, Falcone C, De Santis P, Antonelli M. Accuracy of plethysmographic indices as predictors of fluid responsiveness in mechanically ventilated adults: a systematic review and meta-analysis. Intensive Care Med. 2012;38:1429–37.
23. Biais M, Cottenceau V, Petit L, Masson F, Cochard JF, Sztark F. Impact of norepinephrine on the relationship between pleth variability index and pulse pressure variations in ICU adult patients. Crit Care. 2011;15:R168.
24. Monnet X, Guerin L, Jozwiak M, Bataille A, Julien F, Richard C, Teboul JL. Pleth variability index is a weak predictor of fluid responsiveness in patients receiving norepinephrine. Br J Anaesth. 2013;110:207–13.
25. Monnet X, Bleibtreu A, Ferré A, Dres M, Gharbi R, Richard C, Teboul JL. Passive leg raising and end-expiratory occlusion tests perform better than pulse pressure variation in patients with low respiratory system compliance. Crit Care Med. 2012;40:152–7.
26. Myatra SN, Prabu NR, Divatia JV, Monnet X, Kulkarni AP, Teboul JL. The changes in pulse pressure variation or stroke volume variation after a "tidal volume challenge" reliably predict fluid responsiveness during low tidal volume ventilation. Crit Care Med. 2017;45:415–21.
27. Diaz F, Erranz B, Donoso A, Salomon T, Cruces P. Influence of tidal volume on pulse pressure variation and stroke volume variation during experimental intra-abdominal hypertension. BMC Anesthesiol. 2015;15:127.
28. Duperret S, Lhuillier F, Piriou V, Vivier E, Metton O, Branche P, Annat G, Bendjelid K, Viale JP. Increased intra-abdominal pressure affects respiratory variations in arterial pressure in normovolaemic and hypovolaemic mechanically ventilated healthy pigs. Intensive Care Med. 2007;33:163–71.
29. Mahjoub Y, Pila C, Friggeri A, Zogheib E, Lobjoie E, Tinturier F, Galy C, Slama M, Dupont H. Assessing fluid responsiveness in critically ill patients: False-positive pulse pressure variation is detected by Doppler echocardiographic evaluation of the right ventricle. Crit Care Med. 2009;37:2570–5.
30. Fischer MO, Dechanet F, du Cheyron D, Gerard JL, Hanouz JL, Fellahi JL. Evaluation of the knowledge base of French intensivists and anaesthesiologists as concerns the interpretation of respiratory arterial pulse pressure variation. Anaesth Crit Care Pain Med. 2015;34:29–34.
31. Vieillard-Baron A, Chergui K, Rabiller A, Peyrouset O, Page B, Beauchet A, Jardin F. Superior vena caval collapsibility as a gauge of volume status in ventilated septic patients. Intensive Care Med. 2004;30:1734–9.
32. Zhang Z, Xu X, Ye S, Xu L. Ultrasonographic measurement of the respiratory variation in the inferior vena cava diameter is predictive of fluid responsiveness in critically ill patients: systematic review and meta-analysis. Ultrasound Med Biol. 2014;40:845–53.
33. Vignon P, Repesse X, Begot E, Leger J, Jacob C, Bouferrache K, Slama M, Prat G, Vieillard-Baron A. Comparison of echocardiographic indices used to predict fluid responsiveness in ventilated patients. Am J Respir Crit Care Med. 2017;195:1022–32.
34. Corl K, Napoli AM, Gardiner F. Bedside sonographic measurement of the inferior vena cava caval index is a poor predictor of fluid responsiveness in emergency department patients. Emerg Med Australas. 2012;24:534–9.
35. Airapetian N, Maizel J, Alyamani O, Mahjoub Y, Lorne E, Levrard M, Ammenouche N, Seydi A, Tinturier F, Lobjoie E, Dupont H, Slama M. Does inferior vena cava respiratory variability predict fluid responsiveness in spontaneously breathing patients. Crit Care. 2015;19:400.

36. Guerin L, Teboul JL, Persichini R, Dres M, Richard C, Monnet X. Effects of passive leg raising and volume expansion on mean systemic pressure and venous return in shock in humans. Crit Care. 2015;19:411.
37. Boulain T, Achard JM, Teboul JL, Richard C, Perrotin D, Ginies G. Changes in BP induced by passive leg raising predict response to fluid loading in critically ill patients. Chest. 2002;121:1245–52.
38. Jabot J, Teboul JL, Richard C, Monnet X. Passive leg raising for predicting fluid responsiveness: importance of the postural change. Intensive Care Med. 2009;35:85–90.
39. Monnet X, Marik P, Teboul JL. Passive leg raising for predicting fluid responsiveness: a systematic review and meta-analysis. Intensive Care Med. 2016;42:1935–47.
40. Monnet X, Rienzo M, Osman D, Anguel N, Richard C, Pinsky MR, Teboul JL. Passive leg raising predicts fluid responsiveness in the critically ill. Crit Care Med. 2006;34:1402–7.
41. Cherpanath TG, Hirsch A, Geerts BF, Lagrand WK, Leeflang MM, Schultz MJ, Groeneveld AB. Predicting fluid responsiveness by passive leg raising: a systematic review and meta-analysis of 23 clinical trials. Crit Care Med. 2016;44:981–91.
42. Cecconi M, De Backer D, Antonelli M, Beale R, Bakker J, Hofer C, Jaeschke R, Mebazaa A, Pinsky MR, Teboul JL, Vincent JL, Rhodes A. Consensus on circulatory shock and hemodynamic monitoring. Task force of the European Society of Intensive Care Medicine. Intensive Care Med. 2014;40:1795–815.
43. Monnet X, Teboul JL. Passive leg raising: five rules, not a drop of fluid! Crit Care. 2015;19:18.
44. Pierrakos C, Velissaris D, Scolletta S, Heenen S, De Backer D, Vincent JL. Can changes in arterial pressure be used to detect changes in cardiac index during fluid challenge in patients with septic shock? Intensive Care Med. 2012;38:422–8.
45. Monnet X, Letierce A, Hamzaoui O, Chemla D, Anguel N, Osman D, Richard C, Teboul JL. Arterial pressure allows monitoring the changes in cardiac output induced by volume expansion but not by norepinephrine*. Crit Care Med. 2011;39:1394–9.
46. Young A, Marik PE, Sibole S, Grooms D, Levitov A. Changes in end-tidal carbon dioxide and volumetric carbon dioxide as predictors of volume responsiveness in hemodynamically unstable patients. J Cardiothorac Vasc Anesth. 2013;27:681–4.
47. Monnet X, Bataille A, Magalhaes E, Barrois J, Le Corre M, Gosset C, Guerin L, Richard C, Teboul JL. End-tidal carbon dioxide is better than arterial pressure for predicting volume responsiveness by the passive leg raising test. Intensive Care Med. 2013;39:93–100.
48. Monge Garcia MI, Gil Cano A, Gracia Romero M, Monterroso Pintado R, Perez Madueno V, Diaz Monrove JC. Non-invasive assessment of fluid responsiveness by changes in partial end-tidal CO2 pressure during a passive leg-raising maneuver. Ann Intensive Care. 2012;2:9.
49. Malbrain ML, Reuter DA. Assessing fluid responsiveness with the passive leg raising maneuver in patients with increased intra-abdominal pressure: be aware that not all blood returns. Crit Care Med. 2010;38:1912–5.
50. Monnet X, Osman D, Ridel C, Lamia B, Richard C, Teboul JL. Predicting volume responsiveness by using the end-expiratory occlusion in mechanically ventilated intensive care unit patients. Crit Care Med. 2009;37:951–6.
51. Jozwiak M, Depret F, Teboul JL, Alphonsine JE, Lai C, Richard C, Monnet X. Predicting fluid responsiveness in critically Ill patients by using combined end-expiratory and end-inspiratory occlusions with echocardiography. Crit Care Med. 2017;11:e1131–8.
52. Silva S, Teboul JL. Defining the adequate arterial pressure target during septic shock: not a 'micro' issue but the microcirculation can help. Crit Care. 2011;15:1004.
53. Tusman G, Groisman I, Maidana GA, Scandurra A, Arca JM, Bohm SH, Suarez-Sipmann F. The sensitivity and specificity of pulmonary carbon dioxide elimination for noninvasive assessment of fluid responsiveness. Anesth Analg. 2015;122:1404–11.
54. Preisman S, Kogan S, Berkenstadt H, Perel A. Predicting fluid responsiveness in patients undergoing cardiac surgery: functional haemodynamic parameters including the Respiratory Systolic Variation Test and static preload indicators. Br J Anaesth. 2005;95:746–55.
55. Muller L, Toumi M, Bousquet PJ, Riu-Poulenc B, Louart G, Candela D, Zoric L, Suehs C, de La Coussaye JE, Molinari N, Lefrant JY. An increase in aortic blood flow after an infusion of 100 ml colloid over 1 minute can predict fluid responsiveness: the mini-fluid challenge study. Anesthesiology. 2011;115:541–7.
56. Aya HD, Rhodes A, Ster IC, Cecconi M. Haemodynamic effect of different doses of fluids for a fluid challenge: a quasi-randomised controlled study. Crit Care Med. 2016;45:e161–8.
57. Wu Y, Zhou S, Zhou Z, Liu B. A 10-second fluid challenge guided by transthoracic echocardiography can predict fluid responsiveness. Crit Care. 2014;18:R108.
58. Jozwiak M, Monnet X, Teboul JL. Pressure waveform analysis. Anesth Analg. 2018;126:1930–3.

Pulmonary Artery Catheter

Ina Filipović-Grčić and Didier Payen

M. R. Pinsky et al. (eds.), *Hemodynamic Monitoring*, Lessons from the ICU,
https://doi.org/10.1007/978-3-319-69269-2_25

Beware of false knowledge; it is more dangerous than ignorance.

–George Bernard Shaw

Learning Objectives

The pulmonary arterial catheter (PAC) was used for almost five decades to monitor patients with severe hemodynamic situations or at high risk of hemodynamic complications. The development of less invasive technologies, mainly ultrasound, had replaced several indications of PAC, but not all. The added parameters on PAC offered the possibility to continuously measure cardiac output (CO), pulmonary pressures (PAP), left and right filling pressures, and mixed venous oxygen saturation (SvO_2). PAC is said to estimate cardiac function, guide volume resuscitation, maintain adequacy of oxygen delivery, and assess the coupling or interdependence between right and left circulation.

In this chapter we will describe and discuss the interest for each parameter given by PAC monitoring: Pra measurements for (1) detecting hypovolemia or cardiac dysfunction and (2) to diagnose venous congestion leading to a reduction in diastolic perfusion pressure; PAP values as the main determinant of right ventricle (RV) function that may precipitate RV dysfunction when PAP rises; the filling right and left heart pressures as surrogate of preload; lung hydrostatic pressure PAP-LV filling pressure; CO and SV, even they have been replaced by less or noninvasive methods; and SvO_2 as a surrogate of adequacy for tissue perfusion.

25.1 Introduction

Integrating the work of Drs. Swan, Ganz, and Forrester, almost 50 years ago was introduced to clinical practice a balloon tipped thermodilution catheter called the pulmonary artery catheter (PAC) [1]. Inserted by invasive procedure via the large veins and floated into pulmonary artery, with the risk of complications (bleeding, PA rupture, arrhythmia, infection, thrombus, air emboli, etc.) still remains the main tool for direct and derived hemodynamic measurements to diagnose and manage the therapy in selected critically ill patients in the early resuscitation phase. Despite the fact that early data showed increased mortality and strongly suggested its withdrawal [2], further studies confirmed that PAC, as a device, does not impair the outcome [3, 4]. Detailed evaluation of the available studies, in terms of appropriate patient population, timing of insertion and resuscitation, interpretation of hemodynamic values and shapes, goals of study, and applied treatments, leads to use the PAC less frequently than in the past but wisely and accurately when hemodynamic situations are complex and when ultrasound technology is limited. This chapter aims to clarify the information derived from PAC and to guide individually the therapeutic end points in a complex patient.

Since providing the continuous information on the right side of the circulation remains a challenge for echocardiography [5], PAC remains important among the wide range of hemodynamic tools, especially the less invasive one implemented in day-to-day care. Considering the intravascular intrathoracic pressure, cardiac output, and mixed venous oxygen saturation with other derived variables, the use of PAC as a diagnostic tool should, by the consensus statement of the American College of Cardiology, offer the data about shock states, differentiation of high versus low pressure pulmonary edema, primary pulmonary hypertension, valvular disease, intracardiac shunts, cardiac tamponade, and pulmonary embolism, monitoring and management of complicated acute myocardial infarction, assessing hemodynamic response to therapies, management of multiorgan failure in severe sepsis, severe burns, and hemodynamic instability after cardiac surgery, assessment of response to treatment in patients with primary pulmonary hypertension,

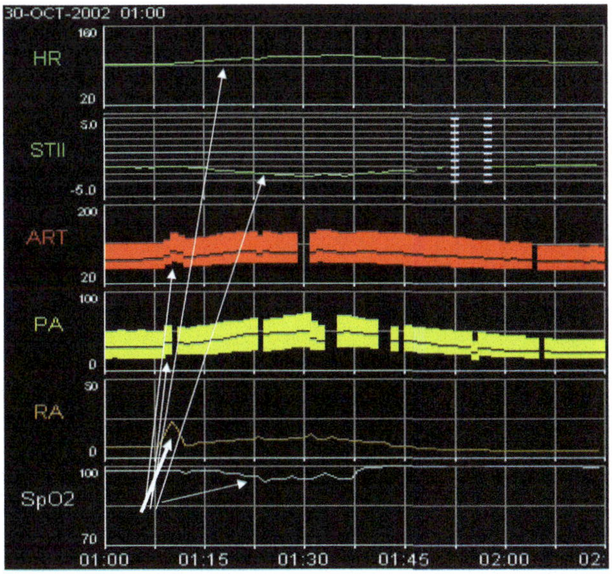

Fig. 25.1 Chronologic modifications of different hemodynamic parameters during pulmonary embolism occurring in intensive care patient. Note the right side parameters provided by PAC (*RA* right atrium, *PA* pulmonary artery pressure) associated with other monitored parameters (*HR* heart rate, *STII* S-T segment registered in the DII ECG derivation, *SpO2* arterial saturation given by pulse oximetry, *ART* arterial blood pressure from radial catheter). Pressure in the right atrium (RA) was the first modified parameter as expected, rapidly followed by an elevation of PA. ART increased after a short delay that maintains the coronary perfusion pressure for right ventricle. Then tachycardia and negativity of STII occurred simultaneously followed by a delayed decrease in SpO2. Interestingly, all two of these modifications were transient, coming back to baseline value after 1 h. This observation validates the concept that one pulmonary embolism is rarely the cause of death, but it is the repetition of emboli that may put the patient at risk

and aspiration of air emboli as the therapeutic tool. If thermodilution is not a beat-by-beat cardiac output (CO) measurement since a measurement requires thermic clearance over several cardiac beats that repeated to average several measurements to obtain one value, the other parameters given by the PAC can be analyzed in beat-by-beat basis, a unique advantage when compared with other techniques (Fig. 25.1).

However, considering that PAC is available in practice since almost five decades, we still miss protocols to guide therapy accordingly to the set of information obtained with this device [6], mainly because of the heterogeneity of the cause for unstable circulation and of context in critically ill patients having multiple comorbidities [7].

25.2 Hemodynamic Information from PAC Measurements

Many studies competed to target hemodynamic values higher than physiological range and showed no benefit, leading to conclude that individual therapeutic targets defined by PAC monitoring are the trace that should be promoted. Based on the regular data observed with PAC, the information about right atrial and ventricular pressures, pulmonary artery pressure, pulmonary artery occlusion pressure, cardiac output, and mixed venous oxygen saturation and the interplay of them in the variety of clinical conditions can be hold.

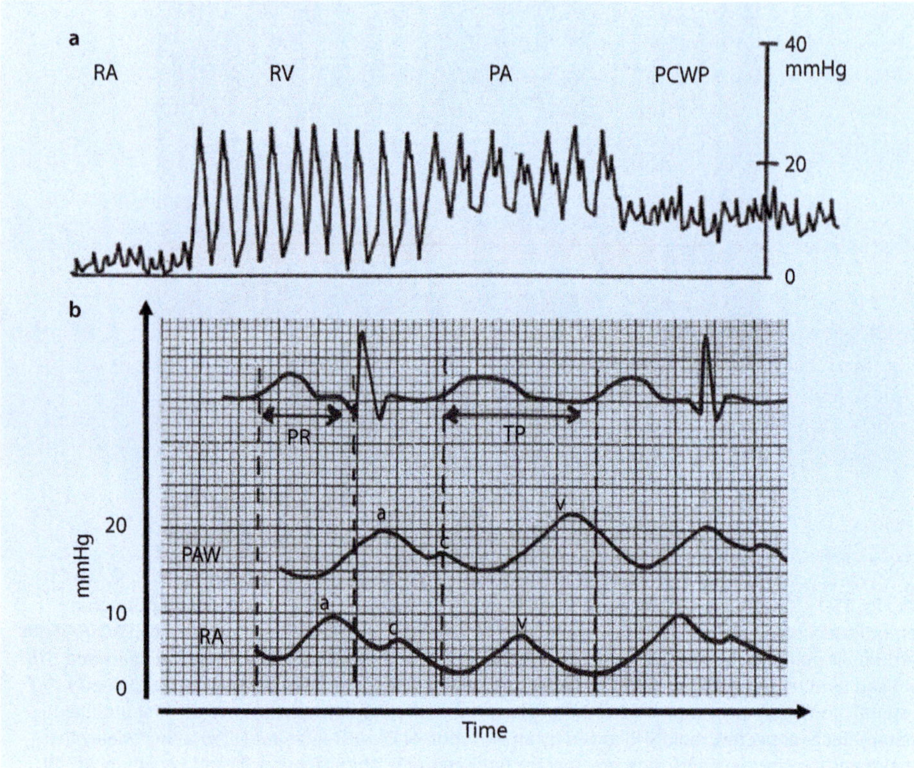

Fig. 25.2 (**a**) Pulmonary artery catheter tip pressure tracings during placement. (Modified from Mihm and Rosenthal MH [44]). (**b**) A typical tracing of right atrial (RA) and of pulmonary artery wedge (PAW) or pulmonary capillary wedge (PCWP) pressures. Note that both curves have similar "accidents" even with a delay and with higher values for PAW

25.2.1 Right Atrial and Ventricular Pressures (Fig. 25.2a, b)

Right atrial pressure (Pra) had lost its interest to be monitored mainly because of its elusive information to guide the volume loading [8, 9]. However, it is informative for other contexts mostly related to the risk of venous congestion and in many other circumstances out of severe sepsis or systemic inflammation [10, 11].

25.2.1.1 Venous Congestion

Although poorly investigated as a negative factor for organ perfusion, some reports have emphasized the negative role of venous congestion for organs, especially the liver and the kidney [12–15]. Pra has to be considered as the back pressure for venous return and not as an indicator of the right ventricle filling. That implies that all conditions that increase Pra, primarily right ventricular dysfunction, tamponade, and elevation in intrathoracic pressure during mechanical ventilation might induce an elevation in Pra. Then the upstream venous pressure has to increase proportionally to keep the venous return perfusion pressure gradient: $Pv_{peripheral}$ – Pra around 3 or 4 mmHg [16]. This may raise the tissue venous pressure up to 12–16 mmHg or more. Such $Pv_{peripheral}$ may then impair the organ perfusion pressure, especially in organs where the veins do not have venous anti-reflux valves as in the liver [15] or kidney [14]. The direct consequence of this congestion is an increase in organ volume with elevated interstitial pressure. In organs having a surrounding non-compliant envelope, when the serosa stress volume is reached, the interstitial pressure increases and may collapse the intra-organ veins, amplifying the congestion and the tissue ischemia. In organs with autoregulated blood flow, the venous congestion reduces perfusion pressure especially in diastole, a crucial phase for diastolic perfusion. The Pra level continuously given by PAC may alarm about the risk of organ congestion. Recently, it was shown in retrospective cohort a linear relation between the level of Pra and the incidence or the persistence of acute kidney injury [12]. This had been confirmed by prospective studies, especially in a context of the right ventricle dysfunction [17]. It is well known by the clinician that hepatic congestion induces a large elevation of plasma lactate level, frequently over 10 mMole/L. [18] The resolution of congestion leads to a rapid decline in lactate level, which indicates the liver recovery of lactate clearance.

25.2.1.2 Pra Use for Volume Resuscitation

The Pra value to guide volume resuscitation was shown useless if the absolute number is taken [19]. That is not surprising since Pra cannot reflect the RV preload (volume) if surrounding pressure of the cardiac cavities differs from atmospheric pressure. In this condition, only the transmural Pra can inform on the RV preload (volume). Because the extra-cardiac pressure is difficult to measure routinely, transmural pressures cannot be used in clinical practice. The analysis of the trends or variations in Pra after a fluid challenge (even not well standardized) may inform on the change in RV preload combined with RV function in combination with stroke volume measurements [20]. Several observed scenarios can be clarified only by the use of PAC: increase in Pra with no change in CO, indicating the RV dysfunction; large Pra increase with a moderate increase in CO indicates a moderate RV dysfunction that may alarm on the risk of congestion if fluid therapy continues; and moderate increase in Pra with large increase in CO indicates an adequate RV and LV function. Very few reports have been published on such a relation between changes in Pra and CO to ascertain the different scenarios supporting the benefit to use PAC data.

25.2.2 Pulmonary Artery Pressure (PAP) (▫ Fig. 25.2a)

PAP is largely lower than aortic pressure for the same CO, which implies a lower pulmonary vascular resistance (PVR) and a higher pulmonary vessel compliance [21]. This characteristic supports the concept that the thin-walled RV is not a resistive pump but furtherly more of a volume pump that generates flow at low level of pressure compared to the left side. It is then vulnerable to any acute rise in wall stress, such as acute PAP elevation [22]. Due to both right and left share of myocardial muscle fibers and interventricular septum, 20–40% of RV systolic performance can be attributed to LV contraction, which may partly explain the complexity to analyze RV in presence of LV failure [23]. Because of a low pulmonary vessel elastance and resistance, the RV P/flow relation shows modest PVR changes when CO increases. The classic approach to calculate resistance by the direct ratio P/flow supposes that (1) the P/flow relationship is linear and (2) the extrapolation to x-axis (zero flow pressure) equals the left atrium pressure. In fact this extrapolated pressure (effective outflow pressure) frequently exceeds the left atrium pressure. Consequently, the vascular tone is better described by the slope of the linear relation between P/flow [24], easily obtained with the PAC. This approach allows to better adapt the resuscitation when PAP increase from flow increase or from increase in pulmonary vascular tone. Practically, an acute rise in PAP may result from an increase in resistance, a reduced vessel compliance, and increase in pulmonary blood flow. Such a pulmonary hypertension should be treated according to the mechanism involved: if PVR is increased, pulmonary vasodilators (prostaglandins or inhaled nitric oxide) should be used, knowing they better coupled RV function to the pulmonary vasculature; if CO rise is the main determinant of PAP increase, only a flow reduction will reduce PAP and then RV afterload. Resistance increase may result from vasoconstriction but also from obstruction and compression. The later can be easily modified by changing the setup of the ventilator. In acute inflammation as observed in sepsis, the use of PAC allows to test the P/F relationship when PAP increased, since both flow may increase with fluid therapy and resistance increases in relation to microemboli. PAC could then inform on the main mechanism involved. In such acute condition, the inflammatory-induced aortic pressure drop with a PAP increase may reduce the systolic and diastolic coronary perfusion pressure for RV. Myocardium of the RV might be then ischemic with a limited oxygen delivery and an increase O2 demand related to RV afterload increase. Only the PAC provides continuous information on RV myocardial perfusion by estimating the coronary perfusion pressure (CPP):

25

$$CPP = CPP_{syst} \text{ and } CPP_{diast}$$

$$CPP_{syst} = PAo_{syst} - PAP_{syst}$$

$$CPP_{diast} = PAo_{diast} - RVP_{diast}$$

Where RVP_{diast} is similar to Pra (given by the PAC). Such systolic and diastolic CPP has to be sufficient to overcome the coronary vascular resistance, frequently elevated in patient with coronary artery disease. Again the PAC allows to monitor both, the stroke volume and CO, with concomitant evaluation of CPP. A frequent clinical scenario of septic shock patient having a PAC is an aortic pressure reduced to 80/40 mmHg and an elevated PAP_{syst} at 30 with a Pra around 20 mmHg. Then CPP is 80–30 = 50 mmHg for systole and 40–20 = 20 mmHg for diastole, which might be insufficient to generate an adequate coronary blood flow for increased myocardial oxygen consumption. The 2D Echo-Doppler can easily assess the acute cor pulmonale [25]; the therapeutic benefit will be better assessed by the PAC, especially if there is a limited window for Echo or if echocardiography is not available or trained operator is not present.

25.2.3 Pulmonary Artery Occlusion Pressure (PAoP) (Fig. 25.2a)

PAoP wave is similar to Pra pressure but with higher pressure delayed in the cardiac cycle considering QRS complex. The mean PAoP is lower than end-diastolic pulmonary pressure with a difference that does not exceed 5 mmHg. In this case the end-diastolic pulmonary pressure can be used in place of PAoP. When a continuous fluid column between the distal tip of catheter after balloon inflation and the left atrium exists, PAoP is considered as a good reflect of left atrial pressure and LV diastolic pressure. Pulmonary vessels being collapsible vessels when surrounding pressure overcomes intravascular pressure, the PAoP may represent different pressures, according to the concept of West Zones [26]. When the tip of PAC is located in a zone where alveolar pressure is higher than PAoP (West Zone 1), PAoP represents mainly alveolar pressure [27]. Only when PAoP is largely above the alveolar pressure (West Zone 3) it represents the left atrial pressure and LV diastolic pressure. Although commonly assumed to indicate LV preload, PAoP is far from identical to LV end-diastolic volume but can be used as a surrogate, especially when variations more than absolute values are considered. As for Pra wave, PAoP wave contains similar "accidents" than those observed for Pra. The "v" wave particularly allows to diagnose mitral regurgitation; even 2D Echo-Doppler does not observe mitral regurgitation if transmitral pressure gradient is small.

25.2.4 Cardiac Output (CO)

The fast resistance on the tip of PAC catheter allows to measure cardiac output (CO) by the thermodilution method based on the Steward-Hamilton equation. Even the technique for thermodilution methods evolved along time from cold bolus injection to "continuous" method; the principle remained similar. The quicker the rate of change in blood temperature, the greater is the CO. Different conditions may jeopardize the accuracy of flow measurements that have been reviewed recently [28]. The most frequently encountered critical conditions are tricuspid regurgitation and/or intracardiac shunt, use of intermittent compression system, hypothermia, etc. Stroke volume (SV) is then computed dividing the CO by heart rate. When cardiac dysfunction (right and/or left) is suspected and/or documented, PAC allows to construct ventricular function curves plotting SV in vertical axis and ventricular filling pressure on the horizontal axis. The impact of used therapy or the evolution of ventricular dysfunction can then be assessed from time to time in critically ill patients. SV and CO are key values to interpret systemic hemodynamic situation, since SV integrates the cardiac and vascular functions, while CO is an adapted item that varies always under reflex modifications and metabolic requirements. Such variations can be altered when cardiac function and/or volemic status are abnormal. If both variables can be obtained with less invasive techniques such as Doppler devices [29] or pulse contour methods [30], the other parameters given by the PAC cannot.

25.2.5 Mixed Venous Oxygen Saturation (SvO_2)

Based on physiological background, when hemoglobin concentration is stable and adequate, the oxygen requirement (O_2 consumption) is covered by oxygen delivery (mainly CO) and oxygen peripheral extraction ($D_{a\text{-}v}O_2$). If arterial O_2 content is maintained (adequate [Hb] and PaO_2), then mixed SvO_2 reflects well the adequacy of delivery for the requirement. As a consequence, a SvO_2 decrease below 70% indicates an insufficient O_2 delivery for O_2 needs. In the contrary, the "normal" or elevated SvO_2 does not imply an adequate balance between demand and delivery. SvO_2 can be maintained high in the presence of microvascular shunt, which has been well documented in septic shock [31, 32]. Even the superior vena cava $ScvO_2$ had been proposed as a surrogate of mixed venous

SvO_2 measurement [33]; the only tool providing simultaneously and almost continuously CO and mixed SvO_2 is the PAC. Recently, Squara nicely reviewed the physiology and interpretation of SvO_2 [34]. This report highlighted the integrative nature of this parameter, which has to be analyzed on a case-to-case basis having the four main determinants in mind ([Hb], CO, oxygen consumption, PaO_2). The PAC is the best tool to guide therapy to correct a low SvO_2 with transfusion, reduction in pulmonary VA/Q mismatch, decrease in oxygen consumption, improvement of cardiac function, or treatment of hypovolemia. At least at the early phase of acute circulatory failure, low value of SvO_2 warns the clinician about cardiocirculatory and/or metabolic impairment, whereas normal or high values do not rule out persistent tissue hypoxia [35].

25.2.6 Indications for PAC in Anesthesiology or Intensive Care

To propose the reasonable indications for PAC use in critically ill patients, three questions might be answered: (1) Does PAC insertion carry a significant risk of complications, questioning the benefit/risk ratio? (2) Can the data from the PAC improve outcomes in critically ill patients, at least at the early phase? (3) How to define the type of patients or conditions for which PAC may improve quality of care and outcomes?

For the last 50 years, the context for hemodynamic monitoring based on PAC had changed. Safety concern of this invasive technique associated with the development of less or noninvasive techniques to measure CO (SV) or characterize ventricular functions had challenged the use of PAC. The paper of Connors et al. [2] suggesting in a retrospective analysis that PAC use might increase mortality with an impressive list of complications related to PAC strongly pushed clinicians to reduce the PAC use. As mentioned in "point of view" published in 2008 [7], many studies or trials have excluded PAC use for specific patients undergoing cardiac surgery and failed to show any impact on outcome or mortality. Even the global sense is to decrease the PAC use; the lack of evidence showing a mortality reduction is not a solid argument to abandon the PAC. If this argument is taken, then almost all monitoring devices should be abandoned since none of them have been shown to reduce mortality, including the cardiac 2D Echo-Doppler. Accordingly, PAC should be used in critically ill patients who are the most likely to benefit.

In 2000, a meta-analysis of the effectiveness of the PAC reported a total of 1610 patients enrolled in 12 trials [36]. The authors found a lower mortality when PAC is used, with a relative risk ratio of 0.8 (corresponding to $P < 0.02$). Despite the limitations of these meta-analyses, it at least confirmed the safety of PAC use in ICU patients and suggested potential benefit. It was also demonstrated in a prospective, descriptive cohort study a change in therapy after insertion of the PAC in shocked patients who did not respond to standard therapy [37]. This therapeutic strategy modification was statistically associated with better morbidity. The five randomized trials that investigated the effectiveness of PAC use in critically ill patients failed to show an impact on outcome and morbidity compared to the control group. Conversely, none of these trails could demonstrate a benefit in term of outcome for patients having severe cardiovascular disease, sepsis or septic shock, or acute lung injury. In the context of congestive heart failure, the use of PAC seems to largely differ from center to center in the absence of consensus on safety and effectiveness. The ESCAPE study randomized 433 patients comparing the resolution of pulmonary congestion between clinically driven therapy and clinic + PAC assessed by days alive out of hospital over the first 6 months [38]. The PAC use did not affect the primary end point, with a trend for better exercise capacity as a secondary end point. In any case, removal of the PAC as early as possible after the acute phase is a proactive decision that may limit the potential complications [38]. In anesthesiology context, there is a gap between the evidence for the benefit of optimization protocol and the technologies used, such as the PAC or other methods, as reported in North America and Europe survey [39]. The use of PAC is now limited to the high-risk patients having heavy surgical procedures. Among the monitored parameters, Pra obtained from central catheter or PAC associated with clinical experience, urine output and blood pressure were considered as the indicators for volume expansion.

Practical Guidelines for Use of PAC

From the above statement, it seems clear that PAC has neither positive nor negative effects on outcome. It appears useful for individualized medicine in specific and complex patient, which is then difficult to prove in a large trial. Using properly the data obtained might improve the treatment strategy and the recovery conditions. This has been shown in high-risk surgical patients that improved their outcome even in absence of a clear algorithm [40]. In ICU patients, it seems clear that routine use of PAC should be avoided. PAC use has to be restricted to complex hemodynamic situations, especially with merged abnormalities for both the heart and vessels and for right and left ventricle dysfunctions. This aspect has been recently published as a format of "Consensus on circulatory shock and hemodynamic monitoring" published in 2014 [41]. The task force suggested to additionally use pulmonary artery catheterization in complex patients on top of cardiac Echo-Doppler to understand the shock mechanism(s) and elaborate the therapeutic strategy. Among the recommended parameters to be measured in these complex patients, CO and SV are important to evaluate the treatment response such as fluid loading and/or pressors. This recommendation is of particular interest for patients in shock with a complex interaction between vascular failure and RV dysfunction. This context is more frequent in acute respiratory failure with shock state, frequently related to severe sepsis. As mentioned before, the task force did not recommend the routine use of PAC. To better use all the information coming from PAC, a solid background on hemodynamic physiology and pathophysiology is essential. Such a background can better come from the use of PAC under the umbrella of well-experienced senior, helping to clarify the patterns obtained useful to make a therapeutic decision. Such issue has been nicely demonstrated when a classic case was presented to members of the three major societies of critical care. The first vote for therapeutic proposals was made with the clinical story without hemodynamic monitoring by PAC. A large dispersion and contradictory of attitude were proposed within the members of these three societies, including in so-called experts. Such heterogeneity disappeared when the PAC data have been given, especially CO and Pwp, confirming that measurements first with adequate interpretation may lead to a better therapeutic decision [20]. The difficulty to achieve a sufficient background at time of less invasive techniques or imaging is difficult to solve. Potentially, the development of expert software and artificial intelligence might be the best proposed solution [42, 43].

25

Take-Home Message

- Although being invasive, the PAC technique is almost safe, but itself does not change patients' outcome. Only protocols based on PAC data might improve the outcome.
- Acute hemodynamic situations in ICU include mainly right circulation problems such as RV dysfunction, pulmonary hypertension, venous congestion, high lung hydrostatic pressure, and edema. All situations can be worsened when fluid is given and positive pressure breathing is applied.
- Pra and PAP continuously measured help to evaluate the tissue congestion and hypoperfusion or the increase in RV afterload precipitating RV dysfunction.
- CO and SV can be obtained by other methods being less or noninvasive.
- SvO_2 is useful to detect hypoperfusion when it is below 65%, but higher level does not imply an adequate tissue oxygenation.

References

1. Swan HJ, Ganz W, Forrester J, Marcus H, Diamond G, Chonette D. Catheterization of the heart in man with use of a flow-directed balloon-tipped catheter. N Engl J Med. 1970;283:447–51.
2. Connors AF Jr, Speroff T, Dawson NV, Thomas C, Harrell FE Jr, Wagner D, Desbiens N, Goldman L, Wu AW, Califf RM, Fulkerson WJ Jr, Vidaillet H, Broste S, Bellamy P, Lynn J, Knaus WA. The effectiveness of right heart catheterization in the initial care of critically ill patients. SUPPORT investigators. JAMA. 1996;276:889–97.
3. Richard C, Warszawski J, Anguel N, Deye N, Combes A, Barnoud D, Boulain T, Lefort Y, Fartoukh M, Baud F, Boyer A, Brochard L, Teboul JL, French Pulmonary Artery Catheter Study G. Early use of the pulmonary artery catheter and outcomes in patients with shock and acute respiratory distress syndrome: a randomized controlled trial. JAMA. 2003;290:2713–20.
4. Sandham JD, Hull RD, Brant RF, Knox L, Pineo GF, Doig CJ, Laporta DP, Viner S, Passerini L, Devitt H, Kirby A, Jacka M, Canadian Critical Care Clinical Trials G. A randomized, controlled trial of the use of pulmonary-artery catheters in high-risk surgical patients. N Engl J Med. 2003;348:5–14.
5. Bossone E, Nanda NC, Naeije R. Imaging the right heart: a challenging road map. Echocardiography. 2015;32(Suppl 1):S1–2.
6. Pinsky MR, Vincent JL. Let us use the pulmonary artery catheter correctly and only when we need it. Crit Care Med. 2005;33:1119–22.
7. Vincent JL, Pinsky MR, Sprung CL, Levy M, Marini JJ, Payen D, Rhodes A, Takala J. The pulmonary artery catheter: in medio virtus. Crit Care Med. 2008;36:3093–6.
8. Marik PE, Monnet X, Teboul JL. Hemodynamic parameters to guide fluid therapy. Ann Intensive Care. 2011;1:1.
9. Kumar A, Anel R, Bunnell E, Habet K, Zanotti S, Marshall S, Neumann A, Ali A, Cheang M, Kavinsky C, Parrillo JE. Pulmonary artery occlusion pressure and central venous pressure fail to predict ventricular filling volume, cardiac performance, or the response to volume infusion in normal subjects. Crit Care Med. 2004;32:691–9.
10. Rosenkranz S, Preston IR. Right heart catheterisation: best practice and pitfalls in pulmonary hypertension. Eur Respir Rev. 2015;24:642–52.
11. Payen D, Gayat E. Which general intensive care unit patients can benefit from placement of the pulmonary artery catheter? Crit Care. 2006;10(Suppl 3):S7.
12. Legrand M, Dupuis C, Simon C, Gayat E, Mateo J, Lukaszewicz AC, Payen D. Association between systemic hemodynamics and septic acute kidney injury in critically ill patients: a retrospective observational study. Crit Care. 2013;17:R278.
13. Testani JM, Damman K. Venous congestion and renal function in heart failure ... it's complicated. Eur J Heart Fail. 2013;15:599–601.
14. Rajendram R, Prowle JR. Venous congestion: are we adding insult to kidney injury in sepsis? Crit Care. 2014;18:104.

15. Tapper EB, Sengupta N, Bonder A. The incidence and outcomes of ischemic hepatitis: a systematic review with meta-analysis. Am J Med. 2015;128:1314–21.
16. Guyton A, Jones C, Coleman T Circulatory physiology: cardiac output and its regulation. 1973, pp 1–10.
17. Tarvasmaki T, Haapio M, Mebazaa A, Sionis A, Silva-Cardoso J, Tolppanen H, Lindholm MG, Pulkki K, Parissis J, Harjola VP, Lassus J, CardShock Study I. Acute kidney injury in cardiogenic shock: definitions, incidence, haemodynamic alterations, and mortality. Eur J Heart Fail. 2017:572–81.
18. Waseem N, Chen PH. Hypoxic hepatitis: a review and clinical update. J Clin Transl Hepatol. 2016;4:263–8.
19. Monnet X, Marik PE, Teboul JL. Prediction of fluid responsiveness: an update. Ann Intensive Care. 2016;6:111.
20. Squara P, Bennett D, Perret C. Pulmonary artery catheter: does the problem lie in the users? Chest. 2002;121:2009–15.
21. Naeije R, Brimioulle S, Dewachter L. Biomechanics of the right ventricle in health and disease (2013 Grover conference series). Pulm Circ. 2014;4:395–406.
22. Naeije R, Manes A. The right ventricle in pulmonary arterial hypertension. Eur Respir Rev. 2014;23: 476–87.
23. Haddad F, Hunt SA, Rosenthal DN, Murphy DJ. Right ventricular function in cardiovascular disease, part I: anatomy, physiology, aging, and functional assessment of the right ventricle. Circulation. 2008;117:1436–48.
24. Leeman M, Lejeune P, Melot C, Naeije R. Pulmonary vascular pressure-flow plots in canine oleic acid pulmonary edema. Effects of prostaglandin E1 and nitroprusside. Am Rev Respir Dis. 1988;138:362–7.
25. Repesse X, Charron C, Vieillard-Baron A. Acute cor pulmonale in ARDS: rationale for protecting the right ventricle. Chest. 2015;147:259–65.
26. West JB. Blood-flow, ventilation, and gas exchange in the lung. Lancet. 1963;2:1055–8.
27. West JB. The beginnings of cardiac catheterization and the resulting impact on pulmonary medicine. Am J Physiol Lung Cell Mol Physiol. 2017;313:L651–8.
28. Gidwani UK, Mohanty B, Chatterjee K. The pulmonary artery catheter: a critical reappraisal. Cardiol Clin. 2013;31:545–565, viii.
29. Valtier B, Cholley BP, Belot JP, de la Coussaye JE, Mateo J, Payen DM. Noninvasive monitoring of cardiac output in critically ill patients using transesophageal Doppler. Am J Respir Crit Care Med. 1998;158:77–83.
30. Scolletta S, Franchi F, Romagnoli S, Carla R, Donati A, Fabbri LP, Forfori F, Alonso-Inigo JM, Laviola S, Mangani V, Maj G, Martinelli G, Mirabella L, Morelli A, Persona P, Payen D, Pulse wave analysis Cardiac Output validation G. Comparison between Doppler-echocardiography and uncalibrated pulse contour method for cardiac output measurement: a multicenter observational study. Crit Care Med. 2016;44:1370–9.
31. Hernandez G, Bruhn A, Ince C. Microcirculation in sepsis: new perspectives. Curr Vasc Pharmacol. 2013;11:161–9.
32. Kanoore Edul VS, Ince C, Dubin A. What is microcirculatory shock? Curr Opin Crit Care. 2015;21:245–52.
33. Sinaasappel M, van Iterson M, Ince C. Microvascular oxygen pressure in the pig intestine during haemorrhagic shock and resuscitation. J Physiol. 1999;514(Pt 1):245–53.
34. Squara P. Central venous oxygenation: when physiology explains apparent discrepancies. Crit Care. 2014;18:579.
35. Caille V, Squara P. Oxygen uptake-to-delivery relationship: a way to assess adequate flow. Crit Care. 2006;10(Suppl 3):S4.
36. Ivanov R, Allen J, Calvin JE. The incidence of major morbidity in critically ill patients managed with pulmonary artery catheters: a meta-analysis. Crit Care Med. 2000;28:615–9.
37. Mimoz O, Rauss A, Rekik N, Brun-Buisson C, Lemaire F, Brochard L. Pulmonary artery catheterization in critically ill patients: a prospective analysis of outcome changes associated with catheter-prompted changes in therapy. Crit Care Med. 1994;22:573–9.
38. Binanay C, Califf RM, Hasselblad V, O'Connor CM, Shah MR, Sopko G, Stevenson LW, Francis GS, Leier CV, Miller LW, Investigators E, Coordinators ES. Evaluation study of congestive heart failure and pulmonary artery catheterization effectiveness: the ESCAPE trial. JAMA. 2005;294:1625–33.
39. Cannesson M, Pestel G, Ricks C, Hoeft A, Perel A. Hemodynamic monitoring and management in patients undergoing high risk surgery: a survey among north American and European anesthesiologists. Crit Care. 2011;15:R197.
40. Scheeren TW, Wiesenack C, Gerlach H, Marx G. Goal-directed intraoperative fluid therapy guided by stroke volume and its variation in high-risk surgical patients: a prospective randomized multicentre study. J Clin Monit Comput. 2013;27:225–33.

41. Cecconi M, De Backer D, Antonelli M, Beale R, Bakker J, Hofer C, Jaeschke R, Mebazaa A, Pinsky MR, Teboul JL, Vincent JL, Rhodes A. Consensus on circulatory shock and hemodynamic monitoring. Task force of the European Society of Intensive Care Medicine. Intensive Care Med. 2014;40:1795–815.
42. Michard F, Cannesson M, Vallet B. Perioperative hemodynamic therapy: quality improvement programs should help to resolve our uncertainty. Crit Care. 2011;15:445.
43. Squara P, Fourquet E, Jacquet L, Broccard A, Uhlig T, Rhodes A, Bakker J, Perret C. A computer program for interpreting pulmonary artery catheterization data: results of the European HEMODYN resident study. Intensive Care Med. 2003;29:735–41.
44. Mihm FG, Rosenthal MH. Pulmonary artery catheterization. In: Benito JL, editor. Clinical procedures in anesthesia and intensive care. Philadelphia: JB Lippincott; 1994. p. 416.

Arterial Pressure Waveform Analysis on Cardiac Output Monitoring

Manuel Ignacio Monge García and Arnoldo Santos

M. R. Pinsky et al. (eds.), *Hemodynamic Monitoring*, Lessons from the ICU,
https://doi.org/10.1007/978-3-319-69269-2_26

Learning Objectives
- To briefly describe the determinants of arterial pressure and the physiological relationship between arterial pressure and blood flow
- To apply this pressure-flow relationship for defining the common assumptions and limitations of the APWA methods for estimating stroke volume from the arterial pressure waveform
- To provide a physiological rationale to determine why and when to calibrate the APWA-based systems
- To provide a practical recommendation for selecting the adequate patient for monitoring using the APWA method according to its potential benefits and limitations

26.1 Introduction

Cardiac output (CO) is one of the major determinants of the oxygen delivery to the tissues and an important parameter used to evaluate heart function. In consequence, CO monitoring has become an essential component of the hemodynamic assessment of critically ill patients.

Many methods have been developed for estimating CO over the last years. However, because of its apparent simplicity and ease applicability, arterial pressure waveform analysis (APWA) is currently one of the most widely used. This technique allows the continuous estimation of the stroke volume (SV) and CO analyzing the characteristics of the arterial pressure waveform.

The common premise for all APWA algorithms is that there is a proportional and predictable relationship between arterial pressure and SV. As the arterial pressure is the result of interaction between the blood flow ejected by the heart and the arterial system, assessment of the arterial system is necessary to establish a valid SV estimation from the blood pressure waveform. Therefore, how the arterial system is characterized ultimately defines each particular APWA algorithm. However, under this same premise, all APWA algorithms also share some common features and limitations.

In this chapter, we will describe the physiological basis of pressure-volume relationship to understand the underlying assumptions shared by most of the available APWA algorithms. We will not, however, compare proprietary algorithms or specific questions related to commercial devices. Knowledge of these common physiological assumptions will allow the physician to understand the benefits and limitations of this technology and thus use it appropriately to improve patient care.

26.2 Physiological Basis of the Arterial Pressure Waveform Analysis: The Arterial Pressure-Volume Relationship

Essentially, APWA-based monitoring systems aim to estimate SV from the analysis of the characteristics of the arterial pressure waveform. From this estimation, other clinically relevant parameters can also be derived, such as cardiac output or dynamic indexes of preload responsiveness. Since the arterial pressure is a biological signal that can be easily measured at the bedside, even continuously or noninvasively, estimating SV from the arterial pressure provides a beat-to-beat monitoring of CO and could represent a significant improvement over other traditional CO monitoring techniques.

The APWA monitoring method is primarily based on the physiological assumption that the arterial pressure is proportional to SV. Therefore, there is a relationship between arterial pressure and SV that can be determined and quantified. Interestingly, although this assumption was proposed for such a purpose more than one century ago [1], its validity is still applicable for current and sophisticated hemodynamic APWA-based monitoring systems. However, understanding how the SV can be derived from the blood pressure requires first defining the physiological determinants of arterial pressure, since the relationship between arterial pressure and SV is complex and not easily predictable [2].

Blood pressure represents the product of the interaction between the flow ejected by the heart and the arterial system (◘ Fig. 26.1) [3]. Arterial pressure, therefore, depends on both the SV and the arterial system, which involves different elements, such as resistance, compliance, characteristic impedance, arterial wave reflections, etc., brought together under the term *arterial load* [3]. Consequently, the arterial system modulates the pressure-volume relationship and eventually defines the arterial pressure for a given SV. For that reason, if the arterial system changes, the pressure-volume relationship will change too, and arterial pressure will poorly reflect SV changes. Therefore, blood pressure changes could reflect variations in SV, arterial system, or both [2]. Moreover, the relationship between pressure and SV is nonlinear but also pressure-dependent. That means that as the

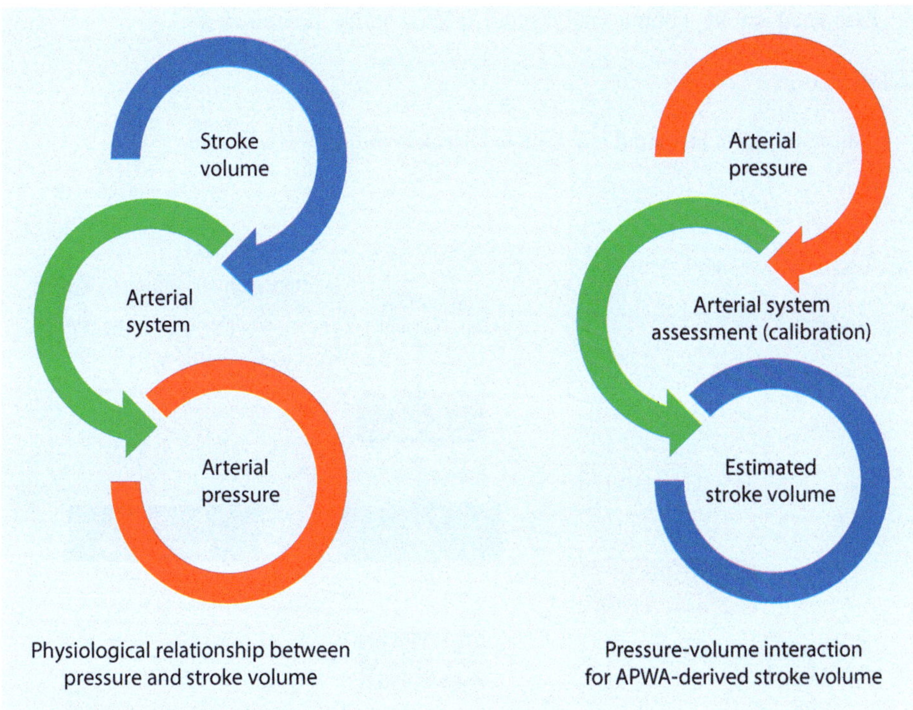

◘ **Fig. 26.1** The pressure-volume relationship in normal physiology and arterial pressure waveform analysis (APWA). Physiologically, the arterial pressure is the product of the combined effects of the blood flow ejected by the heart and the arterial system, which compromises both the mechanical properties of the arteries and the effects of arterial wave reflections. Arterial pressure waveform analysis aims to estimate the stroke volume from the arterial pressure, so the arterial system must be characterized to establish a valid pressure-volume relationship and a reliable stroke volume estimation stroke volume increases, the distensibility of the aortic wall progressively decreases, and the arterial pressure rises more quickly [4]. Such nonlinear behavior of the arterial system precludes any simple method for estimating SV from arterial pressure. So, the apparent simplicity of the pressure-volume relationship and the physiological assumption of the APWA method is just that: *apparent*.

26.3 Applying the Physiological Basis of Pressure-Volume Relationship for Determining When and Why to Calibrate

26

To accurately interpret arterial pressure waveform and make reliable SV estimations, it is necessary to establish a valid relationship between arterial pressure and SV. Therefore, to correctly use the arterial pressure for estimating SV, one must also simultaneously define the current status of the arterial system. This is the purpose of the calibration process (◘ Fig. 26.2).

Initial calibration represents the procedure by which the APWA algorithm adjusts the relation between pressure and SV, determining the state of the arterial system in a sort of scaling factor. Let's call this factor *X*. Thus, for a given arterial pulse pressure, the SV will be as follows:

$$\text{Estimated stroke volume} = \text{Measured arterial pulse pressure} \times X$$

and therefore:

$$\text{Estimated cardiac output} = \text{Estimated stroke volume} \times \text{Heart rate}$$

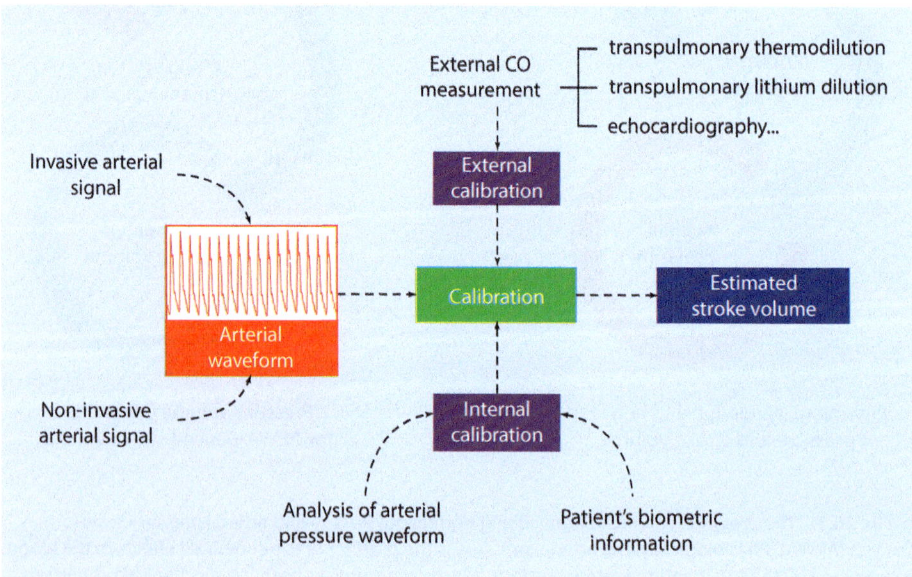

◘ **Fig. 26.2** Arterial pressure waveform analysis. Schematic representation of the internal process of arterial pressure waveform analysis

This calibration factor is usually obtained from an external measure of cardiac output, as obtained by using the transpulmonary thermo- or lithium dilution methods [5] or echocardiography [6]. It can also be internally estimated from individual patient's biometric information, as the method described by Langewouters [4], or from the analysis of the morphological characteristics of the arterial pressure curve [7, 8]. It is important to note that, in both cases, a calibration process needs to be performed; otherwise, the algorithm would be unable to establish the initial conditions of the arterial system for estimating SV. So, what is usually referred as uncalibrated systems, because no external calibration is performed, should be correctly named as self-calibrated or internally calibrated APWA systems (◘ Table 26.1).

While this initial calibration provides a starting point from which to begin monitoring SV, the system has however to compensate the frequent disturbances that occur in the status of the arterial system. Many physiologic and pathophysiologic processes can alter the relation between arterial pulse pressure and left ventricular SV. Regrettably most of these processes are commonly seen in the critically ill patients at baseline and in response to vasoactive therapies. If the arterial system changes, as during vasopressor therapy or changes in patient's condition [9–12], then the primary assumptions about the interaction between SV and blood pressure also vary, and the validity of a specific APWA algorithm may be significantly affected. This is, therefore, the cornerstone of the APWA method: the way the arterial system is characterized ultimately defines the specific strength of each algorithm but also the intrinsic limitations of this technique [13, 14]. Accordingly, situations in which arterial system is frequently and profoundly altered, such as septic shock or the use of vasoactive agents, are the worst scenario for APWA [9–12, 15–17]. On the contrary, during isolated changes in preload and relatively stable arterial conditions, as during the passive leg raising maneuver or a fluid challenge, SV becomes the main determinant

◘ Table 26.1 Autocalibrated (or self-calibrated) and externally calibrated arterial pressure waveform analysis (APWA) methods commercially available for estimating stroke volume and cardiac output from the arterial pressure

Autocalibrated (or self-calibrated) APWA methods		Vigileo/FloTrac (Edwards Lifesciences)
		MostCare (Vygon)
		LiDCOrapid (LiDCO)
		Nexfin/ClearSight (Edwards Lifesciences)
		PulsioFlex/ProAQT (Pulsion)[a]
		CNAP system (CNSystem)[a]
Externally calibrated APWA methods	Transpulmonary thermodilution	EV1000 (Edwards Lifesciences)
		PiCCO$_2$ (Pulsion)
	Transpulmonary lithium dilution	LiDCO plus (LiDCO)
	Esophageal Doppler	CardioQ-ODM+ (Deltex Medical)

[a]Optionally, they can be calibrated using an external cardiac output value

of the blood pressure, and the APWA method would provide a reliable estimation of SV changes [18, 19].

Recalibration represents then the process by which the APWA algorithm aims to readapt the relation between arterial pressure and SV to the current status of the arterial system. Recalibration process can be intermittently performed using a new external calibration (e.g., performing a new thermodilution and obtaining a new independent measure of CO) or continuously by using an internal analysis based on mathematical models of the arterial system, such as the classical Windkessel model [20, 21]. In modern APWA algorithms, these models of the arterial circulation should involve not only the mere analysis of mechanical properties of the arterial system, such as arterial compliance or resistance, but also more complex factors related to the nonuniform and finite nature of the arterial system [22]. If these factors are ignored, for example, the impact of the physiological pulse pressure amplification from the aorta to the radial artery and thus the site where blood pressure is measured could significantly affect to the SV estimation (◘ Fig. 26.3).

Because of the ever-changing nature of the pressure-volume relationship, in those systems with the ability to perform an external calibration, the decision of when to perform a recalibration should be therefore based on the suspicion of a significant change in the arterial system status, rather than on a fixed time interval criterion [23, 24]. Moreover, this external calibration also brings relevant and complementary information concerning the patient's clinical status, such as volumetric data, cardiac function, extravascular lung water, etc.

In the monitoring systems without external calibration, or self-calibrated, the reliability of SV estimations however will depend only on the ability of the internal APWA algorithm to compensate the arterial system changes, which in turn will be determined by the

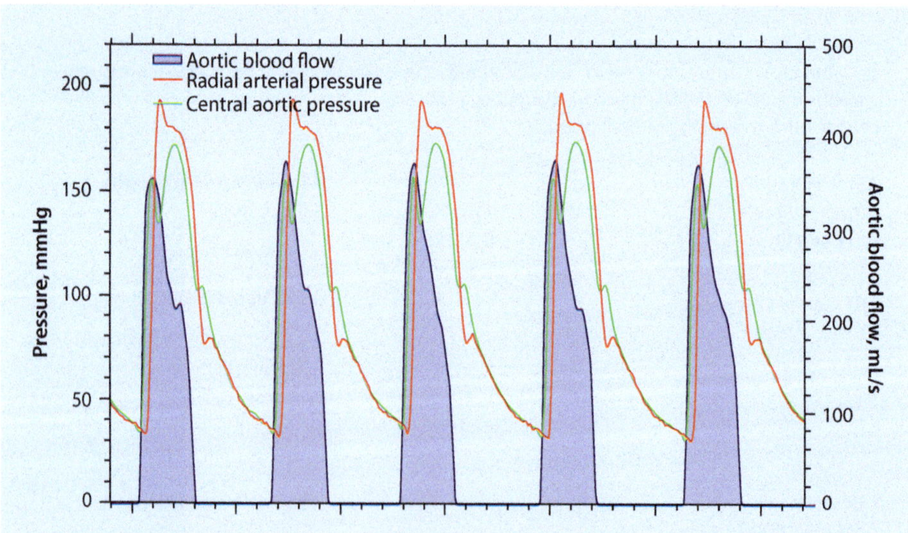

◘ **Fig. 26.3** The relationship between radial pressure (red line, obtained from an invasive arterial line), central aortic pressure (green line, estimated by a generalized transfer function), and aortic blood flow (blue shade area, obtained from an esophageal Doppler). Differences in morphology and height of both blood pressure waveforms are due to the impact of arterial wave reflections and the physiological pulse pressure amplification phenomenon. Analysis of these two arterial waveforms will produce different stroke volume values if these differences in the same patient are not considered validity of its assumptions about the arterial system [10, 23, 25, 26]. This is not a trivial point. To demonstrate the robustness of a specific continuous APWA algorithm, they should be tested not only in stable conditions but also during significant changes in the arterial system. Only during unstable hemodynamic conditions, the mathematical assumptions about the arterial system of a specific APWA algorithm can be challenged.

26.4 Other Potential Factors Affecting APWA CO Reliability

Besides the limitations described above, it is important to note that the reliability of APWA for estimating SV ultimately depends on the signal quality of the arterial pressure waveform. As most of the critically ill patients are instrumented with a fluid-filled catheter-transducer system, aspects such as damping, calibration, and zeroing should be carefully assessed [27, 28]. Moreover, considering that the occurrence of underdamping/resonance artifacts is present in about one-third of critically ill patients [29], ensuring routinely an adequate damping of the intra-arterial pressure using the fast-flush test is strongly encouraged. Similarly, in the situations in which the arterial pressure curve is artificially or pathologically distorted, as during the use of intra-aortic balloon pump or severe aortic regurgitation, the primary assumptions of APWA are not valid, and the continuous SV estimation from the arterial pressure is not feasible.

With APWA systems using continuous noninvasive measurements of blood pressure, such as the volume-clamp method [30], the reliability of the SV estimation not only depends on the strength of the APWA algorithm but also on the validation of the blood pressure measurements and the quality of the estimated blood pressure waveform [18]. Factors such as an impaired peripheral perfusion, as frequently observed during the use of high doses of vasoconstrictors or in the presence of the sepsis-related microcirculatory abnormalities, could affect to the SV estimation, limiting this noninvasive APWA method for the less compromised patients or in the perioperative setting [31, 32].

Practical Implications

At the time of deciding when to use an APWA-based CO monitoring, it is essential to remember the primary objective for monitoring and the particular clinical situation. In this regard, we should decide if the primary monitoring target is (a) to know the absolute value of CO, (b) to track trends and changes in CO and be warned about them, or (c) to monitor dynamic indexes, such as SV variation or pulse pressure variation. The specific indications of any of these options are out of the scope of this chapter. However, the interpretation and limitations of APWA-based CO monitoring will depend on them as follows [33]:

1. *Reliability of the absolute CO value measurement (accuracy).* This could be the main pitfall of the APWA methods. If the algorithm we are using applies a population-based calibration (internal calibration), absolute CO values will be reliable only if the patient demographic characteristics are similar to the population used to calibrate the APWA algorithm. As most of the populations used in algorithm calibrations represent people in stable or healthy conditions, this precludes the absolute values of most of the devices. In the other hand, if an external calibration

is used (as thermodilution), two aspects should be assured for a reliable CO absolute value measurement: (1) the hemodynamic conditions present at the time of the calibration remains, and (2) the calibration was performed under stable conditions.

2. *Reliability of CO changes detection (trending ability)*. In the other hand, tracking CO changes could be the main application of APWA CO monitoring. As long as the arterial system conditions do not drastically vary, the relative changes in the arterial pressure should be proportional to the stroke volume and could reliably act as a valid surrogate of it. However, based on the possible pitfalls in the related absolute measurement value describe above, if these detected changes are huge, a new recalibration is recommended.
3. *Reliability of dynamic SV changes measurement*. For the interpretation and reliability of this measurement, the pitfalls are more related to the limitations of dynamic indexes itself instead of the limitations for the measurement of the SV based on the APWF. In this regard, once the conditions for the application of a dynamic index are fulfilled [34], APWF algorithms appear as practical and usable tools to guide clinical decisions based on functional monitoring. This is due to the reliability of APWF algorithms to track changes in SV in a short-term scale [13].

Conclusions

APWA methods provide a continuous estimation of the cardiac output from the analysis of the characteristics of the arterial pressure waveform. The understanding of the physiological basis of the pressure-volume relationship may help to recognize the main advantages and limitation of this technique. The integration of the modern computational technology and a better knowledge of the arterial circulation physiology have led to the development of improved APWA algorithms and more reliable monitoring systems. In this regard, APWA seems to be a promising and evolving technology.

Take-Home Messages

- All APWA algorithms depend on the same physiological assumption: a predictable relation exists between arterial pressure and SV. However, since the arterial pressure is the result of the interaction between the volume ejected by the heart and the arterial system, the relationship between arterial pressure and SV is also defined by the arterial system. Consequently, how the arterial system is evaluated will ultimately determine the strength and weakness of each APWA algorithm.
- The calibration process (external or internal) allows defining the status of the arterial system for establishing the current rules of the pressure-volume relationship and obtaining a reliable SV estimation. Whenever a significant change in the arterial system is suspected (by introduction or change in vasoactive agents or a change in the patient's condition), a new calibration should be performed to reestablish a valid relationship between arterial pressure and SV.
- As in any other monitoring systems, a key aspect in deciding whether to use an APWF CO monitoring system is the patient's clinical situation and clearly defining

the main question or problem that must be solved. This is valid not only for deciding whether or not using an APWF-based monitor but also for interpretation and clinical decision making. In this regard, some important questions that should be answered are: is the patient hemodynamically stable? Am I interested on the absolute CO value or do I want to track relative CO changes over time? Does my patient fulfill the criteria for using a dynamic index of preload responsiveness, such as stroke volume variation? Could the arterial properties have changed since my last calibration?

- APWA reliability also depends on the quality of the arterial pressure signal. Under- and overdamping could profoundly affect the pressure waveform shape and the SV estimation. So, damping assessment by fast-flushing the pressure transducer system should be periodically performed to guarantee the quality of the pressure signal.

References

1. Erlanger J, Hooker DR. An experimental study of blood-pressure and of pulse-pressure in man. Johns Hopkins Hosp Rep; 1904.
2. Monnet X, Letierce A, Hamzaoui O, Chemla D, Anguel N, Osman D, Richard C, Teboul JL. Arterial pressure allows monitoring the changes in cardiac output induced by volume expansion but not by norepinephrine. Crit Care Med. 2011;39:1394–9.
3. Monge Garcia MI, Saludes Orduna P, Cecconi M. Understanding arterial load. Intensive Care Med. 2016;42:1625–7.
4. Langewouters GJ, Wesseling KH, Goedhard WJ. The static elastic properties of 45 human thoracic and 20 abdominal aortas in vitro and the parameters of a new model. J Biomech. 1984;17:425–35.
5. Reuter DA, Huang C, Edrich T, Shernan SK, Eltzschig HK. Cardiac output monitoring using indicator-dilution techniques: basics, limits, and perspectives. Anesth Analg. 2010;110:799–811.
6. Monge Garcia MI, Romero MG, Cano AG, Rhodes A, Grounds RM, Cecconi M. Impact of arterial load on the agreement between pulse pressure analysis and esophageal Doppler. Crit Care. 2013;17:R113.
7. Geerts BF, Aarts LP, Jansen JR. Methods in pharmacology: measurement of cardiac output. Br J Clin Pharmacol. 2011;71:316–30.
8. Thiele RH, Durieux ME. Arterial waveform analysis for the anesthesiologist: past, present, and future concepts. Anesth Analg. 2011;113:766–76.
9. Meng L, Tran NP, Alexander BS, Laning K, Chen G, Kain ZN, Cannesson M. The impact of phenylephrine, ephedrine, and increased preload on third-generation Vigileo-FloTrac and esophageal doppler cardiac output measurements. Anesth Analg. 2011;113:751–7.
10. Monnet X, Anguel N, Jozwiak M, Richard C, Teboul JL. Third-generation FloTrac/Vigileo does not reliably track changes in cardiac output induced by norepinephrine in critically ill patients. Br J Anaesth. 2012;108:615.
11. Yamashita K, Nishiyama T, Yokoyama T, Abe H, Manabe M. The effects of vasodilation on cardiac output measured by PiCCO. J Cardiothorac Vasc Anesth. 2008;22:688–92.
12. Johansson A, Chew M. Reliability of continuous pulse contour cardiac output measurement during hemodynamic instability. J Clin Monit Comput. 2007;21:237–42.
13. Pinsky MR. Probing the limits of arterial pulse contour analysis to predict preload responsiveness. Anesth Analg. 2003;96:1245–7.
14. Peyton PJ, Chong SW. Minimally invasive measurement of cardiac output during surgery and critical care: a meta-analysis of accuracy and precision. Anesthesiology. 2010;113:1220–35.
15. Bein B, Meybohm P, Cavus E, Renner J, Tonner PH, Steinfath M, Scholz J, Doerges V. The reliability of pulse contour-derived cardiac output during hemorrhage and after vasopressor administration. Anesth Analg. 2007;105:107–13.

16. De Backer D, Marx G, Tan A, Junker C, Van Nuffelen M, Huter L, Ching W, Michard F, Vincent JL. Arterial pressure-based cardiac output monitoring: a multicenter validation of the third-generation software in septic patients. Intensive Care Med. 2011;37(2):233–40.
17. Biais M, Mazocky E, Stecken L, Pereira B, Sesay M, Roullet S, Quinart A, Sztark F. Impact of systemic vascular resistance on the accuracy of the pulsioflex device. Anesth Analg. 2017;124:487–93.
18. Truijen J, van Lieshout JJ, Wesselink WA, Westerhof BE. Noninvasive continuous hemodynamic monitoring. J Clin Monit Comput. 2012;26:267–78.
19. Cecconi M, Rhodes A. Pulse pressure analysis: to make a long story short. Crit Care. 2010;14:175.
20. Westerhof N, Lankhaar JW, Westerhof BE. The arterial Windkessel. Med Biol Eng Comput. 2009;47:131–41.
21. Montenij LJ, de Waal EE, Buhre WF. Arterial waveform analysis in anesthesia and critical care. Curr Opin Anaesthesiol. 2011;24:651–6.
22. Nichols WW, O'Rourke M. McDonald's blood flow in arteries: theoretical, experimental and clinical principles. London: Oxford University Press; 2005.
23. Gruenewald M, Meybohm P, Renner J, Broch O, Caliebe A, Weiler N, Steinfath M, Scholz J, Bein B. Effect of norepinephrine dosage and calibration frequency on accuracy of pulse contour-derived cardiac output. Crit Care. 2011;15:R22.
24. Hamzaoui O, Monnet X, Richard C, Osman D, Chemla D, Teboul JL. Effects of changes in vascular tone on the agreement between pulse contour and transpulmonary thermodilution cardiac output measurements within an up to 6-hour calibration-free period. Crit Care Med. 2008;36:434–40.
25. Gopal S, Do T, Pooni JS, Martinelli G. Validation of cardiac output studies from the Mostcare compared to a pulmonary artery catheter in septic patients. Minerva Anestesiol. 2014;80:314–23.
26. Eleftheriadis S, Galatoudis Z, Didilis V, Bougioukas I, Schon J, Heinze H, Berger KU, Heringlake M. Variations in arterial blood pressure are associated with parallel changes in FlowTrac/Vigileo-derived cardiac output measurements: a prospective comparison study. Crit Care. 2009;13:R179.
27. Magder S. Invasive intravascular hemodynamic monitoring: technical issues. Crit Care Clin. 2007;23:401–14.
28. He HW, Liu DW, Long Y, Wang XT, Zhao ML, Lai XL. The effect of variable arterial transducer level on the accuracy of pulse contour waveform-derived measurements in critically ill patients. J Clin Monit Comput. 2016;30:569–75.
29. Romagnoli S, Ricci Z, Quattrone D, Tofani L, Tujjar O, Villa G, Romano SM, De Gaudio AR. Accuracy of invasive arterial pressure monitoring in cardiovascular patients: an observational study. Crit Care. 2014;18:644.
30. Penaz J. Criteria for set point estimation in the volume clamp method of blood pressure measurement. Physiol Res. 1992;41:5–10.
31. Monnet X, Picard F, Lidzborski E, Mesnil M, Duranteau J, Richard C, Teboul JL. The estimation of cardiac output by the Nexfin device is of poor reliability for tracking the effects of a fluid challenge. Crit Care. 2012;16:R212.
32. Fischer MO, Avram R, Carjaliu I, Massetti M, Gerard JL, Hanouz JL, Fellahi JL. Non-invasive continuous arterial pressure and cardiac index monitoring with Nexfin after cardiac surgery. Br J Anaesth. 2012;109:514–21.
33. Cecconi M, Malbrain ML. Cardiac output obtained by pulse pressure analysis: to calibrate or not to calibrate may not be the only question when used properly. Intensive Care Med. 2013;39:787–9.
34. Monnet X, Marik PE, Teboul JL. Prediction of fluid responsiveness: an update. Ann Intensive Care. 2016;6:111.

Oesophageal Doppler

Jonathan Lacey and Monty Mythen

M. R. Pinsky et al. (eds.), *Hemodynamic Monitoring*, Lessons from the ICU,
https://doi.org/10.1007/978-3-319-69269-2_27

Learning Objectives

This chapter will discuss the historical and scientific context to the development of the oesophageal Doppler monitor. We will explain the Doppler principle and how it is applied to the use of ultrasound in measuring blood flow. We will discuss the practicalities and clinical applications of the oesophageal Doppler as well as exploring the impact of its use on patient outcome. This chapter aims to equip the clinician with the knowledge and evidence base to ensure appropriate and effective use of this important clinical tool.

27.1 Introduction

27

Central to the role of the intensivist is the maintenance of adequate organ perfusion to ensure sufficient oxygen delivery, thereby mitigating sequelae of oxygen deficit. More often than not, resuscitative efforts are dictated by easily obtained blood *pressure* parameters, which are unreliable surrogate markers of the more important measures of *flow* [1, 2]. In a seminal paper, Shoemaker and colleagues demonstrated that targeting supranormal macrocirculatory blood flow and oxygen delivery in high-risk surgical patients significantly reduced mortality, post-operative complications and critical care stay [3]. Similar outcomes of augmented oxygen delivery in the perioperative period were seen in subsequent studies [4–6]. A strong body of evidence was developed, underlining the importance of goal-directed therapy in which interventions are manipulated to achieve predetermined *flow*-derived haemodynamic parameters.

However, the 'gold standard' for assessing haemodynamic status requires the use of a pulmonary artery catheter (PAC). This is invasive, requires a highly skilled operator and has become increasingly controversial [7–9]. In the past 20 years, minimally invasive cardiac output monitors, such as the oesophageal Doppler monitor (ODM), have all but superseded the PAC. The ODM provides continuous haemodynamic assessment of aortic blood flow allowing real-time evaluation of fluid and inotropic therapy. It has been pivotal in broadening the application of flow-based monitoring, and its use has been associated with improved patient outcomes, principally in the perioperative setting.

This chapter will explore the scientific principles that underpin the ODM, its clinical applications and the evidence supporting (or contesting) the use of this innovative clinical tool. The CardioQ-ODM device (Deltex Medical, Chichester, UK) is the predominant ODM in clinical practice (and in the literature) so will form the focus of our discussions.

27.2 Physical Principles

27.2.1 The Doppler Effect

In 1842, Christian Doppler first described his theory that *light* waves emitted or reflected from a moving object demonstrate a shift in frequency that is dependent on the relative velocity between that object and the observer [10]. Although there were errors in his scientific assumptions [11], the acceptance of the theory (and its eponymous naming) was cemented by a Dutch mathematician, named Christophorus Buys Ballot, who unequivocally demonstrated the frequency shift in *sound waves* using a moving train and some trumpets [12]! The Doppler effect is actually observed in all forms of waves, and it is the scientific principle upon which myriad innovations have developed within meteorology, astronomy and medicine.

27.2.2 The Doppler Equation

Within medicine, ultrasound has been used with great efficacy to measure arterial and intracardiac blood flow. Ultrasonic waves, emitted from a stationary probe, are reflected off moving red blood cells causing a shift in frequency (Doppler effect). The Doppler equation is used to calculate the velocity of blood flow:

$$V = \frac{c \times f_{\mathrm{d}}}{2 \times f_{\mathrm{T}} \times \cos\theta}$$

where V is velocity of red blood cells; c is speed of sound through body tissues (1540 m/s); f_{d} is frequency shift (Hz); f_{T} is frequency of transmitted ultrasound wave (Hz); and $\cos\theta$ is the cosine of the angle between the direction of blood flow and the sound beam axis (the angle of insonation). In human arteries, peak blood flow velocity will be up to 5–6 ms^{-1} which produces Doppler shift frequencies within the audible frequency range (less than 20 kHz) [13] allowing both visual and auditory Doppler flow assessment. A higher pitched Doppler shift represents higher velocity. It is important to note that the Doppler equation provides the flow *velocity*, not the flow *volume*. Flow volume is the product of the cross-sectional area of the artery and the mean velocity (or mean Doppler shift in frequency). Applying these principles to the aorta is the basis of measuring cardiac output using Doppler ultrasound.

27.2.3 Angle of Insonation

The angle of insonation (or Doppler angle), represented by θ in the Doppler equation, is the angle between the ultrasound beam and the direction of blood flow (■ Fig. 27.1). Under ideal circumstances this should be 0°, that is, the ultrasound beam is directly in line with the direction of blood flow (cos 0 = 1). However, in practice, this is not feasible. The greater the angle of insonation, the greater the potential error in flow measurement, until at 90° the beam is perpendicular to flow and no velocity will be detected (cos 90 = 0). In general, the smallest angle that maintains adequate signal should be used. For clinical use, this angle must be kept below 60°, as above this threshold, the calculation error is considered unacceptably high [14]. Furthermore, consistency of the insonation angle is of obvious importance for reliability in repeated measurements.

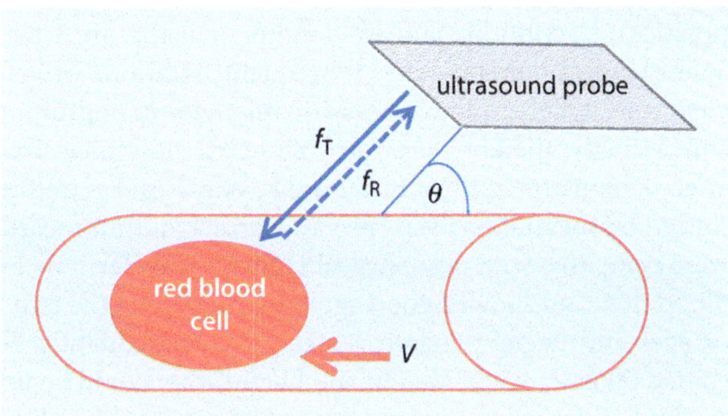

■ **Fig. 27.1** Diagram showing Doppler blood flow measurement. f_{T} is frequency of transmitted ultrasound wave (Hz); f_{R} is reflected frequency (Hz); θ is the angle of insonation; V is velocity of red blood cells. The Doppler shift is the difference between f_{T} and f_{R}

27.2.4 Pulsed and Continuous Wave Doppler

Pulsed wave technique involves a single-element Doppler probe that alternates between transmitting ultrasound and detecting reflected waves. It can be used to only 'listen' for Doppler-shifted waves after a specific time delay, ignoring all other reflected ultrasound, thereby measuring flow at a predetermined depth or location. Pulsed Doppler becomes inaccurate at high velocities, the threshold for which is dependent on the sample depth.

Continuous wave Doppler probe uses two piezoelectric elements, one to transmit and the other to detect reflected ultrasound. Although this technique lacks depth discrimination, it is very accurate over high velocity ranges.

27.2.5 Spectral Display and Doppler Waveforms

During Doppler assessment of pulsatile flow, there will be a spectrum of observed Doppler shift frequencies due to the multiple red blood cells moving at varying velocities. Following fast Fourier transform analysis, a spectral display of velocity over time produces a characteristic triangular-shaped Doppler waveform. The interpretation of this waveform is fundamental to oesophageal Doppler monitoring and will be discussed in more detail in a later section.

27.3 Development of the Oesophageal Doppler

The concept of using Doppler ultrasound to measure arterial blood flow has been applied since the middle part of the twentieth century. In the 1960s and 1970s, studies evaluated aortic blood flow measurement using transcutaneous probes positioned either in the intercostal space or suprasternal notch [15, 16]. Although the transcutaneous route achieved promising results, there were several disadvantages to the technique that limited its use, including difficulty securing position for continuous monitoring and the impact of lung pathology on signal transduction. Alternative Doppler techniques required invasive, surgical procedures using intra-aortic flowmeter catheters [17, 18]. It was recognised that the anatomical position of the oesophagus, in close proximity to the descending aorta, provided great potential for measuring aortic blood flow without the limitations of cutaneous probes. In 1971, Side and Gosling first described the use of a continuous wave Doppler ultrasound oesophageal probe to measure blood velocity in the aortic arch [19]. This was substantiated by Duck et al. in 1974, who provided detailed practical descriptions and limitations of using an 8 MHz continuous wave probe on anaesthetised humans [20]. Subsequent iterations of oesophageal probes incorporated echo transducers to measure aortic diameter in addition to Doppler ultrasound to measure velocity, thereby allowing volumetric flow measurement [21, 22]. In 1989, Singer et al. demonstrated the clinical utility of a 5 MHz continuous wave Doppler probe supported by spectral analysis display. Cardiac output measurements using thermodilution were compared with oesophageal Doppler waveform measurements of descending aortic blood flow and showed good agreement between the two techniques across a wide range of ages and haemodynamic states [23]. Subsequently, Singer developed a nomogram (based on patient age, weight and height) that could be used to convert the Doppler flow readings into estimates for left ventricular stroke volume. This enabled the device to calculate cardiac output without the need for separate echo measurements of the aortic diameter. It is Singer's work that ultimately led to the development of the CardioQ-ODM (Deltex, Chichester, UK). The latest incarnation, the CardioQ-ODM+, incorporates input from an invasive arterial blood pressure monitor to combine flow velocity measurements with pressure waveform analysis.

27.4 The CardioQ-ODM Oesophageal Doppler Monitor

The CardioQ-ODM uses a long flexible probe that is inserted via the mouth (or less commonly via the nose) until it is positioned at the mid-thoracic level. A transducer, at the tip of the probe, consists of a piezoelectric crystal that transmits 4 MHz continuous wave Doppler ultrasound and a second crystal that acts to detect Doppler-shifted ultrasound waves reflected off red blood cells in the aorta. The bevelled tip of the probe is orientated towards the aorta and is designed to provide an angle of insonation of 45°. The probe connects to a monitor to enable real-time spectral display of red cell velocities, and it is this velocity-time waveform that is used to calculate cardiac indices (◻ Fig. 27.2).

27.4.1 Probe Insertion and Positioning

Lubricant gel should be used to aid atraumatic insertion but also to improve signal transmission. Normally patients are anaesthetised, but the device can be used in the awake patient, in which case sedation or local anaesthesia may be used to improve patient tolerance (◻ Fig. 27.3). For most adults, the probe will need to be inserted 35–40 cm

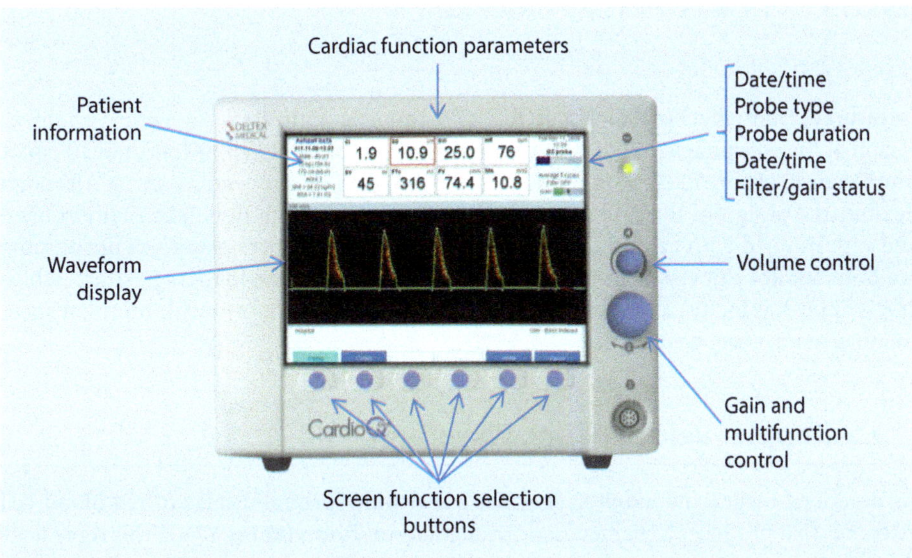

◻ **Fig. 27.2** CardioQ-ODM monitor and spectral display. (Image reproduced with permission of Deltex Medical, UK)

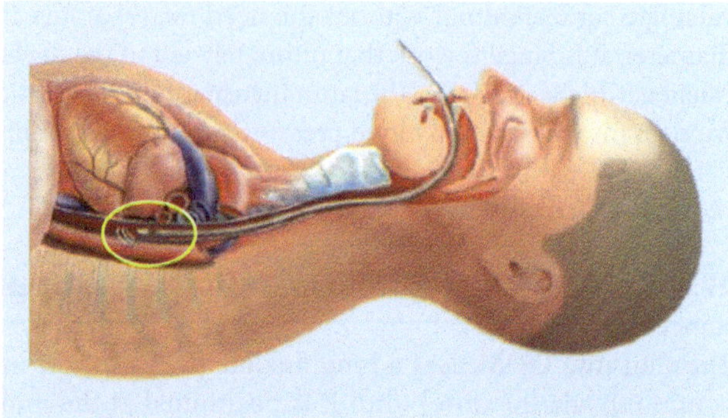

Fig. 27.3 Correctly positioned Doppler probe in the mid-thoracic region of the oesophagus and with tip facing posteriorly towards the aorta. The circled area highlights the relationship between the probe and aortic blood flow that is also represented by the schematic in Fig. 27.1. (*Image reproduced with permission of Deltex Medical, UK*)

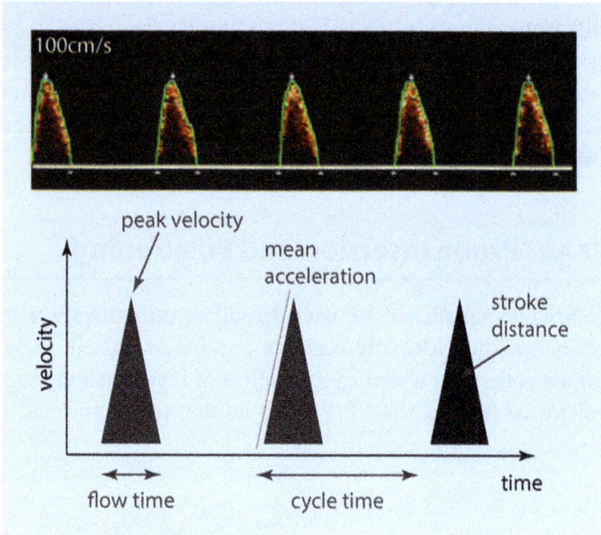

Fig. 27.4 Optimal waveform (top panel) showing the brightest (orange/white) signal at the peripheries and a dark central component; green tracer line neatly follows the waveform with white arrows at the triangular points. A schematic diagram (bottom panel) of the measured Doppler variables. (Top panel image *reproduced with permission of Deltex Medical, UK. Bottom panel reproduced from Esophageal Doppler Monitoring, 2005, Singer M with permission of Springer*)

(measured from the lips) to reach the mid-thoracic (5th–sixth thoracic vertebrae) region of the oesophagus. Note, Doppler waveforms located at depths less than 30 cm or more than 45 cm are likely to be from vessels other than the descending aorta. Although flexible, the design of the probe is such that it is rigid enough to be externally rotated and repositioned with ease to ensure optimal poisition. Features of correct positioning are both auditory (a classical pulsatile Doppler signal with the loudest possible 'whip-crack' at peak velocity) and visual (optimal time-velocity waveform with minimal spectral dispersion – see next section).

27.4.2 Doppler Velocity-Time Waveform

As described earlier, the monitor provides a real-time spectral display of red blood cell velocities that produces a characteristic triangular waveform (Fig. 27.4). This represents the pulsatile aortic flow seen during the cardiac cycle. The probe is positioned to achieve the brightest and tallest waveform possible. When the probe is positioned correctly (and flow is laminar), the majority of red blood cells will be travelling at approximately the same velocity, as such the brightest signal (orange to white) forms a clear spectral envelope to the waveform. If the waveform is small with an ill-defined centre, then there is spectral dispersion and indicates inadequate positioning or turbulent flow.

27.4.3 Measured and Derived Haemodynamic Variables

Stroke distance (SD) is the area under the velocity-time waveform and represents the distance moved by the column of blood within the aorta following left ventricular contraction. It is the SD that is used to generate the nomogram-derived *stroke volume (SV)*. Both measurements are the principal determinants of fluid responsiveness when using the ODM: if there is a less than 10% increase in SV following a fluid challenge, then it can be assumed that preload optimisation has been achieved, and, if required, alternative interventions should be used to correct further haemodynamic abnormality. *Cardiac output (CO)* can be simply calculated as the product of SV and heart rate. These values may be indexed to body surface area to provide *stroke volume index (SVI)* and *cardiac index (CI)*.

The width of the base of the waveform is termed the *flow time (FT)* and represents the duration of systolic blood flow. Systole occupies approximately one-third of the cardiac cycle, and therefore FT will vary significantly with heart rate. Using a derivation of Bazett's formula, FT is corrected to a heart rate of 60 beats per minute, thereby allowing intra-individual comparison independent of changes in heart rate. This *corrected flow time (FTc)* has a normal range of 330–360 ms and is inversely related to systemic vascular resistance. A low FTc (<330 ms) is seen in the vasoconstricted, hypovolaemic patient and a high FTc (>360 ms) during vasoplegic states (e.g. sepsis). The FTc has repeatedly demonstrated equivocal or superior ability to guide optimisation of left ventricular preload when compared to the PAC [24–26].

The maximum height of the waveform is called the *peak velocity (PV)*, and its upstroke gradient is termed the *mean acceleration (MA)*. PV and MA are both proportionate markers of left ventricular contractility, although PV is more often used clinically. Hyperdynamic states (e.g. sepsis and pregnancy) will display high PV, and low contractility states (e.g. systolic cardiac failure) will have a blunted PV. The normal range varies significantly with age, reflecting the loss of intrinsic myocardial contractility: in a 20-year-old, it will be between 90 and 120 cm/s, and this will decrease to only 50–70 cm/s in a 70-year-old.

The ODM will provide visual and numerical feedback to dynamic changes in preload, contractility and afterload and illustrate the complex interplay between these cardiac functions. This affords the clinician real-time haemodynamic assessment regarding the patient's need for *and* response to fluid and inotropic therapy (◘ Figs. 27.5 and 27.6). For the experienced user, the shape of the waveform alone can inform intervention, even before quantitative data is displayed.

27.4.4 Limitations

The CardioQ-ODM incorporates a nomogram, based on data from paired thermodilution and ODM measurements, to translate descending aortic Doppler flow into estimates of left ventricular output. The aortic cross-sectional area is not measured and is considered constant; as such any intra-individual variation in aortic diameter will affect the accuracy of cardiac output calculations. The impact of this appears to be negligible: aortic diameter

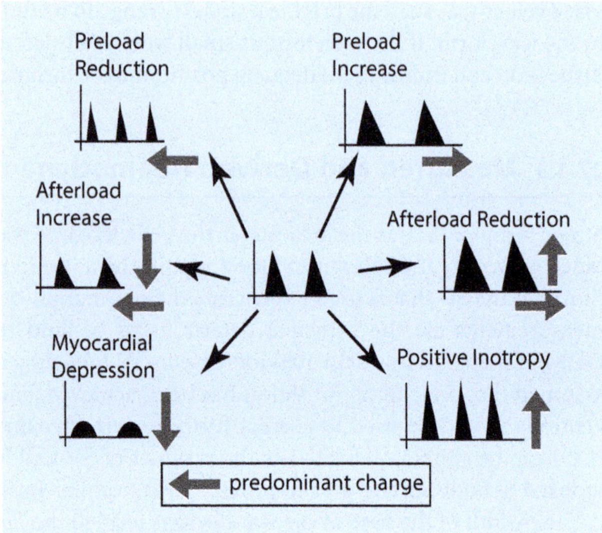

Fig. 27.5 Changes in waveform characteristics in response to changes in haemodynamic state. (*Reproduced from Esophageal Doppler Monitoring, 2005, Singer M with permission of Springer*)

fluctuates very little during the cardiac cycle, and ODM measurements have repeatedly demonstrated strong correlation with thermodilution across a range of clinical scenarios. However, it is worth considering that one small study did show that aorta compliance following fluid resuscitation is such that the response may be underestimated without concomitant aortic diameter measurement [27]. That said, the nomogram is also a key attribute of the ODM in that it obviates the need for separate echocardiographic measurement of the aortic radius, for which even minor inaccuracy can prove significant if the erroneous value is squared to calculate the cross-sectional area [28].

There is also an assumption of a fixed distribution (70%) of cardiac output to the descending aorta. This may limit reliability of use in patients in whom this distribution may be disturbed, notably in pregnancy and neuraxial sympathetic blockade [29, 30]. Increased intra-abdominal pressure during laparoscopic surgery, or due to pathological intra-abdominal hypertension, has significant effects on the cardiovascular system [31, 32] that may also include abnormally cephalad distribution of cardiac output [33]. However, although these scenarios may affect absolute values for the derived SV/CO, the measured Doppler values (e.g. SD and FTc) will be unaffected and remain reliable indices with which to guide fluid therapy. It is also important to note that thresholds and reliability of dynamic indicators of fluid responsiveness (such as stroke volume variation and pulse pressure variation) are affected by changes in thoraco-abdominal pressure: reduced pressures (i.e. open abdomen or thoracotomy) will blunt intrathoracic pressure variations during the respiratory cycle, thereby reducing the variability of these indices, whilst increased cavity pressure will amplify the variation [34–38]. The clinician should be wary of this if using these dynamic indicators in the latest ODM incarnation, the CardioQ-ODM+.

Accuracy of Doppler flow measurement is dependent on knowing the angle of insonation and ensuring this remains constant to allow interpretation of sequential readings. The ODM assumes a parallel anatomical relationship between the aorta and oesophagus; thus the angle of insonation is dictated by the bevelled probe tip and will remain constant at 45°. This is an entirely rational assumption, but it is worth noting that aortic

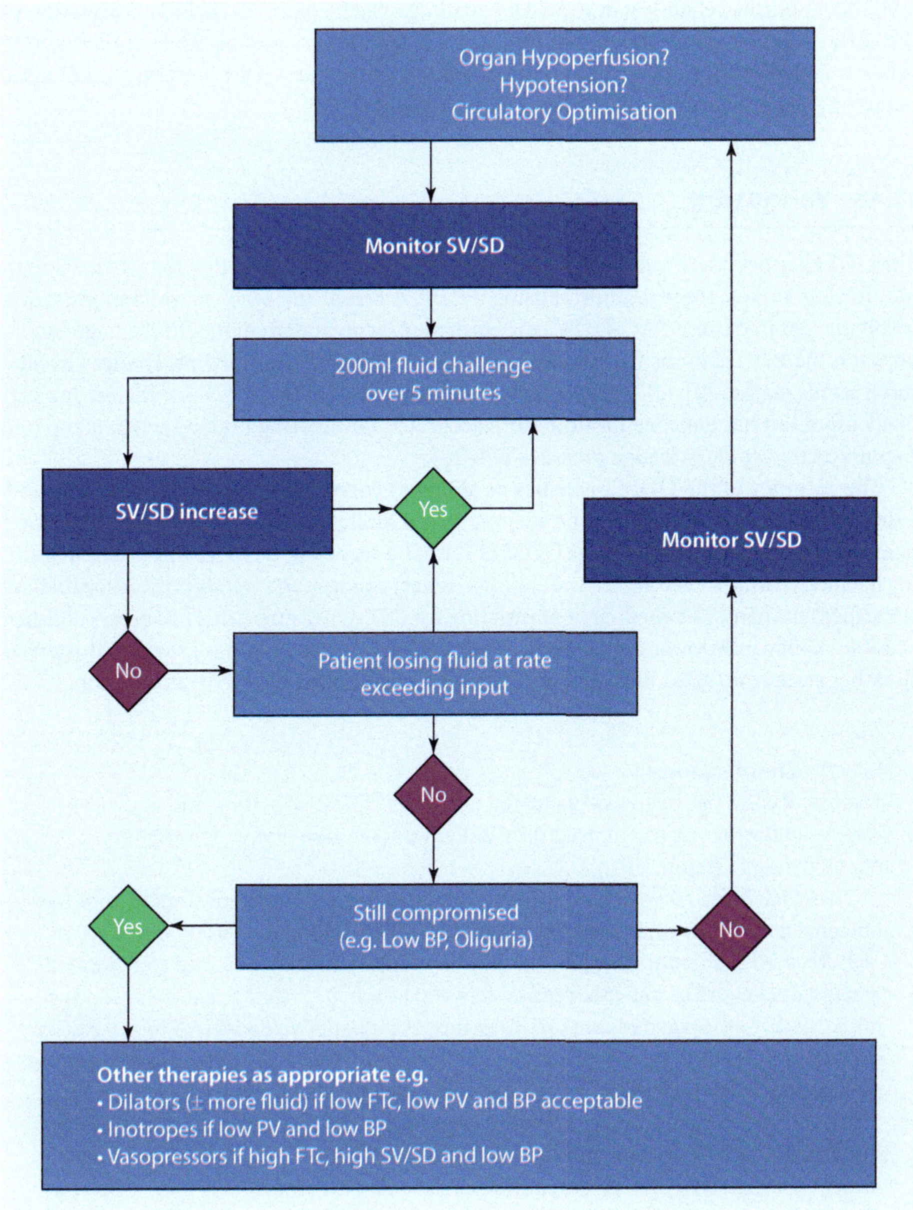

Fig. 27.6 Algorithm to aid decision-making when using oesophageal monitor. SV is stroke volume, SD is stroke distance, FTc is corrected flow time, PV is peak velocity, BP is blood pressure. A 10% or more increase in SV/SD is the typical threshold to determine response to a fluid challenge. (Image reproduced with kind *permission of Deltex Medical, UK*)

displacement and tortuosity will upset this parallel relationship and hence the angle of insonation [39]. Once again, however, the *trend* in values will be unaffected.

Finally, the ODM measurements are dependent on a good Doppler signal and the assumption of lamina blood flow. Therefore any condition that may distort these factors will impact on the reliability of the ODM readings. Such examples include coarctation of the aorta, thoracic aortic aneurysms and intra-aortic balloon pumps. The use of an ODM is best avoided in patients at risk from traumatic insertion of ODM, notably oesophageal pathology (e.g. varices, tumour, stents) and coagulopathy.

27.4.5 Validation

The ODM has been well validated when compared against the yardstick for cardiac output monitoring, that is, thermodilution using a PAC. A recent review of 11 validation studies involving 2400 paired PAC-ODM measurements concluded high clinical agreement between the two methods for measuring cardiac output and in tracking changes in haemodynamic states [40]. ODM not only offers a less invasive technique for measuring cardiac output but has also been found more accurate in evaluating preload when compared to pulmonary capillary wedge pressure [24–26].

27

The accuracy of the ODM describes its ability to correctly calculate the SV or CO and, although well-substantiated, may be affected by the limitations mentioned above. Precision describes the reproducibility of the ODM and can be argued to be more important in guiding haemodynamic intervention: the ability to reflect changes and trends is more useful than static measurement. The coefficient of variation for ODM measurements has been published at 3.8%, significantly lower than simultaneous thermodilution readings [23]. It is this precision that places the ODM in such a well-favoured position to guide SV optimisation.

Practical Implications

The use of ODM has been well validated in the perioperative setting and in critical care, including across multiple surgical patient populations and wide-ranging haemodynamic states.

There have been several randomised controlled trials (RCTs) demonstrating improved outcome for patients who received intraoperative fluid optimisation using the ODM. In 1995, Mythen et al. reported improved gastric mucosal perfusion, reduced complications and reduced length of stay (both critical care and hospital) for cardiac patients receiving intraoperative ODM-guided care [41]. Over the subsequent two decades, a series of RCTs supported these findings with the consistent conclusion that those patients who received intraoperative haemodynamic optimisation using the ODM benefited from improved indices of cardiovascular function, shorter hospital length of stay, improved post-operative gastrointestinal function and a lower overall complication rate [42, 43]. These studies incorporated patients from varied specialities including orthopaedics [44, 45], colorectal [46–50], hepatic [51], spinal [52] and thoracic surgery [53]. Importantly the ODM demonstrated reliability for monitoring in real time the direction and magnitude of change in haemodynamics across a range of clinical states [23, 51, 54].

There have also been RCTs demonstrating the clinical benefit of using the ODM in the post-operative period and critical care. McKendry et al. demonstrated that cardiac surgical patients randomised to a nurse-led post-operative haemodynamic optimisation protocol benefitted from significantly shorter hospital stay [55]. And in 2007, Chytra et al. found that polytrauma patients admitted to intensive care following major haemorrhage suffered lower rates of morbidity and shorter length of stay when they received ODM-guided resuscitation compared to conventional care [56]. Another study reported the potential role that ODM-measured cardiac indices on admission critical care units may have in risk stratifying for adverse outcome [57].

Between 2012 and 2014, several RCTs were published that demonstrated no improved outcome for patients receiving ODM-guided intraoperative fluid therapy. This may represent the impact of other advances in surgical care, most notably enhanced recovery programmes and minimally invasive surgical techniques: the physically fit, pre-optimised, well-hydrated and euvolaemic patient undergoing a laparoscopic procedure is at less risk of suffering from the sequelae of significant fluid shifts and blood loss [58]. Challand et al. demonstrated no difference in readiness for discharge or length of stay for colorectal patients receiving intraoperative ODM-guided care. However, the authors noted that the control group had more laparoscopic and colonic surgery; both factors are known to increase length of stay when compared to open and rectal procedures [59]. In 2013, McKenny et al. carried out the first RCT of intraoperative ODM use in patients undergoing open major gynaecological surgery and reported no difference in morbidity and length of stay [60]. Another RCT conducted by Brandstrup et al. compared SV optimisation using an ODM with a 'zero-balance' approach and showed no effect on post-operative cardiopulmonary morbidity or length of stay in elective colorectal patients [61]. There were similar findings from both Phan et al. and Srinivasa et al., who concluded that within an established enhanced recovery pathway, the use of intraoperative ODM did not improve clinical outcome for colorectal surgical patients [62, 63].

These studies were followed by a systematic review and meta-analysis, also by Srinivasa et al., of ODM-guided fluid optimisation for colorectal patients. This showed a temporal divide, as described above, in which the positive outcome seen in earlier RCTs was not replicated in the more recent trials. It concludes that there is no difference in complication rate or length of stay when ODM-guided therapy is compared with restrictive (zero-balance) fluid regimes or enhanced recovery programmes [64]. This review only included six trials, and since its publication there has been an RCT demonstrating benefit within the colorectal enhanced recovery programme [50] as well as in other surgical cohorts [51–53].

It is important to note that all the trials to date have been small in size and heterogeneous in design. There is strong signal, and physiological sense, that the use of the ODM in perioperative period is associated with improved outcome [65, 66], but, as is so often the case, the conclusive large multicentre RCT remains absent.

Conclusion

The ODM is a minimally invasive, simple to use cardiac output monitor with a rapid learning curve and low incidence of complications. It provides continuous, real-time haemodynamic measurements and imaging of descending aortic blood flow. The ODM has been well validated against the established thermodilution technique and demonstrates good reliability. In clinical scenarios that may affect the accuracy of the nomogram-derived volumetric measurements, Doppler parameters remain dependable for guiding haemodynamic optimisation.

There is a strong body of evidence for cardiac output monitoring to enable flow-derived goal-directed therapy in the major surgical population, in particular the very high-risk patient [65–69]. The ODM is ideally placed to deliver this care, and its use in the perioperative period is supported by numerous trials demonstrating improved patient outcome.

The ODM is a precision tool and its capability as a cardiac output monitor is clear. Recent trials have introduced a healthy dose of equipoise into its impact on patient outcome [70]: in the authors' opinion, this serves to highlight the importance of ensuring that the ODM is reserved for the high-risk, major surgical patient who stands to benefit most.

Take-Home Message

- Oesophageal Doppler monitoring provides continuous and reliable haemodynamic monitoring in the perioperative and critical care environments.
- Its use is most advocated in the comorbid, complex surgical patient who is at risk of (or suffering from) major fluid shifts and blood loss.
- Optimal probe positioning is essential for accurate signal acquisition.
- Doppler-measured variables are reliable even in scenarios when nomogram-adjusted calculations (i.e. volumetric data) may not be.

References

1. Hamilton-Davies C, Mythen MG, Salmon JB, Jacobson D, Shukla A, Webb AR. Comparison of commonly used clinical indicators of hypovolaemia with gastrointestinal tonometry. Intensive Care Med. 1997;23:276–81.
2. Dünser MW, Takala J, Brunauer A, Bakker J. Re-thinking resuscitation: leaving blood pressure cosmetics behind and moving forward to permissive hypotension and a tissue perfusion-based approach. Crit Care. 2013;17:326.
3. Shoemaker WC, Appel PL, Kram HB, Waxman K, Lee TS. Prospective trial of supranormal values of survivors as therapeutic goals in high-risk surgical patients. Chest. 1988;94:1176–86.
4. Boyd O, Grounds RM, Bennett ED. A randomized clinical trial of the effect of deliberate perioperative increase of oxygen delivery on mortality in high-risk surgical patients. JAMA. 1993;270:2699–707.
5. Wilson J, Woods I, Fawcett J, Whall R, Dibb W, Morris C, McManus E. Reducing the risk of major elective surgery: randomised controlled trial of preoperative optimisation of oxygen delivery. BMJ. 1999;318:1099–103.
6. Lobo SM, Salgado PF, Castillo VG, Borim AA, Polachini CA, Palchetti JC, Brienzi SL, de Oliveira GG. Effects of maximizing oxygen delivery on morbidity and mortality in high-risk surgical patients. Crit Care Med. 2000;28:3396–404.
7. Connors AF, Speroff T, Dawson NV, et al. The effectiveness of right heart catheterization in the initial care of critically ill patients. SUPPORT Investigators. JAMA. 1996;276:889–97.
8. Harvey S, Harrison DA, Singer M, et al. Assessment of the clinical effectiveness of pulmonary artery catheters in management of patients in intensive care (PAC-Man): a randomised controlled trial. Lancet. 2005;366:472–7.
9. Wiener RS, Welch HG. Trends in the use of the pulmonary artery catheter in the United States, 1993-2004. JAMA. 2007;298:423–9.
10. Doppler C. Über das farbige Licht der Doppelsterne und einiger anderer Gestirne des Himmels. Abh Königl Böhm Ges Wiss. 1843;2:465–82.
11. Coman I. Christian Andreas Doppler - the man and his legacy. Eur J Echocardiogr. 2005;6:7–10.
12. Buys Ballot C. Akustische Versuche auf der Niederländischen Eisenbahn, nebst gelegentlichen Bemerkungen zur Theorie des Hrn. Prof Doppler Ann der Phys und Chemie. 1845;66:321–51.
13. Hoskins PR. Measurement of arterial blood flow by Doppler ultrasound. Clin Phys Physiol Meas. 1990;11:1–26.
14. Thrush A. Spectral Doppler ultrasound. In: Hoskins PR, Martin K, Thrush A, editors. Diagnostic ultrasound. 2nd ed. Cambridge: Cambridge University Press; 2010. p. 114–5.
15. Light LH. Non-injurious ultrasonic technique for observing flow in the human aorta. Nature. 1969;224:1119–21.

16. Huntsman LL, Gams E, Johnson CC, Fairbanks E. Transcutaneous determination of aortic blood-flow velocities in man. Am Heart J. 1975;89:605–12.
17. Benchimol A, Stegall HF, Maroko PR, Gartlan JL, Leib B. Aortic flow velocity in man during cardiac arrhythmias measured with the Doppler catheter-flowmeter system. Am Heart J. 1969;78:649–59.
18. Benchimol A, Desser KB, Gartlan JL. Bidirectional blood flow velocity in the cardiac chambers and great vessels studied with the Doppler ultrasonic flowmeter. Am J Med. 1972;52:467–73.
19. Side CD, Gosling RG. Non-surgical assessment of cardiac function. Nature. 1971;232:335–6.
20. Duck FA, Hodson CJ, Tomlin PJ. An esophageal Doppler probe for aortic flow velocity monitoring. Ultrasound Med Biol. 1974;1:233–41.
21. Olson RM, Cooke JP. A nondestructive ultrasonic technique to measure diameter and blood flow in arteries. IEEE Trans Biomed Eng. 1974;BME-21:168–71.
22. Lavandier B, Cathignol D, Muchada R, Bui Xuan B, Motin J. Noninvasive aortic blood flow measurement using an intraesophageal probe. Ultrasound Med Biol. 1985;11:451–60.
23. Singer M, Clarke J, Bennett ED. Continuous hemodynamic monitoring by esophageal Doppler. Crit Care Med. 1989;17:447–52.
24. Singer M, Bennett ED. Noninvasive optimization of left ventricular filling using esophageal Doppler. Crit Care Med. 1991;19:1132–7.
25. DiCorte CJ, Latham P, Greilich PE, Cooley MV, Grayburn PA, Jessen ME. Esophageal Doppler monitor determinations of cardiac output and preload during cardiac operations. Ann Thorac Surg. 2000;69:1782–6.
26. Madan AK, UyBarreta VV, Aliabadi-Wahle S, Jesperson R, Hartz RS, Flint LM, Steinberg SM. Esophageal Doppler ultrasound monitor versus pulmonary artery catheter in the hemodynamic management of critically ill surgical patients. J Trauma. 1999;46:607–11–2.
27. Monnet X, Chemla D, Osman D, Anguel N, Richard C, Pinsky MR, Teboul J-L. Measuring aortic diameter improves accuracy of esophageal Doppler in assessing fluid responsiveness. Crit Care Med. 2007;35:477–82.
28. Mark JB, Steinbrook RA, Gugino LD, Maddi R, Hartwell B, Shemin R, DiSesa V, Rida WN. Continuous noninvasive monitoring of cardiac output with esophageal Doppler ultrasound during cardiac surgery. Anesth Analg. 1986;65:1013–20.
29. Penny JA, Anthony J, Shennan AH, de Swiet M, Singer M. A comparison of hemodynamic data derived by pulmonary artery flotation catheter and the esophageal Doppler monitor in preeclampsia. Am J Obstet Gynecol. 2000;183:658–61.
30. Leather HA, Wouters PF. Oesophageal Doppler monitoring overestimates cardiac output during lumbar epidural anaesthesia. Br J Anaesth. 2001;86:794–7.
31. Papavramidis T, Pliakos I, Papavramidou N, Marinis A, Kesisoglou I. Abdominal compartment syndrome – intra-abdominal hypertension: defining, diagnosing, and managing. J Emerg Trauma Shock. 2011;4:279.
32. Odeberg-Wernerman S. Laparoscopic surgery – effects on circulatory and respiratory physiology: an overview. Eur J Surg. 2000;166:4–11.
33. Robotham JL, Wise RA, Bromberger-Barnea B. Effects of changes in abdominal pressure on left ventricular performance and regional blood flow. Crit Care Med. 1985;13:803–9.
34. Reuter DA, Goresch T, Goepfert MSG, Wildhirt SM, Kilger E, Goetz AE. Effects of mid-line thoracotomy on the interaction between mechanical ventilation and cardiac filling during cardiac surgery. Br J Anaesth. 2004;92:808–13.
35. van Lavieren M, Veelenturf J, Hofhuizen C, van der Kolk M, van der Hoeven J, Pickkers P, Lemson J, Lansdorp B. Dynamic preload indicators decrease when the abdomen is opened. BMC Anesthesiol. 2014;14:90.
36. Jacques D, Bendjelid K, Duperret S, Colling J, Piriou V, Viale J-P. Pulse pressure variation and stroke volume variation during increased intra-abdominal pressure: an experimental study. Crit Care. 2011;15:R33.
37. Wyffels PAH, Sergeant P, Wouters PF. The value of pulse pressure and stroke volume variation as predictors of fluid responsiveness during open chest surgery. Anaesthesia. 2010;65:704–9.
38. Koliopanos A, Zografos G, Skiathitis S, Stithos D, Voukena V, Karampinis A, Papastratis G. Esophageal Doppler (ODM II) improves intraoperative hemodynamic monitoring during laparoscopic surgery. Surg Laparosc Endosc Percutan Tech. 2005;15:332–8.
39. Zhang J, Critchley LAH, Huang L. The effect of aorta unfolding and remodelling on oesophageal Doppler readings as probe depth is varied. Br J Anaesth. 2015;115:708–15.

40. Dark PM, Singer M. The validity of trans-esophageal Doppler ultrasonography as a measure of cardiac output in critically ill adults. Intensive Care Med. 2004;30:2060–6.
41. Mythen MG, Webb AR. Perioperative plasma volume expansion reduces the incidence of gut mucosal hypoperfusion during cardiac surgery. Arch Surg. 1995;130:423–9.
42. Abbas SM, Hill AG. Systematic review of the literature for the use of oesophageal Doppler monitor for fluid replacement in major abdominal surgery. Anaesthesia. 2007;63:44–51.
43. Walsh SR, Tang T, Bass S, Gaunt ME. Doppler-guided intra-operative fluid management during major abdominal surgery: systematic review and meta-analysis. Int J Clin Pract. 2007;62:466–70.
44. Sinclair S, James S, Singer M. Intraoperative intravascular volume optimisation and length of hospital stay after repair of proximal femoral fracture: randomised controlled trial. BMJ. 1997;315:909–12.
45. Venn R, Steele A, Richardson P, Poloniecki J, Grounds M, Newman P. Randomized controlled trial to investigate influence of the fluid challenge on duration of hospital stay and perioperative morbidity in patients with hip fractures. Br J Anaesth. 2002;88:65–71.
46. Gan TJ, Soppitt A, Maroof M, El-Moalem H, Robertson KM, Moretti E, Dwane P, Glass PSA. Goal-directed intraoperative fluid administration reduces length of hospital stay after major surgery. Anesthesiology. 2002;97:820–6.
47. Conway DH, Mayall R, Abdul-Latif MS, Gilligan S, Tackaberry C. Randomised controlled trial investigating the influence of intravenous fluid titration using oesophageal Doppler monitoring during bowel surgery. Anaesthesia. 2002;57:845–9.
48. Wakeling HG, McFall MR, Jenkins CS, Woods WGA, Miles WFA, Barclay GR, Fleming SC. Intraoperative oesophageal Doppler guided fluid management shortens postoperative hospital stay after major bowel surgery. Br J Anaesth. 2005;95:634–42.
49. Noblett SE, Snowden CP, Shenton BK, Horgan AF. Randomized clinical trial assessing the effect of Doppler-optimized fluid management on outcome after elective colorectal resection. Br J Surg. 2006;93:1069–76.
50. Zakhaleva J, Tam J, Denoya PI, Bishawi M, Bergamaschi R. The impact of intravenous fluid administration on complication rates in bowel surgery within an enhanced recovery protocol: a randomized controlled trial. Color Dis. 2013;15:892–9.
51. El Sharkawy OA, Refaat EK, Ibraheem AEM, Mahdy WR, Fayed NA, Mourad WS, Abd Elhafez HS, Yassen KA. Transoesophageal Doppler compared to central venous pressure for perioperative hemodynamic monitoring and fluid guidance in liver resection. Saudi J Anaesth. 2013;7:378–86.
52. Picard J, Bedague D, Bouzat P, Ollinet C, Albaladejo P, Bosson J-L, Payen J-F. Oesophageal Doppler to optimize intraoperative haemodynamics during prone position. A randomized controlled trial. Anaesth Crit Care Pain Med. 2016;35:255–60.
53. Kaufmann KB, Stein L, Bogatyreva L, Ulbrich F, Kaifi JT, Hauschke D, Loop T, Goebel U. Oesophageal Doppler guided goal-directed haemodynamic therapy in thoracic surgery – a single centre randomized parallel-arm trial. BJA Br J Anaesth. 2017;118:852–61.
54. Haxby EJ, Gray MR, Rodriguez C, Nott D, Springall M, Mythen M. Assessment of cardiovascular changes during laparoscopic hernia repair using oesophageal Doppler. Br J Anaesth. 1997;78:515–9.
55. McKendry M, McGloin H, Saberi D, Caudwell L, Brady AR, Singer M. Randomised controlled trial assessing the impact of a nurse delivered, flow monitored protocol for optimisation of circulatory status after cardiac surgery. BMJ. 2004;329:258.
56. Chytra I, Pradl R, Bosman R, Pelnár P, Kasal E, Zidková A. Esophageal Doppler-guided fluid management decreases blood lactate levels in multiple-trauma patients: a randomized controlled trial. Crit Care. 2007;11:R24.
57. Poeze M, Ramsay G, Greve JW, Singer M. Prediction of postoperative cardiac surgical morbidity and organ failure within 4 hours of intensive care unit admission using esophageal Doppler ultrasonography. Crit Care Med. 1999;27:1288–94.
58. Srinivasa S, Taylor MHG, Sammour T, Kahokehr AA, Hill AG. Oesophageal Doppler-guided fluid administration in colorectal surgery: critical appraisal of published clinical trials. Acta Anaesthesiol Scand. 2011;55:4–13.
59. Challand C, Struthers R, Sneyd JR, Erasmus PD, Mellor N, Hosie KB, Minto G. Randomized controlled trial of intraoperative goal-directed fluid therapy in aerobically fit and unfit patients having major colorectal surgery. BJA Br J Anaesth. 2012;108:53–62.
60. McKenny M, Conroy P, Wong A, Farren M, Gleeson N, Walsh C, O'Malley C, Dowd N. A randomised prospective trial of intra-operative oesophageal Doppler-guided fluid administration in major gynaecological surgery. Anaesthesia. 2013;68:1224–31.

61. Brandstrup B, Svendsen PE, Rasmussen M, et al. Which goal for fluid therapy during colorectal surgery is followed by the best outcome: near-maximal stroke volume or zero fluid balance? BJA Br J Anaesth. 2012;109:191–9.
62. Srinivasa S, Taylor MHG, Singh PP, Yu T-C, Soop M, Hill AG. Randomized clinical trial of goal-directed fluid therapy within an enhanced recovery protocol for elective colectomy. Br J Surg. 2013;100:66–74.
63. Phan TD, D'Souza B, Rattray MJ, Johnston MJ, Cowie BS. A randomised controlled trial of fluid restriction compared to oesophageal Doppler-guided goal-directed fluid therapy in elective major colorectal surgery within an Enhanced Recovery After Surgery program. Anaesth Intensive Care. 2014;42:752–60.
64. Srinivasa S, Lemanu DP, Singh PP, Taylor MHG, Hill AG. Systematic review and meta-analysis of oesophageal Doppler-guided fluid management in colorectal surgery. Br J Surg. 2013;100:1701–8.
65. Mowatt G, Houston G, Hernández R, de Verteuil R, Fraser C, Cuthbertson B, Vale L. Systematic review of the clinical effectiveness and cost-effectiveness of oesophageal Doppler monitoring in critically ill and high-risk surgical patients. Health Technol Assess (Rockv). 2009;13:iii–iv, ix–xii, 1–95.
66. Bundgaard-Nielsen M, Holte K, Secher NH, Kehlet H. Monitoring of peri-operative fluid administration by individualized goal-directed therapy. Acta Anaesthesiol Scand. 2007;51:331–40.
67. Cecconi M, Corredor C, Arulkumaran N, Abuella G, Ball J, Grounds RM, Hamilton M, Rhodes A. Clinical review: goal-directed therapy-what is the evidence in surgical patients? The effect on different risk groups. Crit Care. 2013;17:209.
68. Grocott MPW, Dushianthan A, Hamilton MA, Mythen MG, Harrison D, Rowan K. Perioperative increase in global blood flow to explicit defined goals and outcomes after surgery: a Cochrane systematic review. Br J Anaesth. 2013;111:535–48.
69. Hamilton MA, Cecconi M, Rhodes A. A systematic review and meta-analysis on the use of preemptive hemodynamic intervention to improve postoperative outcomes in moderate and high-risk surgical patients. Anesth Analg. 2011;112:1392–402.
70. Morris C. Oesophageal Doppler monitoring, doubt and equipoise: evidence based medicine means change. Anaesthesia. 2013;68:684–8.

Additional Resources

The Deltex Medical website (http://www.deltexmedical.com/) provides excellent educational training resources for the use and interpretation of CardioQ-ODM monitors.

Bioimpedance and Bioreactance

Lee S. Nguyen and Pierre Squara

M. R. Pinsky et al. (eds.), *Hemodynamic Monitoring*, Lessons from the ICU,
https://doi.org/10.1007/978-3-319-69269-2_28

Learning Objectives

This chapter covers:

- How the bioimpedance and bioreactance signals are generated
- Which hypotheses allow the thoracic fluid content, stroke volume, and cardiac output from the signal to be estimated
- How the principle was validated in studies and, subsequently, what metrologic performance can be expected from these technologies

28.1 Introduction

Bioimpedance (*Z*) refers to the response of biological tissues to the application of a sine wave electric current. Physically, it is composed of a constant resistance (*R*) and a time-varying reactance (*X*). *Z* and *X* differ in their sensing and filtering methods but share the same model and assumptions to derive stroke volume (SV) and cardiac output (CO) from the electric signal.

Although it was recognized in the late nineteenth century that biological tissues had specific electric impedance, correlations with cardiac activity only started in the 1930s [1–3] and correlations with body water, in the 1960s [4, 5]. A huge leap in the understanding of thoracic impedance was made when the National Aeronautics and Space Administration (NASA) looked into continuous monitoring of the hemodynamic status of spacecraft pilots. Subsequent investigations described the model by which SV could be derived from the electric signal [6–9]. Additional lines of research in various medical fields including cardiac surgery and nephrology also started using thoracic impedance for estimating thoracic blood volume [10–12].

Although these technologies are probably the most promising truly noninvasive methods for CO monitoring and despite half a century of development [13–16], their metrological performance remains controversial and their practical use limited to hemodynamic maneuvers (i.e., intraindividual changes). This limitation raises questions about the model assumptions and the signal calibration, requiring further developments.

28.2 Signal Acquisition

Although electrical impedance is the opposition that a circuit presents to a current when a voltage is applied, standard bioimpedance and bioreactance systems apply a high-frequency electrical calibrated current across the thorax and measure changes in output voltage (explained below). The ratio between voltage and current amplitudes is generically referred to as impedance and varies in inverse proportion to the amount of fluid in the thorax. In addition to changing the amplitude of an electrical signal passing through the thorax, changes in thoracic blood volume also modify the electrical capacitive and inductive (i.e., reactance) properties of the electrical signal. This time-varying bioreactance can be detected as a change in frequency or phase of the received signal. Traditionally, techniques for the measurement of frequency modulation (FM) are inherently less prone to noise than techniques to measure changes in signal amplitudes (AM). There is a direct analogy here with the difference between AM and FM radio.

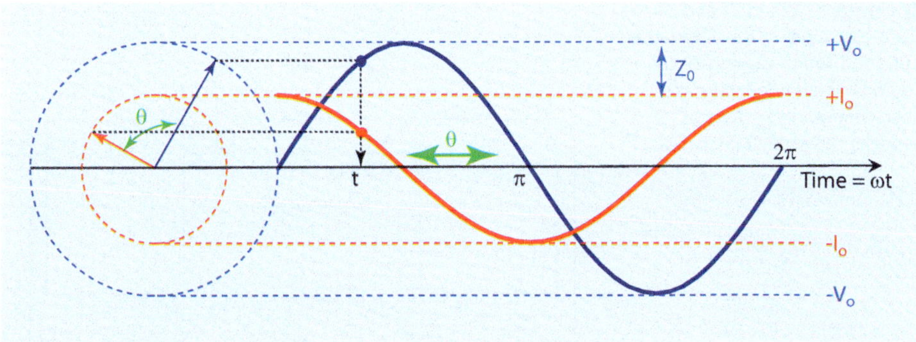

Fig. 28.1 Trigonometric cycle and corresponding sine wave voltage with phase set to zero (in blue) and current response (in red). The blue arrow represents the amplitude ratio $Z_0 = V_o/I_o$. The green arrows show a phase lag set to 90° in this example for clarity. The blue and red plots show the value of V and I at time t, respectively. The black arrow shows the value of $V(t)$

28.2.1 Electrical Principle at Steady State

The response of an electric circuit to a sine wave voltage V, oscillating at a frequency $F = \omega/2\pi$, corresponds to a sine wave current I oscillating at the same frequency but with a phase shift θ (see Fig. 28.1). At any time, the ratio V/I is equal to impedance Z. These relations can be symbolized mathematically by the traditional set of equations:

$$V = V_o \sin \omega t \quad \text{or} \quad V = V_o \cdot e^{j\omega t}$$

$$I = I_o \sin(\omega t - \theta) \quad \text{or} \quad I = I_o \cdot e^{j(\omega t - \theta)}$$

$$Z = V / I \quad \text{or} \quad Z = V_o / I_o \cdot e^{j\theta}$$

Using Euler's formula, $A \cdot e^{j\phi} = A \cdot (\cos \phi + j \sin \phi)$,

$$Z = V_o / I_o \cdot (\cos \theta + j \sin \theta) \tag{28.1}$$

$$\text{and conventionally } Z_0 = V_o / I_o \tag{28.2}$$

where V_o is the amplitude of the oscillating voltage in volts, I_o is the amplitude of the oscillating current in amperes, Z is in ohms, ω is in radians/s, F is in Hz, and θ is in radians. Z is composed of a resistance (R), its real part, and of a reactance (X), its time-varying part. According to $Z = R + jX$, (28.1) can be decomposed into $R = V_o/I_o \cos \theta$ and $X = V_o/I_o \sin \theta$. Since $j = e^{j\pi/2}$, j is indicative that R and X are in 90° of phase.

28.2.2 Electrical Principle During Transient Changes

The above relationships are valid under steady-state conditions when the impact of transient changes is negligible, allowing Z_0 to be derived. However, during transient changes, for example, when Z varies following heart ejection, the frequency and phase also change transiently. The formulas linking Z, V_o, I_o, and θ then become complex, and simply

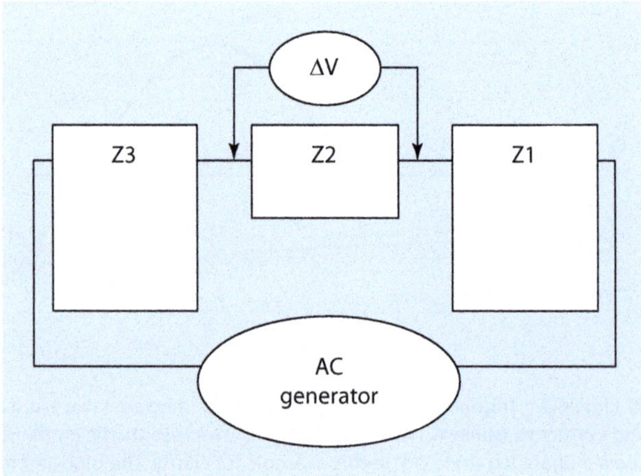

Fig. 28.2 When $Z1$ and $Z3 >> Z2$, the changes in the alternative current through varying $Z2$ can be considered negligible, and then changes in V_o (ΔV) are representative of $Z2$ changes

28

recalculating Z from V and I measurements is not possible anymore. To circumvent this issue, a different circuit can be created (Fig. 28.2) to make the change in I_o negligible in a given part of the circuit. Then, from this constant I_o, changes in V_o and θ can be measured in order to calculate Z.

In this double circuit, the current going through $Z2$ and the voltage across $Z2$ are represented by the following equations, if ΔV is the specific change in V_o for a given period T and if we set the steady-state phase to zero.

$$I = I_o \cdot e^{j\omega t} \quad V = V_o \cdot e^{j\omega t} + \Delta V \cdot e^{j(\omega t + \Delta\omega t + \theta)} \text{ then,}$$

$$V = \left[V_o + \Delta V \cdot e^{j(\Delta\omega t + \theta)} \right] \cdot e^{j\omega t}$$

$$\text{Leading to } \Delta Z = \Delta V / I_o \cdot e^{j(\Delta\omega t + \theta)}$$

The sum of all periods T ($k = 1$ to end) gives a final set of equations

$$V(t) = \left[V_o + \Sigma_k \Delta V_k \cdot e^{j(\Delta\omega k t + \theta k)} \right] \cdot e^{j\omega t} \tag{28.3}$$

$$\text{Leading to } Z(t) = \Sigma_k \Delta V_k / I_o \cdot e^{j(\Delta\omega k t + \theta k)} \tag{28.4}$$

$$\text{or } Z(t) = \Sigma_k \Delta V_k / I_o \cdot [\cos(\Delta\omega_k t + \theta_k) + j \sin(\Delta\omega_k t + \theta_k)]$$

Since $Z(t) = R(t) + jX(t)$ then

$$R(t) = \Sigma_k \Delta V_k / I_o \cdot \cos(\Delta\omega_k t + \theta_k) \text{ and}$$

$$X(t) = \Sigma_k \Delta V_k / I_o \cdot \sin(\Delta\omega_k t + \theta_k) \tag{28.5}$$

This shows the physical links between $Z(t)$, the time change in Z, its amplitude modulation (AM) component as seen by detecting the V_o envelope $\Delta V(t)$, and its frequency modulation (FM) component, as seen by detecting $\Delta\omega(t)$ (Fig. 28.3). As a consequence, the AM signal and the FM signal, as seen on the receive side, have the same shape.

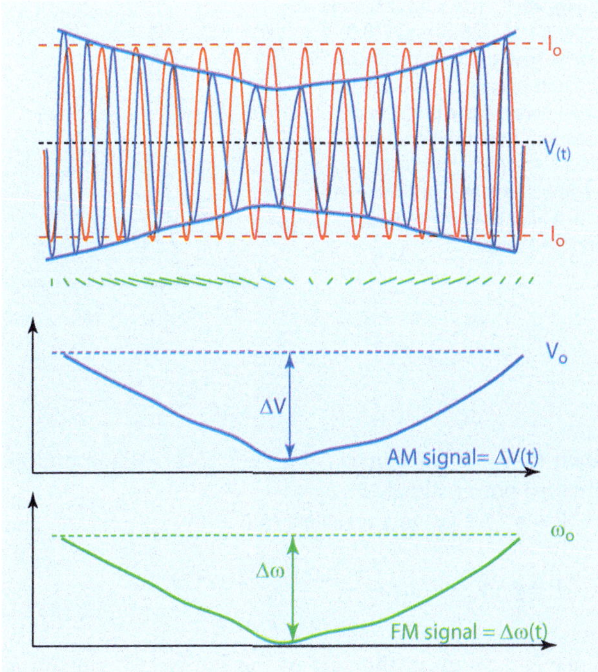

Fig. 28.3 Upper part, in red the input constant alternating current: I_o = 5 mA, frequency 75 kHz (ω = 150,000π radians/s.). In blue the output voltage. $V(t)$ = 200 ± 2 mVolts, frequency $F(t)$ = 75 kHz ± 5 Hz. The instantaneous changes in phase are figured in green. In the middle, the V_o envelope (AM component) is extracted from the envelope of ΔV = 4 mV, corresponding to ΔZ = 4/5 = 0.8 Ω. The lower part shows the corresponding changes in frequency as obtained by the sum of instant phase shift (FM signal) figuring ΔF = 10 Hz ($\Delta\omega$ = 20π radians/s.). Using appropriate scaling, the shape of the AM and FM signals is the same

28.2.3 Bioimpedance and Bioreactance

For estimating CO, the chest can be considered as varying impedance as shown in Fig. 28.3 [6].

Standard bioimpedance-based medical systems apply a high-frequency electrical current of known amplitude and frequency across the chest via two electrodes and measure the resulting changes in voltage using two other electrodes placed in adjacent regions. Two or more different circuits can be used and averaged. The ratio V_0/I_0 is a measure of the steady-state transthoracic impedance Z_0 when there is no blood flow and is used to estimate baseline chest fluid. In the presence of flow through the aorta, $Z(t)$ decreases periodically from Z_0 following Eq. (28.4) proportionally to the increase of water and iron in the thorax (i.e., blood volume).

Traditional bioimpedance systems use the AM signal $\Delta V(t)$ (28.3). Bioreactance systems use the FM signal $\Delta\omega(t)$ (28.5). Although the curves depicting AM and FM depending on time have the same shape after appropriate scaling, FM analysis yields a better signal-to-noise ratio. As the probability of interference (noise due to other electronic devices) is proportional to the bandwidth, in an AM signal as shown in (28.3), $V(t)$ is a high-frequency signal ($\omega = 2\pi F$ = 150,000π radians/s associated with a high level of noise. Conversely, the FM component in (28.5) with $\Delta\omega = 20\pi$ radians.s^{-1}) is associated with a lower level of noise (Fig. 28.4).

In practice, the FM signal is extracted from the autocorrelation method, by multiplying the input current carrier by the received voltage signal. First, a limiter is applied on the output voltage (28.3) saturating the real part of the signal. To magnify the FM component, when multiplying voltage by current, the current carrier phase is shifted to an angle of 90°.

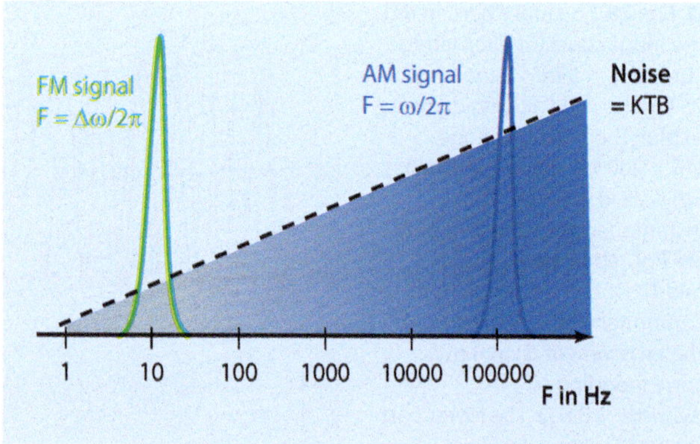

Fig. 28.4 The output signals coming from (28.3) and (28.5) can be seen using an oscillator. The noise power (*N*) is given by KTB where *K* is the Boltzmann's constant, *T* the temperature in Kelvin, and *B* the bandwidth in Hz. AM is located in a bandwidth with a high level of noise as opposed to FM

Then $I = I_o \cdot e^{j\omega t}$ becomes $I = I_o \cdot e^{j(\omega t + \pi/2)}$. When multiplying by the output voltage, we obtain a power signal (P):

$P = V \cdot I = [V_o + \Delta V \cdot e^{j(\Delta\omega t + \theta)}] \cdot e^{j\omega t} \cdot I_o \cdot e^{j(\omega t + \pi/2)}$ that can be rearranged as

28

$$P = \left[I_o V_o + I_o \Delta V \cdot e^{j(\Delta\omega t + \theta)} \right] \cdot e^{j(2\omega t + \pi/2)} \tag{28.6}$$

Since $2\omega t >> \Delta\omega t$, the part of the Eq. (28.6) containing $2\omega t$ can be filtered, to better decrease the noise (Fig. 28.4). If the low-pass filter rejects frequencies near $2\omega t$, the filtered output becomes:

$P = I_o \Delta V \cdot e^{j(\Delta\omega t + \theta)}$ and for the sum of $T(k = 1$ to end),

$$P(t) = \Sigma_k I_o \Delta V_k \cdot e^{j(\Delta\omega k t + \theta k)}$$

And again, from Euler's formula, this can be written

$$P(t) = \Sigma_k I_o \Delta V_k \cdot \left[\cos(\Delta\omega_k t + \theta_k) + j \sin(\Delta\omega_k t + \theta_k) \right]$$

When divided by the known value I_o^2, this signal is equivalent to $Z(t)$ as shown in (28.4) with a real part, R, and an imaginary part, X. The limiter, applied before entering $V(t)$ in the multiplier, has saturated the real part of the signal, $\Sigma_k \Delta V_k / I_o \cdot \cos(\Delta\omega_k t + \theta_k)$, and has then fixed it to a constant envelope C that can also be filtered ($F = 0$ Hz). The final signal, formulated $\Sigma_k \Delta V_k / I_o \cdot \sin(\Delta\omega_k t + \theta_k)$, is that of the bioreactance signal $X(t)$ seen in (28.5) and schematized in the lower part of Fig. 28.3

28.3 From the Signal to the Cardiac Output

Bioimpedance and bioreactance systems are based on the same general physical model linking the change in aortic volume and the change in chest impedance [6, 17]. This model is based on the impedance law applied to the aorta considered as a conductor $Z = \rho L / A$, where ρ = specific resistivity, L = length, and A = cross-sectional area of the tube. Twelve assumptions and mathematical simplifications are necessary to derive the stroke volume (SV) from the change in impedance ΔZ.

1. If we simultaneously emit and receive across and around the chest an alternating current, a change in thoracic impedance might be due to a change in blood flow (volume/time).
2. The effect of ventilation on the blood flow can be averaged.
3. The blood volume of low-pressure vessels (veins) is relatively constant.
4. The thickness of myocardial walls electrically isolates intraventricle blood volumes. These four first assumptions allow us to consider that a change in thoracic impedance may be mostly due to variations of aortic blood volume. Variation of impedance that is not due to variation of aortic blood volume (i.e., pulmonary artery) is also linked to stroke volume. Therefore, a coefficient of proportionality can be determined to interrelate changes in impedance with changes in aortic blood volume.
5. The aorta can be considered as a cylinder with a constant length.
6. Blood resistivity is constant so that the hemoglobin concentration is stable during the measurements. When hemoglobin is out of the normal range but stable, the impact of high or low hemoglobin concentrations can be corrected.

Then, from these six assumptions and from $Z = \rho L/A$, we can write, $Z(t) = \rho L/A(t)$, where $A(t)$ is the time aortic expansion. Since $A(t) = V_a(t)/L$, where $V_a(t)$ is the instantaneous aortic volume, $Z(t) = \rho L^2/V_a(t)$ and at any time:

$$V_a(t) = \rho L^2 / Z(t) \tag{28.7}$$

It is impossible to measure the change in aortic impedance $Z(t)$ noninvasively. We can only measure easily the change in thoracic impedance $Z_T(t)$. Deriving $Z(t)$ from $Z_T(t)$ requires three other assumptions.

7. The resistivity ρ of blood and thoracic tissues are similar.
8. The thorax can be considered as a cylinder.
9. The thorax can be considered as a unique chamber C in parallel with the aorta with constant impedance Z_C.

With these new assumptions, $1/Z_T(t) = 1/Z_C + 1/Z(t)$. Solving this for $Z(t)$ gives:

$$Z(t) = Z_T(t) \bullet Z_C / [Z_C - Z_T(t)] \tag{28.8}$$

Two additional assumptions are required to derive the cardiac output from impedance measurement:

10. If the aortic impedance is small as compared to the tissue impedance, $Z_T(t)$ is close to Z_C and to the basic impedance Z_0. Then, $Z_T(t) \times Z_C \approx Z_0^2$. Similarly, the denominator $[Z_C - Z_T(t)]$ would be zero. As this is impossible, the assumption is:
11. $Z_C - Z_T(t) \approx Z_0 - Z_T(t) = \Delta Z(t)$. Then (28.8) can be written $Z(t) = Z_0^2/\Delta Z(t)$ and (28.7) becomes $V_a(t) = \rho L^2/Z_0^2 \times \Delta Z(t)$.
    From the end of filling to the end of ejection, $\Delta V_a = \rho L^2/Z_0^2 \cdot \Delta Z$. Pulsatile change of aortic volume ΔV_a is linked to SV by ΔV_a = SV – the aortic output flow. Because the output flow is unknown, it is necessary to extrapolate SV using another assumption. One approach requires apnea and an independent assessment of aortic valve closure, which is not possible in clinical practice. An alternative method requires the final assumption.
12. ΔV_{ae} (change in aortic volume that would occur if there was no output flow) can be extrapolated according to SV = $\Delta V_{ae} = \rho L^2/Z_0^2 \cdot \Delta Z_{ae}$.

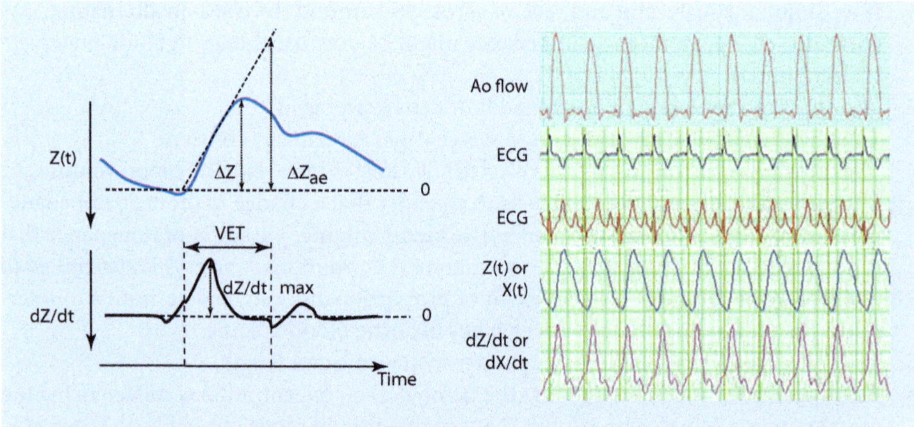

Fig. 28.5 Left, the upper part shows ΔZ_{ae}, the extrapolation in *Z*(*t*) if the aorta was a capacitor without output flow. This value can be estimated by the product of the maximum *Z*(*t*) slope (in Ω/sec.) by its duration (in sec.). The duration to reach ΔZ_{ae} is the left ventricle ejection time (VET) identified from characteristic points on the dZ/dt curve (lower panel), and the maximum *Z*(*t*) slope is the point of its maximum time derivative (dZ/dt max). Then $\Delta Z_{ae} = \text{VET} \cdot \text{dZ/dt max}$. In this figure, the x axis is conventionally inverted so that the bioimpedance signal mimics the aortic pressure curve. On the right, impedance and reactance (lower curves) are in phase with the ECG and flow signals

28

Substituting ΔZ_{ae} with VET dZ/dt_{max} (see Fig. 28.5) allows us to reach the final formula for SV:

$$\text{SV} = \rho L^2 / Z_0^{\ 2} \bullet \text{VET} \bullet \text{dZ} / \text{dt}_{max}. \tag{28.9}$$

In both bioimpedance- and bioreactance-based systems, the assumptions are the same. We have seen that the shape of the AM and FM signal is the same, so dZ/dt_{max} can be replaced by dX/dt_{max}. A transformation constant *C* is simply added to ρL^2 which is also constant for each individual patient, so that the final bioreactance formula for SV is:

$$\text{SV} = C\rho L^2 / Z_0^{\ 2} \bullet \text{VET} \bullet \text{dX} / \text{dt}_{max} \tag{28.10}$$

and CO = heart rate $\cdot\ C\rho L^2/Z_0^{\ 2} \cdot \text{VET} \cdot \text{dX/dt}_{max}$.

Several approaches have been suggested to limit the impact of these 12 assumptions and to improve the reliability of CO estimation. For example, a truncated cone has been suggested instead of a cylinder to model the thorax [8]. More generally, each of the assumptions may lead to individual discordances. To address this issue, a multivariate calibration factor (CF) is required using a reference method based on age, gender, height, weight, body surface area, body mass index, and, if available, hematocrit and pulmonary artery pressure. This CF derived from a specific population raises the question of its "generalizability" to all populations of patients. The final practical bioimpedance/bioreactance formulas for SV are then:

$$\text{SV} = \text{CF} / Z_0^{\ 2} \bullet \text{VET} \bullet \text{dZ} / \text{dt}_{max} \tag{28.11}$$

$$\text{SV} = \text{CF} / Z_0^{\ 2} \bullet \text{VET} \bullet \text{dX} / \text{dt}_{max} \tag{28.12}$$

28.4 Validation Studies

28.4.1 Experimental Data

One may be skeptical about the reliability of bioimpedance and/or bioreactance- derived CO due to the number of underlying assumptions and simplifications. However, bioimpedance-based systems have proven their interest in various settings. Moreover, bioreactance can be considered an improved form of bioimpedance based on similar assumptions and simplifications but giving a better signal-to-noise ratio.

The following example of an animal study shows that the assumptions required to derive CO from the bioimpedance and bioreactance signal may be most often valid [13]. In open-chest pigs, total cardiac output was controlled using an extracorporeal cardiopulmonary bypass pump while maintaining pulsatility in the pulmonary artery and aorta. Adjusting the pump allowed the CO to vary. Results from one animal are shown in ◘ Fig. 28.6 (upper). The bioreactance-derived CO closely and quite immediately matched the output set by the pump. Inter-animal variability of the results was moderate, and the overall results from nine animals in this series showed strong correlation between bioreactance CO and CPB: $r = 0.90 \pm 0.09$, range 0.75–0.99. The other experiment was done under the same conditions but comparing bioreactance-derived CO with that of a Transonic® ultrasound flow probe positioned directly around the pulmonary artery. CO variation was performed by sequential increases and decreases of dobutamine infusion. Results from one animal are shown in ◘ Fig. 28.6 (lower). Again, bioreactance-derived CO closely tracked the reference CO. The overall results of nine animals showed a strong correlation between these two modalities of CO measurement: $r = 0.64 \pm 0.19$, range 0.41–0.96.

However, in these experimental studies, bioreactance CO did not include any calibration factor (CF). The initial CO value was simply adjusted to the baseline CO of the reference method. Therefore, only relative changes in CO were analyzed. The dismaying results observed in some animals may be attributable to the different assumptions and mathematic simplifications of the model. Indeed, each assumption may be more or less valid for each individual and may occasionally introduce errors. This mandates further development to improve our understanding of the origin of the signal.

28.4.2 Clinical Data

Metrologic parameters for measurements (accuracy, trueness, reproducibility, repeatability, etc.) and for devices (sensitivity, linearity, selectivity, resolution, stability, step response time, etc.) are neither reported nor standardized in medicine [18, 19].

Unfortunately, validation studies are often limited to the evaluation of the accuracy through an averaged bias of measurements and its inter-patient variability or percentage error, often improperly qualified "precision."

This paragraph will review the available data regarding (1) systematic errors of measurements, qualifying the *untrueness*, and (2) random errors of measurements, qualifying the *imprecision*, either for the same device and same patient (*repeatability*) or for different devices and different patients (*reproducibility*), from which are derived the *resolution* (i.e., identifying small changes) and the *step response time* of any monitoring device. Without other specification, the *inaccuracy* of a measurement combines *untrueness* and *imprecision*.

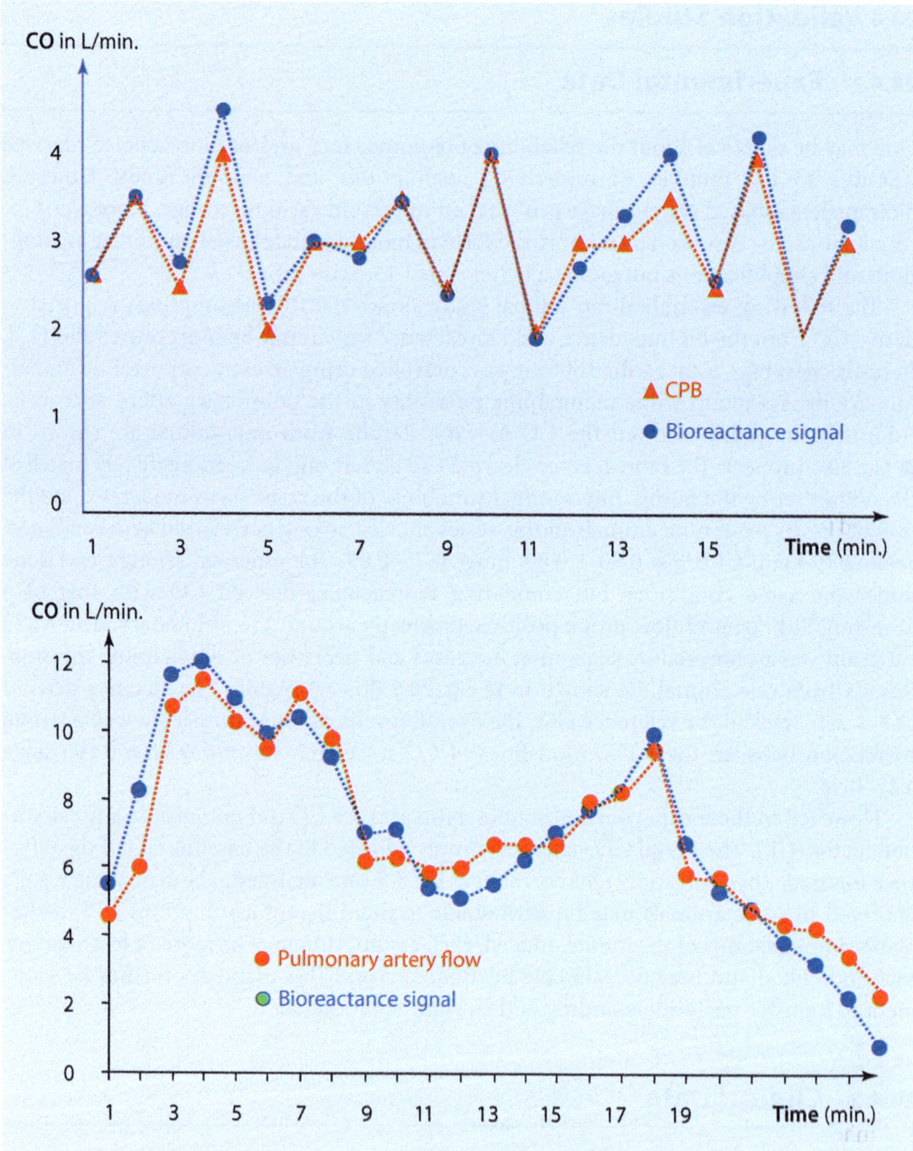

Fig. 28.6 Upper panel, bioreactance CO versus cardiopulmonary bypass (CPB). Lower panel, bioreactance CO versus Transonic® flow probe. (Reprinted from Ref. [13])

28.4.2.1 Baseline Impedance for Thoracic Fluid Content Assessment

In all devices based on bioimpedance or bioreactance, static impedance Z_0 as seen in (28.2) can be derived without assumptions. For any device tested, whatever the setting, studies showed that $1/Z_0$ co-varies with thoracic blood water and blood volume [20–29]. Similarly to time-dependent varying variables (impedance and reactance), an autocalibration is mandatory to adjust for chest anatomic characteristics [30]. Hence, patients act as their own reference and only intraindividual relative changes are estimated. On the other hand, absolute measurements are of poor interest [31], whereas when taking a patient as his own reference, there is no systematic error. Although less studied, fluctuation due to random errors (imprecision) was reported to be low after appropriate averaging, with 2 SE/mean estimated <2% [32, 33], allowing a resolution <3% when using the least significant change ($2\sqrt{2}$SE) as indicator [18, 19], and a step response time of 1 min.

28.4.2.2 Time-Varying Impedance for SV and CO Assessment

When used to estimate SV and CO, bioimpedance-based technologies – also referred to as electrical impedance plethysmography, impedance cardiography, electric cardiometry, integral rheography, or thoracic electrical bioimpedance – have been used in different products: NCCOM (Bomed Medical, Irvine CA), BioZ (CardioDynamics, San Diego, CA), NICCOMO (MEDIS, Ilmenau, Germany), ICON (Osypka Cardiotronic, Berlin, Germany), ICG (Philips Medical Systems, Andover, MA), NICOMON (Larsen and Toubro Ltd., Mumbai, India), the CSM3000 (Cheers Sails Medical, Shenzhen, China), and PhysioFlow (Manatec Biomedical, Paris, France).

The NICaS system (NI Medical, Petah-Tikva, Israel) uses the same principles but applied to the whole body. An alternating current is applied in a wrist-to-ankle configuration, and then the electrical current is assumed to seek the path of least resistance (Kirchhoff's laws) and to flow through the blood. The way SV is derived from the signal uses a proprietary algorithm linking the signal, not only with the change in the aortic volume but also with the change of the whole arterial system volume.

In the ECOM system (Ecom Medical, San Juan Capistrano, CA), the transmitting and receiving electrodes are located on the cuff of an endotracheal tube, therefore close to the ascending aorta, in order to minimize the impact of analogous signals from other cardiac structures.

The inductance thoracocardiography or respiratory inductive plethysmography (LifeShirt, Vivometrics, Ventura, CA) is not in the scope of the chapter. It is a different technology based on the analysis of ventricular volume curves recorded by an inductive plethysmographic transducer encircling the chest at the level of the heart.

Although early studies in controlled settings yielded interesting results, and despite the development of progressively more complex algorithms [14, 15], more recent studies showed conflicting results concerning the individual accuracy of bioimpedance-based measurements. Discrepancies were more frequent in papers studying patients hospitalized in intensive care and postoperative care units [34–40] where percentage errors >50% have been observed. The lack of consistent accuracy shown by these studies may be due to the inherently low signal-to-noise ratio of this approach but also to inherent discordances between the reference population used to derive the CF and individual patients in specific populations. Consequently, despite the wide array of available products, this technology is not widely used in ICU for estimating the absolute value of CO. However, monitoring capabilities are not only based on trueness but also on precision. Although the real precision (intra-patient variability due to random error) was only reported in one validation study [36], it is estimated to be good with a 2SD/mean around 15% [41]. Hence, the resolution is around 20%, and few elementary measurements are averaged before displaying a value [19], providing a fast step response time, close to 1 min [40, 42]. These features broadly explain the results reported in situations such as exercise testing [43, 44]. Indeed, whether or not the CO value is true, its variation can be tracked, and any significant change can be detected and quantified as exemplified in ◘ Fig. 28.6 [41].

28.4.2.3 Time-Varying Reactance for SV Assessment

Bioreactance technology is limited to two products (NICOM and Starling) from the same company (Cheetah Medical, Newton Center, MA). Two initial validation studies were performed in post-cardiac surgical patients in the same population of patients from which the CF was derived. The first study included a cohort of 119 patients, and the bioreactance device (NICOM) was compared to continuous thermodilution (PAC-CCO) [16]. In the first study, bias was optimally analyzed during 40 periods of stable PAC-CCO to minimize the effects of both natural changes in CO and time responsiveness differences of the two devices. This part of the study included more than 9000 minute-by-minute CO values. The inter-patient-averaged bias was negligible (0.16 L/min), and the variability of the biases (2SD) was close to 1 L/min (see Fig. 28.7). Regarding all the CO minute-by-minute values, 80.4% of them had a bias <20%.

The random errors of measurements were assessed by the variability of measurements around the CO trend line slope. It was systematically higher for the bioreactance device (2SD/mean = 12 ± 7% vs. 14 ± 4%) as compared to continuous thermodilution. After hemodynamic challenge, the time responsiveness of the bioreactance was 3 min faster than continuous thermodilution, and the amplitude of response was comparable. Finally, the sensitivity for detecting significant CO directional changes was 93% and specificity was 93%.

28

In a second study including 29 patients, bioreactance was compared to PAC-CCO and to a pulse-contour system using autocalibration (Vigileo) [45]. This study showed similar correlations between bioreactance and pulse contour, taking PAC-CCO as reference. During recording periods when PAC-CCO was stable, including 4100 minute-by-minute CO values, the averaged bias was negligible for both bioreactance and pulse contour (0.0 and − 0.1 L/min., respectively). When CO values were averaged during all periods of PAC-CCO stability, the relationship between bioreactance and pulse contour was closer than between continuous thermodilution and pulse contour. Precision was not significantly different between the two modalities of measurement. Responsiveness was not

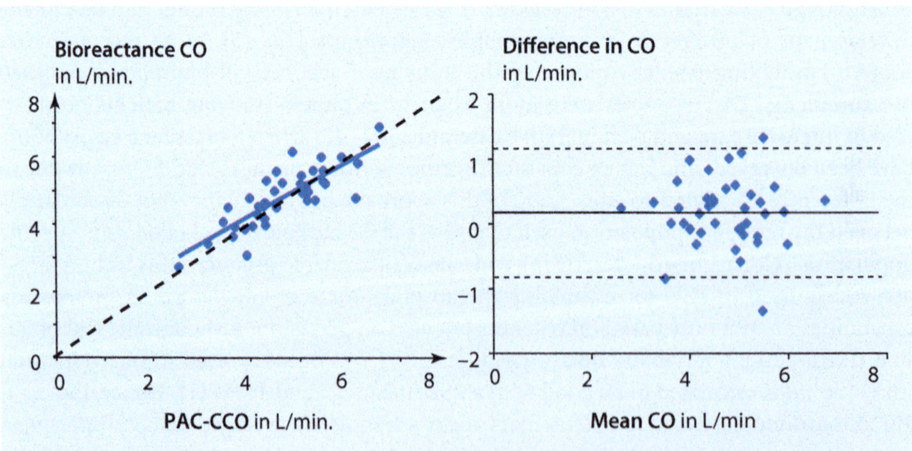

Fig. 28.7 On the left panel, the relationship between a bioreactance device and continuous thermodilution (in L/min), $r = 0.87$, NS from the identity line (dotted line). The right panel shows the corresponding Bland & Altman representation. Upper and lower limits: 2SD = 1.0 L/min. Mean bias =0.16 L/min. In 37/40 (92.5% of cases), the bias was <1 L/min. (Reprinted from Ref. [16])

significantly different in amplitude, although pulse contour was mildly faster (1.10 ± 0.3 min. vs. 1.35 ± 0.3 min.).

Although the inter-patient-averaged bias was negligible, these two first studies showed that individual systematic error (bias >20%) may be found in 20% of the patients, despite the fact that they were designed in the same population of patients from which the CF was derived. These limitations were amplified in other settings, and bioreactance CO were not found acceptable in more heterogeneous populations of patients [46–50]. However, the good precision allows a resolution <20% and step response time close to 1 min, proving to be useful with homogeneous populations of patients [51–56] and when a given patient can be taken as his own reference, such as for pacemaker optimization [57–59], or hemodynamic challenges [45, 60–63].

Limitations and Perspectives

All bioimpedance and bioreactance products share a need for initial calibration through either an independent reference or an autocalibration process. The objective is to determine the CF value seen in formulas (28.9, 28.10, 28.11, and 28.12). The CF determinants and formulas are established by regressions analyses between the measurements and the values of a reference method. In other words, the CF is created to adjust the indications obtained by the tested device to the reference values. The CF is generally based on various preliminary internal measurements and on demographic and morphologic parameters such as age, gender, height, and weight, from which other parameters can then be derived (i.e., body surface area or body mass index). Hematocrit may also be used to optimize the CF. Moreover, the specific patients' setting and the reference method by which the CF are derived are not usually reported. This might sometimes explain the large discrepancies observed between the results of different clinical studies.

Indeed, random results are likely to be observed when the assumptions made to derive CO from chest impedance and reactance variations are no longer valid. This is especially the case when the relationship between changes in aortic volume and stroke volume is very different from what is expected, as in patients with modified aortic compliance (atheroma, prosthesis, large thoracic aortic aneurysm and/or dissection, mediastinal collections, etc.). Other limitations may come from aortic valve diseases, abnormal hematocrit [64], obesity, severe overhydration, or dehydration. The model assumes several hypotheses. First, a complete electrical isolation of heart chambers may depend on myocardium wall thickness. Therefore, a significant proportion of the signal may be due to their volume changes. Second, although of smaller magnitude, pulmonary expansion may also create a change in the thoracic response similarly to the aortic expansion [65]. According to how these noises hamper the aortic signal, it affects necessarily either the VET or the maximal time derivative of the signal change dZ/dt_{max} and dX/dt_{max}, as seen in formulas (28.9, 28.10, 28.11, and 28.12). Therefore, compensation obtained by the CF may not be generalizable to all patients. Clinical studies have confirmed these suspected limitations. They also allowed compensatory factors to be determined (i.e., pulmonary artery pressure, hematocrit). Moreover, other electrical signals such as pacemaker-induced stimulations have to be added to the list of these perturbators. To put it in a nutshell, significant limitations remain shared by all noninvasive technologies regarding CO evaluation [66, 67].

Perspectives may come from a better understanding of the signal composition, isolation of its aortic part, current flow modeling using new tools such as sensors with the active shield, and/or measurement of tissue impedance layers with local electrode arrays.

Practical Implications

1. Bioimpedance and bioreactance technologies represent a totally safe and noninvasive method for assessing thoracic fluid content, SV, and CO.
2. Their calibration remains an issue. Although appropriate autocalibration processes may provide a negligible inter-patient-averaged bias, statistical adjustments cannot fit with all patients, and individual untrueness are frequently unacceptable (systematic measurement error > 20%).
3. In contrast, these technologies yield acceptable precision (fluctuation of measurements due to random errors in a single patient ≈ 10%), allowing good resolution (ability to detect changes around 15%) and fast step response time (≈ 1 min).
4. As of today, these technologies are more useful for tracking changes in CO rather than measuring absolute values.
5. Further developments are necessary to better understand the signal composition and the means for improving it. Indeed, continuous noninvasive hemodynamic monitoring remains a quite respectable goal given its potential advantages.

Conclusion

Bioreactance is rapidly becoming an accepted bedside modality to assess cardiac output non-invasively and continuously at the bedside. Its ease of use and lack of monitoring of an arterial pressure signal make it an attractive alternative to more invasive measures of cardiac output.

Take-Home Messages

Bioimpedance and mostly bioreactance are promising technologies for noninvasive cardiac output assessment. The validation studies are currently discordant. Further researches are needed for better understanding the signal composition.

Conflicts of Interest Pierre Squara was a consultant for Cheetah Medical between 2005 and 2010.

References

1. Altzer E, Lehmann G. Uber ein neues Verfarhen zur Darstellung der Herztätigkreit (Dielecktrogaphie). Arbeitsphysiologie. 1932;5:636–80.
2. Nyboer J, Bango S, Barnett A, Halsey R. Radiocardiograms: electrical impedance changes of the heart in relation to electrocardiograms and heart sounds. J Clin Invest. 1940;19:773.
3. Bonjer FH, Van Den Berg J, Dirken MN. The origin of the variations of body impedance occurring during the cardiac cycle. Circulation. 1952;6:415–20.
4. Thomasset A. Bio-electrical properties of tissue impedance measurements. Lyon Med. 1962;207:107–18.
5. Hoffer EC, Meador CK, Simpson DC. Correlation of whole-body impedance with total body water volume. J Appl Physiol. 1969;27:531–4.
6. Kubicek W, Patterson R, Witsoe D. Development and evaluation of an impedance cardiac output system. Aerospace Med. 1966;37:1208–12.

7. Tishchenko MI, Smirnov AD, Danilov LN, Aleksandrov AL. Characteristics and clinical use of integral rheography--a new method of measuring the stroke volume. Kardiologiia. 1973;13:54–62.
8. Sramek B. Non-invasive technique for measurements of cardiac output by mean of electrical impedance. Proceedings of the Fifth International Conference on Electrical Bioimpedance, Tokyo , Japan 1981, p. 39–42.
9. Bernstein DP. A new stroke volume equation for thoracic electrical bioimpedance: theory and rationale. Crit Care Med. 1986;14:904–9.
10. Perko G, Perko MJ, Jansen E, Secher NH. Thoracic impedance as an index of body fluid balance during cardiac surgery. Acta Anaesthesiol Scand. 1991;35:568–71.
11. Pomerantz M, Baumgartner R, Lauridson J, Eiseman B. Transthoracic electrical impedance for the early detection of pulmonary edema. Surgery. 1969;66:260–8.
12. Graziani G, Badalamenti S, Como G, Ambroso G, Gazzano G, Finazzi S, Mangiarotti R, Morganti A. Validation study of thoracic fluid bioimpedance for assessing the haemodialysis-induced changes in total body fluids. Blood Purif. 1994;12:106–12.
13. Keren H, Burkhoff D, Squara P. Evaluation of a noninvasive continuous cardiac output monitoring system based on thoracic bioreactance. Am J Physiol Heart Circ Physiol. 2007;293:H583–9.
14. Barin E, Haryadi D, Schookin S, Westenskow D, Zubenko V, Beliaev K, Morozov A. Evaluation of a thoracic bioimpedance cardiac output monitor during cardiac catheterization. Crit Care Med. 2000;28:698–702.
15. Spiess B, Patel M, Soltow L, Wright I. Comparison of bioimpedance versus thermodilution cardiac output during cardiac surgery: evaluation of a second-generation bioimpedance device. J Cardiothorac Vasc Anesth. 2001;15:567–73.
16. Squara P, Denjean D, Estagnasie P, Brusset A, Dib JC, Dubois C. Noninvasive cardiac output monitoring (NICOM): a clinical validation. Intensive Care Med. 2007;33:1191–4.
17. Bernstein DP. Continuous noninvasive real-time monitoring of stroke volume and cardiac output by thoracic electrical bioimpedance. Crit Care Med. 1986;14:898–901.
18. Squara P, Cecconi M, Rhodes A, Singer M, Chiche JD. Tracking changes in cardiac output: methodological considerations for the validation of monitoring devices. Intensive Care Med. 2009;35:1801–8.
19. Squara P, Imhoff M, Cecconi M. Metrology in medicine: from measurements to decision, with specific reference to anesthesia and intensive care. Anesth Analg. 2015;120:66–75.
20. Nierman DM, Eisen DI, Fein ED, Hannon E, Mechanick JI, Benjamin E. Transthoracic bioimpedance can measure extravascular lung water in acute lung injury. J Surg Res. 1996;65:101–8.
21. Newman RB, Pierre H, Scardo J. Thoracic-fluid conductivity in peripartum women with pulmonary edema. Obstet Gynecol. 1999;94:48–51.
22. Saunders CE. The use of transthoracic electrical bioimpedance in assessing thoracic fluid status in emergency department patients. Am J Emerg Med. 1998;6:337–40.
23. Metry G, Mallmin H, Wikstrom B, Danielson BG. Proportional changes in body fluid with hemodialysis evaluated by dual-energy X-ray absorptiometry and transthoracic bioimpedance with particular emphasis on the thoracic region. Artif Organs. 1997;21:969–76.
24. Zerahn B, Jensen BV, Olsen F, Petersen JR, Kanstrup IL. The effect of thoracentesis on lung function and transthoracic electrical bioimpedance. Respir Med. 1999;93:196–201.
25. Peacock WI, Albert NM, Kies P, White RD, Emerman CL. Bioimpedance monitoring: better than chest x-ray for predicting abnormal pulmonary fluid? Congest Heart Fail. 2000;6:86–9.
26. Moharram EE, El Attar AM, Kamel MA. The impact of anesthesia on hemodynamic and volume changes in operative hysteroscopy: a bioimpedance randomized study. J Clin Anesth. 2017;38:59–67.
27. Malfatto G, Blengino S, Perego GB, Branzi G, Villani A, Facchini M, Parati G. Transthoracic impedance accurately estimates pulmonary wedge pressure in patients with decompensated chronic heart failure. Congest Heart Fail. 2012;18:25–31.
28. Cagini L, Capozzi R, Tassi V, Savignani C, Quintaliani G, Reboldi G, Puma F. Fluid and electrolyte balance after major thoracic surgery by bioimpedance and endocrine evaluation. Eur J Cardiothorac Surg. 2011;40:e71–6.
29. Malfatto G, Branzi G, Giglio A, Villani A, Facchini C, Ciambellotti F, Facchini M, Parati G. Transthoracic bioimpedance and brain natriuretic peptide levels accurately indicate additional diastolic dysfunction in patients with chronic advanced systolic heart failure. Eur J Heart Fail. 2010;12:928–35.
30. Cuba-Gyllensten I, Gastelurrutia P, Bonomi AG, Riistama J, Bayes-Genis A, Aarts RM. A method to adapt thoracic impedance based on chest geometry and composition to assess congestion in heart failure patients. Med Eng Phys. 2016;38:538–46.

31. Kamath SA, Drazner MH, Tasissa G, Rogers JG, Stevenson LW, Yancy CW. Correlation of impedance cardiography with invasive hemodynamic measurements in patients with advanced heart failure: the BioImpedance CardioGraphy (BIG) substudy of the Evaluation Study of Congestive Heart Failure and Pulmonary Artery Catheterization Effectiveness (ESCAPE) Trial. Am Heart J. 2009;158:217–23.
32. Kossari N, Hufnagel G, Squara P. Bioreactance: a new tool for cardiac output and thoracic fluid content monitoring during hemodialysis. Hemodial Int. 2009;13:512–7.
33. Nescolarde L, Bogonez P, Calpe J, Hernandez R, Donate T, Rosell J. Whole-body and thoracic bio-impedance measurement: hypertension and hyperhydration in hemodialysis patients. Conf Proc IEEE Eng Med Biol Soc. 2007;2007:3593–6.
34. Genoni M, Pelosi P, Romand JA, Pedoto A, Moccetti T, Malacrida R. Determination of cardiac output during mechanical ventilation by electrical bioimpedance or thermodilution in patients with acute lung injury: effects of positive end-expiratory pressure. Crit Care Med. 1998;26:1441–5.
35. Leslien S, McKee S, Newby D, Webb D, Denvir M. Non-invasive measurement of cardiac output in patients with chronic heart failure. Blood Press Monit. 2004;9:277–80.
36. Engoren M, Barbee D. Comparison of cardiac output determined by bioimpedance, thermodilution, and the Fick method. Am J Crit Care. 2005;14:40–5.
37. Heringlake M, Handke U, Hanke T, Eberhardt F, Schumacher J, Gehring H, Heinze H. Lack of agreement between thermodilution and electrical velocimetry cardiac output measurements. Intensive Care Med. 2007;33:2168–72.
38. Taylor K, Manlhiot C, McCrindle B, Grosse-Wortmann L, Holtby H. Poor accuracy of noninvasive cardiac output monitoring using bioimpedance cardiography [PhysioFlow(R)] compared to magnetic resonance imaging in pediatric patients. Anesth Analg. 2012;114:771–5.
39. Thonnerieux M, Alexander B, Binet C, Obadia JF, Bastien O, Desebbe O. The ability of esCCO and ECOM monitors to measure trends in cardiac output during alveolar recruitment maneuver after cardiac surgery: a comparison with the pulmonary thermodilution method. Anesth Analg. 2015;121:383–91.
40. Magliocca A, Rezoagli E, Anderson TA, Burns SM, Ichinose F, Chitilian HV. Cardiac output measurements based on the pulse wave transit time and thoracic impedance exhibit limited agreement with thermodilution method during orthotopic liver transplantation. Anesth Analg. 2017; https://doi.org/10.1213/ANE.0000000000002171.
41. Boldt J, Kling D, Thiel A, Hempelmann G. Non-invasive versus invasive cardiovascular monitoring. Determination of stroke volume and pulmonary hydration using a new bioimpedance monitor. Anaesthesist. 1988;37:218–23.
42. Ram M, Lavie A, Lev S, Blecher Y, Amikam U, Shulman Y, Avnon T, Weiner E, Many A. Cardiac hemodynamics before, during and after elective cesarean section under spinal anesthesia in low-risk women. J Perinatol. 2017; https://doi.org/10.1038/jp.2017.53.
43. Keramidas ME, Kolegard R, Mekjavic IB, Eiken O. PlanHab: hypoxia exaggerates the bed-rest-induced reduction in peak oxygen uptake during upright cycle ergometry. Am J Physiol Heart Circ Physiol. 2016;311:H453–64.
44. Gayda M, Normandin E, Meyer P, Juneau M, Haykowsky M, Nigam A. Central hemodynamic responses during acute high-intensity interval exercise and moderate continuous exercise in patients with heart failure. Applied Physiology, Nutrition, and Metabolism = Physiologie Appliquee. Nutrition et Metabolisme. 2012;37:1171–8.
45. Marqué S, Cariou A, Chiche J, Squara P. Non Invasive Cardiac Output Monitoring (NICOM) compared to minimally invasive monitoring (VIGILEO). Crit Care. 2009;13(3):R73.
46. De Pascale G, Singer M, Brealey D. Comparison of stroke volume measurement between non-invasive bioreactance and esophageal Doppler in patients undergoing major abdominal-pelvic surgery. J Anesth. 2017;31:545–51.
47. Fagnoul D, Vincent JL. Backer de D, Cardiac output measurements using the bioreactance technique in critically ill patients. Crit Care. 2012;16:460.
48. Conway DH, Hussain OA, Gall I. A comparison of noninvasive bioreactance with oesophageal Doppler estimation of stroke volume during open abdominal surgery: an observational study. Eur J Anaesthesiol. 2013;30:501–8.
49. Trinkmann F, Schneider C, Michels JD, Stach K, Doesch C, Schoenberg SO, Borggrefe M, Saur J, Papavassiliu T. Comparison of bioreactance non-invasive cardiac output measurements with cardiac magnetic resonance imaging. Anaesth Intensive Care. 2016;44:769–76.

50. Huang L, Critchley LA, Zhang J. Major upper abdominal surgery alters the calibration of bioreactance cardiac output readings, the NICOM, when comparisons are made against suprasternal and esophageal Doppler intraoperatively. Anesth Analg. 2015;121:936–45.
51. Rosenblum H, Helmke S, Williams P, Teruya S, Jones M, Burkhoff D, Mancini D, Maurer MS. Peak cardiac power measured noninvasively with a bioreactance technique is a predictor of adverse outcomes in patients with advanced heart failure. Congest Heart Fail. 2010;16:254–8.
52. Myers J, Gujja P, Neelagaru S, Burkhoff D. Cardiac output and cardiopulmonary responses to exercise in heart failure: application of a new bio-reactance device. J Card Fail. 2007;13:629–36.
53. Doherty A, El-Khuffash A, Monteith C, McSweeney L, Breatnach C, Kent E, Tully E, Malone F, Thornton P. Comparison of bioreactance and echocardiographic non-invasive cardiac output monitoring and myocardial function assessment in primagravida women. Br J Anaesth. 2017;118:527–32.
54. Rich JD, Archer SL, Rich S. Noninvasive cardiac output measurements in patients with pulmonary hypertension. Eur Respir J. 2013;42:125–33.
55. Engineer RS, Benoit JL, Hicks CW, Kolattukudy SJ, Burkhoff D, Peacock WF. Hemodynamic changes as a diagnostic tool in acute heart failure--a pilot study. Am J Emerg Med. 2012;30:174–80.
56. Elliott A, Hull JH, Nunan D, Jakovljevic DG, Brodie D, Ansley L. Application of bioreactance for cardiac output assessment during exercise in healthy individuals. Eur J Appl Physiol. 2010;109:945–51.
57. Khan FZ, Virdee MS, Hutchinson J, Smith B, Pugh PJ, Read PA, Fynn SP, Dutka DP. Cardiac resynchronization therapy optimization using noninvasive cardiac output measurement. Pacing Clin Electrophysiol. 2011;34:1527–36.
58. Jones MA, Khiani R, Foley P, Webster D, Qureshi N, Wong KC, Rajappan K, Bashir Y, Betts TR. Inter- and intravein differences in cardiac output with cardiac resynchronization pacing using a multipolar LV pacing lead. Pacing Clin Electrophysiol. 2015;38:267–74.
59. Wang JS, Wu MH, Mao TY, Fu TC, Hsu CC. Effects of normoxic and hypoxic exercise regimens on cardiac, muscular, and cerebral hemodynamics suppressed by severe hypoxia in humans. J Appl Physiol. 1985;109:219–29.
60. Benomar B, Ouattara A, Estagnasie P, Brusset A, Squara P. Fluid responsiveness predicted by noninvasive bioreactance-based passive leg raise test. Intensive Care Med. 2010;36:1875–81.
61. Marik PE, Levitov A, Young A, Andrews L. The use of bioreactance and carotid Doppler to determine volume responsiveness and blood flow redistribution following passive leg raising in hemodynamically unstable patients. Chest. 2013;143:364–70.
62. Okwose NC, Chowdhury S, Houghton D, Trenell MI, Eggett C, Bates M, MacGowan GA, Jakovljevic DG. Comparison of cardiac output estimates by bioreactance and inert gas rebreathing methods during cardiopulmonary exercise testing. Clin Physiol Funct Imaging. 2017; https://doi.org/10.1111/cpf.12442.
63. Min JJ, Lee JH, Hong KY, Choi SJ. Utility of stroke volume variation measured using non-invasive bioreactance as a predictor of fluid responsiveness in the prone position. J Clin Monit Comput. 2017;31:397–405.
64. Tremper KK, Hufstedler SM, Barker SJ, Zaccari J, Harris D, Anderson S, Roohk V. Continuous noninvasive estimation of cardiac output by electrical bioimpedance: an experimental study in dogs. Crit Care Med. 1986;14:231–3.
65. Panagiotou M, Vogiatzis I, Jayasekera G, Louvaris Z, Mackenzie A, McGlinchey N, Baker JS, Church AC, Peacock AJ, Johnson MK. Validation of impedance cardiography in pulmonary arterial hypertension. Clin Physiol Funct Imaging. 2017; https://doi.org/10.1111/cpf.12408.
66. Peyton PJ, Chong SW. Minimally invasive measurement of cardiac output during surgery and critical care: a meta-analysis of accuracy and precision. Anesthesiology. 2010;113:1220–35.
67. Joosten A, Desebbe O, Suehiro K, Murphy LS, Essiet M, Alexander B, Fischer MO, Barvais L, Van Obbergh L, Maucort-Boulch D, Cannesson M. Accuracy and precision of non-invasive cardiac output monitoring devices in perioperative medicine: a systematic review and meta-analysis. Br J Anaesth. 2017;118:298–310.

Basic Goals in Clinical Practice

Contents

Blood Pressure Targets in the Initial Stabilization

Julien Demiselle, Peter Radermacher, and Pierre Asfar

M. R. Pinsky et al. (eds.), *Hemodynamic Monitoring*, Lessons from the ICU,
https://doi.org/10.1007/978-3-319-69269-2_29

Learning Objectives

In this chapter, students will:

- Understand the potential benefits and harm of increasing blood pressure.
- Learn the knowledge regarding low- and high-pressure threshold according to what is known from the literature.
- Understand the prerequisites and the difficulties of an individual approach for blood pressure targets.

29.1 Introduction

Circulatory shock is defined as the imbalance between oxygen delivery and demand and may be associated with systemic arterial hypotension (systolic arterial pressure less than 90 mm Hg or mean arterial pressure less than 70 mm Hg), clinical signs of hypoperfusion, and increase in arterial lactate [1]. Physiologically, cardiac output and systemic arterial pressures are pulsatile. The physiological role of the arterial bed is to demodulate the pulsatile flow via resistive arteries and to decrease arterial blood pressure in order to perfuse capillaries with the lowest acceptable intraluminal pressure. The adequacy of peripheral perfusion blood pressure and the microcirculatory blood flow is maintained only within the range of physiological mean arterial pressure. When MAP decreases below a critical threshold value, organ blood flow becomes dependent from perfusion pressure. This leads to organ hypoperfusion and then to organ dysfunction and ultimately to organ failure. Some organs (heart, brain, and kidneys) have an adaptive mechanism to blood pressure variations called autoregulation. Autoregulation is the ability of organs to keep the blood flow rate constant entering the organ, no matter what the perfusion pressure is, over a range of values that is the "autoregulation range" [2]. The autoregulation relationship is presented in ◘ Fig. 29.1. Autoregulation threshold values vary among organs as well as between individuals [3–5], for example, kidney circulation has the highest autoregulation threshold values [3]. In addition, autoregulation thresholds differ in accordance with patient's comorbidities, especially in case of chronic hypertension.

It must be emphasized that a low systemic pressure is associated with decreased microcirculatory blood flow and that the correction of MAP does not necessarily improve microcirculatory blood flow, as many other mechanisms are involved in the microcirculatory blood flow dysfunction (endothelial dysfunction, impaired inter-cell communication, altered glycocalyx, adhesion and rolling of white blood cells as well as platelets, and altered red blood cell deformability) [6].

The determinants of MAP are cardiac output, systemic arterial resistance, and venous return. During shock, one or more of these determinants fail, and MAP decreases when physiological compensatory mechanisms are overwhelmed. MAP is commonly accepted as a surrogate of organ perfusion pressures and is therefore a main target for hemodynamic resuscitation. To increase MAP and obtain the target MAP, fluids (in shock states with decreased venous return) and vasopressors are required. Norepinephrine is the first recommended vasoactive drug and stimulates alpha- and beta-receptors. Consequently, norepinephrine increases both systemic vascular resistances and cardiac output. A high target of MAP requires a higher load of vasopressor drug and may induce excessive arterial systemic vasoconstriction, which in turn may induce organ ischemia.

Consequently, the main challenge for the clinician driving the early hemodynamic resuscitation phase of patients with shock is to set the vasopressor infusion rate to target

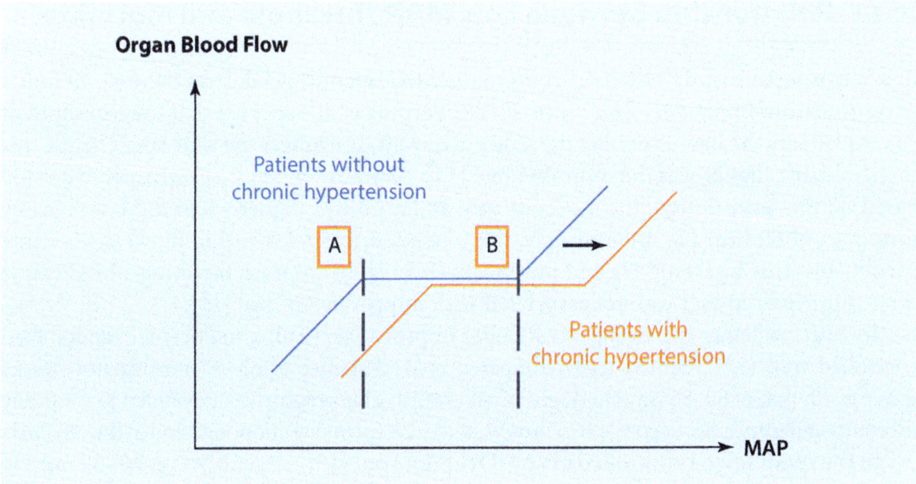

Fig. 29.1 MAP, mean arterial pressure; A, lower critical value of MAP; B, higher critical value of MAP. The autoregulation zone is between the vertical lines. When MAP fall under a critical perfusion pressure (point A), organ blood flow becomes dependent on pressure level, and this relationship was reported in the heart, brain, and kidney [2–4]. On the right side of the autoregulation zone, organ blood flow is dependent on pressure level and was reported in the brain circulation [5]. In case of chronic hypertension, the relationship between MAP and blood flow is right-shifted, as presented with the black arrow [5]

MAP within the adequate pressure range to avoid from one hand a low perfusion pressure and, from the other hand, excessive vasoconstriction and other side effects due to vasoactive drug such as arrhythmias.

Currently, for resuscitation of hemorrhagic shock, there is no available data supporting specific blood pressure targets as stated by the recommendations [7, 8]. The only randomized controlled trial focusing on systolic arterial pressure in patients with hemorrhagic shock and without traumatic brain injuries aimed at comparing early aggressive fluid resuscitation to maintain systolic blood pressure above 100 mm Hg versus delayed fluid administration with permissive low systolic blood pressure until bleeding control. The aggressive fluid resuscitation strategy was associated with higher mortality rate [9]. Therefore, the European guidelines suggest to tolerate a lower level of blood pressure in patients with uncontrolled bleeding without severe head injury with a recommendation of weak level with low quality of evidence [8].

In the setting of cardiogenic shock, it should be underlined that currently, no clinical studies so far have attempted to assess the optimal blood pressure level [8, 10]. This may explain the absence of formal recommendations.

Therefore, in this chapter, we will focus on the blood pressure targets in the initial resuscitation of patients with septic shock.

29.2 MAP Target in the Initial Stabilization: Is There a Low Threshold?

Many retrospective, observational, and interventional studies investigated whether a specific MAP level was associated with main outcomes such as mortality and/or acute kidney injury.

29.2.1 Relationship Between Low MAP Threshold and Mortality

In a retrospective study based on continuous MAP recordings during the first 48 hours of resuscitation in patients with septic shock, Varpula et al. reported that the threshold of 65 mm Hg was the best to predict mortality at day 30. The longer the time spent below this threshold, the higher was the mortality rate [11]. Similarly, in another retrospective study based on the same design, the mortality rate at day 28 was higher when MAP was below threshold of 60 mm Hg. Interestingly, there was a linear relationship between the time spent below this threshold Hg and mortality rate [12]. In contrast, targeting a MAP value of 70 mm Hg or higher was not associated with improved survival [13].

To assess whether increasing MAP target improves survival, a multicenter randomized controlled trial (SEPSISPAM trial) compared a MAP target of 65–70 mmHg (low-target group) with that of 80–85 mmHg (high-target group). This pragmatic study failed to show any mortality difference between the two groups at day 28 (primary endpoint) and at day 90 [14].

In the randomized controlled OVATION pilot trial [15], target MAP of 60–65 mmHg was compared to a target MAP of 75–80 mmHg with no difference in mortality at day 28. Interestingly, in the subgroup of patients aged 75 years and older, a lower MAP target was associated with reduced mortality.

29.2.2 Relationship Between Low MAP Threshold and Kidney Function

In the literature, the impact of MAP target on organ function has been studied only through the evaluation of kidney function. A retrospective study suggests that a higher MAP target could be mandatory to prevent acute kidney injury (AKI) occurrence [12].

The impact of MAP level in the first hours of resuscitation regarding kidney failure occurrence is a key point. Two observational studies reported that in patients with septic shock with early AKI, those who experienced persistent or worsened AKI had lower MAP during their initial hemodynamic management [16, 17].

Three prospective studies, all only recruiting a small number of patients, have tested the effects on renal function of incremental thresholds of MAP, achieved by increasing norepinephrine infusion. MAP was increased from 65 to 75 and then 85 mm Hg. None of these studies demonstrated any beneficial effect on renal function. It should be noticed that in these studies, the timing of the intervention was not mentioned and, hence, delayed intervention after initial stabilization cannot be ruled out (fluids administration and vasopressors infusion) [18–20]. The results of these studies are presented in ◘ Table 29.1.

The incidence of renal failure was a secondary outcome in the SEPSISPAM trial. There was no difference in renal outcomes (renal replacement therapy requirement, doubling in serum creatinine level) between the low- and high-target groups [14]. In the predefined subgroup of chronic hypertensive patients, the high-target group required less renal replacement therapy as compared with low-pressure target patients. Conversely to the abovementioned short-term studies, SEPSISPAM trial recruited patients very early within the 6 first hours after initiation of norepinephrine infusion. This may have favorably impacted the renal failure and may suggest a reversibility part of renal dysfunction in the early phase of septic shock.

Table 29.1 Prospective studies assessing the effects of an increase in MAP on kidney function

Study	Patients (*n*)	Target MAP (mm Hg)	Experimentation duration (hours)	Creatinine clearance	Urine output	Renal resistive index
Ledoux [19]	10	Incremental increase in MAP from 65, 75, 85 mm hg	3*1 h45	NA	No change	NA
Bourgoin [20]	2×14	65 versus 85 mm hg in two groups	8 h	No change	No change	NA
Deruddre [18]	11	Incremental increase in MAP from 65, 75, 85 mm hg	3*2 h	No change	65->75: ↑ 75->85: No change	65->75: ↓ 75->85: No change

29.3 MAP Target in the Initial Stabilization: Is There a High Threshold?

An accurate analysis of the randomized controlled trials, where MAP was reported in patients with septic shock, shows that MAP raised up to 80 mm Hg in studies aimed at comparing vasoactive drugs in patients with septic shock (CATS, comparison of epinephrine versus the association of dobutamine and norepinephrine [21]; VASST, comparison of vasopressin versus norepinephrine [22]; SOAP 2, comparison of dopamine versus norepinephrine [23]). None of these studies reported excessive incidence of ischemic events.

Conversely in 2004, Lopez et al. reported the results of a randomized controlled trial aimed at comparing L-NMMA, a nitric oxide synthase inhibitor, versus norepinephrine, in patients with septic shock. The trial was stopped prematurely for excess in mortality in L-NMMA-treated patients. Interestingly, patients treated with L-NMMA had a higher MAP, and 25% of the patients even had MAP values higher than 90 mm Hg. Whether the higher mortality rate was related to the high MAP level and/or the drug per se remained open.

The direct comparison of two levels of MAP in patients with septic shock in the SEPSISPAM and OVATION trials did not report a significant benefit in favor of the higher MAP targets. In contrast, increasing MAP in patients with septic shock was associated with significantly more frequent arrhythmias, e.g., new onset atrial fibrillation. In turn, de novo atrial fibrillation was reported to be associated with higher mortality in patients with severe sepsis [24]. In that study, Walkey et al. assessed the impact of new onset atrial fibrillation in the setting of severe sepsis: on the 49,082 septic patients included in this study, new onset atrial fibrillation occurred in 5.9% of patients and was associated with significantly higher mortality (56% versus 36%).

29.4 MAP Target in the Initial Stabilization: An Individual Approach for MAP Target?

The recent version of the surviving Sepsis campaign guidelines recommends adaptating MAP target to the patient's condition, using an individualized approach [8, 25]. However, in the daily life, this approach may be challenging for clinicians.

First, outside the intensive care unit setting, the SPRINT randomized controlled trial compared a maximal target of 120 mmHg (intensive treatment) for systolic arterial pressure (SAP) with that of a target of 140 mmHg (standard treatment) in nondiabetic patients with cardiovascular comorbidities. The primary outcome was a composite of significant cardiovascular events (myocardial infarction, stroke, heart failure, and/or death from cardiovascular causes). Albeit the primary composite outcome and mortality were lower in the intensive treatment group, serious adverse events were significantly more frequent in these patients, and especially AKI occurred more frequently [26]. Outside the intensive care unit, lowering blood pressure is apparently beneficial when regarding cardiovascular outcome and mortality, but this therapeutic strategy remains at risk for renal function. Altogether, the results of the SPRINT and SEPSISPAM trials suggest that kidney function may benefit from higher range of blood pressure in patients with chronic hypertension. Nevertheless, a "kidney-centered" resuscitation should be balanced with side effects such as arrhythmias as well as survival outcome related to the timing of norepinephrine infusion. Indeed, the most recent individual patient data meta-analysis showed that increasing MAP after 6 h of norepinephrine infusion start was associated with significant higher mortality rates and thus confirmed the significantly higher rate of cardiac side effects in the high MAP target group [27].

29

Hence, the individualization of blood pressure targets is complex. Age [15], chronic hypertension [14], and delay of vasopressor start [27] have been reported to impact mortality and renal outcomes. These clinical features should be balanced with the risk of new onset arrhythmias (please refer to ◘ Table 29.2).

- At the initial phase of hemodynamic management in patients with septic shock, according to available data as well as the most recent guidelines, a MAP target of 65 mm Hg is recommended [8, 25].
- In particular situation, e.g., chronic hypertension, a higher MAP target could be considered but requires a higher vasopressor load which may be associated with cardiovascular side effects. Therefore, increasing MAP target above 65 mm Hg must be cautiously weighted.

◘ **Table 29.2** Impact of high MAP target according to patients and clinical situation characteristics

Baseline characteristics reported to impact outcomes	Effect of high MAP target
Age over 75 years	Increase in mortality [15]
Chronic hypertension	Reduction of renal failure [14]
Start of vasopressors >6 h	Increase in mortality [27]
Side effects	Higher rate of cardiac arrhythmias [14, 15]

Conclusion

To date, blood pressure target remains a controversial subject during the initial resuscitation of patients with septic shock. A MAP target of 65 mm Hg is recommended. Some patients may benefit from higher targets, but such increases in MAP may be associated with a higher vasopressor load and more frequent cardiac side effects.

Take-Home Messages

- In the initial resuscitation, relevant blood pressure target is MAP.
- The objective of resuscitation is to restore MAP into autoregulation range.
- In clinical practice, MAP target is 65 mmHg.
- MAP target should be individualized taking in account the benefit risk ratio of high vasopressor load.

References

1. Finfer SR, Vincent J-L, Vincent J-L, De Backer D. Circulatory shock. N Engl J Med. 2013;369:1726–34.
2. Johnson PC. Autoregulation of blood flow. Circ Res. 1986;59:483–95.
3. Bellomo R, Wan L, May C. Vasoactive drugs and acute kidney injury. Crit Care Med. 2008;36:S179–86.
4. Cupples WA, Braam B. Assessment of renal autoregulation. Am J Physiol Renal Physiol. 2007;292: F1105–23.
5. Strandgaard S, Olesen J, Skinhoj E, Lassen NA. Autoregulation of brain circulation in severe arterial hypertension. Br Med J. 1973;1:507–10.
6. De Backer D, Donadello K, Taccone F, Ospina-Tascon G, Salgado D, Vincent J-L. Microcirculatory alterations: potential mechanisms and implications for therapy. Ann Intensive Care. 2011;1:27.
7. Rochwerg B, Hylands M, Møller MH, et al. CCCS-SSAI WikiRecs clinical practice guideline: vasopressor blood pressure targets in critically ill adults with hypotension and vasopressor use in early traumatic shock. Intensive Care Med. 2017;43:1062–4.
8. Cecconi M, De Backer D, Antonelli M, et al. Consensus on circulatory shock and hemodynamic monitoring. Task force of the European Society of Intensive Care Medicine. Intensive Care Med. 2014;40:1795–815.
9. Bickell WH, Wall MJ, Pepe PE, Martin RR, Ginger VF, Allen MK, Mattox KL. Immediate versus delayed fluid resuscitation for hypotensive patients with penetrating torso injuries. N Engl J Med. 1994;331:1105–9.
10. O'Gara PT, Kushner FG, Ascheim DD, et al. 2013 ACCF/AHA guideline for the management of ST-elevation myocardial infarction: a report of the American College of Cardiology Foundation/American Heart Association Task Force on Practice Guidelines. Circulation. 2013;127:e362–425.
11. Varpula M, Tallgren M, Saukkonen K, Voipio-Pulkki L-M, Pettilä V. Hemodynamic variables related to outcome in septic shock. Intensive Care Med. 2005;31:1066–71.
12. Dünser MW, Takala J, Ulmer H, Mayr VD, Luckner G, Jochberger S, Daudel F, Lepper P, Hasibeder WR, Jakob SM. Arterial blood pressure during early sepsis and outcome. Intensive Care Med. 2009;35: 1225–33.
13. Dünser MW, Ruokonen E, Pettilä V, Ulmer H, Torgersen C, Schmittinger CA, Jakob S, Takala J. Association of arterial blood pressure and vasopressor load with septic shock mortality: a post hoc analysis of a multicenter trial. Crit Care. 2009;13:R181.
14. Asfar P, Meziani F, Hamel J-F, et al. High versus low blood-pressure target in patients with septic shock. N Engl J Med. 2014;370:1583–93.
15. Canadian Critical Care Trials Group, Lamontagne F, Meade MO, et al. Higher versus lower blood pressure targets for vasopressor therapy in shock: a multicentre pilot randomized controlled trial. Intensive Care Med. 2016;42:542–50.
16. Badin J, Boulain T, Ehrmann S, et al. Relation between mean arterial pressure and renal function in the early phase of shock: a prospective, explorative cohort study. Crit Care. 2011;15:R135.

17. Poukkanen M, Wilkman E, Vaara ST, et al. Hemodynamic variables and progression of acute kidney injury in critically ill patients with severe sepsis: data from the prospective observational FINNAKI study. Crit Care Lond Engl. 2013;17:R295.
18. Deruddre S, Cheisson G, Mazoit J-X, Vicaut E, Benhamou D, Duranteau J. Renal arterial resistance in septic shock: effects of increasing mean arterial pressure with norepinephrine on the renal resistive index assessed with Doppler ultrasonography. Intensive Care Med. 2007;33:1557–62.
19. LeDoux D, Astiz ME, Carpati CM, Rackow EC. Effects of perfusion pressure on tissue perfusion in septic shock. Crit Care Med. 2000;28:2729–32.
20. Bourgoin A, Leone M, Delmas A, Garnier F, Albanèse J, Martin C. Increasing mean arterial pressure in patients with septic shock: effects on oxygen variables and renal function*. Crit Care Med. 2005;33:780–6.
21. Annane D, Vignon P, Renault A, et al. Norepinephrine plus dobutamine versus epinephrine alone for management of septic shock: a randomised trial. Lancet Lond Engl. 2007;370:676–84.
22. Russell JA, Walley KR, Singer J, et al. Vasopressin versus norepinephrine infusion in patients with septic shock. N Engl J Med. 2008;358:877–87.
23. De Backer D, Biston P, Devriendt J, et al. Comparison of dopamine and norepinephrine in the treatment of shock. N Engl J Med. 2010;362:779–89.
24. Walkey AJ, Wiener RS, Ghobrial JM, Curtis LH, Benjamin EJ. Incident stroke and mortality associated with new-onset atrial fibrillation in patients hospitalized with severe Sepsis. JAMA. 2011; https://doi.org/10.1001/jama.2011.1615.
25. Rhodes A, Evans LE, Alhazzani W, et al. Surviving sepsis campaign: international guidelines for management of sepsis and septic shock: 2016. Intensive Care Med. 2017;43:304–77.
26. The SPRINT Research Group. A randomized trial of intensive versus standard blood-pressure control. N Engl J Med. 2015;373:2103–16.
27. Lamontagne F, Day AG, Meade MO, et al. Pooled analysis of higher versus lower blood pressure targets for vasopressor therapy septic and vasodilatory shock. Intensive Care Med. 2018;44:12–21.

Lessons from the ICU: Choosing the Right Vasopressor

Francesco Fiorini, David Antcliffe, and Anthony C. Gordon

M. R. Pinsky et al. (eds.), *Hemodynamic Monitoring*, Lessons from the ICU,
https://doi.org/10.1007/978-3-319-69269-2_30

Learning Objectives

Vasopressors are a potent class of pharmacological agents used to produce vasoconstriction in critically ill patients. Since vascular resistance is an important determinant of mean arterial pressure (MAP), vasopressors have a direct effect on it and are widely used for cardiovascular support.

This chapter outlines the main vasoconstrictors used in current practice, their mechanisms of action, advantages, pitfalls and clinical applications with up-to-date medical evidence where available. This will equip the reader with the knowledge to appreciate the choice of vasopressors in the ICU, based on clinical indication, desired effect and side-effect profile.

30.1 Introduction

The main role of vasopressors is to improve mean arterial pressure (MAP), and thereby tissue perfusion, by increasing arterial vasomotor tone, given that:

$$\text{MAP} = \text{cardiac output} \times \text{total peripheral resistance}$$

There may be a need to increase MAP for a number of reasons including management of shock, maintenance of cerebral perfusion in brain injury and optimisation of renal perfusion in acute kidney injury (AKI) and hepato-renal syndrome.

The main distinction between vasopressors and inotropes lies in their lack of a *direct* effect on cardiac output (CO), though *indirect* 'reflex' cardiovascular changes often occur. In addition to this, several drugs display both inotropic and vasopressor characteristics. Vasoconstriction can be mediated by various classes of receptors, and vasopressors can be classified based on their action on adrenergic or other receptors.

30

Some essential concepts should be considered with all vasoactive agents:

- Prior to initiating vasoconstrictive therapy, adequate fluid resuscitation must be carried out to restore circulating volume, improve CO and optimise peripheral perfusion.
- Most vasopressors follow variable dose-response relationships, and their effects depend on concentration and patient factors. This is especially relevant given the complications that may ensue, which are discussed later in this chapter.
- The dosing of vasopressors can be challenging. As a rule of thumb, it may be appropriate to administer low initial doses and gradually titrate up. This should be based on patient response, desired outcome and monitoring for side effects, rather than aiming for a predetermined infusion dose. Most vasopressors have a relatively short half-life and their dosage can be adjusted as necessary.
- Administration is generally through centrally inserted venous access. Peripheral routes are more prone to extravasation, which can result in devastating necrosis of local tissue.

30.2 Adrenergic Vasopressors

Adrenoceptors are G protein-coupled receptors found throughout the human body; the most relevant ones within the cardiovascular system include alpha- and beta-receptors. Postsynaptic alpha-1 and to a lesser extent alpha-2 receptors lead to vasoconstriction by direct stimulation of vascular smooth muscle. In the myocardium, alpha-1 receptors have also been shown to have a mild inotropic but not chronotropic effect [1, 2]. Moreover, presynaptic alpha-2 receptors are part of a negative feedback loop that inhibits the release of noradrenaline.

Beta-1 receptors are most abundant in the myocardium, where they produce both direct inotropic and chronotropic effects, without significantly affecting vascular calibre. They also lead to increased renin release and bladder relaxation. Their beta-2 counterparts are responsible for smooth muscle relaxation, with resulting bronchodilation and vasodilation. Within these receptor classes, several further subtypes have been identified, though their clinical relevance is uncertain given that no subtype-specific drugs currently exist.

Polymorphisms of adrenergic receptor genes have been characterised particularly in chronic illnesses such as hypertension, coronary artery disease and heart failure. While they're unlikely to play a causative role in their pathogenesis, they might affect the pharmacodynamics of adrenergic drugs [3]. The importance of this in ICU patients is not yet clear and will require further studies targeted specifically at this population. In septic shock, a beta-2 polymorphism has been linked to increased mortality and noradrenaline requirements [4].

Adrenergic vasopressors include endogenous catecholamines such as noradrenaline, adrenaline and dopamine and synthetic ones, commonly phenylephrine, ephedrine and metaraminol.

Noradrenaline An endogenous catecholamine and neurotransmitter, noradrenaline is primarily a direct alpha-1 agonist with modest beta-1 and beta-2 action in the cardiovascular system. Overall, it produces significant systemic vasoconstriction with minimal impact on heart rate; its mild beta-agonist effect is counteracted by a reflex bradycardia from increased afterload. The rise in MAP and consequently in diastolic pressure is thought to improve coronary artery blood flow, which together with beta-1 activation can result in a modest increase in stroke volume. However, cardiac output is variable and might actually decrease because of greater afterload and reflex bradycardia. The half-life of exogenous noradrenaline is 1.5 min [5].

Noradrenaline's principal application is in septic shock, where current international guidelines advocate for its use as a first-line vasopressor [6]. Noradrenaline is associated with lower mortality rates and lower incidence of tachyarrhythmia compared to dopamine [7, 8], while adrenaline is more likely to lead to tachycardia [9]. Interestingly, a national noradrenaline shortage period in the United States was met by a rise in phenylephrine use for the treatment of septic shock at affected centres, corresponding with greater inpatient mortality [10].

Noradrenaline may also be used in other causes of shock. In cardiogenic shock, vasoactive therapy can help maintain MAP and improve coronary blood flow as a supportive bridge to definitive diagnosis and treatment. Noradrenaline might often need to be used in combination with dobutamine in this situation [11]. It is associated with a lower incidence of tachycardia, hyperlactataemia and arrhythmia compared to adrenaline [12] and lower mortality than dopamine [13].

Noradrenaline also has a role in critical hypotension from traumatic haemorrhagic shock, while volume replacement is being achieved: in addition to its systemic effect, venoconstriction particularly at the splanchnic level is thought to help divert more volume into the arterial circulation [14, 15].

Additionally, it can be used in type 1 hepato-renal syndrome (HRS) if terlipressin is contraindicated [16] and in acute brain injury to achieve a target MAP for the desired cerebral perfusion pressure (CPP) [17]. Hypertensive therapy with noradrenaline can be trialled as part of haemodynamic augmentation in the treatment and prevention of vasospasm following subarachnoid haemorrhage (SAH).

Adrenaline The pharmacology of adrenaline is broader than that of its immediate precursor noradrenaline, with preferential activation of beta-1 and beta-2 receptors over alpha-1 receptors.

At lower doses, it exerts predominantly a beta-1 agonist function with minimal change to vascular tone, as beta-2 and alpha-1 stimulation in vascular smooth muscle counteract one another. This results in direct inotropy and chronotropy, thus increasing cardiac output. At higher doses, its alpha-agonist properties prevail, resulting in vasoconstriction. The half-life of adrenaline is 2–3 min given intravenously.

The use of adrenaline is currently recommended in international resuscitation guidelines for cardiac arrest [18, 19], mainly because of its alpha-adrenergic effect. However, evidence is limited and largely drawn from out-of-hospital events, and while some studies have found a greater likelihood of return of spontaneous circulation with adrenaline, it may not improve survival nor neurological outcome at discharge [20]. Moreover, early administration (<2 min from first defibrillation) in shockable rhythms is associated with worse prognosis [21]. Its role in out-of-hospital cardiac arrest is being investigated in the PARAMEDIC-2 trial [22].

Adrenaline remains a suitable second-line agent in septic shock if noradrenaline alone is not sufficient to achieve the target MAP [6]. However, it may cause hyperlactataemia which may not be related to any adverse effect but can complicate the use of serum lactate as a resuscitation target.

In cardiogenic shock, the combination of noradrenaline and dobutamine is preferred to adrenaline because of the greater risk of tachycardia and the hyperlactataemia associated with the latter [11, 12].

Intramuscular/intravenous adrenaline is considered the first-line agent for use in anaphylactic shock [23], with its benefits being linked to beta-2-mediated bronchodilation in addition to vasoconstriction.

Dopamine Dopamine is a direct precursor to noradrenaline, and, unlike the other endogenous catecholamines, its agonist action extends beyond adrenergic receptors. It is a potent activator of dopamine receptors, as well as beta- and alpha-adrenoceptors. Dopaminergic receptors too are G protein-coupled and various subtypes exist; these can be grouped into D1- and D2-like, though dopamine is an unselective agonist of both. Their activation in myocardial tissue produces a degree of inotropy and chronotropy, less pronounced than that from adrenoceptors. In the vascular system, the overall effect is of vasodilation particularly in the renal, mesenteric and splanchnic circulations [24].

The physiological effects of dopamine on various receptor classes are largely dose-dependent [25, 26] and at some concentrations can act almost purely as a vasopressor. This must be considered when selecting the initial dose and especially before up-titrating it.

- *Low-dose* dopamine (<3 μg/kg/min) exerts mainly a dopaminergic effect, with consequent reduction in vascular tone and mild increase in cardiac output. Moreover, in the kidneys it acts as a natriuretic hormone reducing sodium reabsorption in the proximal convoluted tubule and increasing water excretion [27].
- *Intermediate doses* (<10 μg/kg/min) lead to activation of beta-1 receptors and greater inotropic effect, usually accompanied by an increase in heart rate.
- At *higher doses* (>10 μg/kg/min), dopamine is more akin to a vasoconstrictor with predominantly alpha-1 effects.

The plasma concentration of dopamine can be very variable and is often not reflected by the infusion rates described above, particularly in the critically ill where its clearance is less predictable. The titration of dopamine should therefore be guided by its desired use and clinical effect. Its half-life given intravenously is approximately 2 min.

The applications of dopamine in the ICU setting have become somewhat limited. In septic shock, because of greater mortality and incidence of tachyarrhythmia, it has been superseded by noradrenaline [7, 8]. Its role in this population is confined to those with bradycardia and low risk of arrhythmia [6]. Moreover, the concept of 'renal-dose' dopamine in critical care has been largely abandoned, as there is no proven benefit to renal function in this group of patients [28, 29]. The increase in diuresis sometimes reported with low-dose dopamine is likely to be mediated by its natriuretic effect rather than any improvement in glomerular filtration, given its unselective vasodilation of both afferent and efferent arterioles. In cardiogenic shock, dopamine is associated with increased mortality and arrhythmic events compared to noradrenaline [13].

Phenylephrine This synthetic selective alpha-1 agonist has virtually no beta-activity. Because of this, the resulting increase in afterload can lead to unopposed reflex bradycardia and reduction in cardiac output.

Phenylephrine can be used as a bolus in the rapid correction of hypotension of abrupt onset or in case of concomitant pre-existing tachycardia. Further applications include severe hypotension in fixed output states such as aortic stenosis and hypertrophic obstructive cardiomyopathy to reduce the left ventricular outflow tract gradient. As detailed above, the rise in mortality seen with increased phenylephrine use during a national noradrenaline shortage would suggest caution against more widespread use [10].

Ephedrine Similar to adrenaline, ephedrine is a direct alpha- and beta-agonist, though a weaker one. Its main effect is instead via an indirect mechanism, acting on peripheral sympathetic neurons as a noradrenaline-releasing agent and to inhibit its reuptake [30]. This can lead to pronounced tachyphylaxis, limiting its usefulness particularly in critically ill patients with a generally depleted pool of catecholamines. It is used in boluses to correct transient hypotension in anaesthetic practice.

Metaraminol Though mostly a vasoconstrictor through alpha-agonist effects, metaraminol too is a modest noradrenaline-releasing agent. In the ICU setting, bolus doses can help reverse or prevent hypotension during endotracheal intubation. It can also be administered peripherally during the initial stabilisation of an unwell patient, such as in the emergency department, or before central venous access is obtained.

30.3 Non-adrenergic Vasopressors

Catecholamines can be associated with an increase in myocardial oxygen demand and tachyarrhythmia; thus non-adrenergic compounds have gained attention as possible adjunctive vasopressor agents. However, it is unclear whether they confer any improvement in overall mortality [31]. The main non-adrenergic vasopressors are discussed here.

Vasopressin Vasopressin is an endogenous stress hormone released by the posterior pituitary gland mainly in response to increased serum osmolality, hypovolaemia and hypotension. Stimulation of vasopressin receptors leads to several effects, including vasoconstriction especially in the muscle, skin and splanchnic vessels (V1a receptors) and vasodilation in pulmonary and coronary circulation; water retention (V2 receptors); and release of ACTH from the anterior pituitary (V1b receptors) [32]. The use of vasopressin in critical care stems from evidence that its levels are significantly decreased in patients with septic shock receiving catecholamines [33]. In health, the effects of vasopressin on the circulatory system are not dramatic. However, in shock states it leads to vasoconstriction, an effect reinforced by its blockade of potassium-dependent ATP channels [34].

In septic shock, vasopressin can be added to noradrenaline as a second-line agent for hypotension unresponsive to catecholamine therapy or to reduce the dose of noradrenaline [6]. In a large randomised controlled trial, vasopressin reduced mortality in less severe shock (those that required lower noradrenaline doses initially) [35]. Early administration was also associated with a decreased requirement for renal replacement therapy (although there was no impact on renal failure outcomes), and a sparing effect on noradrenaline dose is consistently seen [36, 37].

Terlipressin Terlipressin is a synthetic prodrug and vasopressin analogue with a longer duration of action and slightly greater selectivity for V1a receptors [38]; its longer half-life means that it can be administered as intravenous boluses.

In upper GI variceal haemorrhage, terlipressin is used as complementary treatment at presentation until definitive haemostasis is achieved [39]. It is more effective than vasopressin and similar to balloon tamponade in controlling the bleeding [40, 41], with mortality rates similar to octreotide and somatostatin [39].

30

In addition to this, terlipressin may be of benefit in hepato-renal syndrome (HRS), given in combination with albumin, to counteract splanchnic vasodilation and improve renal function [16]. The evidence for this is largely confined to type 1 HRS and without concurrent sepsis, and it has no advantage over noradrenaline when the patient is managed in an area where the latter can be safely administered.

Angiotensin II The renin-angiotensin-aldosterone system is one of several physiological rescue mechanisms activated in response to hypotension. The vasoactive properties of angiotensin II are mediated largely via AT-1 receptors; they include increased vascular tone, aldosterone secretion, salt and water retention and vasopressin release. It also has roles in coagulation and the pro-inflammatory response [42]. Angiotensin-converting enzyme in the pulmonary circulation converts angiotensin I into angiotensin II, and it is thought that vasodilatory shock can impair this process due to insults to the pulmonary vasculature.

In vasodilatory shock, exogenous angiotensin II in addition to high-dose vasopressors can achieve an early (in the first 3 h) improvement in MAP with a sparing effect on background vasopressor dose and no significant adverse events [43]. However, more evidence is required to fully understand its effect on important clinical outcomes.

30.4 Adverse Events

Therapy with vasopressors must be monitored closely, not least because their cardiovascular effects can produce serious adverse events, including tissue hypoperfusion, tachyarrhythmia and myocardial infarction.

Excessive vasoconstriction can impair circulation to the peripheries, particularly skin and digits. While this typically develops gradually, rarely sudden arterial occlusion may occur and threaten limb or bowel perfusion. It is unclear whether vasopressors are exclusively responsible for this, since advanced circulatory shock itself will significantly impair peripheral blood flow. Therefore, maintaining a satisfactory MAP is still likely to be of greater benefit overall. The incidence of such events in cardiovascular shock has been reported at 6.5% with noradrenaline and 9.2% with dopamine, the majority being mild skin ischaemia [13]. While it is true that adding vasopressin has a sparing effect on noradrenaline, it is still a vasoconstrictor and does not alter the incidence of these events [35]. If peripheral hypoperfusion is suspected, it is important to reassess the patient thoroughly and establish whether they are appropriately fluid resuscitated or excessively vasoconstricted or perhaps have developed a superimposed element of cardiogenic shock.

Vasopressors can also be associated with tachyarrhythmia, likely due to a combination of changes to vascular physiology and myocardial excitability. Agents that act directly on the myocardium via beta-1 stimulation are generally thought to be more prone to this, with significantly higher rates of arrhythmias seen, for instance, with dopamine (24.1%) compared to noradrenaline (12.4%) [13]. The cause for a tachyarrhythmia should be investigated as usual before attributing it to vasopressor therapy. In addition to treating the abnormal rhythm, fluid and electrolyte status should be optimised and consideration given to switching to a less arrhythmogenic alpha-selective or vasopressin agent.

The haemodynamic changes produced by vasoactive agents can increase myocardial oxygen demand [12], especially if tachycardia ensues. In the context of a critically ill patient, this can be associated with myocardial infarction. It is therefore important to obtain continuous cardiac monitoring when administering vasoconstrictors and perform 12-lead electrocardiograms (ECGs) in case of deterioration.

Activation of beta-1 receptors can reduce insulin sensitivity leading to hyperglycaemia [26], while the absorption of exogenous insulin and other subcutaneous drugs may be diminished because of local vasoconstriction. Uncontrolled plasma glucose is associated with worse outcomes in the critically ill and should be closely monitored.

Locally, extravasation of vasopressors leads to excessive vasoconstriction and tissue necrosis. The risk of this is reduced by administration via centrally sited venous access, which should be positioned and secured appropriately before use. If extravasation does occur, the vasopressor infusion should be moved to a different, centrally located venous port. Local administration of subcutaneous phentolamine (a selective alpha-antagonist) may help reverse the excessive vasoconstriction, and plastic surgery input should be sought.

Practical Implications

The main vasopressors for specific clinical situations (◘ Table 30.1) and commonly encountered adult doses (◘ Table 30.2) are listed below. This is only an indicative summary, and in medical practice these decisions will be influenced by several aspects including clinical indication, experience, patient factors and relevant up-to-date guidelines and evidence.

Table 30.1 Summary of the main vasopressors used in specific clinical situations

Clinical situation	Vasopressors
Septic shock	Noradrenaline is first line Add vasopressin or adrenaline if necessary to increase MAP Add vasopressin if necessary to reduce noradrenaline dose Consider adding dobutamine if persistent hypoperfusion
Cardiogenic shock	Noradrenaline and/or dobutamine
Anaphylaxis	Adrenaline (IM, unless experience with IV use)
Upper GI bleed	Terlipressin if variceal source suspected
Type 1 HRS	Terlipressin Consider noradrenaline if in the appropriate care setting and/or terlipressin contraindicated
Cardiac arrest	Adrenaline if non-shockable or persistent shockable rhythm
Brain injury	Noradrenaline if appropriate

GI gastrointestinal, *HRS* hepato-renal syndrome

Table 30.2 Indicative common adult doses for widely used vasopressors

Vasopressor	Typical dose
Noradrenaline	0–1.0 µg/kg/min IV infusion
Adrenaline	0–0.5 µg/kg/min IV infusion 1 mg IV bolus (*cardiac arrest*) 0.5 mg IM bolus (*anaphylaxis*)
Dopamine	0–20 µg/kg/min IV infusion
Phenylephrine	0.1–0.5 mg slow IV bolus
Ephedrine	3–6 mg slow IV bolus
Metaraminol	0–10 mg/h IV infusion 0.5–5 mg slow IV bolus
Vasopressin	0–0.03 U/min IV infusion (up to 0.06 U/min in some studies)
Terlipressin	1–2 mg IV bolus

Conclusions

Vasopressors are an important therapy for cardiovascular support in the ICU.

Catecholamines are widely used for this purpose, and their action is mediated predominantly via alpha-adrenergic vasoconstriction and beta-agonist inotropy and chronotropy.

Non-adrenergic agents are gaining interest in the hope to reduce complications associated with catecholamines and provide further support when catecholamine doses rise. They have been shown to have an adrenergic-sparing action and in certain circumstances comparable effects. As their function is further investigated, they are likely to find increasing applications in the ICU alongside adrenergic vasopressors.

In addition to this, genetic polymorphisms can affect response to vasopressors, and a better understanding will help tailor individual therapy in the future.

Take-Home Messages

- Vasopressors are used predominantly to increase mean arterial pressure by increasing vascular tone.
- Appropriate fluid resuscitation should be ensured when starting vasopressor therapy.
- Establishing the cause for haemodynamic instability will help guide the choice of vasopressor (e.g. noradrenaline in septic shock).
- Serious complications can occur with vasopressors, and close monitoring is essential to detect and act on them early.

References

1. Landzberg JS, Parker JD, Gauthier DF, Colucci WS. Effects of myocardial alpha 1-adrenergic receptor stimulation and blockade on contractility in humans. Circulation. 1991;84:1608–14.
2. Williamson AP, Seifen E, Lindemann JP, Kennedy RH. WB4101- and CEC-sensitive positive inotropic actions of phenylephrine in rat cardiac muscle. Am J Phys. 1994;266:H2462–7.
3. Brodde O-E. Beta1- and beta2-adrenoceptor polymorphisms and cardiovascular diseases. Fundam Clin Pharmacol. 2008;22:107–25.
4. Nakada T, Russell JA, Boyd JH, Aguirre-Hernandez R, Thain KR, Thair SA, Nakada E, McConechy M, Walley KR. Beta2-Adrenergic receptor gene polymorphism Is associated with mortality in septic shock. Am J Respir Crit Care Med. 2010;181:143–9.
5. Benedict CR, Fillenz M, Stanford C. Changes in plasma noradrenaline concentration as a measure of release rate. Br J Pharmacol. 1978;64:305–9.
6. Rhodes A, Evans LE, Alhazzani W, et al. Surviving sepsis campaign. Crit Care Med. 2017;45:486–552.
7. Avni T, Lador A, Lev S, Leibovici L, Paul M, Grossman A. Vasopressors for the treatment of septic shock: systematic review and meta-analysis. PLoS One. 2015;10:1–17.
8. Gamper G, Havel C, Arrich J, Losert H, Pace NL, Müllner M, Herkner H. Vasopressors for hypotensive shock. Cochrane Database Syst Rev. 2016; https://doi.org/10.1002/14651858.CD003709.pub4.
9. Myburgh JA, Higgins A, Jovanovska A, Lipman J, Ramakrishnan N, Santamaria J. A comparison of epinephrine and norepinephrine in critically ill patients. Intensive Care Med. 2008;34:2226–34.
10. Vail E, Gershengorn HB, Hua M, Walkey AJ, Rubenfeld G, Wunsch H. Association between US norepinephrine shortage and mortality among patients with septic shock. JAMA. 2017;317:1433.

11. Levy B, Bastien O, Karim B, et al. Experts' recommendations for the management of adult patients with cardiogenic shock. Ann Intensive Care. 2015;5:17.
12. Levy B, Perez P, Perny J, Thivilier C, Gerard A. Comparison of norepinephrine-dobutamine to epinephrine for hemodynamics, lactate metabolism, and organ function variables in cardiogenic shock. A prospective, randomized pilot study. Crit Care Med. 2011;39:450–5.
13. De Backer DP, Biston P, Devriendt J, Madl C. Comparison of dopamine and norepinephrine in the treatment of shock. N Engl J Med 2010;362:779–89.
14. Rossaint R, Bouillon B, Cerny V, et al. The European guideline on management of major bleeding and coagulopathy following trauma: fourth edition. Crit Care. 2016;20:100.
15. Gelman S, Mushlin P. Catecholamine-induced changes in the splanchnic circulation affecting systemic hemodynamics. Anesthesiology. 2004;100:434–9.
16. Ginès P, Angeli P, Lenz K, et al. EASL clinical practice guidelines on the management of ascites, spontaneous bacterial peritonitis, and hepatorenal syndrome in cirrhosis. J Hepatol. 2010;53:397–417.
17. Bratton SL, Chestnut RM, Ghajar J, et al. Cerebral perfusion thresholds. J Neurotrauma. 2007;24:S-59–64.
18. Soar J, Nolan JP, Böttiger BW, et al. European Resuscitation Council Guidelines for Resuscitation 2015. Section 3. Adult advanced life support. Resuscitation. 2015;95:100–47.
19. Link MS, Berkow LC, Kudenchuk PJ, et al. Part 7: adult advanced cardiovascular life support: 2015 American Heart Association guidelines update for cardiopulmonary resuscitation and emergency cardiovascular care. Circulation. 2015;132:S444–64.
20. Long B, Koyfman A. Emergency medicine myths: epinephrine in cardiac arrest. J Emerg Med. 2017;52:809–14.
21. Andersen LW, Kurth T, Chase M, Berg KM, Cocchi MN, Callaway C, Donnino MW. Early administration of epinephrine (adrenaline) in patients with cardiac arrest with initial shockable rhythm in hospital: propensity score matched analysis. BMJ. 2016;353:i1577.
22. Perkins GD, Quinn T, Deakin CD, et al. Pre-hospital assessment of the role of adrenaline: measuring the effectiveness of drug administration in cardiac arrest (PARAMEDIC-2): trial protocol. Resuscitation. 2016;108:75–81.
23. Truhlář A, Deakin CD, Soar J, et al. European Resuscitation Council Guidelines for Resuscitation 2015. Section 4. Cardiac arrest in special circumstances. Resuscitation. 2015;95:148–201.
24. Bangash MN, Kong ML, Pearse RM. Use of inotropes and vasopressor agents in critically ill patients. Br J Pharmacol. 2012;165:2015–33.
25. Calabrese EJ. Dopamine: biphasic dose responses. Crit Rev Toxicol. 2001;31:563–83.
26. Jentzer JC, Coons JC, Link CB, Schmidhofer M. Pharmacotherapy update on the use of vasopressors and inotropes in the intensive care unit. J Cardiovasc Pharmacol Ther. 2015;20:249–60.
27. Denton MD, Chertow GM, Brady HR. "Renal-dose" dopamine for the treatment of acute renal failure: scientific rationale, experimental studies and clinical trials. Kidney Int. 1996;50:4–14.
28. Marik PE. Low-dose dopamine: a systematic review. Intensive Care Med. 2002;28:877–83.
29. Kellum JA, Decker JM. Use of dopamine in acute renal failure: a meta-analysis. Crit Care Med. 2001;29:1526–31.
30. Kobayashi S, Endou M, Sakuraya F, Matsuda N, Zhang X-H, Azuma M, Echigo N, Kemmotsu O, Hattori Y, Gando S. The sympathomimetic actions of l-ephedrine and d-pseudoephedrine: direct receptor activation or norepinephrine release? Anesth Analg. 2003;97:1239–45.
31. Belletti A, Musu M, Silvetti S, et al. Non-adrenergic vasopressors in patients with or at risk for vasodilatory shock. A systematic review and meta-analysis of randomized trials. PLoS One. 2015;10:1–13.
32. Russell JA. Bench-to-bedside review: Vasopressin in the management of septic shock. Crit Care. 2011;15:226.
33. Landry DW, Levin HR, Gallant EM, Ashton RC, Seo S, D'Alessandro D, Oz MC, Oliver JA. Vasopressin deficiency contributes to the vasodilation of septic shock. Circulation. 1997;95:1122–5.
34. Holmes CL, Patel BM, Russell JA, Walley KR. Physiology of vasopressin relevant to management of septic shock. Chest. 2001;120:989–1002.
35. Russell JA, Walley KR, Singer J, et al. Vasopressin versus norepinephrine infusion in patients with septic shock. N Engl J Med. 2008;358:877–87.
36. Gordon AC, Mason AJ, Thirunavukkarasu N, et al. Effect of early vasopressin vs norepinephrine on kidney failure in patients with septic shock: the VANISH randomized clinical trial. JAMA. 2017;316:509–18.
37. Polito A, Parisini E, Ricci Z, Picardo S, Annane D. Vasopressin for treatment of vasodilatory shock: An ESICM systematic review and meta-analysis. Intensive Care Med. 2012;38:9–19.

38. Bernadich C, Bandi JC, Melin P, Bosch J. Effects of F-180, a new selective vasoconstrictor peptide, compared with terlipressin and vasopressin on systemic and splanchnic hemodynamics in a rat model of portal hypertension. Hepatology. 1998;27:351–6.
39. National Institute for Health and Clinical Excellence. Management of acute upper gastrointestinal bleeding. (Clinical guideline 141.) 2012. http://guidance.nice.org.uk/CG141.
40. Freeman JG, Cobden I, Lishman AH, Record CO. Controlled trial of terlipressin ('Glypressin') versus vasopressin in the early treatment of oesophageal varices. Lancet. 1982;2:66–8.
41. Fort E, Sautereau D, Silvain C, Ingrand P, Pillegand B, Beauchant M. A randomized trial of terlipressin plus nitroglycerin vs. balloon tamponade in the control of acute variceal hemorrhage. Hepatology. 1990;11:678–81.
42. Corrêa TD, Takala J, Jakob SM. Angiotensin II in septic shock. Crit Care. 2015;19:98.
43. Khanna A, English SW, Wang XS, et al. Angiotensin II for the treatment of vasodilatory shock. N Engl J Med. 2017;377:419–30.

Fluid Resuscitation

Peter Buhl Hjortrup and Anders Perner

M. R. Pinsky et al. (eds.), *Hemodynamic Monitoring*, Lessons from the ICU,
https://doi.org/10.1007/978-3-319-69269-2_31

Learning Objectives

In this chapter we will analyse different aspects of fluid resuscitation in order to inform decision-making. This will include an analysis of the rationale for fluid resuscitation, assessing different types of fluid compounds, and provide an applicable approach to fluid therapy based on available evidence.

31.1 Introduction

Fluid resuscitation is a very frequent intervention in critical care and has been used for almost two centuries. Fluid resuscitation lacks a uniformly recognized definition but may be defined as intravenous fluid administration with the aim of improving the circulation in the case of shock. Most intravenous fluid compounds are cheap and readily available.

The main mechanism by which intravenous fluid may improve the circulation is by increasing stroke volume through increased preload and, in turn, cardiac output. However, intravenous fluid administration also carries potential adverse effects, including electrolyte derangements and organ and peripheral oedema that may lead to impaired ventilation, kidney function and circulation. The balance between benefits and harms is presently not fully elucidated, and clinicians must, thereby, base their decisions concerning fluid resuscitation mostly on patient history and pathophysiology and lower quality of evidence.

31.2 Physiological Rationale for Intravenous Fluid Resuscitation

The first documented use of intravenous fluid resuscitation was performed in 1832 when Dr. Thomas Latta treated severely dehydrated cholera patients with large amounts of saline fluids intravenously [1]. Fluid administration was somewhat paradigm challenging since the predominant treatments at the time were laxatives, emetics and venesection [2]; since then, few have questioned the administration of fluids in replacement of severe losses. The concept of administering intravenous fluids beyond replacement of losses is based on the findings of early twentieth-century physiologists Ernest Starling and Otto frank, who gave name to the "frank-Starling mechanism" that states when all other variables are constant, a larger end-diastolic volume increases the stroke volume until a certain point where the heart becomes over-distended and the stroke volume decreases. Thus, the idea of fluid resuscitation is to increase the venous return and preload and in turn increasing stroke volume and cardiac output.

31.2.1 Fluid Responsiveness

The term "fluid responder" is rooted in the frank-Starling mechanism and is used when a patient responds to a fluid challenge with an increase in stroke volume and/or cardiac output – Usually a 10–15% increase. Conversely, if the stroke volume/cardiac output does not increase, the term "nonresponder" is used. The fluid challenge can either be performed by administering a fixed amount of intravenous fluid or by mobilizing venous blood by a passive leg raising test [3]. Numerous invasive and noninvasive techniques have been proposed to assess stroke volume/cardiac output. Importantly, regardless of the validity of the technique used, a "positive" fluid response does not necessarily infer that the patient will benefit from fluid administration – Only that the stroke volume/cardiac output will increase.

31.2.2 Adverse Effects

All medical interventions are associated with potential beneficial effects and potential adverse effects; intravenous fluids are no exception. Increased fluid balance has been associated with worse outcome in several observational studies [4–6]. Organ oedema impeding diffusion of oxygen into the tissue including – but not restricted to – the lungs are likely to contribute to these findings. High fluid input also increases the risk of electrolyte derangements, especially in case of acute kidney injury (AKI) with impaired excretion. Hypernatraemia is not uncommon following high-volume fluid administration, and restoring plasma sodium to acceptable values in presence of AKI represents a substantial challenge for clinicians. Despite the long history of using intravenous fluids, there may also be potential adverse effects that are not yet fully understood. The FEAST randomized clinical trial was stopped early due to increased mortality in febrile children with impaired circulation receiving either a saline bolus or an albumin bolus as compared with those receiving no fluid bolus [7]. A subsequent analysis of the observed increase in mortality suggested cardiovascular collapse rather than respiratory failure to be the driving cause of death indicating that the physiology of fluid resuscitation is not yet fully understood by the medical community [8].

31.3 When to Administer Fluids?

The decision on whether to administer intravenous fluids is a perpetual challenge for clinicians and is still a matter of discussion. Unfortunately, the available evidence do not allow for clear and easy-to-apply recommendations. Two seemingly simple clinical questions are important to answer to inform decision-making.

1. Do we have to intervene?
2. If so, is fluid likely beneficial?

▪ Do we have to intervene?

Whether or not to intervene on circulatory comprise is in some cases obvious (e.g. septic shock with mean arterial pressure (MAP) 40 mmHg, heart rate 150 beats/min, lactate 10 mmol/l) but in many cases less clear (e.g. sepsis with MAP 62 mmHg, heart rate 110 beats/min, lactate 1,9 mmol/l). To inform the decision on whether to intervene, doing a thorough clinical exam and gathering available haemodynamic measurements are needed (◘ Fig. 31.1). Markers of hypoperfusion such as lactate and mottling are likely to be superior to surrogate markers such as heart rate, blood pressure and, especially in sepsis, urinary output, because they are suggestive of a circulation unable to fulfil the supply/demand of the organs. Advanced invasive haemodynamic monitoring using pulmonary artery catheter (PAC) has not suggested benefit compared to less invasive monitoring [9]. Accordingly, observational studies have shown that the majority of clinicians use simple markers rather than advanced haemodynamic measurements when assessing indication for fluid resuscitation – the most frequent being hypotension/high-dose vasopressor, oli-

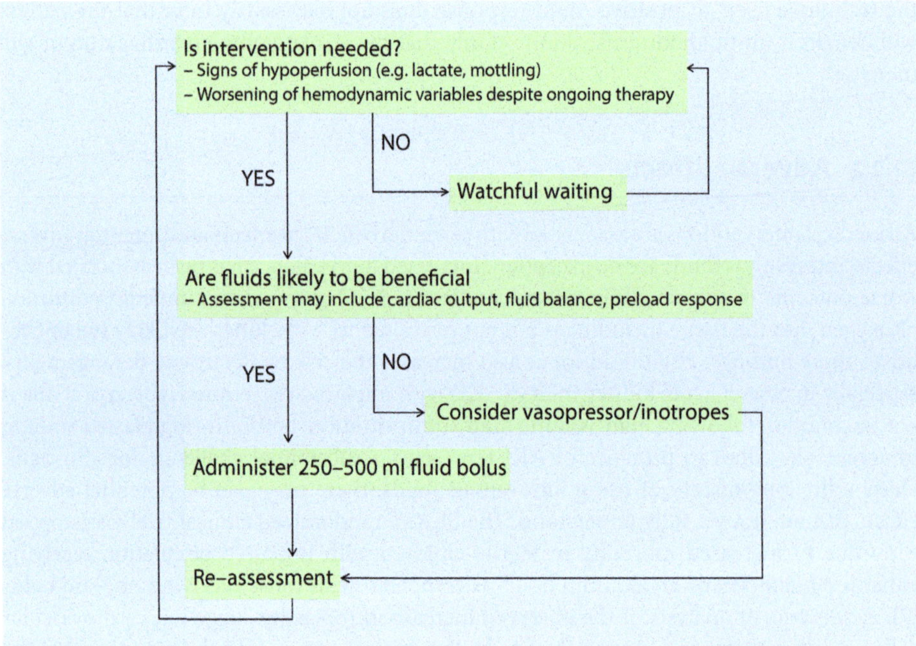

Fig. 31.1 Flow chart for clinicians assessing patients with haemodynamic compromise

31

guria and high plasma lactate [10, 11]. Also, simple clinical exam findings such as mottling and capillary refill time have been associated with increased mortality [12, 13]; however, association with worse outcome does not infer that intervening will benefit patients, and trials assessing benefit vs. harm with interventions on these markers of haemodynamic compromise are lacking.

▪ If so, is fluid likely beneficial?

Facing a patient with haemodynamic compromise, clinicians are basically presented with three options: fluid administration, vasopressor/inotropic therapy or watchful waiting. If watchful waiting is not deemed pertinent (see above), then an assessment of whether fluid is likely to be beneficial is needed (Fig. 31.1). Since the potential benefit of fluid resuscitation is to increase cardiac output, first clinicians must estimate whether cardiac output/stroke volume is insufficient. The clinical gold standard for measuring cardiac output is using invasive thermodilution, but the routine use of this technique has not been shown to improve outcome [14, 15]. Less invasive markers of cardiac output have been suggested, including pulse contour analysis and echocardiography [16, 17], none of which have been sufficiently validated in shocked patients. Simple markers such as central venous oxygen saturation [18], temperature gradients on the extremities or temperature of the great toe may be easy and readily available alternatives [19].

If an increase in cardiac output is deemed indicated, an assessment whether fluid resuscitation is likely to do so is needed. Several advanced techniques of assessing fluid responsiveness have been proposed with and without administering fluids, but both precise and accurate less invasive methods that may be used in the majority of patients have

Table 31.1 Ranking of clinical variables favouring and opposing fluid resuscitation, respectively

	Favours fluid resuscitation	Oppose fluid resuscitation
Strong	Documented fluid loss	Pulmonary oedema
		No effect by a previous fluid bolus
Moderate	Mottling	
	Low $ScvO_2/SvO_2$	Peripheral oedemas
	Low cardiac output	Known cardiac failure
	Elongated capillary refill time	Negative preload response
	High plasma lactate, e.g. >4 mmol/l	Established AKI with low urinary output
	Temperature gradients on arms and legs	
Weak	Low CVP	High CVP
	Low MAP	
	High heart rate	
	Low urinary output	
	Higher vasopressor dose	
	Positive preload response	

Abbreviations: *$ScvO_2$* central venous oxygen saturation, *SvO_2* mixed venous oxygen saturation, *CVP* central venous pressure, *MAP* mean arterial pressure

not yet been found. The passive leg raising test has shown promising predictive values for fluid response but needs an estimate of changes in stroke volume to assess fluid response [20]. A meticulous fluid balance history with in- and outputs may provide important information along a clinical examination. A high positive fluid balance, considerable peripheral oedemas and established AKI with low urinary output should be cause for concern for further fluid input (Table 31.1). On the other hand, a low fluid balance and documented fluid losses from gut or drains should advocate fluid administration. Fluid resuscitation aimed at increasing central venous pressure (CVP) has previously been promoted by international guidelines [21], but the predictive value of CVP for fluid response is low, and fluid administration aiming at increasing CVP should no longer be used as standard practice [22].

If a decision to administer fluid is taken, it is of paramount importance to reassess the patient after the administration. In order to allow a meaningful reassessment, the fluid administration can be performed with a fixed amount (e.g. 250–500 ml) bolus administration. The most important observations in this regard are the values/observations that led to the fluid administration, but signs of adverse effects such as worsening respiratory function should be assessed and plasma electrolyte concentrations monitored regularly.

31.4 Effects of Fluid Resuscitation

Knowledge on the balance between benefits and harms with a medical intervention is necessary in order to provide recommendation for its use. Patient-important outcomes such as survival and quality of life are of special interest, because they inherently assess the balance between beneficial effects and harmful effects. Results from randomized trials on fluid volumes are presently limited. A recent meta-analysis of fluid volumes in ARDS and sepsis included only 11 trials, and the results were therefore imprecise due to the limited sample [23]. Although the point estimate for mortality favoured fluid restriction, the results were not statistically significant. Fluid restriction was associated with reduced use of mechanical ventilation, but this result was largely driven by the FACTT trial done in patients with acute lung injury [14]. Other potential harm has been suggested. Fluid bolus in African children with impaired perfusion was associated with increased mortality compared with no bolus [7], and in a small trial of patients with septic shock, a restrictive fluid resuscitation strategy was associated with less AKI compared to standard care [24].

In case of fluid resuscitation, the haemodynamic effects are often measured immediately following administration, but the adverse effects may accumulate during a longer period of time. Traditionally, the term fluid responder is used when the patient has an immediate response to fluids (<30 min), but the sustained effect is less studied, and suggestions on a transient effect have been reported in fluid responders where the initial increase in cardiac output following a fluid bolus returned to baseline within 90 minutes [25]. In concordance with this, in a post hoc analysis of the CLASSIC randomized trial, no apparent effects of increased fluid resuscitation volume were observed on urinary output, vasopressor dose or plasma lactate levels in patients with septic shock [24]. Thus, sustained haemodynamic effects have not been established, and repeated episodes of fluid resuscitation following a "positive" fluid challenge may carry the risk of longer-term adverse effects.

31.4.1 Fluid Resuscitation and AKI

Low urinary output is one of the most frequently reported indications for fluid resuscitation, but there are limited data to support this practice. The rationale for this practice is likely that low urinary output is interpreted as prerenal AKI caused by decreased blood flow to the kidneys. This notion may be an oversimplification, especially in case of sepsis where AKI has been associated with increased renal blood flow [26–28]. Albeit not strong evidence, there are data to suggest that fluid resuscitation may aggravate rather mitigate AKI [23, 24, 29]. If fluid resuscitation is administered due to low urinary output, special vigilance to the response is pertinent. In the case of a modest response in urinary output to fluid resuscitation, it may take several days to excrete the additional fluid without further interventions.

31.5 Choosing Type of Fluid

Choosing type of fluid is another intensely discussed topic when it comes to fluid resuscitation. Basically the choice stands between crystalloids, either saline or buffered salt solutions, and colloids, either human albumin or synthetic colloids. Synthetic colloids, with hydroxyethyl starches being the most studied, have been associated with increased mortality and use of renal replacement therapy and should not be used [30–32]. Human albumin solutions appear safe and have a potential volume-reducing effect of around a factor 1.3 compared to crystalloids, but firm evidence of benefit has not been shown, and albumin is an expensive and limited resource [33, 34].

Isotonic saline has been used for decades but has been increasingly replaced by buffered salt solutions such as Ringer's lactate/acetate [35]. Use of chloride-rich solutions such as saline has been associated with AKI [36], but firm evidence on causality is lacking. Buffered salt solutions, the euphemism "balanced crystalloids" often used, are crystalloids which are buffered with anions like lactate, acetate, gluconate and/or malate to lower the chloride content as compared to saline. The effects of these nonphysiological concentrations of anions are currently unknown. Of note, the buffered salt solutions often contain lower concentrations of sodium (around 130 mmol/l), which may reduce patient sodium levels compared to saline [37]. On the other hand, there is still a risk of hypernatraemia with the buffered solutions if the renal excretion of sodium is lower than the infused quantity. The best available evidence on saline vs. buffered salt solutions is the results of the SPLIT trial. In this cluster randomized trial, ICU patients with relatively low illness severity were allocated to either saline or a buffered salt solution. No differences were observed between the two groups in the main outcomes including marker of AKI and mortality [38]. Large randomized trials comparing buffered salt solutions and saline are currently ongoing; until the results of these are reported, both saline and buffered salt solutions are viable choices. Changes in plasma sodium and base excess should, however, be observed during the care because of risks of dysnatremia and hyperchloremic acidosis with buffered solutions and saline, respectively [37].

Conclusions

Fluid resuscitation has been one of the most frequent interventions performed in critical care for decades, and most types of fluids are cheap and readily available, but the effects including haemodynamic effects beyond an initial response are not yet fully understood. Moreover, harm has been suggested with higher fluid inputs within the range of standard practice. Initiation and especially continued fluid resuscitation should be based on thorough clinical exam and assessment of available haemodynamic values and vigilant monitoring of signs of adverse effects to fluids.

Take-Home Messages

- Fluids are drugs, and administration of fluids is only indicated when the potential beneficial effects are judged to outweigh the potential harmful effects. In order to make this assessment a careful medical history, clinical exam and evaluation of available haemodynamic variables are needed.
- In case of haemodynamic compromise, two clinical questions should be answered [1]. Is any intervention needed? And [2] if yes, are fluids likely to be beneficial?
- Following fluid administration, a reassessment is pivotal in order to assess the potential need for further fluid administration.

31.6 Questions

1. A test finding a patient to be a fluid responder tells us that the patient needs fluids.
2. Buffered crystalloid solutions may lower plasma sodium levels.
3. The first documented use of intravenous fluid administration was aimed at maximizing cardiac output.
4. The frank-Starling mechanism states that a larger end-diastolic volume increases the stroke volume until a certain point.
5. The most commonly used indication for fluid administration is a low cardiac output measurement.
6. Organ failure due to increased diffusion path due to organ oedema is a potential risk with higher fluid balance.
7. Fluid resuscitation based on advanced haemodynamic monitoring has been shown to benefit intensive care patients compared to simple haemodynamic variables.
8. The temperature gradient on the extremities may be used as a surrogate for cardiac output.

9. Central venous pressure has high predicted value for fluid response.
10. Slow continuous fluid administration will improve the ability to assess the haemodynamic effects compared to bolus therapy.
11. Infusion of large volumes of buffered salt solutions with a sodium content of 130 mmol/l may cause hypernatraemia (plasma sodium >145 mmol/litre).
12. Infusion of 1 litre of colloid solution has the same potency as 3 litres of crystalloids.
13. Increased mean arterial pressure following a passive leg raising test is a strong predictor of fluid responsiveness.
14. Buffered salt solutions such as Ringer's solutions contain bicarbonate anions mimicking plasma values.
15. A plasma lactate >4 mmol/L suggests impaired perfusion.
16. Pulse contour analysis is the gold standard for measuring cardiac output.
17. Reassessment following fluid resuscitation is important.
18. Low urinary output is always due to decreased renal blood flow.

19. Watchful waiting can be a valid choice instead of intervening with fluids and/or vasopressors.

20. Synthetic colloids may cause kidney failure.

31.7 Answers

1. N
2. Y
3. N
4. Y
5. N
6. Y
7. N
8. Y
9. N
10. N
11. Y
12. N
13. N
14. N
15. Y
16. N
17. Y
18. N
19. Y
20. Y

References

1. Latta T. Malignant Cholera. Lancet. 1832;18(460):274–80.
2. Mackintosh J. Principles of pathology and practice of physic. 3rd ed. Philadelphia: Key & Briddle; 1836.
3. Vincent J-L, Weil MH. Fluid challenge revisited. Crit Care Med. 2006;34(5):1333–7.
4. Boyd JH, Forbes J, Nakada T-A, Walley KR, Russell JA. Fluid resuscitation in septic shock: a positive fluid balance and elevated central venous pressure are associated with increased mortality. Crit Care Med. 2011;39(2):259–65.
5. Vaara ST, Korhonen A-M, Kaukonen K-M, Nisula S, Inkinen O, Hoppu S, et al. Fluid overload is associated with an increased risk for 90-day mortality in critically ill patients with renal replacement therapy: data from the prospective FINNAKI study. Crit Care. 2012;16(5):R197-R.
6. Acheampong A, Vincent J-L. A positive fluid balance is an independent prognostic factor in patients with sepsis. Crit Care. 2015;19(1):251.
7. Maitland K, Kiguli S, Opoka RO, Engoru C, Olupot-Olupot P, Akech SO, et al. Mortality after fluid bolus in African children with severe infection. N Engl J Med. 2011;364(26):2483–95.
8. Maitland K, George EC, Evans JA, Kiguli S, Olupot-Olupot P, Akech SO, et al. Exploring mechanisms of excess mortality with early fluid resuscitation: insights from the FEAST trial. BMC Med. 2013;11:68.
9. Wheeler AP, Bernard GR, Thompson BT, Schoenfeld D, et al. Pulmonary-artery versus central venous catheter to guide treatment of acute lung injury. N Engl J Med. 2006;354(21):2213–24.
10. Bihari S, Baldwin CE, Bersten AD, Ou J, Holt AW, Prakash S, et al. Post resuscitation fluid boluses in severe sepsis or septic shock: prevalence and efficacy (price study). Crit Care Resusc. 2013;12(1):66–70.
11. Cecconi M, Hofer C, Teboul J-L, Pettila V, Wilkman E, Molnar Z, et al. Fluid challenges in intensive care: the FENICE study: a global inception cohort study. Intensive Care Med. 2015;41(9):1529–37.
12. Ait-Oufella H, Lemoinne S, Boelle PY, Galbois A, Baudel JL, Lemant J, et al. Mottling score predicts survival in septic shock. Intensive Care Med. 2011;37(5):801–7.
13. Ait-Oufella H, Bige N, Boelle PY, Pichereau C, Alves M, Bertinchamp R, et al. Capillary refill time exploration during septic shock. Intensive Care Med. 2014;40:958–64.
14. Wiedemann HP, Wheeler AP, Bernard GR, Thompson BT, Hayden D, DeBoisblanc B, et al. Comparison of two fluid-management strategies in acute lung injury. N Engl J Med. 2006;354(24):2564–75.
15. Harvey S, Harrison DA, Singer M, Ashcroft J, Jones CM, Elbourne D, et al. Assessment of the clinical effectiveness of pulmonary artery catheters in management of patients in intensive care (PAC-Man): a randomised controlled trial. Lancet. 2005;366(9484):472–7.
16. Mehta Y, Arora D. Newer methods of cardiac output monitoring. World J Cardiol. 2014;6(9):1022–9.
17. Wetterslev M, Moller-Sorensen H, Johansen RR, Perner A. Systematic review of cardiac output measurements by echocardiography vs. thermodilution: the techniques are not interchangeable. Intensive Care Med. 2016;42(8):1223–33.
18. Perner A, Haase N, Wiis J, White JO, Delaney A. Central venous oxygen saturation for the diagnosis of low cardiac output in septic shock patients. Acta Anaesthesiol Scand. 2010;54(1):98–102.
19. Joly HR, Weil MH. Temperature of the great toe as an indication of the severity of shock. Circulation. 1969;39(1):131–8.
20. Cavallaro F, Sandroni C, Marano C, La Torre G, Mannocci A, De Waure C, et al. Diagnostic accuracy of passive leg raising for prediction of fluid responsiveness in adults: systematic review and meta-analysis of clinical studies. Intensive Care Med. 2010;36(9):1475–83.
21. Bone RC, Balk RA, Cerra FB, Dellinger RP, Fein AM, Knaus WA, et al. Definitions for sepsis and organ failure and guidelines for the use of innovative therapies in sepsis. The ACCP/SCCM Consensus Conference Committee. American College of Chest Physicians/Society of Critical Care Medicine. Chest. 1992;101(6):1644–55.
22. Eskesen TG, Wetterslev M, Perner A. Systematic review including re-analyses of 1148 individual data sets of central venous pressure as a predictor of fluid responsiveness. Intensive Care Med. 2016;42(3):324–32.
23. Silversides JA, Major E, Ferguson AJ, Mann EE, McAuley DF, Marshall JC, Blackwood B, Fan E. Conservative fluid management or deresuscitation for patients with sepsis or acute respiratory distress syndrome following the resuscitation phase of critical illness: a systematic review and meta-analysis. Intensive Care Med. 2016;43(2):155–70.
24. Hjortrup PB, Haase N, Bundgaard H, Thomsen SL, Winding R, Pettila V, et al. Restricting volumes of resuscitation fluid in adults with septic shock after initial management: the CLASSIC randomised, parallel-group, multicentre feasibility trial. Intensive Care Med. 2016;42(11):1695–705.

25. Nunes TS, Ladeira RT, Bafi AT, de Azevedo LC, Machado FR, Freitas FG. Duration of hemodynamic effects of crystalloids in patients with circulatory shock after initial resuscitation. Ann Intensive Care. 2014;4:25.
26. Langenberg C, Bellomo R, May C, Wan L, Egi M, Morgera S. Renal blood flow in sepsis. Crit Care. 2005;9(4):R363–74.
27. Langenberg C, Bellomo R, May CN, Egi M, Wan L, Morgera S. Renal vascular resistance in sepsis. Nephron Physiol. 2006;104(1):1–11.
28. Brenner M, Schaer GL, Mallory DL, Suffredini AF, Parrillo JE. Detection of renal blood flow abnormalities in septic and critically ill patients using a newly designed indwelling thermodilution renal vein catheter. Chest. 1990;98(1):170–9.
29. Perner A, Prowle J, Joannidis M, Young P, Hjortrup PB, Pettila V. Fluid management in acute kidney injury. Intensive Care Med. 2017;43(6):807–15.
30. Perner A, Haase N, Guttormsen AB, Tenhunen J, Klemenzson G, Åneman A, et al. Hydroxyethyl Starch 130/0.42 versus Ringer's acetate in severe sepsis. N Engl J Med. 2012;367(2):124–34.
31. Haase N, Perner A, Hennings LI, Siegemund M, Lauridsen B, Wetterslev M, et al. Hydroxyethyl starch 130/0.38–0.45 versus crystalloid or albumin in patients with sepsis: systematic review with meta-analysis and trial sequential analysis. BMJ. 2013;346:f839.
32. Myburgh JA, Finfer S, Bellomo R, Billot L, Cass A, Gattas D, et al. Hydroxyethyl starch or saline for fluid resuscitation in intensive care. N Engl J Med. 2012;367(20):1901–11.
33. Finfer S, Bellomo R, Boyce N, French J, Myburgh J, Norton R. A comparison of albumin and saline for fluid resuscitation in the intensive care unit. N Engl J Med. 2004;350(22):2247–56.
34. Caironi P, Tognoni G, Masson S, Fumagalli R, Pesenti A, Romero M, et al. Albumin replacement in patients with severe sepsis or septic shock. N Engl J Med. 2014;370(15):1412–21.
35. Hammond NE, Taylor C, Finfer S, Machado FR, An Y, Billot L, et al. Patterns of intravenous fluid resuscitation use in adult intensive care patients between 2007 and 2014: an international cross-sectional study. PLoS One. 2017;12(5):e0176292.
36. Yunos NM, Bellomo R, Glassford N, Sutcliffe H, Lam Q, Bailey M. Chloride-liberal vs. chloride-restrictive intravenous fluid administration and acute kidney injury: an extended analysis. Intensive Care Med. 2014;41(2):257–64.
37. Bampoe S, Odor PM, Dushianthan A, Bennett-Guerrero E, Cro S, Gan TJ, et al. Perioperative administration of buffered versus non-buffered crystalloid intravenous fluid to improve outcomes following adult surgical procedures. Cochrane Database Syst Rev. 2017;9:CD004089.
38. Young P, Bailey M, Beasley R, Henderson S, Mackle D, McArthur C, et al. Effect of a buffered crystalloid solution vs saline on acute kidney injury among patients in the intensive care unit: the SPLIT randomized clinical trial. JAMA. 2015;314(16):1701–10.

Choosing the Right Hemodynamic Therapy

Contents

Choosing the Ideal Hemodynamic Therapy in Acute Right and Left Heart Failure

Alexa Hollinger and Alexandre Mebazaa

M. R. Pinsky et al. (eds.), *Hemodynamic Monitoring*, Lessons from the ICU,
https://doi.org/10.1007/978-3-319-69269-2_32

Learning Objectives

Learning objectives start revising the main symptoms of acute right and left heart failures (▶ Sect. 32.2), etiologies and differential diagnoses of AHF (▶ Sect. 32.3), and the current practice of therapy of acute right and left heart failure (▶ Sect. 32.4).

32.1 Introduction

AHF refers to both new and rapid presentation of acute heart failure or deterioration of known heart failure [1]. Signs of acute heart failure (see ▶ Sect. 32.2) should raise immediate attention to this potentially life-threatening condition. AHF causes a high burden of mortality, morbidity, as well as repeated hospitalizations. Thereby it also accounts for a multiplier of overall health costs. Multidisciplinary practical guidance and handling are warranted for tailored and focused treatment approaches that can be applied to the various types and different clinical appearances of AHF [2].

32.2 Signs and Symptoms of Acute Heart Failure

Right and left ventricular failure are both life-threatening entities that are not always easy to detect and therefore have to be suspected based on clinical findings. Signs and symptoms of acute right and left heart failure are shown in ◘ Table 32.1.

The mentioned symptoms may dramatically worsen into respiratory failure and hemodynamic compromise. Due to inadequate blood supply, AHF can rapidly affect proper functioning of all vital organs.

Diagnosis of heart failure is confirmed by BNP (brain natriuretic peptide) > 400 pg/ml or NT-proBNP (N-terminal pro-brain natriuretic peptide) >1200 pg/ml.

32

◘ **Table 32.1** Signs and symptoms of acute right and left heart failure

Acute right ventricular failure [3]	Acute left ventricular failure
Signs of systemic congestion: jugular venous distension, hepatojugular reflux, peripheral edema, pericardial effusion, congestive hepatosplenomegaly, ascites, anasarca[a]	Signs of pulmonary congestion: dyspnea, orthopnea, pink frothy sputum, persistent cough or wheezing
Signs of right ventricular dysfunction: third heart sound, systolic murmur of tricuspid regurgitation, hepatic pulse, signs of concomitant left ventricular dysfunction, paradoxical pulse[b]	Signs of left ventricular dysfunction: new-onset arrhythmia, mitral regurgitation
Signs of low cardiac output state: central nervous system abnormalities, exercise intolerance, weakness or fatigue of acute onset, hypotension, tachycardia, angor, oliguria, cool extremities	
Others: Hypoxemia, Kussmaul sign[c]	Others: hypoxemia

[a]Particularly in acute decompensation of chronic RV failure
[b]Abnormally high decrease in systolic pressure and amplitude of pulse wave during inspiration
[c]Increase in jugular venous pressure on inspiration (e.g., RV infarction, constrictive pericarditis)

Table 32.2 Etiologies and differential diagnoses of right and left ventricular failure

Right ventricular failure [3]	Left ventricular failure
Acute left ventricular failure	Acute right ventricular failure
Right ventricular ischemia/infarction	Left ventricular ischemia/infarction
Sepsis	
Chronic pulmonary hypertension (groups 1–5) [4]	Chronic arterial hypertension
Arrhythmias (supraventricular or ventricular tachycardia)	Arrhythmias (supraventricular or ventricular tachycardia)
Congenital heart disease (e.g., atrial or ventricular septal defect, Ebstein's anomaly)	Congenital heart disease (e.g., bicuspid aortic valves, mitral valve prolapse)
Valvulopathies (e.g., tricuspid valve regurgitation, pulmonary valve stenosis)	Valvulopathies (e.g., mitral valve regurgitation, aortic valve regurgitation or stenosis)
Cardiomyopathies (e.g., arrhythmogenic right ventricular dysplasia, peripartum/postpartum, [5–7] familial, idiopathic)	Cardiomyopathies (e.g., peripartum/postpartum, familial, idiopathic)
Myocarditis or other inflammatory diseases	
Cardiac surgery (e.g., cardiac transplant or left ventricular assist device implantation)	Cardiac surgery (e.g., cardiac transplant, valve replacement) [8]
Hematological disorders (e.g., acute chest syndrome in sickle cell disease, polycythemia)	Hematological disorders (e.g., left ventricular diastolic dysfunction in sickle cell disease, polycythemia)
Acute pulmonary embolism	Tako-tsubo or tako-tsubo-like left ventricular dysfunction [9]
Chronic diseases (e.g., diabetes, HIV, hyperthyroidism, hypothyroidism, hemochromatosis, amyloidosis)	
Exacerbation of chronic lung disease and/or hypoxia	
Acute lung injury or respiratory distress syndrome	
Pericardial disease (tamponade)	

32.3 Causes and Differential Diagnoses of Acute Right and Left Ventricular Failure

Acute right and left ventricular heart failure reveal numerous etiologies that have to be kept in mind during the diagnostic work-up (Table 32.2):

32.4 Therapy [2, 3]

Diagnosis of AHF should be completed in a timely manner to start early therapy and prevent death. A high index of suspicion is warranted and should be based on the following clinical findings:

- Chest discomfort.
- Signs of pulmonary (dyspnea, increased respiratory rate, orthopnea, rales on auscultation) and systemic (jugular vein distension, hepatomegaly, peripheral edema) congestion.
- Signs of hypoperfusion (cold periphery, clammy or mottled skin, cyanosis, confusion, oliguria, hyperlactatemia).

Early recognition of AHF is crucial since the first hours after symptom onset are characterized by a high complication rate which includes death [10]. This is substantiated by the fact that earlier diagnosis, triage, and initiation of specific treatment for AHF are associated with reduced mortality and shorter lengths of hospital stay [11–14]. Lung ultrasound is an easy-to-use, inexpensive, noninvasive, reliable, and reproducible method that should be used already in the emergency department: B-line evaluation identifies extravascular lung water [15]. Studies confirm a better outcome after immediate intravenous administration of nitrates and noninvasive positive-pressure ventilation [13, 16, 17]. Special attention is also warranted on precipitating factors like acute coronary syndrome, pulmonary infection, or atrial fibrillation that need specific therapies. A therapy overview is provided at the end of the chapter (◘ Table 32.4).

32.4.1 Choosing the Ideal Therapy in the Prehospital Setting

Prehospital treatment should be based upon the patient's symptoms and vital signs. Oxygen therapy should be started in case of SpO_2 below 90%. In cases of respiratory distress or pulmonary edema, noninvasive ventilation (NIV) should be initiated immediately as it was shown that immediate application of CPAP alone in the prehospital setting improves physiological variables (e.g., PaO_2) and symptoms (e.g., dyspnea) and reduces

32

incidence of tracheal intubation [15]. When findings of congestion are assessed, intravenous diuretics (i.e., furosemide 0.5 mg/kg or the double home dose of loop diuretic) should be administered. Normal or high blood pressure should be treated with intravenous/sublingual/spray nitrates. A careful fluid challenge (i.e., 4 ml/kg or 250 ml) is recommended when the patient is hypotensive or shows signs of hypoperfusion (see above).

32.4.2 Choosing the Ideal Therapy Within the First 2 h in AHF Without Cardiogenic Shock

When "time is muscle," efficient management is crucial. Diuretics, vasodilators, and administration of oxygen or (non-)invasive ventilation represent the main therapeutics for the first 2 h in the hospital. Early administration of intravenous loop diuretics has been shown to be associated with reduced in-hospital mortality in AHF [18]. Target SpO_2 is recommended between 92% and 95% [19–21]. In a recent investigation, routine use of intravenous morphine in AHF has been questioned and was suggested to correlate with increased 30-day mortality in these patients [22].

A loop diuretic (i.e., furosemide; for dosage, see ▸ 32.4.1) should be administered within 30 min after admission if not already done in the prehospital setting [15]. Furosemide (40 mg i.v.) may have two beneficial effects: immediate venodilation and subsequent diuretic effect. This should be repeated if respiratory distress persists after 2 h. In case of oliguria, dosage should be increased. In some patients additional administration of thiazide or other classes of diuretics might be the key to success [23, 24]. A missing response can sometimes be attributed to diuretic resistance. The mechanism of which is unknown to date. Other therapeutic strategies (e.g., tolvaptan, a vasopressin v2 receptor antagonist, sequential nephron blockade) [25, 26] might be promising but did not gain sufficient importance to be integrated into the management guidelines of AHF. (Early) ultrafiltration demonstrates no superiority to pharmacotherapy [27] but has not been studied in this specific cohort [23].

When APE appears with abrupt hypertension, systemic volume overload is usually absent, and high-dose diuretics (i.e., >1 mg/kg) in this case are not recommended. In this situation, vasodilators and NIV represent first-line therapies. Overall, vasodilators are used in 30% of AHF [28]. They should be used with respect to close blood pressure monitoring due to their potential to produce severe hypotension. Their safety and benefit on outcome have been investigated in several trials. Vasodilators can be safely administered in systolic blood pressure >100 mmHg [29]. Nitrates serve as venodilators and arteriodilators at the same time and have been evidenced to be safe and effective even in high doses in severe APE [17]. In addition, high-dose treatment with nitroglycerin was shown to diminish rates of endotracheal intubation and ICU admission [30]. Overall, following the European Society of Cardiology (ESC) and American guidelines, the use of nitrates is strongly recommended [29, 31]. Contraindications of vasodilators are state of shock and significant mitral or aortic valve stenosis, and they should be used with caution in predominant right ventricular failure due to the risk of reduced coronary perfusion pressure.

Even though routine use of opiates is not recommended, morphine can be and is often used in anxious patients with acute respiratory distress [29].

Oxygen therapy and mechanical ventilation are indicated in APE which affects roughly 20% of AHF patients [32]. Depending on the severity of APE, conventional oxygen therapy can be sufficient to treat mild hypoxemia. In case of respiratory failure, NIV is indicated. Contraindications to install NIV therapy are a significantly altered mental state, poor cooperation, apnea, hypotension, vomiting, and possible pneumothorax [2]. In case of fatigue, weakness, obtundation, or failure of NIV, the patient should be intubated.

◻ Figure 32.1 discloses the recommended approach to early diagnosis, management, and treatment of AHF for the first 2 h after hospital admission [2].

32.4.3 Choosing the Ideal Therapy in Cardiogenic Shock

The state of cardiogenic shock is the most severe form of appearance of AHF. CS is characterized by hypotension and signs of organ hypoperfusion due to severe circulatory failure of cardiac origin. It accounts for less than 5% of AHF cases in the western world [32] and is caused by acute coronary syndrome in 80% of cases [33]. Other etiologies include severe decompensation of chronic heart failure, valvular disease, myocarditis, and takotsubo syndrome [2].

All shock patients need urgent ECG, troponin essay, and prompt coronary angiogram if the shock state is not explained elsehow (◻ Fig. 32.2). Urgent revascularization has been proven for benefit [34] and is recommended in the guidelines [35]. After revascularization controlled hypothermia is advocated [36]. For hemodynamic monitoring, echocardiography should be performed immediately and repeatedly used for surveillance of the patient's clinical condition. Inotropes and/or vasopressors should be installed only in

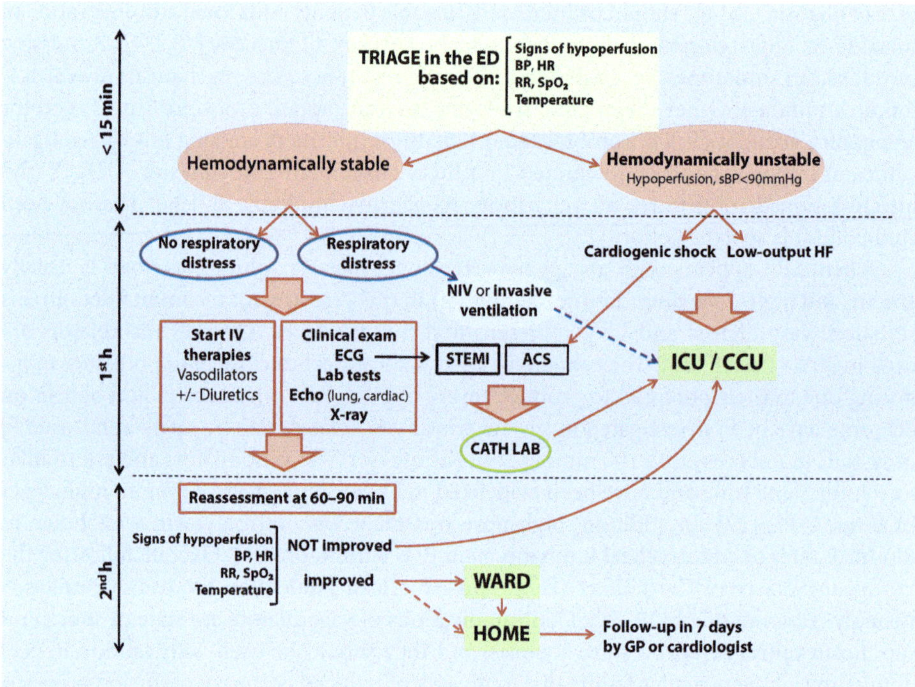

Fig. 32.1 The hospital management of patients with suspected acute heart failure. ED emergency department, BP blood pressure, HR heart rate, RR respiratory rate, SpO2 peripheral capillary oxygen saturation, Temp body temperature, NIV non-invasive ventilation, IV intravenous, ECG electrocardiogram, lab tests laboratory tests, echo ultrasound (lung ± cardiac), ACS acute coronary syndrome, STEMI ST segment elevation myocardial infarction, cath lab cardiac catheterization laboratory, ICU intensive care unit, CCU cardiac care unit, HF heart failure, GP general practitioner. Low output HF systolic <90 mmHg without signs of tissue hypoperfusion, usually in patients with end-stage heart disease

32

evidence of hypoperfusion. Inotropes and/or vasopressors should be administered in the lowest possible dose and for the shortest possible duration to achieve targeted perfusion pressure to minimize their side effects [37]. They should be applied over a central venous catheter (CVC) preferentially. The insertion of a CVC also allows to analyze $ScvO_2$ for the assessment of the ratio of global oxygen demand and supply, hence response to therapy. Dobutamine or levosimendan composes first-line therapy. Levosimendan might be preferred in the history of chronic heart failure or postinterventional myocardial stunning. Milrinone can be proposed before levosimendan in cases of concomitant pulmonary artery pressure as both reduce cardiac filling pressures, but also pulmonary vascular resistance [38]. Epinephrine has little or no indication due to higher incidence of side effects (e.g., arrhythmia, lactic acidosis) [39] and evidence of independent association with excess mortality in cardiogenic shock [40]. Norepinephrine, added to an inotrope, is the ideal vasopressor in CS [41, 42].

An arterial catheter should be inserted as soon as possible. This allows frequent uncomplicated bloodwork to monitor respiratory and hemodynamic support (e.g., lactate) [43, 44]. If the patient doesn't respond to therapy, the insertion of a pulmonary artery catheter (PAC) should be considered [29]. Early echocardiography is not only helpful in establishing a diagnosis but also in speeding up triage to ideal treatment and estimate prognosis (e.g., ejection fraction, right and left ventricular function). Follow-up echocardiography may evaluate treatment response.

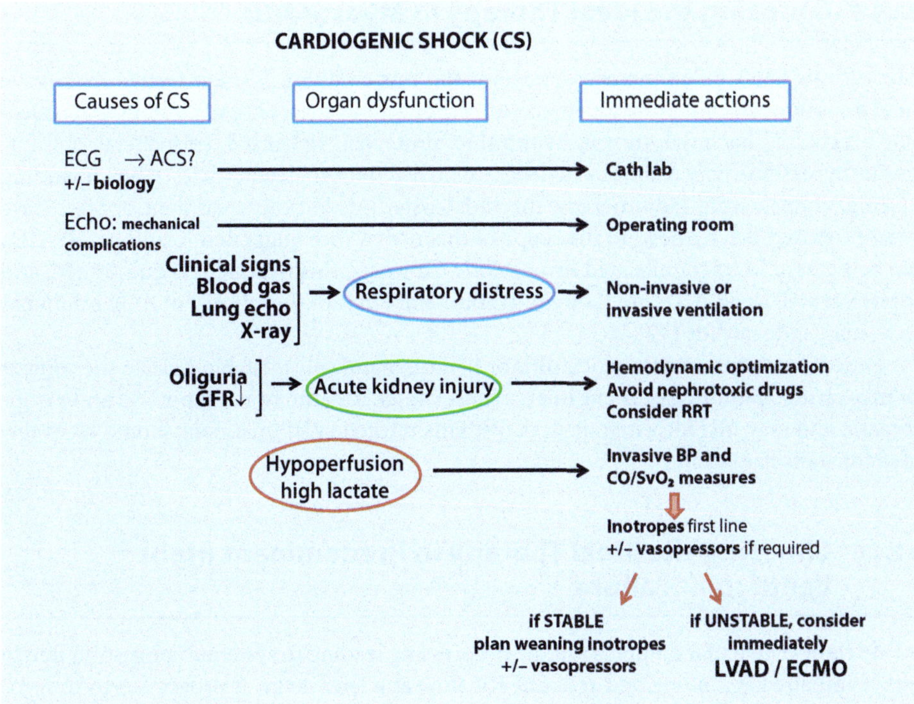

Fig. 32.2 All forms of cardiogenic shock need urgent ECG, troponin essay, and prompt coronary angiogram if the shock etiology is not otherwise explained. Immediate actions can be listed by the specific organ system failure

In selected cases advanced cardiovascular support is needed, such as device therapy. The intra-aortic balloon pump might be indicated for prophylactic reasons (e.g., profound ventricular dysfunction, critical left main disease) or when the patient cannot be weaned from the aforecited medical hemodynamic support [45]. However, no mortality benefit has been shown to date [46, 47]. Guidelines recommend left ventricular assist device (LVAD) or extracorporeal membrane oxygenation (ECMO) without preference in case of required temporary circulatory support [35, 48].

32.4.4 Choosing the Ideal Therapy in AHF with Acute Coronary Syndrome

AHF in this setting is usually a consequence of larger ischemia and myocardial dysfunction, and acute coronary syndrome is one of the main precipitating factors for AHF. The indications of emergency invasive evaluation and revascularization include:

- AHF with STEMI
- AHF with other high-risk ECG signs (e.g., ST-segment elevation in lead aVR, persistent deep precordial T-waves, ST-segment depression)
- ACS associated with persistent chest pain
- ACS with unstable AHF
- ACS with CS

32.4.5 Choosing the Ideal Therapy in Myocarditis

Myocarditis is an inflammatory disease of the myocardium. It often results from viral infections or post-viral immune-mediated responses but shares broad etiology (i.e., infectious including bacterial, fungal, helminthic, protozoal, rickettsial, spirochetal; autoimmune; hypersensitivity reactions to drugs; toxic reactions to drugs; toxic; others including arsenic, copper, iron, radiotherapy, thyrotoxicosis) [3]. Various treatment options have been proposed but are beyond the scope of this review (see Suggested Reading). NSAIDs are being used in uncomplicated myocarditis. However, this treatment is questioned, and aspirin as well as NSAIDs are thought to counteract part of the efficacy of ACE inhibitors in human endocarditis [49].

Patients with fulminant myocarditis or hemodynamically unstable AHF in the context of myocarditis require treatment in an expert center. Treatment is supportive and symptomatic and may include assist devices. Patients refractory to treatment should be evaluated for transplantation.

32.4.6 Choosing the Ideal Therapy in Predominant Right Ventricular Failure

Acute right ventricular failure is rapidly progressing leading to systemic congestion due to either impaired RV filling and reduced RV flow at a later stage. It progresses to dyssynchrony and eventually asynchrony of right and left ventricular performance causing systemic hypotension. This is based on the concept of systolic and diastolic ventricular interdependence where functioning of the left ventricle affects the right ventricle and vice versa.

Four aspects are important in the therapy of right ventricular failure:

1. Volume optimization
2. Vasopressor administration first, and inotrope if needed
3. Mechanical circulatory support
4. Therapy of specific clinical scenarios

32.4.6.1 Volume Optimization

Cautious volume loading based on central venous pressure monitoring is crucial. Even though patients with right ventricular failure can be preload dependent, it is important to not overdistend the right ventricle by volume overloading. Volume overload increases wall tension, decreases contractility, aggravates tricuspid regurgitation, increases ventricular interdependence, impairs left ventricular filling, and ultimately reduces systemic cardiac output.

32.4.6.2 Vasopressor and/or Inotrope Treatment

Norepinephrine is first indicated when hemodynamic instability is present. It is used to restore organ perfusion, especially the coronary and cerebral. A major advantage would be the improvement of systemic hemodynamics without a change in pulmonary vascular resistance.

Inotropes will be administered in case of evidence of low cardiac output. Dobutamine, levosimendan, and phosphodiesterase III inhibitors improve contractility and increase cardiac output. In pulmonary hypertension caused by left heart disease, levosimendan and phosphodiesterase III inhibitors may be preferred over dobutamine.

32.4.6.3 Mechanical Circulatory Support

Mechanical circulatory support may be indicated in RV myocardial infarction, acute PE, following left ventricular assist device implantation, or primary graft failure after heart transplantation.

ECMO and other forms of extracorporeal life support (ECLS) can be chosen for short-term mechanical support. Alternatively, catheter-mounted microaxial pumps can be used (i.e., Impella RP). The problem here is the limited maximum pump capacity. Other right ventricular assist devices such as RVADs can even be used for months but are officially approved for up to 4 weeks. When needed, they can be combined with oxygenators. Rarely, RV function is not restored, and the insertion of an implantable continuous-flow assist device or even heart transplantation has to be considered.

32.4.6.4 Therapeutic Aspects in Specific Clinical Scenarios

Pulmonary Embolism

Acute pulmonary embolism (PE) is one of the most frequent causes of acute right ventricular failure. Early detection and initiation of therapy is pivotal. Choosing the right therapeutic management is mainly based on the patient's condition. The solely, widely accepted indication for systemic thrombolysis is persistent hypotension or shock (i.e., a systolic blood pressure <90 mmHg or a decrease in the systolic blood pressure of ≥40 mmHg from baseline) following acute pulmonary embolism. In hemodynamically stable patients, the hemorrhagic risks of thrombolysis appear to outweigh the clinical benefits. But they should be monitored over the first 2–3 days for consideration of rescue thrombolysis in case of subsequent deterioration.

If thrombolysis is contraindicated or has failed and the patient is hemodynamically unstable, surgical pulmonary embolectomy should be deliberated. Imminent hemodynamic decompensation in combination with anticipated high bleeding risk under thrombolysis is another indication for surgical intervention [50].

Various catheter-directed techniques for the removal of obstructing thrombi from the main pulmonary arteries have been developed over the past years:

- Thrombus fragmentation with pigtail or balloon catheter
- Rheolytic thrombectomy with hydrodynamic catheter devices
- Suction thrombectomy with aspiration catheters
- Rotational thrombectomy

"Purely interventional" options are reserved for patients with absolute contraindications.

Endovascular treatment such as EKOS™ can be used for PE, deep vein thrombosis (DVT), and peripheral arterial occlusion (PAO). EKOS™ represents an ultrasound-enhanced lysis system. The EKOS™ System's targeted ultrasound waves accelerate thrombus dissolution by unwinding the fibrin matrix. Studies reveal lower patient risk and higher procedure predictability when compared to systemic thrombolysis [51, 52].

Pulmonary Hypertension

Right ventricular function is the major determinant of morbidity and mortality in pulmonary hypertension. Looking at the high number of causes of this condition (see Suggested Reading), the diagnostic work-up and the identification of triggers are somewhat time-consuming but also important [53–56]. However, the most frequent cause is infection, and as anticipated, sepsis is known to increase mortality significantly [55]. PH can become

Table 32.3 Most important symptoms of PH and therapies to be considered

Sign/symptom/course	Therapy
Supraventricular arrhythmia	Electrical cardioversion
Anemia	Correction
Hypoxia	Oxygen therapy (arterial oxygen saturation > 90%)
Hypercapnia/acidosis	NIV
Hypothermia	Correction
Venous congestion	Diuretics
Diuretic resistance	RRT
Elevated RV afterload	Intravenous prostacyclin, epoprostenol, inhaled nitric oxide or prostacyclin
Severe PAH but right atrial pressure ≤20 mmHg and arterial oxygen saturation ≥85% on room air	Balloon atrio-septostomy (high-risk technique, not in emergency)
Unresponsive	Bridge to recovery or lung transplant: Impella, ECMO, RVAD

clinically noticeable due to various symptoms. The most important signs and symptoms of PH and therapy considerations are addressed in the following table (Table 32.3).

Concerning correction of anemia, no optimal value for hemoglobin or hematocrit has been determined in patients with RV failure. Focus on correction of hypoxia, hypercapnia, acidosis, and hypothermia is essential as these promote or aggravate pulmonary vasoconstriction. Fluid status should be closely monitored (i.e., cardiac ultrasound, pulmonary artery catheter) due to the aforementioned matters.

Right Ventricular Infarction

Usually, acute inferior wall myocardial infarction (MI) caused by occlusion of the proximal right coronary artery is responsible for right ventricular infarction [57]. The right ventricle tolerates ischemic injury better than the left ventricle due to the following reasons [58, 59]:

- Lower oxygen demand
- Greater oxygen extraction reserve capability during stress
- Dual anatomical supply from the right and the left coronary arteries
- Relatively homogenous transmural perfusion across the cardiac cycle
- Increased propensity to acute collateral development

Treatment includes early myocardial reperfusion, evaluation of inotropic support, correction of bradycardia by atropine or aminophylline, AV sequential pacing in case of high-grade AV block, and reversion of acute atrial fibrillation. In right ventricular infarction as opposed to predominant left ventricular involvement, treatments comprising RV preload such as nitrates or diuretics must be used with caution as they may be deleterious. Treatment of cardiogenic shock has been described above.

Tamponade

Cardiac tamponade mimics acute RV failure and should be considered as differential diagnosis. Urgent percutaneous or surgical pericardial drainage is mandatory and possibly has to be preceded by vasopressor therapy [60].

Acute Right Ventricular Failure in the Intensive Care Setting

Acute RV failure is frequently seen in the ICU [61, 62], and ARDS represents the main cause. Protective ventilation strategy (i.e., plateau pressure < 27cmH_2O, $PaCO_2$ < 8 kPa, adapting PEEP to RV function, considering prone positioning for PaO_2/FiO_2 < 20 kPa/150 mmHg) for prevention or amelioration of its complications is adviced.

Valvular Disease

Acute RV dysfunction develops in both left-sided and right-sided valvular heart diseases. Surgery is recommended in valvular disease with right heart failure, severe tricuspid regurgitation and poor response to diuretics, infective endocarditis difficult to eradicate, large vegetations, and recurrent emboli [63].

Surgery

RV failure can develop after non-cardiac surgery and after cardiac surgery. In non-cardiac surgery, it most often develops secondary to increased right ventricular afterload following acute pulmonary hypertension. In cardiac surgery, it is frequently provoked by volume overload, myocardial ischemia, pre-existing RV dysfunction, or arrhythmia. Therapy should focus on the underlying cause including intolerance of sternal closure after cardiac surgery.

32.5 General Aspects and Long-Term Treatment

When the patient's situation is under control, he or she should be interrogated for cardiac risk factors if not done in the first place. Lifestyle changes (e.g., stop smoking) should now be addressed as a priority. Heart failure medication should be started or adjusted with respect to the installed therapy before acute decompensation. ACE inhibitors are indicated even in asymptomatic patients and should be commenced as soon as possible. Their beneficial effect on outcome including mortality in patients with severe congestive heart failure had been confirmed already in 1987 [64] and was confirmed in studies that were performed after [65, 66]. In 1996, the advantageous effects of beta-blockers (carvedilol) on outcome including mortality in patients with heart failure were confirmed [67]. A recently published paper revealed that the administration of metoprolol can even prevent infarct size [68]. Heart failure medication can be extended to aldosterone blockers (synonym: mineralocorticoid receptor antagonists) and hydralazine or nitrates if hypertensive blood pressure cannot be sufficiently controlled by an ACE inhibitor and a beta-blocker. In case of intolerance of ACE inhibitors, angiotensin 1 receptor antagonists should be considered. Recent findings demonstrate a significant mortality benefit in patients with heart failure with reduced injection fraction when treated with sacubitril plus valsartan (Entresto®), also when compared to an ACE inhibitor alone [18, 19]. More detailed information on heart failure medication is beyond the scope of this chapter but is easily accessible.

Another aspect for the prevention of severe future deterioration of the patient's clinical condition is to explain the nature of this disease to the patient and to emphasize the importance of heart failure medication intake. Comorbidities (e.g., COPD, sleep apnea, anemia, depression, and memory disorders) [2] should not be missed here. The patient should be instructed to see his family doctor every semester initially for documentation of further evolution and continuing adjustment of therapy if indicated.

In summary, the management for prevention of rehospitalization for heart failure includes the following actions [2]:

1. Continuation or initiation of long-lasting therapies of heart failure
2. Optimal management of underlying heart diseases
3. Optimal management of comorbidities
4. Patient education on water and salt restrictions
5. Nutritional support
6. Careful patient education

Conclusion

Acute heart failure is a complex and heterogeneous clinical syndrome. It can be a serious life-threatening condition that in some cases needs urgent and aggressive treatment to achieve patient stabilization [29]. Despite therapeutic advances, the prognosis of AHF remains poor [2, 70]. However, earlier diagnosis, triage, and initiation of specific treatment for AHF are associated with reduced mortality and shorter length of hospital stay.

Take-Home Messages

- Organ congestion is a frequent acute or subacute feature in AHF.
- Early initiation of treatment leads to better outcome.
- Perform intubation and install controlled mechanical ventilation rather early in respiratory deterioration.
- In case of hemodynamic instability, start with inotropes in the left ventricular dysfunction and with vasopressors in the right ventricular dysfunction.
- Ventricular interdependence is an important pathophysiological mechanism in right ventricular failure.
- A multidisciplinary approach is warranted to improve outcome including prevention of rehospitalization.
- AHF management consists of situation-adjusted therapeutical procedures that are summarized in the following ◘ Table 32.4.

Table 32.4 Overview of clinical signs and adequate therapy in AHF

	Clinical signs	Hemodynamic therapy
Prehospital setting[a]	Signs of congestion Signs of right or left ventricular dysfunction Signs of low cardiac output	NIV Diuretics Nitrates Fluid challenge CPR
First 2 h[a]	Warm/wet AHF [29, 69] Dry/cold AHF (CS)	Diuretics Vasodilators Oxygen NIV (APE) Fluid challenge Inotropes Vasopressors
AHF in coronary syndrome	Signs of AHF Angor (may be absent)	Coronary angiogram Supportive therapy based on clinical symptoms Heart failure medication
Myocarditis	Signs of AHF	Supportive therapy based on clinical symptoms
Predominant right ventricular failure[a]	Signs of right ventricular dysfunction, including RV congestion Signs of low cardiac output state Hypoxemia Kussmaul sign	Cautious volume loading Vasopressors and/or inotropes Mechanical circulatory support Etiology-specific treatment
Cardiogenic shock	Hypotension and signs of organ hypoperfusion	Coronary angiogram Inotropes Vasopressors Respiratory support Device therapy

[a]See Table 32.1

To Sum-Up

Key points in acute right and left ventricular heart failure.

Section	Feature	Key points
► 32.2	Main symptoms of acute right heart failure	Jugular venous distension, paradoxical pulse, Kussmaul sign, alteration of mental state, hypotension, tachycardia
	Main symptoms of acute left heart failure	Dyspnea, pink frothy sputum, persistent cough or wheezing, new-onset arrhythmia, alteration of mental state, hypotension, tachycardia
► 32.3	Most common etiologies of right ventricular failure	Acute right ventricular failure, right ventricular ischemia/infarction, sepsis, chronic pulmonary hypertension, arrhythmia

Section	Feature	Key points
	Most common etiologies of left ventricular failure	Acute left ventricular failure, left ventricular ischemia/infarction, sepsis, chronic arterial hypertension, arrhythmia, valvulopathies
▶ 32.4	Current practice of therapy of acute right and left heart failure	Based on etiology (see ◘ Table 32.4)
▶ 32.5	Management for prevention of rehospitalization	Continuation or initiation of long-lasting therapies of heart failure, optimal management of underlying heart diseases, optimal management of comorbidities, patient education on water and salt restrictions, nutritional support, careful patient education

32

References

1. Ponikowski P, Voors AA, Anker SD, et al. 2016 ESC Guidelines for the diagnosis and treatment of acute and chronic heart failure: The Task Force for the diagnosis and treatment of acute and chronic heart failure of the European Society of Cardiology (ESC). Developed with the special contribution of the Heart Failure Association (HFA) of the ESC. Eur J Heart Fail. 2016;18(8):891–975. https://doi.org/10.1002/ejhf.592. [published Online First: Epub Date].
2. Mebazaa A, Tolppanen H, Mueller C, et al. Acute heart failure and cardiogenic shock: a multidisciplinary practical guidance. Intensive Care Med. 2016;42(2):147–63. https://doi.org/10.1007/s00134-015-4041-5. [published Online First: Epub Date].
3. Harjola VP, Mebazaa A, Celutkiene J, et al. Contemporary management of acute right ventricular failure: a statement from the Heart Failure Association and the Working Group on Pulmonary Circulation and Right Ventricular Function of the European Society of Cardiology. Eur J Heart Fail. 2016;18(3):226–41. https://doi.org/10.1002/ejhf.478. [published Online First: Epub Date].
4. Simonneau G, Galie N, Rubin LJ, et al. Clinical classification of pulmonary hypertension. J Am Coll Cardiol. 2004;43(12 Suppl S):5S–12S. https://doi.org/10.1016/j.jacc.2004.02.037. [published Online First: Epub Date].
5. Hilfiker-Kleiner D, Schieffer E, Meyer GP, et al. Postpartum cardiomyopathy: a cardiac emergency for gynecologists, general practitioners, internists, pulmonologists, and cardiologists. Dtsch Arztebl Int. 2008;105(44):751–6. https://doi.org/10.3238/arztebl.2008.0751. [published Online First: Epub Date].
6. Hilfiker-Kleiner D, Haghikia A, Nonhoff J, et al. Peripartum cardiomyopathy: current management and future perspectives. Eur Heart J. 2015;36(18):1090–7. https://doi.org/10.1093/eurheartj/ehv009. [published Online First: Epub Date].
7. Arany Z, Elkayam U. Peripartum Cardiomyopathy. Circulation. 2016;133(14):1397–409. https://doi.org/10.1161/CIRCULATIONAHA.115.020491. [published Online First: Epub Date].
8. Chaliki HP, Mohty D, Avierinos JF, et al. Outcomes after aortic valve replacement in patients with severe aortic regurgitation and markedly reduced left ventricular function. Circulation. 2002;106(21):2687–93.
9. Kurisu S, Sato H, Kawagoe T, et al. Tako-tsubo-like left ventricular dysfunction with ST-segment elevation: a novel cardiac syndrome mimicking acute myocardial infarction. Am Heart J. 2002;143(3):448–55.
10. Zannad F, Mebazaa A, Juilliere Y, et al. Clinical profile, contemporary management and one-year mortality in patients with severe acute heart failure syndromes: The EFICA study. Eur J Heart Fail. 2006;8(7):697–705. https://doi.org/10.1016/j.ejheart.2006.01.001. [published Online First: Epub Date].
11. Wuerz RC, Meador SA. Effects of prehospital medications on mortality and length of stay in congestive heart failure. Ann Emerg Med. 1992;21(6):669–74.
12. Maisel AS, Peacock WF, McMullin N, et al. Timing of immunoreactive B-type natriuretic peptide levels and treatment delay in acute decompensated heart failure: an ADHERE (Acute Decompensated Heart Failure National Registry) analysis. J Am Coll Cardiol. 2008;52(7):534–40. https://doi.org/10.1016/j.jacc.2008.05.010. [published Online First: Epub Date].

13. Peacock WF, Emerman C, Costanzo MR, et al. Early vasoactive drugs improve heart failure outcomes. Congest Heart Fail. 2009;15(6):256–64. https://doi.org/10.1111/j.1751-7133.2009.00112.x. [published Online First: Epub Date].
14. Emerman CL. Treatment of the acute decompensation of heart failure: efficacy and pharmacoeconomics of early initiation of therapy in the emergency department. Rev Cardiovasc Med. 2003;4(Suppl 7):S13–20.
15. Matsue Y, Damman K, Voors AA, et al. Time-to-Furosemide treatment and mortality in patients hospitalized with acute heart failure. J Am Coll Cardiol. 2017;69(25):3042–51. https://doi.org/10.1016/j.jacc.2017.04.042. [published Online First: Epub Date].
16. Gray A, Goodacre S, Newby DE, et al. Noninvasive ventilation in acute cardiogenic pulmonary edema. N Engl J Med. 2008;359(2):142–51. https://doi.org/10.1056/NEJMoa0707992. [published Online First: Epub Date].
17. Cotter G, Metzkor E, Kaluski E, et al. Randomised trial of high-dose isosorbide dinitrate plus low-dose furosemide versus high-dose furosemide plus low-dose isosorbide dinitrate in severe pulmonary oedema. Lancet. 1998;351(9100):389–93. https://doi.org/10.1016/S0140-6736(97)08417-1. [published Online First: Epub Date].
18. Fala L. Entresto (Sacubitril/Valsartan): first-in-class angiotensin receptor neprilysin inhibitor FDA approved for patients with heart failure. Am Health Drug Benefits. 2015;8(6):330–4.
19. Solomon SD, Claggett B, Desai AS, et al. Influence of ejection fraction on outcomes and efficacy of Sacubitril/Valsartan (LCZ696) in heart failure with reduced ejection fraction: the prospective comparison of ARNI with ACEI to determine impact on global mortality and morbidity in heart failure (PARADIGM-HF) trial. Circ Heart Fail. 2016;9(3):e002744. https://doi.org/10.1161/circheartfailure.115.002744. [published Online First: Epub Date].
20. Ural D, Çavuşoğlu Y, Eren M, et al. Diagnosis and management of acute heart failure. Anatol J Cardiol. 2016;15(11):860–89. https://doi.org/10.5152/AnatolJCardiol.2015.6567. [published Online First: Epub Date].
21. Park JH, Balmain S, Berry C, et al. Potentially detrimental cardiovascular effects of oxygen in patients with chronic left ventricular systolic dysfunction. Heart. 2010;96(7):533–8. https://doi.org/10.1136/hrt.2009.175257. [published Online First: Epub Date].
22. Miro O, Gil V, Martin-Sanchez FJ, et al. Morphine use in the ED and outcomes of patients with acute heart failure: a propensity score-matching analysis based on the EAHFE registry. Chest. 2017; https://doi.org/10.1016/j.chest.2017.03.037. [published Online First: Epub Date].
23. ter Maaten JM, Valente MA, Damman K, et al. Diuretic response in acute heart failure-pathophysiology, evaluation, and therapy. Nat Rev Cardiol. 2015;12(3):184–92. https://doi.org/10.1038/nrcardio.2014.215. [published Online First: Epub Date].
24. Channer KS, McLean KA, Lawson-Matthew P, et al. Combination diuretic treatment in severe heart failure: a randomised controlled trial. Br Heart J. 1994;71(2):146–50.
25. Knauf H, Mutschler E. Functional state of the nephron and diuretic dose-response--rationale for low-dose combination therapy. Cardiology. 1994;84(Suppl 2):18–26.
26. Konstam MA, Gheorghiade M, Burnett JC Jr, et al. Effects of oral tolvaptan in patients hospitalized for worsening heart failure: the EVEREST Outcome Trial. JAMA. 2007;297(12):1319–31. https://doi.org/10.1001/jama.297.12.1319. [published Online First: Epub Date].
27. Bart BA, Goldsmith SR, Lee KL, et al. Ultrafiltration in decompensated heart failure with cardiorenal syndrome. N Engl J Med. 2012;367(24):2296–304. https://doi.org/10.1056/NEJMoa1210357. [published Online First: Epub Date].
28. Mebazaa A, Longrois D, Metra M, et al. Agents with vasodilator properties in acute heart failure: how to design successful trials. Eur J Heart Fail. 2015;17(7):652–64. https://doi.org/10.1002/ejhf.294. [published Online First: Epub Date].
29. McMurray JJ, Adamopoulos S, Anker SD, et al. ESC guidelines for the diagnosis and treatment of acute and chronic heart failure 2012: the task force for the diagnosis and treatment of acute and chronic heart failure 2012 of the European Society of Cardiology. Developed in collaboration with the Heart Failure Association (HFA) of the ESC. Eur J Heart Fail. 2012;14(8):803–69. https://doi.org/10.1093/eurjhf/hfs105. [published Online First: Epub Date].
30. Levy P, Compton S, Welch R, et al. Treatment of severe decompensated heart failure with high-dose intravenous nitroglycerin: a feasibility and outcome analysis. Ann Emerg Med. 2007;50(2):144–52. https://doi.org/10.1016/j.annemergmed.2007.02.022. [published Online First: Epub Date].

31. Yancy CW, Jessup M, Bozkurt B, et al. 2013 ACCF/AHA guideline for the management of heart failure: a report of the American College of Cardiology Foundation/American Heart Association Task Force on Practice Guidelines. J Am Coll Cardiol. 2013;62(16):e147–239. https://doi.org/10.1016/j.jacc.2013.05.019. [published Online First: Epub Date].
32. Nieminen MS, Brutsaert D, Dickstein K, et al. EuroHeart Failure Survey II (EHFS II): a survey on hospitalized acute heart failure patients: description of population. Eur Heart J. 2006;27(22):2725–36. https://doi.org/10.1093/eurheartj/ehl193.
33. Harjola VP, Lassus J, Sionis A, et al. Clinical picture and risk prediction of short-term mortality in cardiogenic shock. Eur J Heart Fail. 2015;17(5):501–9. https://doi.org/10.1002/ejhf.260. [published Online First: Epub Date].
34. Hochman JS, Sleeper LA, Webb JG, et al. Early revascularization in acute myocardial infarction complicated by cardiogenic shock. SHOCK Investigators. Should we emergently revascularize occluded coronaries for cardiogenic shock. N Engl J Med. 1999;341(9):625–34. https://doi.org/10.1056/NEJM199908263410901. [published Online First: Epub Date].
35. Authors/Task Force m, Windecker S, Kolh P, et al. 2014 ESC/EACTS guidelines on myocardial revascularization: the task force on myocardial revascularization of the European Society of Cardiology (ESC) and the European Association for Cardio-Thoracic Surgery (EACTS)developed with the special contribution of the European Association of Percutaneous Cardiovascular Interventions (EAPCI). Eur Heart J. 2014;35(37):2541–619. https://doi.org/10.1093/eurheartj/ehu278. [published Online First: Epub Date].
36. Nielsen N, Wetterslev J, Cronberg T, et al. Targeted temperature management at 33 degrees C versus 36 degrees C after cardiac arrest. N Engl J Med. 2013;369(23):2197–206. https://doi.org/10.1056/NEJMoa1310519. [published Online First: Epub Date].
37. Thiele H, Ohman EM, Desch S, et al. Management of cardiogenic shock. Eur Heart J. 2015;36(20):1223–30. https://doi.org/10.1093/eurheartj/ehv051. [published Online First: Epub Date].
38. Arrigo M, Mebazaa A. Understanding the differences among inotropes. Intensive Care Med. 2015;41(5):912–5. https://doi.org/10.1007/s00134-015-3659-7. [published Online First: Epub Date].
39. Levy B, Perez P, Perny J, et al. Comparison of norepinephrine-dobutamine to epinephrine for hemodynamics, lactate metabolism, and organ function variables in cardiogenic shock. A prospective, randomized pilot study. Crit Care Med. 2011;39(3):450–5. https://doi.org/10.1097/CCM.0b013e3181ffe0eb. [published Online First: Epub Date].
40. Ribeiro RA, Restelatto LMF. Increased mortality with the use of adrenaline in shock: the evidence is still limited. Crit Care. 2016;20 https://doi.org/10.1186/s13054-016-1465-4. [published Online First: Epub Date].

32

41. Pirracchio R, Parenica J, Resche Rigon M, et al. The effectiveness of inodilators in reducing short term mortality among patient with severe cardiogenic shock: a propensity-based analysis. PLoS One. 2013;8(8):e71659. https://doi.org/10.1371/journal.pone.0071659. [published Online First: Epub Date].
42. De Backer D, Biston P, Devriendt J, et al. Comparison of dopamine and norepinephrine in the treatment of shock. N Engl J Med. 2010;362(9):779–89. https://doi.org/10.1056/NEJMoa0907118. [published Online First: Epub Date].
43. Levy B, Bastien O, Karim B, et al. Experts' recommendations for the management of adult patients with cardiogenic shock. Ann Intensive Care. 2015;5(1):52. https://doi.org/10.1186/s13613-015-0052-1. [published Online First: Epub Date].
44. Cecconi M, De Backer D, Antonelli M, et al. Consensus on circulatory shock and hemodynamic monitoring. Task force of the European Society of Intensive Care Medicine. Intensive Care Med. 2014;40(12):1795–815. https://doi.org/10.1007/s00134-014-3525-z. [published Online First: Epub Date].
45. Davidson J, Baumgariner F, Omari B, et al. Intra-aortic balloon pump: indications and complications. J Natl Med Assoc. 1998;90(3):137–40.
46. Thiele H, Zeymer U, Neumann FJ, et al. Intra-aortic balloon counterpulsation in acute myocardial infarction complicated by cardiogenic shock (IABP-SHOCK II): final 12 month results of a randomised, open-label trial. Lancet. 2013;382(9905):1638–45. https://doi.org/10.1016/S0140-6736(13)61783-3. [published Online First: Epub Date].
47. Thiele H, Schuler G, Neumann FJ, et al. Intraaortic balloon counterpulsation in acute myocardial infarction complicated by cardiogenic shock: design and rationale of the Intraaortic Balloon Pump in Cardiogenic Shock II (IABP-SHOCK II) trial. Am Heart J. 2012;163(6):938–45. https://doi.org/10.1016/j.ahj.2012.03.012. [published Online First: Epub Date].

48. American College of Emergency P, Society for Cardiovascular A, Interventions, et al. 2013 ACCF/AHA guideline for the management of ST-elevation myocardial infarction: a report of the American College of Cardiology Foundation/American Heart Association Task Force on Practice Guidelines. J Am Coll Cardiol. 2013;61(4):e78–140. https://doi.org/10.1016/j.jacc.2012.11.019. [published Online First: Epub Date].
49. Meune C, Spaulding C, Mahe I, et al. Risks versus benefits of NSAIDs including aspirin in myocarditis: a review of the evidence from animal studies. Drug Saf. 2003;26(13):975–81.
50. Konstantinides SV, Torbicki A, Agnelli G, et al. ESC guidelines on the diagnosis and management of acute pulmonary embolism. Eur Heart J. 2014;35(43):3033–69, 69a-69k. https://doi.org/10.1093/eurheartj/ehu283. [published Online First: Epub Date].
51. James A, Veean S, Keshavamurthy JH, et al. Fibrinolytic administration via EKOS catheter used in pulmonary embolism. Lung India. 2017;34(3):273–4. https://doi.org/10.4103/lungindia.lungindia_342_16. [published Online First: Epub Date].
52. Fuller TJ, Paprzycki CM, Zubair MH, et al. Initial experiences with endovascular management of submassive pulmonary embolism: is it safe? Ann Vasc Surg. 2017;38:158–63. https://doi.org/10.1016/j.avsg.2016.09.002. [published Online First: Epub Date].
53. Green EM, Givertz MM. Management of acute right ventricular failure in the intensive care unit. Curr Heart Fail Rep. 2012;9(3):228–35. https://doi.org/10.1007/s11897-012-0104-x. [published Online First: Epub Date].
54. Gayat E, Mebazaa A. Pulmonary hypertension in critical care. Curr Opin Crit Care. 2011;17(5):439–48. https://doi.org/10.1097/MCC.0b013e32834a7619. [published Online First: Epub Date].
55. Hoeper MM, Granton J. Intensive care unit management of patients with severe pulmonary hypertension and right heart failure. Am J Respir Crit Care Med. 2011;184(10):1114–24. https://doi.org/10.1164/rccm.201104-0662CI. [published Online First: Epub Date].
56. Ventetuolo CE, Klinger JR. Management of acute right ventricular failure in the intensive care unit. Ann Am Thorac Soc. 2014;11(5):811–22. https://doi.org/10.1513/AnnalsATS.201312-446FR. [published Online First: Epub Date].
57. Bowers TR, O'Neill WW, Pica M, et al. Patterns of coronary compromise resulting in acute right ventricular ischemic dysfunction. Circulation. 2002;106(9):1104–9.
58. Laster SB, Shelton TJ, Barzilai B, et al. Determinants of the recovery of right ventricular performance following experimental chronic right coronary artery occlusion. Circulation. 1993;88(2):696–708.
59. Laster SB, Ohnishi Y, Saffitz JE, et al. Effects of reperfusion on ischemic right ventricular dysfunction. Disparate mechanisms of benefit related to duration of ischemia. Circulation. 1994;90(3):1398–409.
60. Bodson L, Bouferrache K, Vieillard-Baron A. Cardiac tamponade. Curr Opin Crit Care. 2011;17(5):416–24. https://doi.org/10.1097/MCC.0b013e3283491f27. [published Online First: Epub Date].
61. Vieillard-Baron A, Price LC, Matthay MA. Acute cor pulmonale in ARDS. Intensive Care Med. 2013;39(10):1836–8. https://doi.org/10.1007/s00134-013-3045-2. [published Online First: Epub Date].
62. Boissier F, Katsahian S, Razazi K, et al. Prevalence and prognosis of cor pulmonale during protective ventilation for acute respiratory distress syndrome. Intensive Care Med. 2013;39(10):1725–33. https://doi.org/10.1007/s00134-013-2941-9. [published Online First: Epub Date].
63. Vahanian A, Alfieri O, Andreotti F, et al. Guidelines on the management of valvular heart disease (version 2012): the Joint Task Force on the Management of Valvular Heart Disease of the European Society of Cardiology (ESC) and the European Association for Cardio-Thoracic Surgery (EACTS). Eur J Cardiothorac Surg. 2012;42(4):S1–44. https://doi.org/10.1093/ejcts/ezs455. [published Online First: Epub Date].
64. Group CTS. Effects of enalapril on mortality in severe congestive heart failure. Results of the Cooperative North Scandinavian Enalapril Survival Study (CONSENSUS). N Engl J Med. 1987;316(23):1429–35. https://doi.org/10.1056/NEJM198706043162301. [published Online First: Epub Date].
65. Investigators S, Yusuf S, Pitt B, et al. Effect of enalapril on survival in patients with reduced left ventricular ejection fractions and congestive heart failure. N Engl J Med. 1991;325(5):293–302. https://doi.org/10.1056/NEJM199108013250501. [published Online First: Epub Date].
66. Sacks CA, Jarcho JA, Curfman GD. Paradigm shifts in heart-failure therapy--a timeline. N Engl J Med. 2014;371(11):989–91. https://doi.org/10.1056/NEJMp1410241. [published Online First: Epub Date].
67. Packer M, Bristow MR, Cohn JN, et al. The effect of carvedilol on morbidity and mortality in patients with chronic heart failure. U.S. Carvedilol Heart Failure Study Group. N Engl J Med. 1996;334(21):1349–55. https://doi.org/10.1056/NEJM199605233342101. [published Online First: Epub Date].

68. Garcia-Prieto J, Villena-Gutierrez R, Gomez M, et al. Neutrophil stunning by metoprolol reduces infarct size. Nat Commun. 2017;8:14780. https://doi.org/10.1038/ncomms14780. [published Online First: Epub Date].
69. Nohria A, Tsang SW, Fang JC, et al. Clinical assessment identifies hemodynamic profiles that predict outcomes in patients admitted with heart failure. J Am Coll Cardiol. 2003;41(10):1797–804.
70. Abraham WT, Adams KF, Fonarow GC, et al. In-hospital mortality in patients with acute decompensated heart failure requiring intravenous vasoactive medications: an analysis from the Acute Decompensated Heart Failure National Registry (ADHERE). J Am Coll Cardiol. 2005;46(1):57–64. https://doi.org/10.1016/j.jacc.2005.03.051. [published Online First: Epub Date].

Suggested Reading

2016 ESC Guidelines for the diagnosis and treatment of acute and chronic heart failure (see reference 1).
Harjola, et al. Contemporary management of acute right ventricular failure: a statement from the Heart Failure Association and the Working Group on Pulmonary Circulation and Right Ventricular Function of the European Society of Cardiology. Eur J Heart Fail. 2016;18:226–41.
Arrigo, et al. Understanding acute heart failure: pathophysiology and diagnosis. Eur Heart J Suppl. 2016;18(Supplement G):G11–8.
Kindermann, et al. Update on myocarditis. J Am Coll Cardiol. 2012;59(9):779–92.
World Health Organization: division of pulmonary hypertension into 5 groups.

Cardiopulmonary Monitoring of Septic Shock

Claude Martin, Gary Duclos, and Marc Leone

M. R. Pinsky et al. (eds.), *Hemodynamic Monitoring*, Lessons from the ICU,
https://doi.org/10.1007/978-3-319-69269-2_33

Learning Objectives

To know in septic patients:
1. The limitations of older hemodynamic methods
2. The advantages, interests, and limitations of newer methods
3. Why prefer dynamic over static parameters for the evaluation of fluid responsiveness
4. Why prefer an integrated approach with bedside ultrasound and invasive techniques

33.1 Introduction

Septic shock is a complex interaction of several hemodynamic abnormalities:
- Absolute hypovolemia
- Relative hypovolemia due to general vasodilatation that coexists with zones of vasoconstriction
- Myocardial dysfunction, even at an earlier stage
- Inadequate oxygen extraction due to intracellular (probably mitochondrial) abnormalities

Septic shock is one subtype of shock states.

33

According to the type of shock, different abnormalities of circulatory parameters are found. Shock is commonly classified into four different subtypes with different pathophysiologies: distributive, cardiogenic, hypovolemic, and obstructive. In ◘ Table 33.1 are described the distinguishing features of the shock states. Septic shock can present one or several of these features. It is of crucial importance to diagnose these hemodynamic abnormalities to select the most appropriate treatments: fluids, vasopressors, inotropic agents, or combination of several [1]. This is always the case in septic shock. Finally, although there is no one best targeted hemodynamic goal in the resuscitations of septic shock patients, optimizing organ blood flow early before end-organ injury develops is usually associated with reduced morbidity and mortality, though no specific endpoints of resuscitations have been validated to be superior.

◘ **Table 33.1** Different hemodynamic features of the causes of shock

	Co	Cardiac filling pressure	SVR	SVO_2
Distributive	Increased (after fluid replacement)	Low or normal	Decreased	Increased or normal
Cardiogenic	Decreased	Increased	Increased	Decreased
Hypovolemic	Decreased	Decreased	Increased	Decreased
Obstructive	Decreased	Decreased (transmural)	Increased	Decreased

CO cardiac output, *SVR* systemic vascular resistance, SvO_2 mixed venous oxygen saturation (central venous can be used as well)

33.2 Monitoring

The goal of hemodynamic monitoring is to assess the adequacy of cardiopulmonary function, blood distribution, and oxygen delivery relative to tissue demand. In septic shock basic hemodynamic assessment (vital signs, physical exam) must be completed by invasive and noninvasive technologies.

33.2.1 Arterial Pressure

Monitoring blood pressure saves lives and the goal of resuscitation must always be tissue perfusion. An arterial catheter is always needed for the monitoring of septic shock patients. The mean arterial pressure should be kept around 60–65 mmHg, but a personalized blood pressure management is needed for each patient. Higher levels may be needed in older, formerly hypertensive patients. Lower levels may be enough in younger patients. A diastolic blood pressure below 40 mmHg is an indication to start immediate vasopressor therapy. Pulse pressure variation is a dynamic tool to evaluate a state of fluid responsiveness (see below).

Add (!) icon Blood pressure is the oldest form of perfusion monitoring. Values targeted during treatment must be individualized.

33.2.2 Prediction of Preload Responsiveness

Static measures can no longer be recommended. The followings do not reliably reflect the left ventricular filling pressure in shock states with pulmonary hypertension or compliance changes:

- Central venous pressure
- Pulmonary occlusion pressure
- Ventricular end-diastolic volumes
- Ventricular diastolic area
- Global end-diastolic volume
- Intrathoracic blood volume

Dynamic measures of fluid responsiveness are recommended instead. Tables 33.2, 33.3, and 33.4 present the parameters to use and the main limitations in their interpretations [2–4]. Ultrasound is useful to reduce the time of diagnostic uncertainty and guide resuscitation. They may be used to assess volume status, ventricular strain, and myocardial dysfunction [5–8]. Passive leg raising test can be used to predict volume responsiveness without giving a single drop of fluid. It should be titrated against changes in CO/SV rather than PP changes (Tables 33.2 and 33.3).

Add (!) icon Dynamic parameters must be preferred over static parameters. Passive leg raising test evaluates the potential efficacy of fluid challenge without using a single drop of fluid.

Table 33.2 Monitoring of fluid challenge (further details for sonography in Table 33.4)

Pulse pressure variation Stroke volume variation	Patient should be sedated, sometimes paralyzed No cardiac arrhythmia No low lung compliance No low tidal volume
Passive leg raising test	Tested against blood flow (preferred) or blood pressure changes
End-expiratory occlusion test	Patients should accept a 15 s pause in ventilation. Maybe invalid at a tidal volume of 6 ml/kg
"Mini" fluid challenge: infusion of 100 ml of fluid Sonography of heart and inferior vena cava (test respiratory variations) (skills needed)	

The first four techniques are validated by many studies and meta-analysis. All parameters are limited by sensitivity and specificity ranging from 75% to 95%
Pulse pressure variation 84% (75–90) sensitivity, 80% (78–96) specificity
Stroke volume variation 82% (74–92) sensitivity, 86% (79–93) specificity
Passive leg raising 88% (80–93) sensitivity, 91% (87–96) specificity

Table 33.3 Cutoff and "gray zone" for parameters

Pulse pressure variation	11 (4–15) mmHg
Stroke volume variation	13 (10–20) mmHg
Passive leg raising (against blood flow)	11 (7–15) mmHg
Inferior vena cava variation (controlled ventilation)	15 (12–21) mmHg

33

Table 33.4 Sonography of heart and inferior vena cava (IVC) to predict preload responsiveness

	Cutoff	Sensitivity	Specificity
Mechanically ventilated patients			
Inferior Vena Cava distensibility	>13%	44%	85%
ΔVmaxAo	>10%	79%	64%
VTI increase after PLR	>10%	97%	94%
VTI increase after MFC	>10%	95%	78%
Spontaneous breathing patients			
IVC collapsibility	>40%	70%	80%
VTI increase after PLR	>12.5%	77%	100%

IVC inferior vena cava, *ΔVmaxAo* respiratory variations of the maximal Doppler velocity in left ventricular outflow tract, *VTI* velocity-time integral, *PLR* passive leg raising, *MFC* mini-fluid challenge

33.2.3 Cardiac Output Monitoring

33.2.3.1 Noninvasive

Indirect measures of CO can be assessed using transesophageal Doppler or thoracic cutaneous bioimpedance or bioreactance (NICOM) for the latter further validation is required in shock state.

33.2.3.2 Invasive and Minimally Invasive Systems [9–11]

The pulmonary artery catheter has still a place and is recommended in the context of refractory shock, severe pulmonary artery hypertension or right ventricular dysfunction [11, 12]. These situations are not rare in septic shock. Other systems are capable to calculate stroke volume (SV) and CO using the pulse contour waveform analysis. They provide real-time, beat-by-beat arterial blood pressure and SV monitoring. The devices provide also parameters for the assessment of fluid responsiveness.

Pulse contour analysis-derived CO: Calibrated devices (PICCO, LIDCO, and volume view) are recommended. Non-calibrated devices (FlowTrac/Vigileo, ProAQT, LiDCO Rapid, MostCare) should not be used in situations where changes in ventricular strain are expected. Calibrated system can use transpulmonary thermodilution (PICCO, volume view) or lithium dilution. Calibration is needed on a regular basis and every time there are significant hemodynamic changes (starting a vasopressor, etc.).

Add (!) icon Transpulmonary thermodilution is the method of choice and should be preferred over non-calibrated methods.

33.2.4 CO and Mixed (Central) O_2 Saturation Monitoring

CO is the vehicle for oxygen and nutriments to the cells. Regardless of the nominal value, CO is either adequate or inadequate to meet the metabolic demand. SVO_2 or $ScVO_2$ is a reasonable indicator of the adequacy of the CO, when it is low or normal. Based on the results of three multicenter studies, a resuscitation protocol targeting a specific value of $ScVO_2$ does not offer survival advantage; the Surviving Sepsis Campaign Guidelines no longer recommend the use of $ScVO_2$ in the management of septic shock patients [13–15]. We believe this is unfortunate because $ScVO_2$ provides valuable information for the interpretation of the adequacy of CO. Anyway, once a central venous catheter is in place, why not draw blood samples for $ScVO_2$ measurements.

Add (!) icon CO and $ScVO_2$ evaluated together are helpful for the management of septic shock.

33.2.5 Microcirculation Monitoring

Sublingual microcirculation monitoring opens a window on the assessment of microcirculation. Persistent abnormalities predict the development of organ dysfunction and subsequent mortality; unfortunately, at the present time, there are no specific strategies to alter the microcirculation [16].

33.2.6 Recommendations for Practice

In ◘ Fig. 33.1 is proposed a two-step protocol for the optimal choice of monitoring septic shock patients.

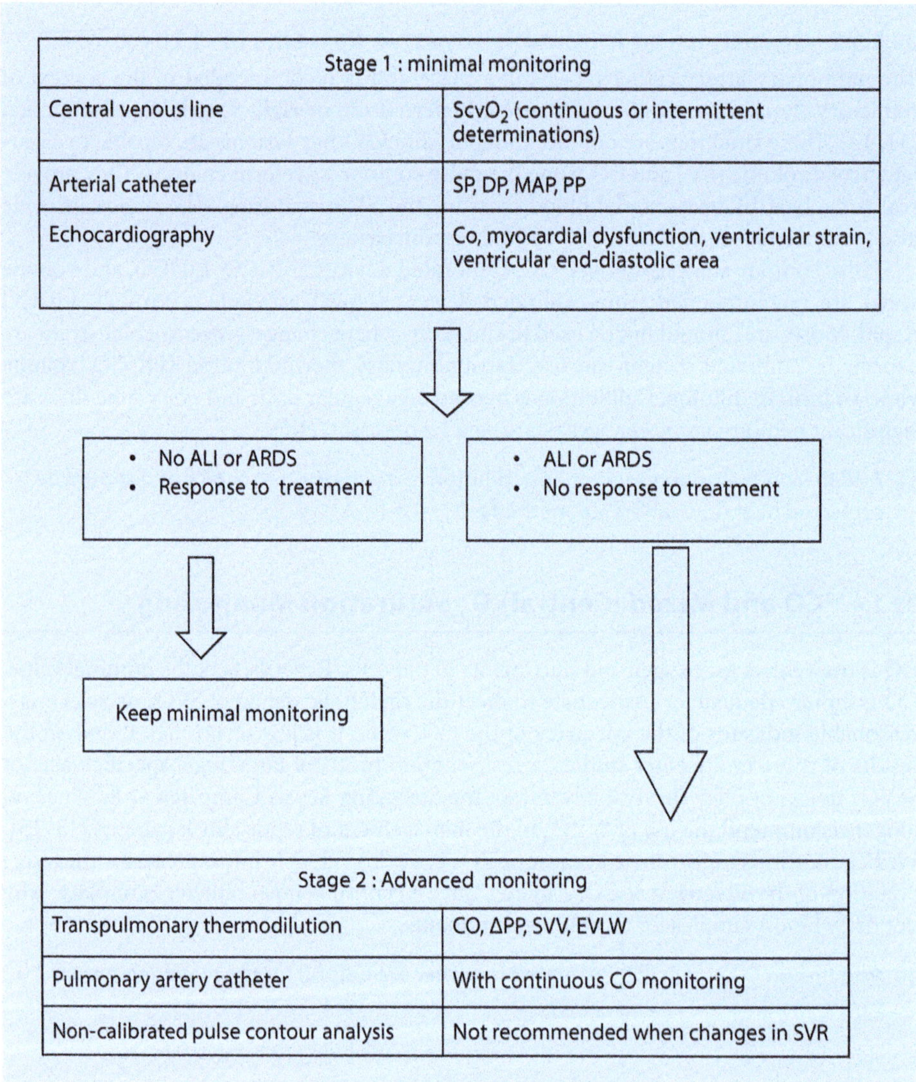

◘ **Fig. 33.1** Minimal or advanced monitoring for the diagnosis and treatment of septic shock. $ScvO_2$ central venous blood oxygen saturation, SP systolic pressure, DP diastolic pressure, MAP mean arterial pressure, PP pulse pressure, ALI acute lung Injury, ARDS acute respiratory distress syndrome, CO cardiac output, ΔPP delta pulse pressure, SVV stroke volume variation, EVLW extravascular lung water, SVR systemic vascular resistance

Conclusion

The ability to monitor the different hemodynamic abnormalities of septic shock, as well as the efficacy of treatments, is of crucial importance to improve outcome. The pathophysiology of septic shock is always complex, but the correct use of monitoring techniques, always in combination, can help prescribe the optimal treatments. There is no one best monitoring modality for septic shock patients. All are subject to measurement errors, and results may be affected by patient pathophysiology or interaction with mechanical ventilation. For the less severe forms of septic shock, minimal monitoring with a central venous line, an arterial catheter, and echocardiography is recommended. For more severe forms, or in case of associated ALI/ARDS, the use of transpulmonary thermodilution, or pulmonary artery catheter, is needed to select and monitor the appropriate treatments.

Take-Home Messages

- Blood pressure is the oldest form of perfusion monitoring. Values targeted during treatment must be individualized.
- Dynamic parameters must be preferred over static parameters. Passive leg raising test evaluates the potential efficacy of fluid challenge without using a single drop of fluid.
- Transpulmonary thermodilution is the method of choice and should be preferred over non-calibrated methods.
- CO and $ScVO_2$ evaluated together are helpful for the management of septic shock.

References

1. Cecconi M, De Backer D, Antonelli M, et al. Consensus on circulatory shock and hemodynamic monitoring. Task force of the European Society of Intensive Care Medicine. Intensive Care Med. 2014;40:1795–815.
2. Marik PE, Cavallazzi R, Vasu T, et al. Dynamic changes in arterial waveform derived variables and fluid responsiveness in mechanically ventilated patients: a systematic review of the literature. Crit Care Med. 2009;37:2642–7.
3. Cavallaro F, Sandroni C, Marano C, et al. Diagnostic accuracy of passive leg raising for prediction of fluid responsiveness in adults: systematic review and meta-analysis of clinical studies. Intensive Care Med. 2010;36:1475–83.
4. Marik PE, Baram M, Vahid B. Does central venous pressure predict fluid responsiveness? A systematic review of the literature and the tale of seven mares. Chest. 2008;134:172.
5. Levitov A, Frankel HL, Blaivas M, et al. Guidelines for the appropriate use of bedside general and cardiac ultrasonography in the evaluation of critically ill patients-part II: cardiac ultrasonography. Crit Care Med. 2016;44:1206–27.
6. Barbier C, Loubières Y, Schmit C, et al. Respiratory changes in inferior vena cava diameter are helpful in predicting fluid responsiveness in ventilated septic patients. Intensive Care Med. 2004;30:1740–6.
7. Spencer KT, Kimura BJ, Korcarz CE, et al. Focused cardiac ultrasound: recommendations from the American Society of Echocardiography. J Am Soc Echocardiogr. 2013;26:567–81.
8. Monnet X, Marik P, Teboul JL. Passive leg raising for predicting fluid responsiveness: a systematic review and meta-analysis. Intensive Care Med. 2016;42:1935–47.
9. Monnet X, Anguel N, Naudin B, et al. Arterial pressure-based cardiac output in septic patients: different accuracy of pulse contour and uncalibrated pressure waveform devices. Crit Care. 2010;14:R109.
10. Monnet X, Teboul JL. Transpulmonary thermodilution: advantages and limits. Crit Care. 2017;21:147.

11. Connors AF Jr, Speroff T, Dawson NV, et al. Support Investigators. The effectiveness of right heart catheterization in the initial care of critically ill patients. JAMA. 1996;276:889–97.
12. Pinsky MR, Vincent JL. Let us use the pulmonary artery catheter correctly and only when we need it. Crit Care Med. 2005;33:1119–22.
13. Rhodes A, Evans LE, Alhazzani W, et al. Surviving sepsis campaign: international guidelines for management of sepsis and septic shock: 2016. Crit Care Med. 2017;45:486–552.
14. The PRISM investigators. Early, goal-directed therapy for septic shock – a patient-level meta-analysis. N Engl J Med. 2017;376:2223–34.
15. Hernandez G, Teboul JL. Fourth surviving sepsis campaign's hemodynamic recommendations: a step forward or a return to chaos? Crit Care. 2017;21:133.
16. Kiyatkin ME, Bakker J. Lactate and microcirculation as suitable targets for hemodynamic optimization resuscitation of circulatory shock. Curr Opin Crit Care. 2017;23:348–54.

In ARDS

Giacomo Grasselli, Nadia Corcione, and Antonio Pesenti

M. R. Pinsky et al. (eds.), *Hemodynamic Monitoring*, Lessons from the ICU,
https://doi.org/10.1007/978-3-319-69269-2_34

Learning Objectives

Monitoring of cardiovascular system function is of cornerstone importance in patients with ARDS either to confirm the diagnosis of the syndrome or to detect any possible hemodynamic impairment. ARDS is by definition a form of non-cardiogenic pulmonary edema. However, heart dysfunction and hypoproteinemia frequently coexist, particularly in septic patients. The resulting hydrostatic edema, superimposed to the increased lung vascular permeability, further worsens oxygenation. Optimization of oxygen delivery, cardiac output, and pulmonary function mandate a cautious fluid management and a careful ventilatory strategy. In the present chapter, we will:

- Summarize the pathophysiology of the most frequent hemodynamic abnormalities seen in ARDS.
- Review indications, advantages, and limits of the available monitoring techniques.
- Provide basic treatment principles to optimize cardiovascular function in these patients.

34.1 Importance of Hemodynamic Monitoring for Diagnosis and Definition of ARDS

Acute respiratory distress syndrome (ARDS) is an inflammatory condition with diffuse injury to the alveolar-capillary barrier leading to capillary congestion, intra-alveolar hemorrhage, hyaline-membrane formation, and alveolar-interstitial edema [1]. ARDS is a form of non-cardiogenic pulmonary edema, since fluid accumulation is not caused by increased hydrostatic capillary filtration pressure secondary to elevated left atrial pressure, but is rather a consequence of impaired permeability of the alveolar-capillary barrier. Exclusion of the cardiogenic origin of respiratory failure is an essential diagnostic criterion for ARDS. In the former American-European Consensus Conference (AECC) definition of ARDS (adopted in 1994), a value of pulmonary artery occlusion pressure (Ppao) lower than 18 mmHg was required to confirm the diagnosis [2]. However, since high Ppao values due to cardiac failure or fluid overload may coexist with ARDS and given the continuous decline in the use of pulmonary artery catheters (PAC), the requirement for a Ppao value has been removed from the currently adopted "Berlin definition" of ARDS [3]. Nevertheless, the Berlin definition states that "respiratory failure must be not fully explained by cardiac failure or fluid overload using all available data" and that "if no ARDS risk factor is apparent, some objective evaluation is required to eliminate the possibility of hydrostatic edema." In conclusion, functional hemodynamic monitoring is essential to exclude the cardiogenic origin of the pulmonary edema and to confirm the diagnosis of the syndrome.

34.2 Frequency and Causes of Hemodynamic Instability in ARDS

The majority of ARDS patients develop hemodynamic instability [4], and more than half of them require infusion of vasopressors [5]. Circulatory failure and need for vasoactive drugs are more strongly associated with the risk of death than the severity of hypoxemia [6]. Several factors contribute to the development of hemodynamic instability in ARDS patients:

1. Direct toxic effect of hypoxemia and acidosis on myocardial function. Oxygen, beyond its essential function in cardiac energy metabolism, is involved in other processes affecting myocardial cell function, such as the modulation of cardiac gene expression and the generation of reactive oxygen species, that may induce irreversible cellular damage [7]. On the other hand, intracellular acidosis is associated with depression of cardiac contractility and may even cause myocardial necrosis [8].
2. Sepsis-associated cardiovascular compromise: sepsis is the most frequent cause of ARDS [9]. Mechanisms of cardiovascular failure during sepsis are distributive shock, altered vascular permeability, increased tissue oxygen demands, and myocardial dysfunction.
3. Pre-existing concomitant cardiovascular diseases.
4. Pulmonary vascular dysfunction and right ventricular (RV) dysfunction.
5. Hemodynamic effects of positive pressure ventilation.

The latter two points, for their clinical and pathophysiological relevance, will be discussed in dedicated paragraphs.

34.2.1 Pulmonary Vascular Dysfunction

ARDS is characterized by injury to the pulmonary circulation leading to destruction of the pulmonary capillaries, increased pulmonary vascular resistance (PVR), and pulmonary hypertension (PH), as first described by Zapol in 1977 [10, 11]. Pulmonary hypertension (PH) is defined by a mean pulmonary artery pressure (mPAP) >25 mmHg [12]. The prognostic value of PH remains unclear: some studies found a significant association of mPAP values with mortality [13], while others did not [14–16]. The term *pulmonary vascular dysfunction* (PVD) has been proposed to indicate an elevation in PVR defined as increased transpulmonary gradient (mPAP-Ppao) [17] and/or pulmonary vascular resistance index (mPAP-Ppao/cardiac index) [18]. Again, data on the association between increased PVR and mortality are conflicting [19]. Bull et al. performed a post hoc analysis of the Fluid and Catheter Treatment Trial (FACTT) and found that, in the subset of 501 patients managed with a PAC, PVD was an independent predictor of adverse outcome. Pulmonary circulation is characterized by high compliance and low resistance to blood flow, and for this reason the relationship between driving pressure and flow is curvilinear, while in the systemic circulation this relationship is linear. This means that in normal conditions an increase in PAP results in a disproportionate increase in pulmonary blood flow due not only to increased driving pressure (i.e., the difference between mPAP and left atrial pressure) but also to distension of the vessels and recruitment of previously closed capillaries. Conversely, a reduction in cardiac output will be associated with higher calculated PVR values, even if the vasomotor tone does not change (◘ Fig. 34.1). In ARDS, things become even more complicated, since the relationship between pulmonary blood flow and PAP changes due to the presence of PVD: hence, changes in calculated PVR values can be particularly difficult to interpret [20, 21].

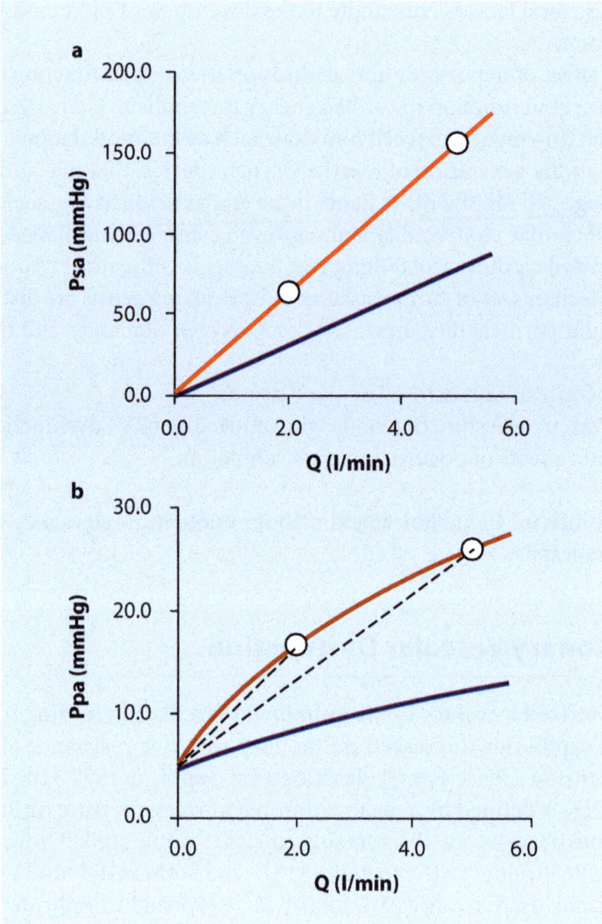

Fig. 34.1 Mean arterial pressure plotted against flow (cardiac output) in the systemic (**a**) and pulmonary (**b**) circulations. The blue curve in each panel represents the formal condition of the circulation, and the red curve a hypertensive condition. (**a**) In the systemic circulation, the mean pressure (P)-flow (Q) plot is well described as a linear (Ohmic) relationship. The two points identified (open circles) show a normal cardiac output and a reduced cardiac output, respectively, in the hypertensive condition. At each of these cardiac outputs, it is clear that the ratio of P to Q is the same and therefore can be used to easily characterize the resistance of the systemic circulation. (**b**) In the pulmonary circulation, the plot of mean pressure against flow is curvilinear with an intercept on the pressure axis that is equal to left atrial pressure. The blue curve represents a normal pressure flow curve (healthy lung), while the red curve represents pressure flow curve in the presence of hypoxic pulmonary hypertension. The two points identified (open circles) show a normal cardiac output and a reduced cardiac output, respectively, in the hypertensive condition. At each cardiac output the pulmonary vascular resistance, Ppa–LAP/Q, is illustrated as the slope of the straight dashed line. Even though the two points are each on the same pressure flow curve, the calculated pulmonary vascular resistance is different at the different cardiac output. Psa, systemic arterial pressure (mean); Ppa, pulmonary arterial pressure (mean); Q, cardiac output (flow)

In patients with ARDS, the following mechanisms contribute to the development of PVD:

1. Hypoxic pulmonary vasoconstriction (HPV). Improvement in oxygenation leads to a decrease in HPV and consequently reduces PVR [22, 23]. Carbon dioxide tension also exerts a significant vasoconstrictive effect on pulmonary vessels [24]: hypercapnia is

associated with increased PVR and consequent higher risk of right ventricular dysfunction [25, 26]. Vasoconstriction is favored also by endothelial damage, causing an imbalance between mediators of vasodilation and vasoconstriction in favor of the latter [27]. It is thereby observed a reduced capacity to accommodate changes in blood flow [4].
2. Depleted capillary reserve, due to thrombosis or compression by interstitial edema of arterial and capillary pulmonary vessels [28]. Endothelial damage in acute lung injury causes local activation of coagulation [27] and fibrinolysis that play a significant prognostic and pathogenetic role in ARDS [29].
3. Fibroproliferation and vascular remodeling (late stages of ARDS).
4. Effects of positive pressure ventilation: airway pressure variations strongly influence pulmonary blood flow by affecting transmural vascular pressure and the distribution of blood flow across different lung zones [30]. The application of positive end-expiratory pressure (PEEP) and the consequent increase in mean airway pressure (Paw) have a profound influence on PAP, mediated by changes in transpulmonary pressure and lung volume. PVR has a U-shaped relationship with lung volume, increasing both at low lung volumes due to compression of extra-alveolar vessels and at very high lung volumes due to stretching of alveolar vessels [31]. Hence, the effect of PEEP on PVR depends on the balance between recruitment of collapsed areas and hyperinflation of already open lung units. If recruitment prevails, distension of extra-alveolar vessels and concomitant reduction of HPV should lead to reduced PVR. If hyperinflation prevails, compression of intra-alveolar capillaries induces West zone 1 and 2 conditions, thereby increasing PVR [30, 32] and RV afterload [33]. Finally, West zone 2 causes a redirection of blood flow toward poorly ventilated alveolar units, worsening gas exchange.

34.2.2 Right Ventricular Functional Impairment

The combined effects of sepsis-induced myocardial depression, hemodynamic effects of positive pressure ventilation, deleterious effects of hypoxemia on myocardial contractility, and PVD may severely affect cardiac function, leading to right ventricular dysfunction (RVD) and acute cor pulmonale (ACP). The RV is very sensitive to changes in afterload: the compliant and thin-walled RV is better suited to lodge significant increases in preload but poorly tolerates acute increases in afterload [34, 35]. In ARDS, the increase in RV afterload results in a mismatch between increased oxygen demand and decreased right coronary artery perfusion pressure [36]. Impairment of RV ejection diminishes pulmonary venous return to the LV, increases end-systolic and end-diastolic RV volume, and decreases, through ventricular interdependence, LV diastolic compliance. The resultant fall of LV ejection leads to a reduction in RV coronary blood flow with consequent RV ischemia: this vicious circle maintains and further amplifies RV dysfunction, ultimately resulting in ACP, which consists in a significant ventriculo-arterial uncoupling between the RV and the pulmonary circulation [24]. The clear-cut result is a drop in cardiac output and a poor volume responsiveness, with risk of fluid overload.

Based on echocardiographic criteria, three sequential steps of RV functional impairment can be identified in ARDS patients:
1. RV dilatation: RV/LV end-diastolic area >0.6.
2. RV dysfunction: tricuspid annular plane systolic excursion <16 mm.
3. Acute cor pulmonale (ACP): association of RV dilatation with paradoxical motion of the interventricular septum at end systole, so-called "D-shape" aspect of LV [37].

34.2.3 Hemodynamic Effects of Positive Pressure Ventilation

The lungs and the heart are situated in the chest cavity and surrounded by intrathoracic pressure (ITP) (pleural and pericardial, respectively). Hemodynamics effects of positive pressure ventilation can be subdivided in "steady state" and "phasic" effects.

1. *Steady state effects* depend both on mechanical and neurohormonal factors, reflecting the impact of sustained alterations of respiratory conditions [38]. They depend on the increase in mean Paw, which is determined by PEEP level (most important), duty cycle duration, and tidal driving pressure [39]. PEEP application is associated with a reduction in cardiac output, which is more evident in presence of hypovolemia. The common explanation is that the increase in ITP translates into an increase in right atrial pressure (Pra), causing a reduction in the gradient for venous return, i.e., the difference between mean systemic filling pressure (Pmsf) and Pra [40]. However, this explanation appears too simplistic. Indeed, it has been demonstrated that PEEP increases not only Pra but also Pmsf through reflex enhancement of venous tone (which causes transfer of blood from unstressed to stressed volume) [41] and through increase in abdominal pressure (with compression of the splanchnic venous reservoir) [42]. This suggests that changes in cardiac output might occur independently of changes in the pressure gradient for venous return [43]. In addition, Marini et al. demonstrated that PEEP has little direct effects on ventricular function [44].
2. *Transient effects* depend on cyclic changes in lung/chest wall volume and in airway/intrathoracic pressures during the respiratory cycle, which are of opposite sign during spontaneous and controlled ventilation. Both during negative and positive pressure inspiration, lung expansion directly compresses the heart in the cardiac fossa, compromising preload. During spontaneous breathing, whether in a ventilated or non-ventilated patient, the decrease in ITP will increase the gradient for venous return (Pmsf – Pra), causing an increase in RV preload and RV dilatation. The latter is associated with decreased LV compliance and filling, which results in decreased LV stroke volume during inspiration, explaining the physiological inspiratory decrease in systolic arterial pressure [45, 46]. On the contrary, positive pressure ventilation induces cyclic increases of ITP and lung volume, both of which decrease venous return. The increase in transpulmonary pressure causes an increase in PVR and then in RV afterload, with reduction of RV stroke volume. Opposite changes will happen on left heart chambers: LV preload tends to increase since the blood is "squeezed out" of the pulmonary vessels, while LV afterload improves due to a decrease in transmural aortic pressure. Hence, LV stroke volume will increase during positive pressure insufflation and decrease upon expiration. The change in pleural pressure for a given change in Paw (i.e., the fraction of Paw increase "transmitted" to ITP) depends on tidal volume and on the compliance of the chest wall (C_{CW}) relative to the compliance of the lung (C_L) [47] according to the formula: $\Delta Ppl/\Delta Paw = C_L/C_L + C_{CW}$ [48]. In normal subjects, since C_L and C_{CW} are similar, ITP should increase of about 50% of the increase in mean Paw [47, 48]. The same increase in Paw will exert completely different effects in a patient with very stiff lungs and normally compliant chest wall (e.g., with primary ARDS) compared with a patient with compliant lungs and stiff chest wall (e.g., with emphysema or intraabdominal hypertension). In the first case, the change in ITP induced by a certain increase in Paw will be modest and will have limited hemodynamic impact; in the second case, the increase in Paw will translate in a much larger increase in ITP with more pronounced hemodynamic effects.

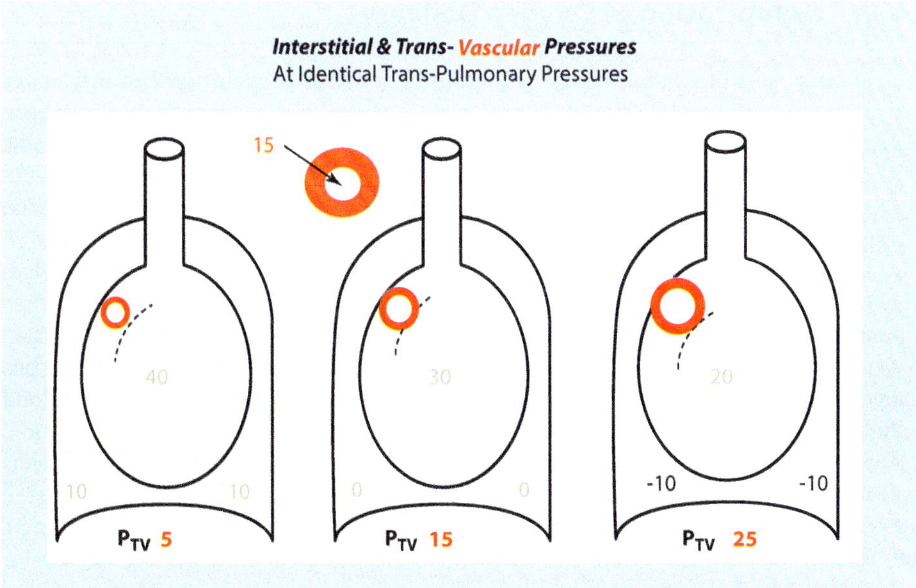

Fig. 34.2 Hypothetical effect of the pleural pressure during controlled and spontaneous breathing on transvascular pressure. In this illustration, the lung distends to the same 30 cmH_2O transpulmonary pressure by three combinations of alveolar and pleural pressure. If the luminal microvascular pressure is equivalent to 15 cmH_2O, and interstitial pressure is assumed equal to pleural pressure, then the fluid-filtering transvascular pressure (P_{TV}) in this extreme example would theoretically range from 5 to 25 cmH_2O

34.2.4 Influence of Spontaneous Breathing Activity

Spontaneously breathing patients with high respiratory drive may generate large negative swings of pleural pressure during inspiratory efforts, resulting in higher transpulmonary pressure changes and increased lung stress and strain [49]. Furthermore, the same change in transpulmonary pressure may be associated with completely different absolute values of alveolar pressure (Palv) [50]. In presence of spontaneous breathing efforts, indeed, Palv may drop well below the end-expiratory pressure value and may even become negative throughout the entire breathing cycle, translating into increased transmural pulmonary vascular pressure (i.e., difference between intravascular capillary pressure and Palv) [51] (Fig. 34.2). This, in presence of increased vascular permeability, causes vascular leakage and interstitial edema, further contributing to worsening and maintenance of lung injury [49].

34.3 Principles of Hemodynamic Management

Hemodynamic management in ARDS patients should be guided by three basic principles, which are all equally important but sometimes difficult to achieve at the same time:

1. Optimization of oxygen delivery
2. Avoidance of fluid overload
3. Prevention of RV functional impairment

34.3.1 Optimization of Oxygen Delivery

The ultimate goal of cardiorespiratory support is to optimize perfusion and delivery of oxygen to the peripheral tissues, in order to meet the metabolic needs of the body. Oxygen delivery (DO_2) is the volume of oxygen delivered to the systemic vascular bed per minute and is the product of arterial oxygen content (CaO_2) and cardiac output (CO): $DO_2 = CaO_2 \times CO$. CaO_2 is defined as the sum of oxygen transported by hemoglobin and of oxygen dissolved in plasma, according to the formula $CaO_2 = (Hb \times 1.39 \times SaO_2) + (PaO_2 \times 0.003)$, where Hb is the hemoglobin level, SaO_2 is the arterial saturation, PaO_2 is the oxygen arterial tension, and 0.003 is the solubility coefficient of oxygen in the human plasma. Since the oxyhemoglobin dissociation curve becomes relatively flat when $SaO_2 > 90\%$, further increases of PaO_2 have relatively little impact on SaO_2 or CaO_2 in this range. In addition, being the amount of dissolved oxygen negligible, once arterial blood is fully saturated, the only way to increase CaO_2 is to increase hemoglobin concentration. Hence, targeting higher hemoglobin levels in more severely hypoxemic ARDS patients will improve CaO_2, increasing the oxygen-carrying capacity of arterial blood (Russell 1999). Extracorporeal Life Support Organization guidelines recommend maintaining a Hb level of 12–14 gr/dL and a normal hematocrit in patients undergoing ECMO for severe hypoxemic respiratory failure [52]. However, several adverse effects of red blood cell transfusions have been reported in patients with acute lung injury [53–55], and the optimal Hb threshold for transfusion remains an open issue. The other component of DO_2 is CO, which is the product of stroke volume (SV) and heart rate (HR): $CO = SV \times HR$. CO can be measured using a variety of invasive devices including PAC and transpulmonary thermodilution systems (e.g., PiCCO or Vigileo) and arterial pressure waveform analysis devices (e.g., LiDCO, PiCCO, FloTrac, MostCare, etc.). Among the noninvasive techniques available to estimate CO, echocardiography is the most popular [56]: a very good agreement between CO estimated by transthoracic echocardiography and that measured by transpulmonary thermodilution has been reported in critically ill, mechanically ventilated patients [57]. However, patients with high PEEP levels may have a poor "acoustic window," and the reliability and reproducibility of echocardiographic findings strongly depend on the operator's expertise. In patients with inadequate CO, each of its physiological determinants (preload, afterload, and contractility) should be assessed. In particular, a crucial step is to understand whether the patient needs fluid infusion for preload optimization. Several methods are available to assess fluid responsiveness (FR):

1. Fluid challenge: adequate assessment of FR requires the integration of cardiac filling pressure (Pra and/or Ppao) variations with CO variations after a fluid challenge (e.g., infusion of 250 mL or 3 mL/Kg of crystalloids over 5 min) [58, 59]. Pra (otherwise called central venous pressure or CVP) and Ppao alone are not accurate indicators of preload and FR [60–62], since their *absolute* values (measured relative to atmospheric pressure) do not necessarily reflect *transmural* pressure, which is the pressure difference between inside and outside the vessels (in this case ITP) and is the relevant pressure for FR. This important distinction is very often neglected. It is the central pressure relative to atmosphere and not the transmural pressure that determines the back pressure for venous return and consequently the hydrostatic capillary filtration pressure in upstream tissues [63]. However, high absolute Pra or Ppao may actually correspond to low transmural pressure values, if ITP is significantly increased. In other words, a patient with high Pra may develop peripheral edema and liver congestion but

still present a significant increase in CO after a fluid bolus [64]. An "alternative version" of a fluid challenge test is the passive leg raising (PLR) test: leg raising causes translocation of venous blood from inferior body district to the thorax, acting as a reversible self-volume challenge. An increase of at least 10% of aortic blood flow or cardiac index is the best cutoff value to detect FR after PLR [65].
2. Dynamic indexes: as previously described, the cyclic variations of ITP during positive pressure ventilation cause concomitant variations of LV stroke volume, which increases during inspiration and decreases upon expiration [66]. The patient's volume status deeply affects the magnitude of these changes, which are more pronounced in presence of hypovolemia. Both pulse pressure variation (PPV) and stroke volume variation (SVV) are used to assess FR. Pulse pressure (PP) is the difference between systolic and diastolic blood pressure, and PPV is calculated by dividing the largest PP by the average PP: a value >13% is a good predictor of FR [67]. SVV is measured by minimally invasive arterial wave from analysis (e.g., LiDCO, PiCCO, FloTrac, MostCare, etc.) or esophageal Doppler and is calculated by dividing the difference between maximum SV and minimum SV by their average in a time window of 30 s. However, some limitations of PPV and SVV are particularly relevant in ARDS patients:
    - They require the absence of spontaneous breathing efforts.
    - Small tidal volumes (<8 mL/Kg) and/or low lung compliance may not induce sufficient changes in ITP [68, 69]. But if either PPV or SVV are >13% with low tidal volume breathing, they still predict FR.
    - PPV poorly predict FR in case of PH because ACP causes its own PPV.
    - They may be less reliable in presence of significant RV dysfunction for the same reason as PH.
3. End-expiratory occlusion (EEO) test: it consists in performing an expiratory pause for 15 s, thus preventing the cyclic impediment to RV and LV filling and functioning as a sort of fluid challenge; the test is independent from the compliance of respiratory system. EEO-induced increase in CO by 5% seems a good predictor of FR in ARDS patients [70].

Once the patient's volume status is adequate, administration of inotropic drugs may be required to improve myocardial contractility and increase CO. Accurate assessment of the adequacy of DO_2 and tissue perfusion is mandatory in each critical patient: clinical and laboratory signs of inadequate oxygen delivery are skin mottling, reduced capillary refilling time, decreased urine output, mixed venous oxygen desaturation, and hyperlactatemia. Mixed venous oxygen saturation (SvO_2) is particularly informative, since it depends on the ratio between DO_2 and oxygen consumption (VO_2): a reduction of SvO_2 below the normal value of 70% may be due to inadequate oxygen delivery, to excessive oxygen consumption, or to both. Hence, in patients with reduced SvO_2, it is crucial not only to improve DO_2 but also to reduce tissue oxygen consumption, e.g., by optimizing sedation and treating fever and pain.

In presence of mixed venous oxygen desaturation and/or hyperlactatemia, accurate hemodynamic monitoring is mandatory.

Two issues must be emphasized:
1. Measurement of the "real" mixed venous oxygen saturation requires placement of a PAC. If a PAC is not in place, oxygen saturation of blood obtained by a central venous catheter placed in the right atrium can be used as surrogate of mixed venous

oxygen saturation. Indeed, while central venous oxygen saturation tends to overestimate mixed venous oxygen saturation, through its variations reliably mirror those of the mixed venous blood [71].
2. In patients with sepsis, oxygen saturation of mixed venous and central venous blood may be misleadingly normal or even elevated. Heterogeneity of microvascular perfusion, opening of microvascular shunts, and mitochondrial dysfunction result in a pathologic uncoupling between macrohemodynamics and microcirculation [72] with reduced capacity to extract and utilize oxygen.

34.3.2 Avoidance of Fluid Overload

As previously mentioned, ARDS is a form of non-cardiogenic, high-permeability pulmonary edema that may be worsened by exogenous fluid infusion. A large body of evidence show that a positive fluid balance *after the initial resuscitation phase* is an independent adverse prognostic factor in critically ill patients [73–75]. An interesting indicator of fluid accumulation within the lung is the extravascular lung water (EVLW), namely, the amount of water contained in the lungs outside the pulmonary vasculature. It corresponds to the sum of interstitial, intracellular, alveolar, and lymphatic fluid, excluding pleural effusion [76]. The normal value of EVLW is <10 mL/Kg [77] and it is strictly regulated by several mechanisms: the lymphatic drainage keeps the tissue matrix dry, while the tight junctions and the active ion transport systems of alveolar cells preserve alveolar spaces by flooding [78]. Starling's law governs the net alveolar and interstitial fluid clearance: an increase in pulmonary capillary hydrostatic pressure or a decrease in oncotic blood pressure induces an increase of EVLW. An increased pulmonary vascular permeability index (PVPI = ratio between EVLW and pulmonary blood volume) is considered a hallmark of ARDS. Pulmonary hypertension, cardiac failure, and water retention due to endocrine influences (i.e., activation of renal-angiotensin-aldosterone system) commonly coexist with ARDS and promote hydrostatic edema superimposed to the original exudate [79]. Finally, fluid therapy (particularly with crystalloids) may also contribute to lung overhydration. In a vicious circle, the fluid overload reduces colloid osmotic pressure in pulmonary capillaries, further worsening lung edema. By definition, in ARDS pulmonary edema is not due to cardiac failure or fluid overload, but for the reasons mentioned above, an increased left ventricular preload does not exclude ARDS. Indeed, studies on animal models of acute lung injury indicate that lung edema is reduced if left atrial pressure is lowered [80] and that infusion of furosemide improves gas exchange, allowing a decrease of PEEP values [81]. It has been reported that the addition of albumin to furosemide therapy in hypoproteinemic patients with ARDS significantly improves oxygenation, with greater net negative fluid balance and better maintenance of hemodynamic stability [82]. While diffuse alveolar damage (DAD), the histopathological hallmark of ARDS, is present only in 45% of patients undergoing autopsy who met the Berlin definition criteria [83], an EVLW value above 15 mL/Kg identifies patients with diffuse alveolar damage with 99% positive predictive value [77]. Hence, assessment of EVLW and PVPI may be useful in patients with acute hypoxemic respiratory failure and pulmonary infiltrates to differentiate ARDS from cardiogenic edema [84, 85] and to guide fluid management [78]. The gold standard for measurement of EVLW is the transpulmonary thermo-dye dilution that requires the simultaneous injection through a central venous catheter of a cold indicator and a colorimetric indicator. However, this complex and expensive technique has been replaced by the transpulmonary thermodilution method that allows estimate of EVLW from global end-diastolic volume (GEDV) (◘ Fig. 34.3). Some significant limitations of EVLW measurement must be acknowledged: EVLW may be underestimated in presence of pulmonary vascular occlusion and pleural effusion, while it may be overestimated in patients with lung resection. Moreover, PEEP has a complex effect on EVLW measurement: high levels of PEEP can squeeze the thin-walled pulmonary vessels, leading to underestimation of lung water [86], while recruitment of atelectatic alveoli with attenuation of hypoxic vasoconstriction may have opposite effects. However, a study in ARDS patients demonstrated a good correlation between EVLW and lung weight measured by computed tomography, independent of the level of PEEP [87].

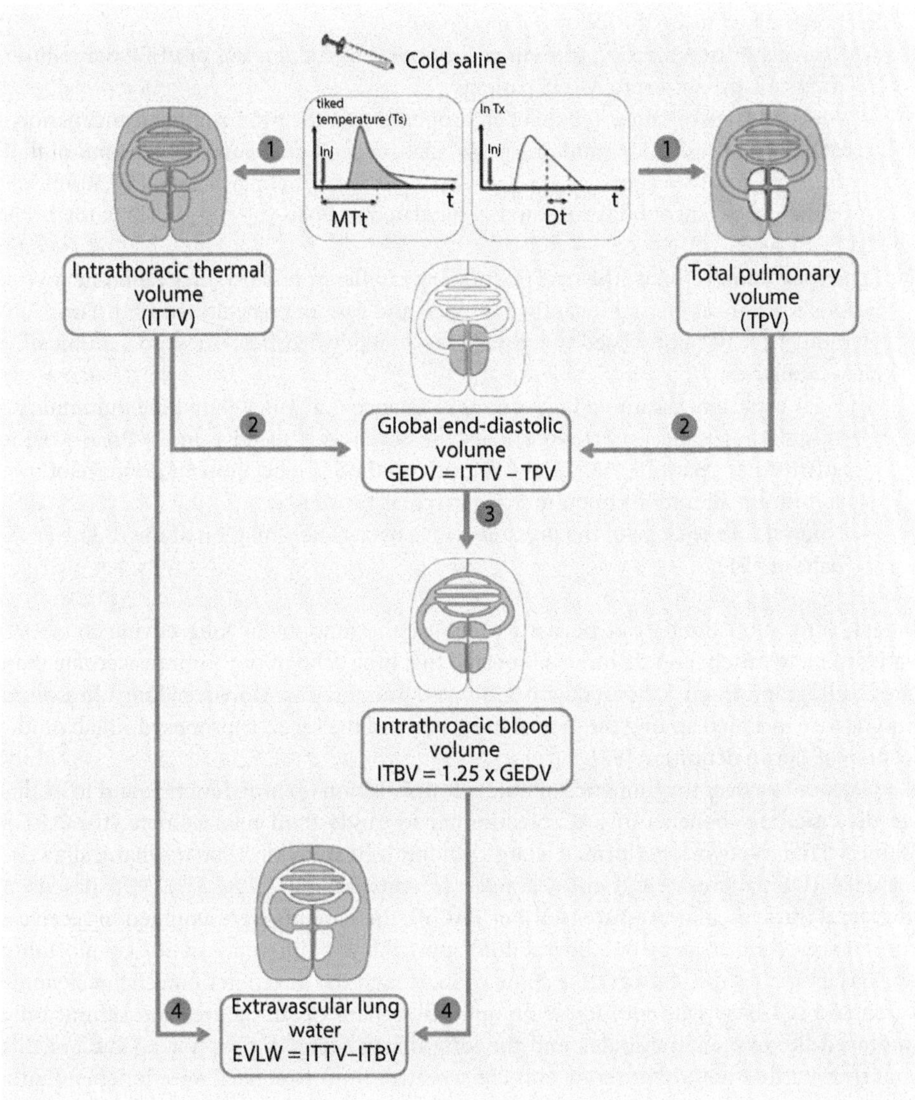

◘ **Fig. 34.3** Measurement of extravascular lung water by single thermal indicator dilution (*MTt* mean transit time, *Dt* downslope time)

Another important parameter for the etiologic evaluation of lung edema is Ppao, with values >18 mmHg suggesting a cardiogenic etiology. PAOP monitoring requires the placement of a PAC and may help to maintain pulmonary vascular pressures at low levels, minimizing lung edema and stress failure to capillary walls. However, many factors (mainly vascular dysfunction, reduced ventricular compliance, and increased ITP) may affect the reliability of measured values of CVP and PAOP as indicators of end-diastolic ventricular volumes (i.e., of the actual cardiac preload). Moreover, in ARDS patients two other limitations of Ppao measurements must be acknowledged:

1. Increase in ITP due to positive pressure ventilation, as reported above, causes an increase in PAOP due to transmission of Paw to vessels. The latter may be quantitatively estimated using the following methods:
   - Transient disconnection from the ventilator (but sudden loss of PEEP may cause lung collapse in severe ARDS patients).
   - Index of transmission: Teboul et al. proposed that the proportional transmission of alveolar pressure to pulmonary vasculature can be accounted by the *index of transmission* IT = $(Ppao_{end\text{-}inspiration} - Ppao_{end\text{-}expiration})/(Pplat - total\ PEEP)$. Hence, the transmural Ppao can be calculated as $Ppao_{end\text{-}expiration} - (IT \times total\ PEEP)$ [88].
2. Ppao may underestimate the true pulmonary capillary pressure since pulmonary venous resistances are significantly increased and cannot be neglected [89]. Two methods have been proposed to estimate the actual hydrostatic pressure in pulmonary capillaries:
   - Gaar equation: assuming that venous resistance is about 40% of total pulmonary vascular resistance, effective capillary pressure is calculated as $Ppc = Ppao + 0.4 \times (mPAP - Ppao)$ [89, 90]. However, this method is inaccurate in presence of significant alterations in pulmonary vascular resistance.
   - Analysis of the slope of the pressure curve decay after inflation of the PAC balloon [91].

Finally, lung ultrasounds can be used to assess the amount of lung edema in ARDS patients: Lichtenstein and coworkers reported that lung echography is more accurate than chest radiograph when compared with computed tomography. Moreover, lung ultrasound findings are included among the diagnostic criteria in the recently proposed Kigali modification of Berlin definition [92].

In order to assess the influence of fluid administration on lung function and to evaluate the risks and benefits of PAC positioning to guide fluid management, the ARDS Clinical Trials Network performed a large randomized study on 1000 mechanically ventilated ARDS patients (Fluid and Catheter Treatment Trial – FACTT) [93]. Based on measured intravascular pressure (CVP or PAOP), the patients were assigned to receive a conservative fluid strategy or a liberal fluid approach. No difference in 60-day mortality was observed, but the conservative strategy shortened the duration of mechanical ventilation and ICU stay without increasing non-pulmonary organ failures and significantly improved the oxygenation index and the lung injury score. A post hoc analysis of this trial showed that both hypoxemia and conservative fluid strategies were independently associated with long-term neuropsychological impairment: since there was no evidence for reduced cerebral perfusion (e.g., cardiac index, systolic blood pressure), it is unclear how conservative fluid management may have caused cognitive impairment [94]. Moreover, no difference in incidence or duration of any type of organ failure nor in the need for organ support (vasopressors, ventilation, renal replacement theray) between PAC-guided and central venous catheter-guided fluid therapy was found; conversely, the PAC group had approximatively twice as many catheter-related complications. However, the Swan-Ganz catheter is a diagnostic, not a therapeutic, tool [95], and the FACTT results indicate that aggressive fluid resuscitation and not the use of PAC per se is the cause of adverse outcome. Ultimately, enhancing the clearance of lung edema with diuretics, hemofiltration, or albumin supplementation results in a better gas exchange and reduces the duration of mechanical ventilation in ARDS patients. However, importantly in ARDS patients, the goal of optimizing DO_2 may be in contrast with the need of fluid restriction, particularly when ARDS occurs in the context of shock and systemic inflammation (e.g., severe sepsis, pancreatitis, burns). In these challenging situations, avoiding the deleterious effects of reduced DO_2 and preserving organ perfusion is certainly more urgent than "keeping the lungs dry" [96, 97], and aggressive fluid resuscitation may be necessary, primarily guided by monitoring of CO and indexes of tissue perfusion (like lactates and mixed venous saturation).

34.3.3 Ventilatory Strategies to Protect the RV

In the era of protective ventilation, the prevalence of ACP has decreased, but it remains around 20–25% [98]. Several studies demonstrate a clear association between mechanical ventilation settings and incidence of ACP. In a retrospective study on 352 patients, Jardin found a linear relationship between the incidence of ACP and Pplat values: ACP was diagnosed in 20% of the patients with Pplat values below 26 cmH_2O, in 39% of those with Pplat of 27–35 cmH_2O, and in 42% of the patients when Pplat exceeded 35 cmH_2O [99]. Since Pplat is a surrogate for transpulmonary pressure, these findings confirm the deleterious effects of increased lung stress on RV afterload. Recent studies suggest that driving pressure (ΔPrs: tidal difference between Pplat and PEEP, which equals the ratio of tidal volume to total respiratory system compliance) is a better indicator of lung stress [100, 101] and is independently associated with mortality and ACP [25]. It has been showed that prone positioning has beneficial effects on hemodynamics by unloading the RV [102]; indeed, patients with severe ARDS undergoing prone position in the PROSEVA trial had lower cardiovascular failure and less cardiac arrest than those in the control group [103]. Prone position allows a significant alveolar recruitment, ameliorating both lung compliance (reduction of transpulmonary pressure) and oxygenation: these effects dramatically reduce RV afterload and consequently RV enlargement and septal dyskinesia [102]. It has been proposed "what is good for the lung is good for right ventricle and vice versa" [5] meaning that mechanical ventilation settings might be guided by RV function assessment. In particular, oxygenation remains a cardinal point for RV protection, since a PaO_2/FiO_2 ratio <100 mmHg is an independent risk factor for ACP. Tidal volume and PEEP should be adjusted to maintain a Pplat <27 cmH_2O and a driving pressure <18 cmH_2O, while $PaCO_2$ should be maintained <48 mmHg [104]: to this end, the combination of extracorporeal CO_2 removal techniques and "ultraprotective" ventilation may be particularly promising to limit the impact of mechanical ventilation on cardiovascular function.

Conclusions

Monitoring of cardiovascular system function is of cornerstone importance in patients with ARDS either to confirm the diagnosis of the syndrome or to detect any possible hemodynamic impairment. Optimization of oxygen delivery, cardiac output, and pulmonary function mandate a cautious fluid management and a careful ventilatory strategy. A group of experts recently reviewed the principles of hemodynamic monitoring and management in ARDS patients [105]: they recommend assessment of PPV in passive patients to evaluate fluid responsiveness and hemodynamic effects of mechanical ventilation. In addition, they suggest placement of a central venous catheter for Pra and $ScVO_2$ monitoring and frequent echocardiographic examination to evaluate RV function and estimate cardiac output. In complex cases, they recommend the insertion of a PAC or the use of a transpulmonary thermodilution system. This algorithm has certainly a strong physiological rationale. However, we would like to underline that, particularly in complex cases, the PAC remains an essential diagnostic tool in severe ARDS patients, since it is the only device allowing continuous monitoring of pulmonary artery pressure, cardiac filling pressures, and "actual" SVO_2; in addition, it allows measurement of cardiac output [106]. These information are crucial both for hemodynamic optimization and for ventilation setting, to improve oxygen delivery while avoiding right heart dysfunction [104].

Take-Home Messages

- Pulmonary hypertension and right ventricular dysfunction negatively affect the prognosis of ARDS patients. Avoidance of fluid overload and reduction of lung distending pressures during mechanical ventilation are reasonable strategies to preserve cardiac output.
- Optimization of oxygen delivery has a key role to prevent the bioenergetic collapse of body tissues: to this end, assessment of intravascular volume status and fluid responsiveness is crucial to guide hemodynamic support while avoiding fluid overload.
- Because of the delicate balance between heart and lung therapeutic needs, a careful hemodynamic monitoring is mandatory: PAC, transpulmonary thermodilution (e.g., PiCCO or Vigileo technology), and echocardiography provide useful information for a rapid and agile shift in medical decision-making.

References

1. Lorente JA, Ballén-Barragán A, Herrero R, Esteban A. Acute respiratory distress syndrome: does histology matter? Crit Care. 2015;19:337.
2. Bernard GR, Artigas A, Brigham KL, Carlet J, Falke K, Hudson L, Lamy M, Legall JR, Morris A, Spragg R. The American-European Consensus Conference on ARDS. Definitions, mechanisms, relevant outcomes, and clinical trial coordination. Am J Respir Crit Care Med. 1994;149(3 Pt 1):818–24.
3. Definition Task Force ARDS, Ranieri VM, Rubenfeld GD, Thompson BT, Ferguson ND, Caldwell E, Fan E, Camporota L, Slutsky AS. Acute respiratory distress syndrome: the Berlin Definition. JAMA. 2012;307(23):2526–33.
4. Vieillard-Baron A, Aneman A. Cardiovascular issues in the ICU: a call for papers. Intensive Care Med. 2017;43(12):1892–3.
5. Repessé X, Charron C, Vieillard-Baron A. Acute respiratory distress syndrome: the heart side of the moon. Curr Opin Crit Care. 2016;22(1):38–44.

6. Vieillard-Baron A, Girou E, Valente E, Brun-Buisson C, Jardin F, Lemaire F, Brochard L. Predictors of mortality in acute respiratory distress syndrome. Focus On the role of right heart catheterization. Am J Respir Crit Care Med. 2000;161(5):1597–601.
7. Davies SW, Wedzicha JA. Hypoxia and the heart. Br Heart J. 1993;69(1):3–5.
8. Poole-Wilson PA. Acidosis and contractility of heart muscle. Ciba Found Symp. 1982;87:58–76.
9. Bellani G, Laffey JG, Pham T, Fan E, Brochard L, Esteban A, Gattinoni L, van Haren F, Larsson A, McAuley DF, Ranieri M, Rubenfeld G, Thompson BT, Wrigge H, Slutsky AS, Pesenti A, LUNG SAFE Investigators; ESICM Trials Group. Epidemiology, patterns of care, and mortality for patients with acute respiratory distress syndrome in intensive care units in 50 countries. JAMA. 2016;315(8): 788–800.
10. Zapol WM, Snider MT. Pulmonary hypertension in severe acute respiratory failure. N Engl J Med. 1977;296(9):476–80.
11. Zapol WM, Kobayashi K, Snider MT, Greene R, Laver MB. Vascular obstruction causes pulmonary hypertension in severe acute respiratory failure. Chest. 1977;71(2 suppl):306–7.
12. Task Force for Diagnosis and Treatment of Pulmonary Hypertension of European Society of Cardiology (ESC); European Respiratory Society (ERS); International Society of Heart and Lung Transplantation (ISHLT), Galiè N, Hoeper MM, Humbert M, Torbicki A, Vachiery JL, Barbera JA, Beghetti M, Corris P, Gaine S, Gibbs JS, Gomez-Sanchez MA, Jondeau G, Klepetko W, Opitz C, Peacock A, Rubin L, Zellweger M, Simonneau G. Guidelines for the diagnosis and treatment of pulmonary hypertension. Eur Respir J. 2009;34(6):1219–63.
13. Osman D, Monnet X, Castelain V, Anguel N, Warszawski J, Teboul JL, Richard C. French Pulmonary Artery Catheter Study Group. Incidence and prognostic value of right ventricular failure in acute respiratory distress syndrome. Intensive Care Med. 2009;35(1):69–76.
14. Villar J, Blazquez MA, Lubillo S, Quintana J, Manzano JL. Pulmonary hypertension in acute respiratory failure. Crit Care Med. 1989;17(6):523–6.
15. Cepkova M, Kapur V, Ren X, Quinn T, Zhuo H, Foster E, Liu KD, Matthay MA. Pulmonary dead space fraction and pulmonary artery systolic pressure as early predictors of clinical outcome in acute lung injury. Chest. 2007;132(3):836–42.
16. Bull TM, Clark B, McFann K, Moss M, National Institutes of Health/National Heart, Lung, and Blood Institute ARDS Network. Pulmonary vascular dysfunction is associated with poor outcomes in patients with acute lung injury. Am J Respir Crit Care Med. 2010;182(9):1123–8.
17. Galiè N, Manes A, Negro L, Palazzini M, Bacchi-Reggiani ML, Branzi A. A meta-analysis of randomized controlled trials in pulmonary arterial hypertension. Eur Heart J. 2009;30(4):394–403.
18. Ryan D, Frohlich S, McLoughlin P. Pulmonary vascular dysfunction in ARDS. Ann Intensive Care. 2014;4:28.
19. Calcaianu G, Calcaianu M, Gschwend A, Canuet M, Meziani F, Kessler R. Hemodynamic profile of pulmonary hypertension (PH) in ARDS. Pulm Circ. 2018;8(1):204589321775341.
20. Versprille A. Pulmonary vascular resistance. A meaningless variable. Intensive Care Med. 1984;10(2):51–3.
21. Naeije R. Pulmonary vascular resistance. A meaningless variable? Intensive Care Med. 2003;29(4): 526–9.
22. Petersson J, Ax M, Frey J, Sánchez-Crespo A, Lindahl SG, Mure M. Positive end-expiratory pressure redistributes regional blood flow and ventilation differently in supine and prone humans. Anesthesiology. 2010;113(6):1361–9.
23. Moudgil R, Michelakis ED, Archer SL. Hypoxic pulmonary vasoconstriction. J Appl Physiol (1985). 2005;98(1):390–403.
24. Repessé X, Charron C, Vieillard-Baron A. Assessment of the effects of inspiratory load on right ventricular function. Curr Opin Crit Care. 2016;22(3):254–9.
25. Boissier F, Katsahian S, Razazi K, Thille AW, Roche-Campo F, Leon R, Vivier E, Brochard L, Vieillard-Baron A, Brun-Buisson C, Mekontso Dessap A. Prevalence and prognosis of cor pulmonale during protective ventilation for acute respiratory distress syndrome. Intensive Care Med. 2013;39(10):1725–33.
26. Lhéritier G, Legras A, Caille A, Lherm T, Mathonnet A, Frat JP, Courte A, Martin-Lefèvre L, Gouëllo JP, Amiel JB, Garot D, Vignon P. Prevalence and prognostic value of acute cor pulmonale and patent foramen ovale in ventilated patients with early acute respiratory distress syndrome: a multicenter study. Intensive Care Med. 2013;39(10):1734–42.

27. Price LC, McAuley DF, Marino PS, Finney SJ, Griffiths MJ, Wort SJ. Pathophysiology of pulmonary hypertension in acute lung injury. Am J Physiol Lung Cell Mol Physiol. 2012;302(9):L803–15.
28. Tomashefski JF Jr, Davies P, Boggis C, Greene R, Zapol WM, Reid LM. The pulmonary vascular lesions of the adult respiratory distress syndrome. Am J Pathol. 1983;112(1):112–26.
29. Ware LB, Koyama T, Zhao Z, Janz DR, Wickersham N, Bernard GR, May AK, Calfee CS, Matthay MA. Biomarkers of lung epithelial injury and inflammation distinguish severe sepsis patients with acute respiratory distress syndrome. Crit Care. 2013;17(5):R253.
30. West JB. Regional differences in the lung. Chest. 1978;74(4):426–37.
31. Whittenberger JL, McGregor M, Berglund E, Borst HG. Influence of state of inflation of the lung on pulmonary vascular resistance. J Appl Physiol. 1960;15:878–82.
32. Permutt S, Bromberger-Barnea B, Bane HN. Alveolar pressure, pulmonary venous pressure, and the vascular waterfall. Med Thorac. 1962;19:239–60.
33. Jardin F. Ventricular interdependence: how does it impact on hemodynamic evaluation in clinical practice? Intensive Care Med. 2003;29(3):361–3.
34. Wauthy P, Pagnamenta A, Vassalli F, Naeije R, Brimioulle S. Right ventricular adaptation to pulmonary hypertension: an interspecies comparison. Am J Physiol Heart Circ Physiol. 2004;286(4):H1441.
35. Mitchell SC, Lelieveldt BP, van der Geest RJ, Bosch HG, Reiber JH, Sonka M. Multistage hybrid active appearance model matching: segmentation of left and right ventricles in cardiac MR images. IEEE Trans Med Imaging. 2001;20(5):415–23.
36. Zochios V, Parhar K, Tunnicliffe W, Roscoe A, Gao F. The right ventricle in ARDS. Chest. 2017;152(1): 181–93.
37. Repessé X, Charron C, Vieillard-Baron A. Acute cor pulmonale in ARDS: rationale for protecting the right ventricle. Chest. 2015;147(1):259–65.
38. Feihl F, Broccard AF. Interactions between respiration and systemic hemodynamics. Part I: basic concepts. Intensive Care Med. 2009;35(1):45–54.
39. Marini JJ, Ravenscraft SA. Mean airway pressure: physiologic determinants and clinical importance--Part 1: physiologic determinants and measurements. Crit Care Med. 1992;20(10):1461–72.
40. Qvist J, Pontoppidan H, Wilson RS, Lowenstein E, Laver MB. Hemodynamic responses to mechanical ventilation with PEEP: the effect of hypervolemia. Anesthesiology. 1975;42(1):45–55.
41. Nanas S, Magder S. Adaptations of the peripheral circulation to PEEP. Am Rev Respir Dis. 1992;146(3):688–93.
42. Maas J, Lagrand WK, Van den Berg PC, Pinsky MR, Jansen JR. Venous return in ICU patients. Crit Care. 2008;12(Suppl 2):P93.
43. Jellinek H, Krenn H, Oczenski W, Veit F, Schwarz S, Fitzgerald RD. Influence of positive airway pressure on the pressure gradient for venous return in humans. J Appl Physiol (1985). 2000;88(3):926–32.
44. Marini JJ, Culver BH, Butler J. Mechanical effect of lung distention with positive pressure on cardiac function. Am Rev Respir Dis. 1981;124(4):382–6.
45. Cherpanath TG, Lagrand WK, Schultz MJ, Groeneveld AB. Cardiopulmonary interactions during mechanical ventilation in critically ill patients. Neth Heart J. 2013;21(4):166–72.
46. Bendjelid K, Schütz N, Suter PM, Romand JA. Continuous cardiac output monitoring after cardiopulmonary bypass: a comparison with bolus thermodilution measurement. Intensive Care Med. 2006;32(6):919–22.
47. Chapin JC, Downs JB, Douglas ME, Murphy EJ, Ruiz BC. Lung expansion, airway pressure transmission, and positive end-expiratory pressure. Arch Surg. 1979;114(10):1193–7.
48. Deal C, Osborn JJ, Ellis E, Gerbode F. Chest wall compliance. Ann Surg. 1968;167(1):73–7.
49. Brochard L, Slutsky A, Pesenti A. Mechanical ventilation to minimize progression of lung injury in acute respiratory failure. Am J Respir Crit Care Med. 2017;195(4):438–42.
50. Bellani G, Grasselli G, Teggia-Droghi M, Mauri T, Coppadoro A, Brochard L, Pesenti A. Do spontaneous and mechanical breathing have similar effects on average transpulmonary and alveolar pressure? A clinical crossover study. Crit Care. 2016;20(1):142.
51. Mauri T, Cambiaghi B, Spinelli E, Langer T, Grasselli G. Spontaneous breathing: a double-edged sword to handle with care. Ann Transl Med. 2017;5(14):292. https://doi.org/10.21037/atm.2017.06.55.
52. ELSO Guidelines 2017.
53. Netzer G, Shah CV, Iwashyna TJ, Lanken PN, Finkel B, Fuchs B, Guo W, Christie JD. Association of RBC transfusion with mortality in patients with acute lung injury. Chest. 2007;132(4):1116–23.
54. Gong MN, Thompson BT, Williams P, Pothier L, Boyce PD, Christiani DC. Clinical predictors of and mortality in acute respiratory distress syndrome: potential role of red cell transfusion. Crit Care Med. 2005;33(6):1191–8.

55. Gaggar A, Patel RP. There is blood in the water: hemolysis, hemoglobin, and heme in acute lung injury. Am J Physiol Lung Cell Mol Physiol. 2016;311(4):L714.
56. Alhashemi JA, Cecconi M, Hofer CK. Cardiac output monitoring: an integrative perspective. Crit Care. 2011;15(2):214.
57. Mercado P, Maizel J, Beyls C, Titeca-Beauport D, Joris M, Kontar L, Riviere A, Bonef O, Soupison T, Tribouilloy C, de Cagny B, Slama M. Transthoracic echocardiography: an accurate and precise method for estimating cardiac output in the critically ill patient. Crit Care. 2017;21(1):136.
58. Vincent JL, Weil MH. Fluid challenge revisited. Crit Care Med. 2006;34(5):1333–7.
59. Carsetti A, Cecconi M, Rhodes A. Fluid bolus therapy: monitoring and predicting fluid responsiveness. Curr Opin Crit Care. 2015;21(5):388–94.
60. Coudray A, Romand JA, Treggiari M, Bendjelid K. Fluid responsiveness in spontaneously breathing patients: a review of indexes used in intensive care. Crit Care Med. 2005;33(12):2757–62.
61. Osman D, Ridel C, Ray P, Monnet X, Anguel N, Richard C, Teboul JL. Cardiac filling pressures are not appropriate to predict hemodynamic response to volume challenge. Crit Care Med. 2007;35(1):64–8.
62. Marik PE. Noninvasive cardiac output monitors: a state-of the-art review. J Cardiothorac Vasc Anesth. 2013;27(1):121–34.
63. Magder S. Central venous pressure monitoring. Curr Opin Crit Care. 2006;12(3):219–27.
64. Hasanin A. Fluid responsiveness in acute circulatory failure. J Intensive Care. 2015;3:50.
65. Monnet X, Rienzo M, Osman D, Anguel N, Richard C, Pinsky MR, Teboul JL. Passive leg raising predicts fluid responsiveness in the critically ill. Crit Care Med. 2006;34(5):1402–7.
66. Saugel B, Bendjelid K, Critchley LAH, Scheeren TWL. Journal of Clinical Monitoring and Computing 2017 end of year summary: cardiovascular and hemodynamic monitoring. J Clin Monit Comput. 2018;32(2):189–96.
67. Zhang D, Song Y, Yang Y, Duan A, Zhang Z, Wang Y. An application of arterial pressure-based cardiac output measurements in fluid management strategies of critically ill patients. Zhonghua Wei Zhong Bing Ji Jiu Yi Xue. 2014;26(9):620–3.
68. Teboul JL. Mean systemic pressure: we can now estimate it, but for what? Intensive Care Med. 2013;39(8):1487–8.
69. Lefrant JY, De Backer D. Can we use pulse pressure variations to predict fluid responsiveness in patients with ARDS? Intensive Care Med. 2009;35(6):966–8.
70. Silva S, Jozwiak M, Teboul JL, Persichini R, Richard C, Monnet X. End-expiratory occlusion test predicts preload responsiveness independently of positive end-expiratory pressure during acute respiratory distress syndrome. Crit Care Med. 2013;41(7):1692–701.
71. Mezger V, Balzer F, Habicher M, Sander M. Venous saturation: between oxygen delivery and consumption. Med Klin Intensivmed Notfmed. 2017;112(6):492–8.
72. López A, Grignola JC, Angulo M, Alvez I, Nin N, Lacuesta G, Baz M, Cardinal P, Prestes I, Bouchacourt JP, Riva J, Ince C, Hurtado FJ. Effects of early hemodynamic resuscitation on left ventricular performance and microcirculatory function during endotoxic shock. Intensive Care Med Exp. 2015;3(1):49.
73. Sakr Y, Rubatto Birri PN, Kotfis K, Nanchal R, Shah B, Kluge S, Schroeder ME, Marshall JC, Vincent JL, Intensive Care Over Nations Investigators. Higher fluid balance increases the risk of death from sepsis: results from a large international audit. Crit Care Med. 2017;45(3):386–94.
74. Bagshaw SM, Brophy PD, Cruz D, Ronco C. Fluid balance as a biomarker: impact of fluid overload on outcome in critically ill patients with acute kidney injury. Crit Care. 2008;12(4):169.
75. Alobaidi R, Morgan C, Basu RK, Stenson E, Featherstone R, Majumdar SR, Bagshaw SM. Association between fluid balance and outcomes in critically ill children: a systematic review and meta-analysis. JAMA Pediatr. 2018;172(3):257–68.
76. Tagami T, Ong MEH. Extravascular lung water measurements in acute respiratory distress syndrome: why, how, and when? Curr Opin Crit Care. 2018;24(3):209–15.
77. Tagami T, Sawabe M, Kushimoto S, Marik PE, Mieno MN, Kawaguchi T, Kusakabe T, Tosa R, Yokota H, Fukuda Y. Quantitative diagnosis of diffuse alveolar damage using extravascular lung water. Crit Care Med. 2013;41(9):2144–50.
78. Jozwiak M, Teboul JL, Monnet X. Extravascular lung water in critical care: recent advances and clinical applications. Ann Intensive Care. 2015;5(1):38.
79. Gattinoni L, Cressoni M, Brazzi L. Fluids in ARDS: from onset through recovery. Curr Opin Crit Care. 2014;20(4):373–7.
80. Prewitt RM, McCarthy J, Wood LD. Treatment of acute low pressure pulmonary edema in dogs: relative effects of hydrostatic and oncotic pressure, nitroprusside, and positive end-expiratory pressure. J Clin Invest. 1981;67(2):409–18.

81. Reising CA, Chendrasekhar A, Wall PL, Paradise NF, Timberlake GA, Moorman DW. Continuous dose furosemide as a therapeutic approach to acute respiratory distress syndrome (ARDS). J Surg Res. 1999;82(1):56–60.
82. Martin GS, Moss M, Wheeler AP, Mealer M, Morris JA, Bernard GR. A randomized, controlled trial of furosemide with or without albumin in hypoproteinemic patients with acute lung injury. Crit Care Med. 2005;33(8):1681–7.
83. Thille AW, Esteban A, Fernández-Segoviano P, Rodriguez JM, Aramburu JA, Peñuelas O, Cortés-Puch I, Cardinal-Fernández P, Lorente JA, Frutos-Vivar F. Comparison of the Berlin definition for acute respiratory distress syndrome with autopsy. Am J Respir Crit Care Med. 2013;187(7):761–7.
84. Kushimoto S, Taira Y, Kitazawa Y, Okuchi K, Sakamoto T, Ishikura H, Endo T, Yamanouchi S, Tagami T, Yamaguchi J, Yoshikawa K, Sugita M, Kase Y, Kanemura T, Takahashi H, Kuroki Y, Izumino H, Rinka H, Seo R, Takatori M, Kaneko T, Nakamura T, Irahara T, Saito N, Watanabe A, PiCCO Pulmonary Edema Study Group. The clinical usefulness of extravascular lung water and pulmonary vascular permeability index to diagnose and characterize pulmonary edema: a prospective multicenter study on the quantitative differential diagnostic definition for acute lung injury/acute respiratory distress syndrome. Crit Care. 2012;16(6):R232.
85. Perel A. Extravascular lung water and the pulmonary vascular permeability index may improve the definition of ARDS. Crit Care. 2013;17(1):108.
86. Carlile PV, Beckett RC, Gray BA. Relationship between CO and transit times for dye and thermal indicators in central circulation. J Appl Physiol (1985). 1986;60(4):1363–72.
87. Patroniti N, Bellani G, Maggioni E, Manfio A, Marcora B, Pesenti A. Measurement of pulmonary edema in patients with acute respiratory distress syndrome. Crit Care Med. 2005;33(11):2547–54.
88. Teboul JL, Pinsky MR, Mercat A, Anguel N, Bernardin G, Achard JM, Boulain T, Richard C. Estimating cardiac filling pressure in mechanically ventilated patients with hyperinflation. Crit Care Med. 2000;28(11):3631–6.
89. Ganter CC, Jakob SM, Takala J. Pulmonary capillary pressure. A review. Minerva Anestesiol. 2006;72(1–2):21–36. Review Erratum in: Minerva Anestesiol 2007 Mar;73(3):XVII.
90. Gaar KA J, Taylor AE, Owens LJ, Guyton AC. Pulmonary capillary pressure and filtration coefficient in the isolated perfused lung. Am J Phys. 1967;213(4):910–4.
91. Takala J. Pulmonary capillary pressure. Intensive Care Med. 2003;29(6):890–3.
92. Riviello ED, Buregeya E, Twagirumugabe T. Diagnosing acute respiratory distress syndrome in resource limited settings: the Kigali modification of the Berlin definition. Curr Opin Crit Care. 2017;23(1):18–23.
93. National Heart, Lung, and Blood Institute Acute Respiratory Distress Syndrome (ARDS) Clinical Trials Network, Wiedemann HP, Wheeler AP, Bernard GR, Thompson BT, Hayden D, de Boisblanc B, Connors AF Jr, Hite RD, Harabin AL. Comparison of two fluid-management strategies in acute lung injury. N Engl J Med. 2006;354(24):2564–75.
94. Mikkelsen ME, Christie JD, Lanken PN, Biester RC, Thompson BT, Bellamy SL, Localio AR, Demissie E, Hopkins RO, Angus DC. The adult respiratory distress syndrome cognitive outcomes study: long-term neuropsychological function in survivors of acute lung injury. Am J Respir Crit Care Med. 2012;185(12):1307–15.
95. Chatterjee K. The Swan-Ganz catheters: past, present, and future. A viewpoint. Circulation. 2009;119(1):147–52.
96. Levy MM, Artigas A, Phillips GS, Rhodes A, Beale R, Osborn T, Vincent JL, Townsend S, Lemeshow S, Dellinger RP. Outcomes of the surviving sepsis campaign in intensive care units in the USA and Europe: a prospective cohort study. Lancet Infect Dis. 2012;12(12):919–24.
97. Tenner S, Baillie J, DeWitt J, Vege SS, American College of Gastroenterology. American College of Gastroenterology guideline: management of acute pancreatitis. Am J Gastroenterol. 2013;108(9):1400–15.
98. Vieillard-Baron A, Schmitt JM, Augarde R, Fellahi JL, Prin S, Page B, Beauchet A, Jardin F. Acute cor pulmonale in acute respiratory distress syndrome submitted to protective ventilation: incidence, clinical implications, and prognosis. Crit Care Med. 2001;29(8):1551–5.
99. Jardin F, Vieillard-Baron A. Right ventricular function and positive pressure ventilation in clinical practice: from hemodynamic subsets to respirator settings. Intensive Care Med. 2003;29(9):1426–34.
100. Mauri T, Lazzeri M, Bellani G, Zanella A, Grasselli G. Respiratory mechanics to understand ARDS and guide mechanical ventilation. Physiol Meas. 2017;38(12):R280–H303.

101. Amato MB, Meade MO, Slutsky AS, Brochard L, Costa EL, Schoenfeld DA, Stewart TE, Briel M, Talmor D, Mercat A, Richard JC, Carvalho CR, Brower RG. Driving pressure and survival in the acute respiratory distress syndrome. N Engl J Med. 2015;372(8):747–55.
102. Vieillard-Baron A, Charron C, Caille V, Belliard G, Page B, Jardin F. Prone positioning unloads the right ventricle in severe ARDS. Chest. 2007;132(5):1440–6.
103. Guérin C, Reignier J, Richard JC, Beuret P, Gacouin A, Boulain T, Mercier E, Badet M, Mercat A, Baudin O, Clavel M, Chatellier D, Jaber S, Rosselli S, Mancebo J, Sirodot M, Hilbert G, Bengler C, Richecoeur J, Gainnier M, Bayle F, Bourdin G, Leray V, Girard R, Baboi L, Ayzac L, PROSEVA Study Group. Prone positioning in severe acute respiratory distress syndrome. N Engl J Med. 2013;368(23):2159–68.
104. Paternot A, Repessé X, Vieillard-Baron A. Rationale and description of right ventricle-protective ventilation in ARDS. Respir Care. 2016;61(10):1391–6.
105. Vieillard-Baron A, Matthay M, Teboul JL, Bein T, Schultz M, Magder S, Marini JJ. Experts' opinion on management of hemodynamics in ARDS patients: focus on the effects of mechanical ventilation. Intensive Care Med. 2016;42(5):739–49.
106. Ventetuolo CE, Klinger JR. Management of acute right ventricular failure in the intensive care unit. Ann Am Thorac Soc. 2014;11:811–22.

In Neurological Emergencies

Ilaria Alice Crippa and Fabio Silvio Taccone

M. R. Pinsky et al. (eds.), *Hemodynamic Monitoring*, Lessons from the ICU,
https://doi.org/10.1007/978-3-319-69269-2_35

Learning Objectives

- At the end of the reading, the reader will be able to:
- Understand fluid and haemodynamic physiology in neurocritically ill patients.
- Integrate physiology into bedside clinical decision-making process in neurological emergencies.
- Understand disease-specific haemodynamic target in neurocritically ill patients.
- Plan haemodynamic therapy in neurological emergencies.

35.1 Introduction

Neurological emergencies are common and frequently devastating. In Europe, millions of people each year experience acute central nervous injuries, either traumatic or non-traumatic, with considerable mortality and long-term disability [1]. The primary goal of the medical therapy of neurological emergencies is to prevent the development of secondary brain injuries [2]. In this setting, optimal haemodynamic management is crucial to optimize cerebral perfusion and oxygenation. Careful choice of fluid therapy and manipulation of blood pressure are cornerstones of therapy in patients with an acute brain injury. In this chapter, we will review physiological evidence, current guidelines and most recent clinical investigations on fluid and haemodynamic management in neurocritically ill patients.

35.2 Fluid Management

A growing body of literature shows that routine fluid management may influence clinical outcomes in general critically ill patients [3]. Most of the current literature on fluid management in brain-injured patients focus on SAH and TBI. However, the clinician should not underestimate the importance of a proper fluid management in other neurological emergencies, such as stroke or post-anoxic brain injury. Brain-injured patients have several distinctive features compared with general critically ill patients. Firstly, the cranial cavity has a peculiar volume-limited structure, which greatly limits the amount of oedema allowed to take place without impacting organ function. Secondly, due to the specific blood-brain barrier structure, in neurocritically ill patients, local effects of fluid take on far
35
greater importance than in peripheral systemic circulation. Thirdly, electrolyte and osmotic disturbances associated with the primary insult itself and administration of hyperosmolar therapy can significantly influence the fluid shift from the intravascular to the cerebral parenchyma space and impact on cerebral haemodynamics.

35.2.1 Pathophysiological Considerations

Plasma and brain interstitial fluid and cerebrospinal fluid (CSF) have equal osmolality under physiological conditions (i.e. 288 ± 5 mOsmol/kg). In the cerebral circulation, water and solute transfer from the intravascular to the extravascular space is regulated by the blood-brain barrier (BBB). BBB basic unit contributes to the so-called neurovascular unit, which is composed of cerebral vascular endothelial cells, surrounding pericytes, basal lamina, perivascular astrocytes and functional neurons [4]. Water can move freely across the BBB, but the tight junctions between endothelial cells prevent solute passage, in contrast to what happens in the peripheral circulation. Thus, while in systemic peripheral circulation, the main driving force for water movement across the wall of the capillaries is the hydrostatic pressure, net water movements in the brain occur mainly in response to imposed osmotic differences across the BBB. Such mechanism is supposed to prevent oedema formation in case of modifications of the intravascular volume and makes the administration of large amounts of isotonic fluids (which have osmolality equals to that of plasma) possible without impacting brain homeostasis [5]. However, this exposes the brain to sudden water transfer in case of administration of non-isotonic fluid. Specifically, hypotonic fluids cause water shifts from the intravascular space to the interstitial space – which in turn equilibrates with intracellular space – whereas hypertonic fluids cause water shifts from the brain (both intracellular and interstitial space) to the intravascular compartment, in order to re-equilibrate the osmotic gradient. The osmotic gradient is restored in few minutes, but equilibration half-times vary depending on the capillary-tissue ratio, the BBB integrity and the characteristics of the hypotonic or hypertonic fluid. Even though this mechanisms can be advantageous in specific conditions (notably in case of administration of hyperosmolar therapy because of intracranial hypertension), acute changes in osmolality should be avoided whenever possible [6]. The neuronal and glial cells can actively compensate for free water shift due to fluctuations in plasma tonicity and normalize intracellular volume, but this mechanism is energy-consuming and has limited compensatory capacity. Moreover, anatomical and functional integrity of BBB in brain-injured patients cannot be easily determined: in case of BBB disruption or energetic impairment of the brain, the ability to maintain fluid and electrolyte homeostasis is compromised.

Learning Box

The occurrence of oedema in the brain can be classified on the basis of the failing homeostatic mechanism: in case of ATP depletion and/or mitochondrial dysfunction, water and solute shift into the cells, thus determining oedema in neurons and astrocytes (cytotoxic oedema); disruption of endothelial tight junctions leads to water and solute shift from the intravascular space to the interstitium (vasogenic oedema). A combination of these two mechanisms leads to ionic oedema: in case of cytotoxic oedema, decreased interstitial osmolality determines compensatory solute and water shifts from the vascular compartment to the interstitium through the intact BBB.

35.2.2 Fluids in Clinical Practice

There is broad consensus that an intravascular volume sufficient to sustain adequate cerebral perfusion and oxygen delivery should be provided in acute phase of brain injury. At the same time, attention should be paid to the amount and physical characteristics of the administered fluid.

35.2.2.1 How Much?

In general, targeting euvolemia is recommended in neurological emergencies. Intravascular volume depletion is frequent in acute stroke, particularly in older adult patients [7]. American Heart Association/American Stroke Association (AHA/ASA) guidelines recommend correction of hypovolemia in acute ischaemic stroke patients regardless of the presence of brain swelling [8]. Fluid management of patients with intraparenchymal haemorrhage (IPH) and traumatic brain injury (TBI) is not discussed in the most recent guidelines by the AHA/ASA and the Brain Trauma Foundation, except in case hyperosmolar therapy is needed [8, 9]. Current guidelines strongly recommend to assure adequate organ and brain perfusion in spinal cord injuries and post-cardiac arrest syndrome [10, 11]. In subarachnoid haemorrhage (SAH), circulating volume expansion is part of the traditional haemodynamic augmentation therapy (or triple-H therapy), which consisted in haemodilution, volume expansion ("hypervolemia") and hypertension [12]. This strategy was believed to increase CBF through different mechanisms, mainly increasing cardiac output and arterial blood pressure through modifications in blood rheology. Triple-H therapy efficacy has been questioned by recent literature on the basis of physiological considerations (haemodilution leads to decreased haematocrit, thus potential decrease in oxygen delivery), clinical observation (volume expansion modestly contributes to increase blood pressure compared to vasopressors used) and observation of higher rate of complications in patients treated with "supranormal" volume expansion [13, 14]. AHA/ASA guidelines recommend that supranormal volume expansion should be avoided in SAH patients, in particular in the absence of diagnosed vasospasm [15], and the Neurocritical Care Society advises against the aggressive administration of fluid in SAH, regardless of the presence of vasospasm [16]. Thus, maintenance of euvolemia and induced hypertension is the preferred strategy now in case of SAH complicated by delayed cerebral ischaemia (DCI) [17]. Unfortunately, precise indications on how to manage neurocritically ill patients after the first few hours are lacking. The most studied paradigms are SAH and TBI, where results from retrospective and prospective studies are conflicting and both positive and negative fluid balance have been alternatively associated with worse outcome.

35.2.2.2 Fluid Composition

Isotonic crystalloids are generally recommended for maintenance and haemodynamic management of acute brain-injured patients [8, 15, 16]. Some guidelines [15] explicitly advise against use of hypotonic fluids. However, the definition of isotonicity requires an in-depth analysis. The correct definitions of osmolarity, osmolality and tonicity should be applied to fluid composition: "osmolarity" represents the sum of all potentially dissociable particles (in mOsmol/L); "osmolality" represents the number of osmotically active solutes (in mOsmol/kg); "tonicity" is the measure of the osmotic pressure gradient between two solutions. Tonicity is a function of osmolality and, unlike osmolarity, is only influenced by solutes that cannot cross the endothelial membrane (i.e. for the brain, BBB). Thus, the clinically relevant variables are the osmolality and the tonicity and not the osmolarity: as an example, "iso-osmolar" solutions can have different tonicity (◘ Table 35.1). A fluid can be considered isotonic when its osmolality approaches the one measured into the plasma; thus it does not determine shift of water in or out the brain even if administered in large amount. Isotonic fluids are commercialized as saline (NaCl 0.9%) or "balanced" solutions, where balanced indicates electrolytes composition close to the plasma [18]. In SAH, the use of more balanced solutions was not inferior to the use of NaCl 0.9% in avoiding hyponatremia and hyposmolality of plasma [19]. Ringer's lactate and Ringer's acetate are hypotonic even if their osmolarity is close to the one of plasma; thus they should be avoided in acute brain-injured patients. Dextrose solutions are isotonic in vitro but hypotonic once infused, because the glucose will be quickly metabolized, thus should be also avoided in brain-injured patients. Hypertonic solutions are generally reserved for emergency treatment of acutely increased intracranial pressure. Synthetic colloids can be isotonic (e.g. Tetraspan 6%), hypotonic (e.g. Gelafundin 4%) or slightly hypertonic (e.g. HES 6%). Low-

Table 35.1 General characteristics of intravenous solutions used in critically ill patients

Solution	mOsm/L	pH	Na	Cl	K	Ca	HCO_3	Lac	Glu	Mg	Acet	Gluco	Tonicity	Oncotic Pressure (mmHg)
Plasma	290	7.4	140	100	4.5	2.3	26	1	60 to 99	1	0	–	=	
Saline 0.9%	308	5.7	154	154	–	–	–	–	–	–	–	–	+	
Saline 0.45%	154	5.6	77	77	–	–	–	–	–	–	–	–	- -	
Saline 3%	1026	5	513	513	–	–	–	–	–	–	–	–	++	
Mannitol 10%	549	4.5[a]	–	–	–	–	–	–	–	–	–	–	++	
Glucose 5%	278	4.5	–	–	–	–	–	–	50	–	–	–	=	
Ringer's Lac	272	6.6	130	109	4	3	–	28[b]	–	–	–	–	–	
PlasmaLyte	294	7.4	140	98	5	–	–	8[b]	–	3	27	23	=	
Albumin 5%	310	7.3	130 to 160	110 to 130	–	–	–	–	–	–	–	–	=	27
Albumin 20%	310	7.3	130 to 160	110 to 130	–	–	–	–	–	–	–	–	=	80
HES 6%[c]	310	5.9	154	154	–	–	–	–	–	–	–	–	=	28
Gelofusine 4%	274		154	120	–	–		–	–	–	–	–	=	34

Lac lactate, *HES* hydroxyethyl starch, *Na* sodium, *Cl* chloride, *K* potassium, *Ca* calcium, *HCO3* bicarbonate, *Mg* magnesium, *Acet* acetate, *Gluco* gluconate, ALL in mEq/L, *Glu* glucose (g/L)

[a]up to 7.0

[b]metabolized to bicarbonate

[c]balanced

concentration human albumin solutions (e.g. albumin solutions 4% and 5%) are hypotonic. The rationale in the use of colloids in brain-injured patients lies in the fact that plasma proteins contribute for up to 80% to the osmotic pressure. However, integrity of BBB must be assumed for colloids to exert their effect. Furthermore, difference in tonicity between specific crystalloids and colloids should not be neglected. In the SAFE study [20], for example, NaCl 0.9% and a solution of human albumin 4% were compared in a subgroup of TBI patients, and the use of colloids was associated with worse 28-day outcome. However, human albumin 4% is hypotonic compared to plasma; thus this result should be interpreted as a negative effect exerted by a hypotonic fluid more than a comparison between crystalloids and colloids. As such, albumin has been also associated with improved outcome or with no additional adverse events after SAH or ischaemic stroke [21–23]. Several clinical studies investigating different fluid therapies in acute neurological conditions are currently registered on ► clinicaltrials.gov and will provide additional high-quality findings on this issue in the next future.

35.3 Blood Pressure Management

Management of blood pressure (BP) in neurological emergencies is challenging: both over- and under-correction of BP are associated with increased morbidity and mortality after TBI [24]. Current guidelines rely on few randomized clinical studies and expert opinions. Based on clinical observation, two phases can be identified with regard to BP management after acute brain injury: the early, emergent phase (from minutes to hours after the injury) and the intensive care phase (from hours to days thereafter). Right after the neurological event has occurred, BP management should take into account the pathophysiology of the central nervous system and the type of injury: in patients with intracranial haemorrhage (ICH) and aneurysmal subarachnoid haemorrhage (SAH), for example, attention should be paid to prevent haemorrhagic progression; in patients with acute ischaemic stroke (AIS), perfusion of the penumbra area at risk of ischaemia should be assured while taking into account the risk of haemorrhagic transformation, in particular after the administration of intravenous thrombolysis; in patients with TBI and post-cardiac arrest syndrome, BP manipulation should focus on assuring adequate brain perfusion because of early cerebral oedema formation. Once the intracranial lesion is relatively stable, BP management should focus on finding the adequate balance between the risk of hypoperfusion (and subsequent ischaemia) and the risk of hyperaemia and subsequent blood-brain barrier and cellular damage.

35.3.1 Pathophysiological Considerations

Cerebral perfusion pressure (CPP) is determined by the pressure gradient across the cerebral circulation (ΔP) and the resistance (R) across the cerebrovascular bed according to the equation: CPP = $\Delta P/R$. The pressure gradient is defined as mean arterial blood pressure (MAP) – intracranial pressure (ICP) or MAP – jugular venous pressure (JVP), whichever is higher. For practical purposes, when ICP and JVP are in the physiological range, CPP is considered to be equivalent to MAP. According to the Hagen-Poiseuille eq. ($R = 8\mu L/\pi r^4$), the radius of the vessel affects the resistance (R) by a factor of four: small changes in vessel lumen diameter have great effects on CBF [25]. Modifications in the diameter of medium-sized cerebral arterioles can be seen in pathological conditions such as vasospasm or intracranial stenosis: the vessel constricts (reduces its diameter), thus increasing R and impairing blood flow, possibly provoking ischaemia. On the opposite, dilation of vessel (increase in diameter) leads to increase in cerebral blood flow (hyperaemia). The first condition is frequent after SAH, while the second one is common after TBI, where hyperaemia due to uncontrolled vasodilation can contribute to brain swelling and high ICP. In physiological condition, the calibre of medium-sized cerebral arterioles is constant, while small cerebral arterioles can constantly modify their diameter. The intrinsic ability of the brain arterioles to modify their calibre in order to maintain constant cerebral blood flow (CBF) despite changes in blood pressure is called "cerebral autoregulation" [26]: in case of increase in CPP, small arterioles constrict so to increase R and keep the ratio constant; vice versa in case of reduction in CPP, small arterioles dilate to reduce the resistance (■ Fig. 35.1a). Traditionally, this mechanism has been thought to work for CPP in the range of about 50–150 mmHg: in this range CBF is maintained constant at around 50 mL/100 g of brain tissue/minute; above and below this limit, autoregulation is lost and CBF becomes directly dependent on CPP, thus on MAP (■ Fig. 35.1b). Under the lower limit of cerebral autoregulation, the maximum vasodilation is reached: for lower value of MAP, small vessels passively collapse, and CBF becomes directly proportional to MAP. The drop in CBF is initially compensated by an increase in oxygen extraction from haemoglobin, but for CBF below 18–20 mL/100 g/min, this compensatory mechanism fails and ischaemic injury occurs. When MAP reaches the upper limit of autoregulation, vasoconstriction is maximal, and cerebral small vessels can no further reduce their calibre, so they passively dilate with subsequent increase in CBF and blood volume. In case of impaired cerebral autoregulation, CBF varies linearly with MAP. Cerebral autoregulation range of efficacy can be affected by several factors, such as chronic comorbidities or, likely, individual variability. In diabetic patients, cerebral autoregulation is frequently impaired early during the disease [27], while in chronically hypertensive patient, the range of efficacy is shifted to the right, so that these patients better tolerate higher than lower arterial pressure [28]. In severely brain-injured patients, cerebral autoregulation curve may be shifted to the right, the range of MAP in which cerebral autoregulation is effective can be reduced or cerebral autoregulation can be completely lost. Cerebral autoregulation is known to be impaired in most acute neurological conditions, such as TBI, SAH, ischaemic stroke and post-cardiac arrest syndrome [29–31]. Each patient is likely to differ from another with regard to baseline cerebral autoregulatory curve and post-injury impairment. Thus, no general rule can be safely applied to every patient with regard to BP management. Each patient probably has an "optimal CPP", i.e. a specific MAP range for which cerebral autoregulation is most effective and cerebral blood flow is optimal. In a recent consensus conference [32], the potential therapeutic implications of manipulation of arterial blood pressure have been largely discussed.

Cerebral autoregulation can be monitored bedside in several ways. Each and every technique relies on the fact that if cerebral autoregulation is intact, CBF should be constant in case of modifications in MAP. This relationship is reflected by the correlation coefficient between two variables: if they are directly related, the correlation coefficient is positive; if they are inversely related, the correlation coefficient is negative; if there is no relationship between the two, the correlation coefficient is 0. In case of intact autoregulation, the correlation coefficient between CBF and MAP should be 0. In clinical practice, a correlation coefficient from negative up to 0.3 is accepted as marker of intact cerebral autoregulation. For correlation coefficient above 0.3, CBF modifications are considered to

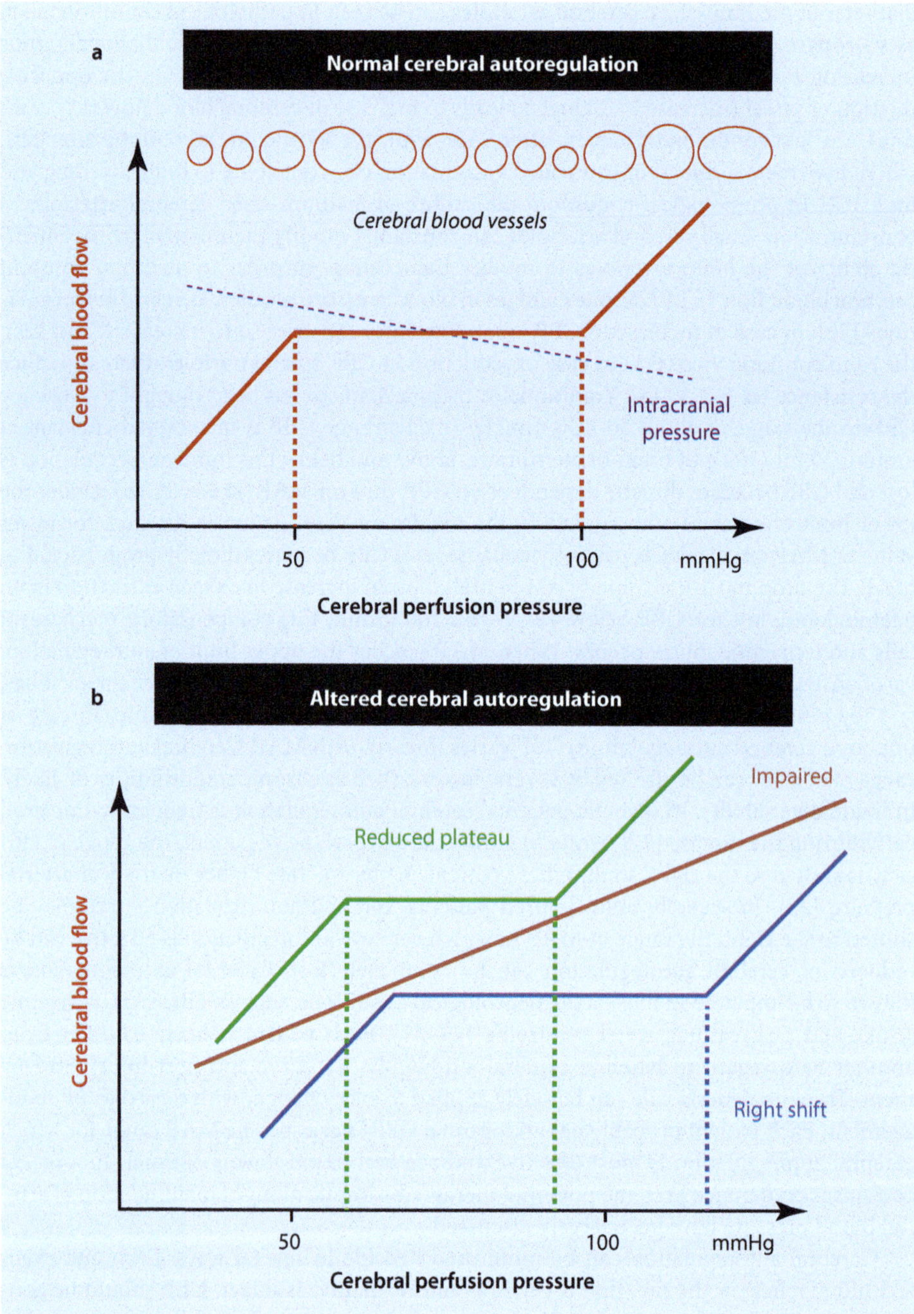

Fig. 35.1 Schematic view of cerebrovascular pressure autoregulation in normal **a** and pathological **b** conditions

parallel those of MAP, i.e. cerebral autoregulation is failing. CBF cannot be easily measured bedside, but there are surrogates that can be used instead. For example, the pressure reactivity index (PRx) calculates the correlation coefficient between MAP and ICP [32]:

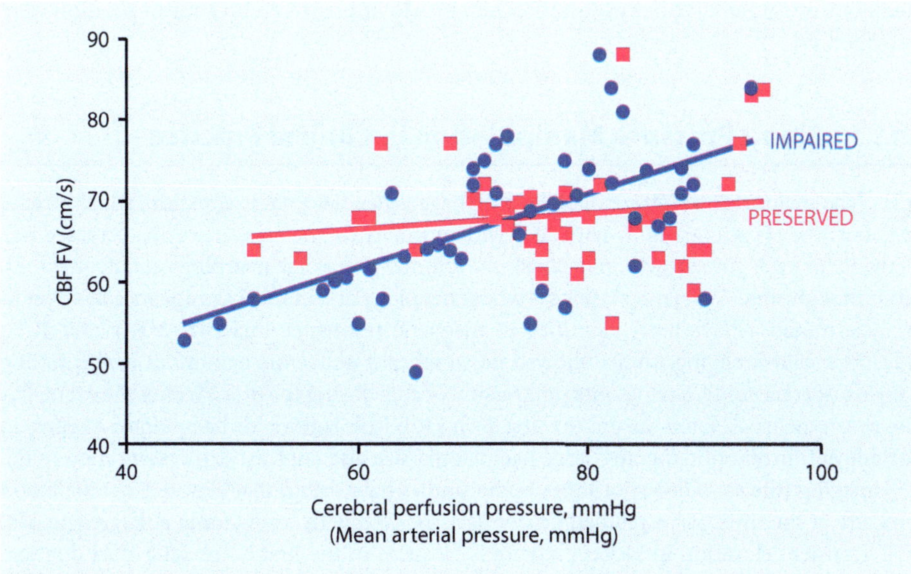

Fig. 35.2 Examples of linear relationship between cerebral blood flow velocities (CBF MV) with cerebral perfusion pressure (or mean arterial pressure) to estimate cerebral autoregulation. If the analysis of the linear relationship shows a coefficient >0.3 (blue line), the autoregulation is considered as "impaired". If the coefficient is ≤0.3, then the autoregulation is considered as "preserved" (pink line). Similar relationship can be analysed using intracranial pressure or brain oxygenation instead of CBF MV

modifications in vessel calibre determine proportional modifications in cerebral blood volume, which in turn is reflected by modification in ICP. In physiological conditions, when MAP decreases, cerebral blood vessels dilate; thus ICP increases. In this case PRx will be negative or close to zero (Fig. 35.2). In contrast, in case of ineffective autoregulation, modifications in ICP follow modifications in MAP and PRx is positive. Clinical studies, predominantly in TBI, have explored the potential benefits of manipulating MAP, specifically targeting PRx close to zero [33, 34]. PRx-based manipulation of MAP is associated with favourable outcome following severe TBI [34]. However, these promising results have not been consistently confirmed, and PRx needs invasive measurement of ICP to be calculated. Tissue oxygenation or blood flow velocities are other available surrogates for CBF [32]. Brain tissue oxygen ($PbtO_2$) can be measured directly by the use of an intraparenchymal probe or indirectly by near-infrared spectroscopy (NIRS), while blood flow velocity (FV) in the intracranial arteries can be non-invasively assessed by the use of transcranial Doppler. The correlation between MAP and $PbtO_2$ is called oxygen reactivity index (ORx); the correlation coefficient between CPP and FV is called mean flow index (Mx); the correlation coefficient between MAP and FV is called mean arterial flow index (Mxa); and the correlation coefficient between MAP and NIRS-derived tissue oxygen content is called tissue oxygenation index (TOx) [32]. Cerebral autoregulation indexes correlate with outcomes in TBI, SAH, ischaemic stroke and ICH [34–37]. However, monitoring of autoregulation does not necessarily mean better therapy and whether strategies aimed at optimizing brain perfusion (e.g. optimal CPP-guided therapy) improves outcome is still uncertain. Last update of Brain Trauma Foundation guidelines on TBI patients acknowledges that cerebral autoregulatory status could have a role in clinical decisions on target CPP, but no specific therapies to improve cerebral autoregulation were provided [9].

35.3.2 Blood Pressure Manipulation in Clinical Practice

ICH The major risk in intracranial haemorrhage is haematoma progression, which occurs in about 30% of patients and is associated with mortality (in the measure of 5% increased risk of dying for each 10% growth in haematoma volume) and worse neurological outcome [38]. Even though small ischaemic lesions – whose aetiology and clinical significance have yet to be determined – have been identified in magnetic resonance imaging (MRI) after ICH, advanced neuroimaging studies showed no significant ischaemic penumbra in this setting [39]. Most commonly, haematoma progression occurs during the first 3 h after the event, but the risk remains elevated during the first 24 h [40]. Risk factors for haematoma expansion include antithrombotic therapy, large haematoma size and contrast extravasation on initial CT imaging (the so-called spot sign). Some studies have found that elevated systolic blood pressure at the time of hospital admission is associated with haematoma enlargement [40, 41]. Transient elevation in blood pressure is frequent in the first hours after ICH due to a variety of factors, including stress, pain, increased ICP or chronic arterial hypertension. Acute hypertensive response in patients with ICH is defined as a systolic blood pressure (SBP) >140 mm Hg or a diastolic blood pressure (DBP) >90 mm Hg on recordings taken over 5 min within the first 24 h from symptoms' onset [42]. It has been shown that systolic blood pressure (SBP) has higher and greater variability than diastolic or mean arterial pressure in the first 24 h after ICH [40]; hence SBP is considered the relevant marker of acute hypertension in patients with ICH. It has been postulated that early correction of hypertensive response could be beneficial; several studies have investigated the safety and potential advantages of lowering blood pressure early after ICH. Animal studies showed no reduction in regional cerebral blood flow with manipulation of BP [43]; these data were confirmed in the clinical setting by the Intracerebral Haemorrhage Acutely Decreasing Arterial Pressure Trial (ICH-ADAPT). On the other hand, small reduction in SBP has been shown to be effective in reducing haematoma expansion, while aggressive blood pressure lowering (>10%) has shown to be deleterious on neurological outcome [44]. The two multicentric Intensive Blood Pressure Reduction in Acute Cerebral Haemorrhage randomized controlled trials (INTERACT and INTERACT-II) enrolled 3243 patients with small ICH (average baseline haematoma volume in INTERACT-II was 11 mL) in which intensive antihypertensive treatment was planned to start within 1 h and continued for 7 days. In both trials, early, intensive lowering of BP to <140 mmHg was not associated with increase in death or serious adverse event rates [45, 46]. INTERACT showed a reduction in expansion rate, and INTERACT-II showed a reduction in the relative growth of haematoma with SBP lowering. The large INTERACT-II trial (2839 patients) showed a better outcome and a trend towards mortality reduction and better neurological outcome in the intensive BP lowering group (SBP < 140 mmHg) compared to the control group (SBP < 180 mmHg). However, more than 30% of the patients in the intensive treatment group did not reach the SBP target, and this could have influenced the negative results with regard to the outcome. The recent ATACH-II multicentric randomized controlled trial showed that lowering BP < 140 mmHg was not associated with survival or better neurological outcome and it was instead associated with a higher rate of renal failure [47]. However, ATACH-II and INTERACT-II differed in many aspects, such as mean BP upon arrival at the emergency department (which was higher in

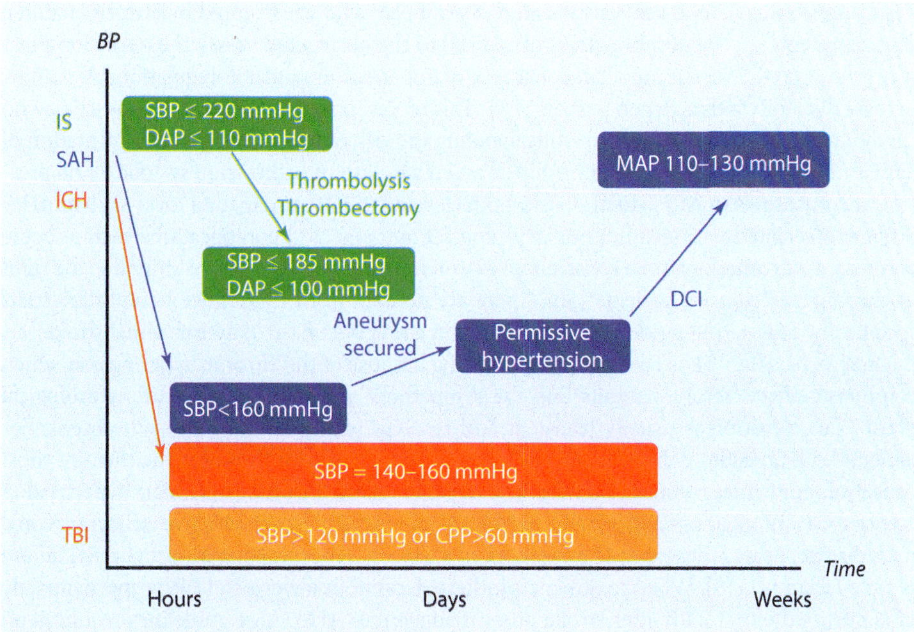

Fig. 35.3 A pragmatic approach to control blood pressure after an acute brain injury. In case of ischaemic stroke (IS, green), the values of systolic (SBP) and diastolic blood pressure (DBP) will depend on the use of thrombolysis and/or thrombectomy. In case of intracerebral haemorrhage (ICH, red), a rapid control of SBP around 140–160 mmHg since the very initial phase after hospital admission is recommended. In patients with a subarachnoid haemorrhage (SAH, blue), blood pressure should be under control until the aneurysm is secured, and then higher values of mean arterial pressure are allowed; in case of delayed cerebral ischaemia, induced hypertension remains the first-line therapy. After a traumatic brain injury (TBI, orange), a minimal requirement of systolic blood pressure or cerebral perfusion pressure (CPP) is required

ATACH-II trial), medication used to control BP, timing of treatment (4 h vs. 6 h in INTERACT) and average BP reached in the intensive treatment group (130 mmHg vs. 146 mmHg in the INTERACT trials). ASA/AHA guidelines suggest acute SBP lowering to 140 mmHg in ICH patients who present with SBP of 150–220 mmHg (if no contraindications to reduction in BP; Class I; level of evidence A) [48]. The European Stroke Organization (ESO) agrees on the BP target but finds this recommendation to be supported only by moderate evidence. Antihypertensive treatment of ICH patient is still uncertain. Given the evidence, we suggest a cautious approach, and we advise against rapid and/or extreme reduction of BP (Fig. 35.3). An active BP control to reduce SBP to 140–160 mmHg within the first 6 h is advised. The use of short-acting intravenous antihypertensive agents, such as labetalol, urapidil or nicardipine, should be associated with oral therapies to avoid wide variations of blood pressure in such patients.

Acute ischaemic stroke The approach to BP management in acute ischaemic stroke is inherently different from the approach in ICH. Most strokes are caused by focal ischaemia, typically involving a single blood vessel. Cells are affected proportionally to the distance from the occluded vessel: the cells closer to the occluded vessel have no access to collateral circulation, so will be most affected; cells which are more distant from the involved vessel will get some perfusion from collateral vessels and can recover if blood flow is restored in a timely manner. This represents the "penumbra". In stroke, distal to the obstructed vessel, the perfusion pressure is low and the vessels are dilated. Because of impaired cerebral autoregulation, blood flow in these dilated vessels is dependent on MAP. This represents a challenge for the physician who should assure adequate perfusion while avoiding the risk of haemorrhagic transformation of damaged tissue. A U-shaped relationship between baseline and admission systolic blood pressure and outcomes in AIS patients exists: both elevated (>200 mmHg) and low (<120 mmHg) SBP are associated with death, poor neurological outcome and complications such as acute coronary syndromes or stroke recurrence [49]. Of note, such relationship is shifted to the right in chronic hypertensive patients [50]. There are no data from randomized controlled trials specifically designed to guide BP management in the acute phase of an ischaemic stroke (i.e. the first 24 h). High BP is common in this setting because of the chronic hypertension which commonly affects stroke patients and the sympathetic response to the acute neurological event. This elevation is usually transient and resolves within 10 days from the event. For patients with an acute ischaemic stroke who are not treated with thrombolytic therapy, most consensus guidelines recommend BP not be treated in the acute phase unless the hypertension is extreme (SBP >220 mmHg or DBP >120 mmHg), or the patient has active ischaemic coronary disease, heart failure, aortic dissection, hypertensive encephalopathy, acute renal failure or pre-/eclampsia [8]. When treatment is indicated, cautious lowering of BP by approximately 15% during the first 24 h after stroke onset is suggested. AHA/ASA guidelines recommend targeting SBP < 185 mmHg and DBP < 110 mmHg before intravenous thrombolysis is administered. BP should be kept at maximum 180/105 mmHg for at least 24 h thereafter [8]. No precise recommendations with respect to BP control in patients who receive endovascular treatment are given in the most recent guidelines, but we suggest to control BP to at least the same threshold than thrombolysis, i.e. SBP < 160–180 mmHg and DBP < 100 mmHg. Optimal BP targets in case of haemorrhagic transformation or haematoma expansion following reperfusion with thrombolysis or thrombectomy are currently uncertain and should be discussed on a case-by-case basis. Guidelines acknowledge that vasopressors may be used to improve cerebral blood flow in rare cases when systemic hypotension is producing neurologic impairment, but this is rarely done in clinical practice in stroke patients. It is reasonable to restart antihypertensive medications 24 h after stroke onset in patients with pre-existing hypertension who are neurologically stable [8]. Reduction in BP should be cautious in patients with extracranial or intracranial large artery stenosis (i.e. over 7–14 days after ischaemic stroke), as some degree of blood pressure elevation may be necessary to maintain an adequate cerebral blood flow.

Aneurysmal subarachnoid haemorrhage Re-bleeding is a major risk after aneurysmal SAH, especially in the first 2–12 h [15]. Aneurysm re-bleeding is associated with mortality and poor neurological prognosis. Risk factors include longer time to aneurysm treatment, worse neurological status on admission, initial loss of consciousness, previous sentinel headaches, larger aneurysm size and possibly SBP >160 mmHg. AHA/ASA guidelines suggest that between the time of aneurysmal SAH onset and aneurysm obliteration, BP should be controlled with a titratable agent to balance the risk of stroke, hypertension-related re-bleeding and maintenance of cerebral perfusion pressure (Class I recommendation), possibly to SBP <160 mmHg (Class II recommendation). However, the possibility of increased intracranial pressure (ICP) and the potential impact on cerebral perfusion should be assessed to determine the haemodynamic targets. In case of DCI, first-line therapy consists to increase gradually MAP, unless blood pressure is elevated at baseline or significant cardiac dysfunction is diagnosed (Class I recommendation) [15]. BP target should be selected considering baseline BP of the patient. In general, SBP 160–180 or MAP 100–110 mmHg is considered appropriate. In symptomatic patients with a reliable clinical examination, the goal is resolution of symptoms. In poor-grade patients with monitored ICP, CPP should be targeted, and efficacy of the treatment should be assessed by multimodality monitoring ($PbtO_2$, EEG, etc.). BP/CPP should be increased stepwise, assessing the efficacy of the treatment for about 30 min before continuing escalating. Current guidelines do not suggest a maximal SBP/MAP or CPP target, but the potentially deleterious effects of hypertension on the other organs should be considered, and close clinical monitoring for complications such as heart failure is mandatory. A limit of CPP around 120 mmHg or MAP around 140 mmHg could be considered reasonable. Norepinephrine, dopamine and phenylephrine all have been demonstrated to be effective in improving CBF and/or cerebral oxygenation [51, 52]. We suggest the use of norepinephrine as the first-line treatment because of the predictable increase in BP and the low frequency of tachycardia. Therapy should be continued for at least 24–48 h and then de-escalated slowly monitoring for recurrence of clinical neurological deficit or alterations in multimodal monitoring.

Traumatic brain injury Hypotension has been known to be associated with worse outcome in TBI patients since at least three decades [51]. Hypotension can be detrimental in several ways: if cerebral autoregulation is intact, a drop in SBP triggers the vasodilation of the cerebral vascular bed, with subsequent increased cerebral blood volume and ICP; if cerebral autoregulation is altered, low BP can cause cerebral ischaemia. Such relationship between cerebral autoregulation, BP, and CPP should be kept in mind when manipulating BP in TBI patients. The adequate BP threshold in TBI patients is still uncertain. Current guidelines from the Brain Trauma Foundation identify different thresholds according to age: SBP should be kept ≥100 mmHg in patients 50–69 years old and ≥110 mmHg in patients 15–49 or over 70 years old (level III recommendation) [9]. Similarly, a cerebral perfusion pressure >60 mmHg should be targeted for patients with ICP monitoring. Recently, a secondary analysis on data derived from the ongoing EPIC study has been published [53]. The EPIC study is a before-after clinical trial designed to evaluate prehospital care for patients with major TBI. A secondary analysis has been conducted on the pre-interventional cohort (3844 patients) that showed a linear association between lowest prehospital systolic blood pressure and mortality (adjusted for severity of trauma) for SBP in the range 40–120 mmHg. Patients with baseline BP <40 mmHg or > 120 mmHg were not included in the analysis. These results suggest that BP threshold for improved outcome in TBI patients could be as high as 120 mmHg and that clinical meaningful hypotension may occur for currently accepted values. Furthermore, this result underlies the difficulties to define a threshold for a continuous parameter such as BP, also considering the interlay mechanisms which mediate CPP. Vasopressors (norepinephrine or phenylephrine) can be used to reach the BP target. In patients with intracranial pressure monitoring, monitoring of cerebral autoregulation and/or oxygenation can be used as accessory information to guide haemodynamic therapy, as described above in this chapter.

Learning Box (■ Fig. 35.3)

- In ICH patients, initial SBP should be reduced around 140–160 mmHg, unless worsening of neurological status or signs of elevated intracranial pressure.
- In SAH patients, initial SBP should be kept below 160 mmHg before the aneurysm has been secured. Thereafter, a more liberal approach is recommended. First-line therapy

of DCI consists in increasing MAP to reverse clinical deficit or improve brain oxygenation/perfusion.
- In patients suffering from an acute stroke, SBP >220 mmHg or DBP >120 mmHg should be maintained. In case of thrombolysis or endovascular thrombectomy, SBP < 185 mmHg and DBP < 110 mmHg are associated with fewer haemorrhagic events.
- In TBI patients, SBP should be kept at least ≥100 mmHg and ideally ≥110–120 mmHg or CPP > 60 mmHg when ICP is monitored.

Conclusions

Haemodynamic therapy in neurological emergencies can be challenging. Isotonic fluid replacement targeting euvolemia should be a priority. BP correction is of utmost importance in both early and late phase after acute brain injury, in order to limit disease progression and prevent secondary brain injury. In patients with intracranial haemorrhage (ICH) and aneurysmal subarachnoid haemorrhage (SAH), attention should be paid to prevent haemorrhagic progression; in patients with acute ischaemic stroke, perfusion of the ischaemic penumbra should be assured while taking into account the risk of haemorrhagic transformation; in patients with TBI, BP manipulation should focus on assuring adequate brain perfusion. Once the intracranial lesion is relatively stable, BP management should focus on finding the adequate balance between the risk of hypoperfusion (and subsequent ischaemia) and the risk of hyperaemia and subsequent blood-brain barrier and cellular damage. In this context, manipulation of BP is a routine practice in the ICU, with the main objective of optimizing cerebral perfusion. BP manipulation should be tailored on individual-specific needs. Cerebral autoregulation is one of the most important physiological mechanisms which protects the brain from hypo- or hyperperfusion. Cerebral autoregulation is frequently altered and is associated with outcome after acute brain injury. Monitoring of cerebral autoregulation can help identifying the range of MAP in which cerebral perfusion is optimal. Management of blood pressure and cerebral perfusion pressure in the neurointensive care unit has evolved towards a paradigm of individualized therapy.

Take Home Messages

- Specific indications on volume management in neurocritically ill patients are lacking. However, in neurocritically ill patient, the possibility of inadequate circulating volume should not be neglected, and intravascular volume adequacy should be carefully assessed in order to prevent secondary brain injury and multiorgan failure.
- Adequate haemodynamic monitoring should be considered when necessary to guide adequate intravascular volume assessment and management, specifically to avoid either hypovolemia or hypervolemia. "Supranormal" volume expansion in case of vasospasm in SAH complicated by DCI is no longer recommended.
- Intravascular volume management with isotonic crystalloids such as NaCl 0.9% or balanced solutions is recommended in neurological emergencies. Hypotonic fluids should be avoided, while use of hypertonic fluids should be

reserved for specific indications (i.e. intracranial hypertension). When prescribing fluid therapy, the clinicians should be aware of the in vivo tonicity of the fluid administered. Systematic use of colloids in neurological emergencies is not recommended.

- Blood pressure targets differ among different forms of brain injury and between the early and late phase of patients' management.
- Individualizing blood pressure targets may be achieved using advanced monitoring tools, such as brain oxygenation or the assessment of cerebral autoregulation. However, there are no data on the impact of such strategies on patients' outcome

References

1. Roozenbeek B, Maas AI, Menon DK. Changing patterns in the epidemiology of traumatic brain injury. Nat Rev Neurol. 2013;9(4):231–6.
2. Gruenbaum SE, Zlotnik A, Gruenbaum BF, Hersey D, Bilotta F. Pharmacologic neuroprotection for functional outcomes after traumatic brain injury: a systematic review of the clinical literature. CNS Drugs. 2016;30(9):791–806.
3. Bednarczyk JM, Fridfinnson JA, Kumar A, Blanchard L, Rabbani R, Bell D, Funk D, Turgeon AF, Abou-Setta AM, Zarychanski R. Incorporating dynamic assessment of fluid responsiveness into goal-directed therapy: a systematic review and meta-analysis. Crit Care Med. 2017;45(9):1538–45.
4. Robertson DS. The physical chemistry of brain and neural cell membranes: an overview. Neurochem Res. 2010;35(5):681–7.
5. Kimelberg HK. Water homeostasis in the brain: basic concepts. Neuroscience. 2004;129(4):851–60. Review.
6. Saw MM, Chamberlain J, Barr M, Morgan MP, Burnett JR, Ho KM. Differential disruption of blood-brain barrier in severe traumatic brain injury. Neurocrit Care. 2014;20(2):209–16.
7. Rodriguez GJ, Cordina SM, Vazquez G, Suri MF, Kirmani JF, Ezzeddine MA, Qureshi AI. The hydration influence on the risk of stroke (THIRST) study. Neurocrit Care. 2009;10(2):187–94.
8. Powers WJ, Rabinstein AA, Ackerson T, Adeoye OM, Bambakidis NC, Becker K, Biller J, Brown M, Demaerschalk BM, Hoh B, Jauch EC, Kidwell CS, Leslie-Mazwi TM, Ovbiagele B, Scott PA, Sheth KN, Southerland AM, Summers DV, Tirschwell DL, American Heart Association Stroke Council. 2018 guidelines for the early management of patients with acute ischemic stroke: a guideline for healthcare professionals from the American Heart Association/American Stroke Association. Stroke. 2018;49:e46–99.
9. Carney N, Totten AM, O'Reilly C, Ullman JS, Hawryluk GW, Bell MJ, Bratton SL, Chesnut R, Harris OA, Kissoon N, Rubiano AM, Shutter L, Tasker RC, Vavilala MS, Wilberger J, Wright DW, Ghajar J. Guidelines for the management of severe traumatic brain injury, fourth edition. Neurosurgery. 2017;80(1):6–15.
10. Callaway CW, Donnino MW, Fink EL, Geocadin RG, Golan E, Kern KB, Leary M, Meurer WJ, Peberdy MA, Thompson TM, Zimmerman JL. Part 8: post-cardiac arrest care: 2015 American Heart Association guidelines update for cardiopulmonary resuscitation and emergency cardiovascular care. Circulation. 2015;132(18 Suppl 2):S465–82.
11. Martin Ginis KA, van der Scheer JW, Latimer-Cheung AE, Barrow A, Bourne C, Carruthers P, Bernardi M, Ditor DS, Gaudet S, de Groot S, Hayes KC, Hicks AL, Leicht CA, Lexell J, Macaluso S, Manns PJ, McBride CB, Noonan VK, Pomerleau P, Rimmer JH, Shaw RB, Smith B, Smith KM, Steeves JD, Tussler D, West CR, Wolfe DL, Goosey-Tolfrey VL. Evidence-based scientific exercise guidelines for adults with spinal cord injury: an update and a new guideline. Spinal Cord. 2018;56:308–21.
12. Dabus G, Nogueira RG. Current options for the management of aneurysmal subarachnoid hemorrhage-induced cerebral vasospasm: a comprehensive review of the literature. Interv Neurol. 2013;2(1):30–51.
13. Sen J, Belli A, Albon H, Morgan L, Petzold A, Kitchen N. Triple-H therapy in the management of aneurysmal subarachnoid haemorrhage. Lancet Neurol. 2003;2(10):614–21.

14. Egge A, Waterloo K, Sjøholm H, Solberg T, Ingebrigtsen T, Romner B. Prophylactic hyperdynamic postoperative fluid therapy after aneurysmal subarachnoid hemorrhage: a clinical, prospective, randomized, controlled study. Neurosurgery. 2001;49(3):593–605.
15. Connolly ES Jr, Rabinstein AA, Carhuapoma JR, Derdeyn CP, Dion J, Higashida RT, Hoh BL, Kirkness CJ, Naidech AM, Ogilvy CS, Patel AB, Thompson BG, Vespa P, American Heart Association Stroke Council; Council on Cardiovascular Radiology and Intervention; Council on Cardiovascular Nursing; Council on Cardiovascular Surgery and Anesthesia; Council on Clinical Cardiology. Guidelines for the management of aneurysmal subarachnoid hemorrhage: a guideline for healthcare professionals from the American Heart Association/American Stroke Association. Stroke. 2012;43(6):1711–37.
16. Diringer MN, Bleck TP, Claude Hemphill J 3rd, Menon D, Shutter L, Vespa P, Bruder N, Connolly ES Jr, Citerio G, Gress D, Hänggi D, Hoh BL, Lanzino G, Le Roux P, Rabinstein A, Schmutzhard E, Stocchetti N, Suarez JI, Treggiari M, Tseng MY, Vergouwen MD, Wolf S, Zipfel G, Neurocritical Care Society. Critical care management of patients following aneurysmal subarachnoid hemorrhage: recommendations from the Neurocritical Care Society's Multidisciplinary Consensus Conference. Neurocrit Care. 2011;15(2):211–40.
17. Muench E, Horn P, Bauhuf C, Roth H, Philipps M, Hermann P, Quintel M, Schmiedek P, Vajkoczy P. Effects of hypervolemia and hypertension on regional cerebral blood flow, intracranial pressure, and brain tissue oxygenation after subarachnoid hemorrhage. Crit Care Med. 2007;35(8):1844–51.
18. Varrier M, Ostermann M. Fluid composition and clinical effects. Crit Care Clin. 2015;31(4):823–37.
19. Lehmann L, Bendel S, Uehlinger DE, Takala J, Schafer M, Reinert M, Jakob SM. Randomized, double-blind trial of the effect of fluid composition on electrolyte, acid-base, and fluid homeostasis in patients early after subarachnoid hemorrhage. Neurocrit Care. 2013;18(1):5–12.
20. Cooper DJ, Myburgh J, Heritier S, Finfer S, Bellomo R, Billot L, Murray L, Vallance S, SAFE-TBI Investigators; Australian and New Zealand Intensive Care Society Clinical Trials Group. Albumin resuscitation for traumatic brain injury: is intracranial hypertension the cause of increased mortality? J Neurotrauma. 2013;30(7):512–8.
21. Palesch YY, Hill MD, Ryckborst KJ, Tamariz D, Ginsberg MD. The ALIAS Pilot Trial: a dose-escalation and safety study of albumin therapy for acute ischemic stroke--II: neurologic outcome and efficacy analysis. Stroke. 2006;37(8):2107–14.
22. Kuwabara K, Fushimi K, Matsuda S, Ishikawa KB, Horiguchi H, Fujimori K. Association of early post-procedure hemodynamic management with the outcomes of subarachnoid hemorrhage patients. J Neurol. 2013;260(3):820–31.
23. Suarez JI, Shannon L, Zaidat OO, Suri MF, Singh G, Lynch G, Selman WR. Effect of human albumin administration on clinical outcome and hospital cost in patients with subarachnoid hemorrhage. J Neurosurg. 2004;100(4):585–90.
24. Maas AI, Murray GD, Roozenbeek B, Lingsma HF, Butcher I, McHugh GS, Weir J, Lu J, Steyerberg EW, International Mission on Prognosis Analysis of Clinical Trials in Traumatic Brain Injury (IMPACT) Study Group. Advancing care for traumatic brain injury: findings from the IMPACT studies and perspectives on future research. Lancet Neurol. 2013;12(12):1200–10.
25. Powers WJ. Cerebral hemodynamics in ischemic cerebrovascular disease. Ann Neurol. 1991;29(3):231–40.
26. Meng L, Hou W, Chui J, Han R, Gelb AW. Cardiac output and cerebral blood flow: the integrated regulation of brain perfusion in adult humans. Anesthesiology. 2015;123(5):1198–208.
27. Pallas F, Larson DF. Cerebral blood flow in the diabetic patient. Perfusion. 1996;11(5):363–70.
28. McBryde FD, Malpas SC, Paton JF. Intracranial mechanisms for preserving brain blood flow in health and disease. Acta Physiol (Oxf). 2017;219(1):274–87.
29. Liu X, Donnelly J, Czosnyka M, Aries MJH, Brady K, Cardim D, Robba C, Cabeleira M, Kim DJ, Haubrich C, Hutchinson PJ, Smielewski P. Cerebrovascular pressure reactivity monitoring using wavelet analysis in traumatic brain injury patients: A retrospective study. PLoS Med. 2017;14(7):e1002348.
30. Budohoski KP, Czosnyka M, Smielewski P, Varsos GV, Kasprowicz M, Brady KM, Pickard JD, Kirkpatrick PJ. Monitoring cerebral autoregulation after subarachnoid hemorrhage. Acta Neurochir Suppl. 2016;122:199–203.
31. Sekhon MS, Smielewski P, Bhate TD, Brasher PM, Foster D, Menon DK, Gupta AK, Czosnyka M, Henderson WR, Gin K, Wong G, Griesdale DE. Using the relationship between brain tissue regional saturation of oxygen and mean arterial pressure to determine the optimal mean arterial pressure in patients following cardiac arrest: a pilot proof-of-concept study. Resuscitation. 2016;106:120–5.
32. Czosnyka M, Miller C, Participants in the International Multidisciplinary Consensus Conference on Multimodality Monitoring. Monitoring of cerebral autoregulation. Neurocrit Care. 2014;21(Suppl 2):S95–102.

33. Howells T, Elf K, Jones PA, Ronne-Engström E, Piper I, Nilsson P, Andrews P, Enblad P. Pressure reactivity as a guide in the treatment of cerebral perfusion pressure in patients with brain trauma. J Neurosurg. 2005;102(2):311–7.
34. Steiner LA, Czosnyka M, Piechnik SK, Smielewski P, Chatfield D, Menon DK, Pickard JD. Continuous monitoring of cerebrovascular pressure reactivity allows determination of optimal cerebral perfusion pressure in patients with traumatic brain injury. Crit Care Med. 2002;30(4):733–8.
35. Jaeger M, Soehle M, Schuhmann MU, Meixensberger J. Clinical significance of impaired cerebrovascular autoregulation after severe aneurysmal subarachnoid hemorrhage. Stroke. 2012;43(8):2097–101.
36. Reinhard M, Rutsch S, Lambeck J, Wihler C, Czosnyka M, Weiller C, Hetzel A. Dynamic cerebral autoregulation associates with infarct size and outcome after ischemic stroke. Acta Neurol Scand. 2012;125(3):156–62.
37. Reinhard M, Neunhoeffer F, Gerds TA, Niesen WD, Buttler KJ, Timmer J, Schmidt B, Czosnyka M, Weiller C, Hetzel A. Secondary decline of cerebral autoregulation is associated with worse outcome after intracerebral hemorrhage. Intensive Care Med. 2010;36(2):264–71.
38. Rodriguez-Luna D, Rubiera M, Ribo M, Coscojuela P, Piñeiro S, Pagola J, Hernandez-Guillamon M, Ibarra B, Romero F, Alvarez-Sabin J, Montaner J, Molina CA. Ultraearly hematoma growth predicts poor outcome after acute intracerebral hemorrhage. Neurology. 2011;77(17):1599–604.
39. Gould B, McCourt R, Asdaghi N, Dowlatshahi D, Jeerakathil T, Kate M, Coutts SB, Hill MD, Demchuk AM, Shuaib A, Emery D, Butcher K, ICH ADAPT Investigators. Autoregulation of cerebral blood flow is preserved in primary intracerebral hemorrhage. Stroke. 2013;44(6):1726–8.
40. Kazui S, Naritomi H, Yamamoto H, Sawada T, Yamaguchi T. Enlargement of spontaneous intracerebral hemorrhage. Incidence and time course. Stroke. 1996;27(10):1783–7.
41. Fujii Y, Takeuchi S, Sasaki O, Minakawa T, Tanaka R. Multivariate analysis of predictors of hematoma enlargement in spontaneous intracerebral hemorrhage. Stroke. 1998;29(6):1160–6.
42. Qureshi AI. Acute hypertensive response in patients with stroke: pathophysiology and management. Circulation. 2008;118(2):176–87.
43. Qureshi AI, Wilson DA, Hanley DF, Traystman RJ. Pharmacologic reduction of mean arterial pressure does not adversely affect regional cerebral blood flow and intracranial pressure in experimental intracerebral hemorrhage. Crit Care Med. 1999;27(5):965–71.
44. Christensen MC, Morris S, Vallejo-Torres L, Vincent C, Mayer SA. Neurological impairment among survivors of intracerebral hemorrhage: the FAST trial. Neurocrit Care. 2012;16(2):224–31.
45. Anderson CS, Huang Y, Wang JG, Arima H, Neal B, Peng B, et al. Intensive blood pressure reduction in acute cerebral haemorrhage trial (INTERACT): a randomised pilot trial. Lancet Neurol. 2008;7: 391–9.
46. Anderson CS, Heeley E, Huang Y, Wang J, Stapf C, Delcourt C, et al. Rapid blood-pressure lowering in patients with acute intracerebral hemorrhage. N Engl J Med. 2013;368:2355–65.
47. Qureshi AI, Palesch YY, Barsan WG, Hanley DF, Hsu CY, Martin RL, et al. Intensive blood-pressure lowering in patients with acute cerebral hemorrhage. N Engl J Med. 2016;375:1033–43.
48. Hemphill JC 3rd, Greenberg SM, Anderson CS, Becker K, Bendok BR, Cushman M, et al. Guidelines for the management of spontaneous intracerebral hemorrhage: a guideline for healthcare professionals from the American Heart Association/American Stroke Association. Stroke. 2015;46:2032–60.
49. Leonardi-Bee J, Bath PM, Phillips SJ, Sandercock PA, IST Collaborative Group. Blood pressure and clinical outcomes in the International Stroke Trial. Stroke. 2002;33(5):1315–20.
50. Okumura K, Ohya Y, Maehara A, Wakugami K, Iseki K, Takishita S. Effects of blood pressure levels on case fatality after acute stroke. J Hypertens. 2005;23(6):1217–23.
51. Rose JC, Mayer SA. Optimizing blood pressure in neurological emergencies. Neurocrit Care. 2004;1(3):287–99.
52. Chesnut RM, Marshall LF, Klauber MR, Blunt BA, Baldwin N, Eisenberg HM, et al. The role of secondary brain injury in determining outcome from severe head injury. J Trauma. 1993;34:216–22.
53. Spaite DW, Hu C, Bobrow BJ, Chikani V, Sherrill D, Barnhart B, Gaither JB, Denninghoff KR, Viscusi C, Mullins T, Adelson PD. Mortality and prehospital blood pressure in patients with major traumatic brain injury: implications for the hypotension threshold. JAMA Surg. 2017;152(4):360–8.

Perioperative Haemodynamic Optimisation

Mark R. Edwards and Rupert M. Pearse

M. R. Pinsky et al. (eds.), *Hemodynamic Monitoring*, Lessons from the ICU,
https://doi.org/10.1007/978-3-319-69269-2_36

Learning Objectives

- To understand the importance of fluid and vasoactive drug therapies in achieving successful post-operative outcomes
- To be aware of the problematic nature of the evidence base in this area
- To be familiar with the primary approaches to fluid and vasoactive drug therapy for the surgical patient

36.1 Introduction

Estimates suggest that over 300 million patients undergo surgery worldwide each year with post-operative mortality reported between 1 and 4% [1, 2]. Complications and deaths are most frequent among high-risk patients, those who are older or have co-morbid disease and undergo major gastrointestinal or vascular surgery. Importantly, patients who develop complications, but survive to leave hospital, suffer reduced long-term survival. It is accepted that intravenous fluid and inotropic drugs have an important effect on patient outcomes, in particular following major surgery. Yet they are commonly prescribed to subjective criteria leading to wide variation in clinical practice. One possible solution is the use of cardiac output monitoring to guide intravenous fluid and inotropic drugs as part of a haemodynamic therapy algorithm.

Trauma, major surgery and severe sepsis are commonly associated with life-threatening hypovolaemia and reductions in myocardial contractility and vascular tone. The optimal therapeutic approach to the treatment of these disease processes undoubtedly includes intravenous fluid therapy and vasoactive drugs. However, the optimal approach to the use of these therapies remains controversial. Clearly, such treatments have benefits as well as risks. The concept of 'optimisation' of haemodynamics evolved following the early work by Clowes and then Shoemaker [3, 4]. These observational studies suggested that when routine parameters, such as blood pressure and urine output, were stabilised in all patients, survivors had consistently higher cardiac output, oxygen delivery (DO_2) and oxygen consumption (VO_2) than those who subsequently died. This observation led to the proposed use of fluid and inotropes to achieve predefined targets for these global haemodynamic variables. This approach has been given many names including 'goal-directed haemodynamic therapy' and 'flow-guided therapy', but for the purposes of this chapter, we will use the term 'haemodynamic optimisation'. A large number of clinical trials have been conducted over the last 40 years, but the inconsistent findings of these diverse trials have been hotly debated. This issue has also become confused with a separate debate about the safety of the pulmonary artery catheter, a matter which has now been resolved [5–7]. In this chapter, we describe the physiological basis for the optimisation of cardiac output-related variables, explore possible mechanisms of biological effect and discuss the current evidence base for this treatment approach.

36

36.2 Physiology

Global or systemic oxygen delivery (DO_2) is determined by cardiac output and the oxygen content of arterial blood (Equation). Adequate tissue oxygen delivery therefore depends upon the adequacy of both respiratory and cardiovascular function. Strategies to optimise

DO_2 have therefore involved a variety of treatment approaches including intravenous fluid, blood transfusion and inotropic therapy [8].

$$DO_2 = CO \times \left[(SaO_2 \times Hb \times 1.36) + (0.02 \times PaO_2) \right]$$

Equation: Determinants of tissue oxygen delivery

DO_2, oxygen delivery; CO, cardiac output; SaO_2, arterial oxygen saturation; Hb, haemoglobin concentration; PaO_2, arterial partial pressure of oxygen

36.3 Therapies Used to Achieve Haemodynamic Goals

A number of alternative haemodynamic goals have been utilised in clinical trials of optimisation strategies. These include oxygen delivery, cardiac output, stroke volume, venous saturation as well as markers of preload variability. All of these goals relate in some way to cardiac output, and in each case, the apparent simplicity of a single variable has the potential to mislead. In terms of intravenous fluid, it is generally agreed that sequential fluid challenges should be administered with the objective of achieving a sustained rise in stroke volume for at least 20 min. This is based on the application of Starling's Law of the heart (Fig. 36.1). In some cases the maximal value of stroke volume achieved may then be used as a goal throughout the intervention period. Although this approach has a very robust physiological basis, the identification of a stroke volume response to fluid is inevitably slightly subjective. Alternatively, studies have shown that pulse pressure, systolic pressure and stroke volume variation during the respiratory cycle may also predict fluid responsiveness. These variables have been termed dynamic markers of preload responsiveness and have the potential to simplify the potentially subjective use of stroke volume as a haemodynamic end point. However, changes in global haemodynamics are influenced by a range of factors that may represent significant confounders. In particular, the effect of spontaneous ventilation on the accuracy of dynamic markers of preload responsiveness is a significant limitation. At present, these variables are useful in identifying patients who clearly do not require fluid resuscitation but are less specific when it comes

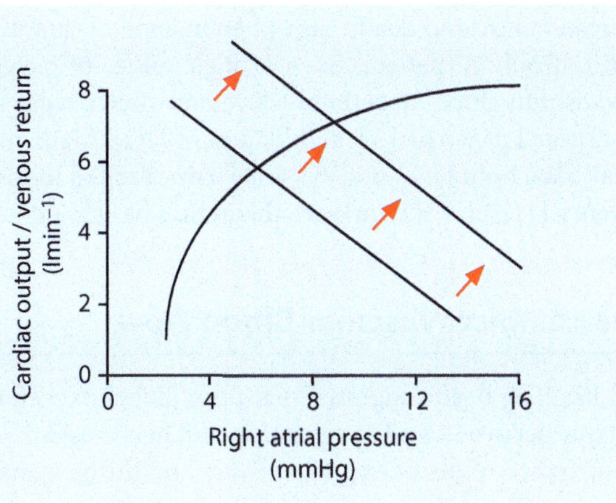

Fig. 36.1 Starling's curve. The increase in venous return due to intravenous fluid (red arrows) increases stroke volume in responsive patients. At maximal stroke volume (horizontal part of curve), the absence of a response indicates fluid is not required

to more marginal fluid treatment decisions [9]. Once fluid resuscitation is under way, there may also be an indication for vasopressor or inotropic therapy. A number of haemodynamic goals have been used to determine the dose of inotropic therapy. In this case, the challenge is to select an appropriate target value for the variable concerned. The use of high or 'supranormal' goals for oxygen delivery and cardiac output has raised concerns in the past. In particular, myocardial ischaemia may be significantly more frequent where vasoactive agents are used in high doses to achieve goals in patients who may fail to respond. Emerging evidence suggests the use of inotropic therapy in more judicious doses may lead to clinical benefit whilst avoiding many of the harmful effects of these agents. Mention should be made of the use of central ($ScvO_2$) and mixed venous oxygen saturation (SvO_2) in optimisation strategies. These variables refer to the haemoglobin saturation of blood in the superior vena cava and proximal pulmonary artery, respectively. Venous oxygen content is determined by arterial oxygen content, oxygen consumption and cardiac output. Venous oxygen saturation does not simply indicate DO_2 but the balance between DO_2 and VO_2 [10].

36.4 Biological Mechanisms of Benefit

An important limitation of the current evidence base for optimisation of oxygen delivery is a lack of a clear mechanistic explanation for any therapeutic benefit. One aspect of this problem may be the lack of suitable biomarkers which might be utilised as indicators of improved resuscitation.

36.4.1 Tissue Oxygen Delivery and Consumption

In his early work, Shoemaker proposed specific values for cardiac output, oxygen delivery and oxygen consumption as haemodynamic goals for all patients [4]. The term 'supranormal' has been used to describe these values, although they were in fact the median values achieved by surviving patients. Shoemaker's theory was based on the observation that an imbalance between global oxygen delivery and consumption was particularly common during critical illness and after major surgery. Originally, it was believed that inadequate oxygen delivery resulted in an oxygen debt which, if unchecked, would eventually lead to organ failure and death. This phenomenon of 'supply dependency' was thought to occur in critically ill patients even at high values of oxygen delivery (◘ Fig. 36.2). However, whilst this situation certainly develops when oxygen delivery is low, it has not been demonstrated at normal or high values of DO_2. Mathematical coupling of variables used to calculate both DO_2 and VO_2 may have resulted in the false observation of supply dependency [11], and Shoemaker's theoretical basis is no longer widely accepted.

36.4.2 Microvascular Blood Flow

It has long been suggested that poor global oxygen delivery is associated with reduced tissue perfusion and oxygenation and hence organ failure. This theory fits logically with current concepts of oxygen delivery and the oxygen cascade (◘ Fig. 36.3). The microcirculation is the principal site of oxygen exchange between blood and underlying tissues,

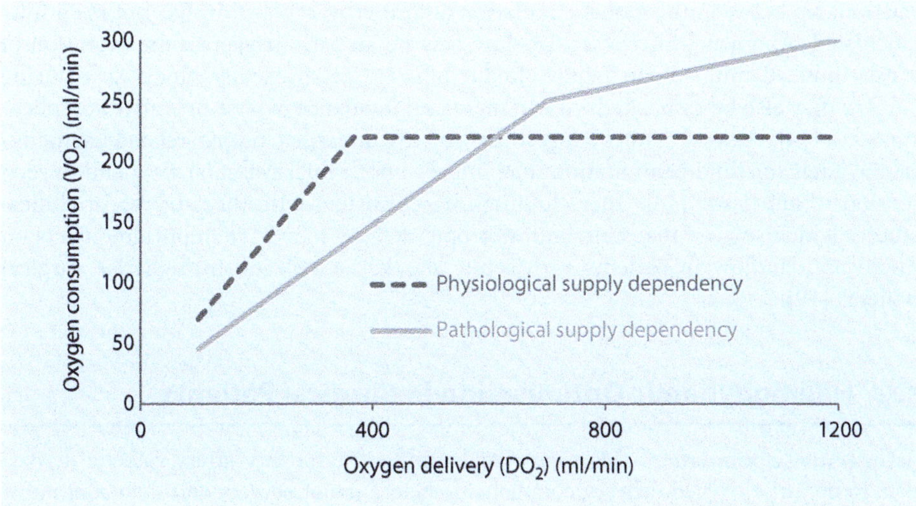

Fig. 36.2 Oxygen supply dependency. Proposed model of oxygen supply dependency. In healthy states (dotted line), oxygen consumption is maintained at a plateau value in the face of falling oxygen delivery – due to increased peripheral oxygen extraction – until this compensatory mechanism is exhausted. It was previously thought that in pathological states (solid line), these compensatory mechanisms fail, and therefore oxygen uptake is more dependent on oxygen delivery across a wide range of values (supply dependency)

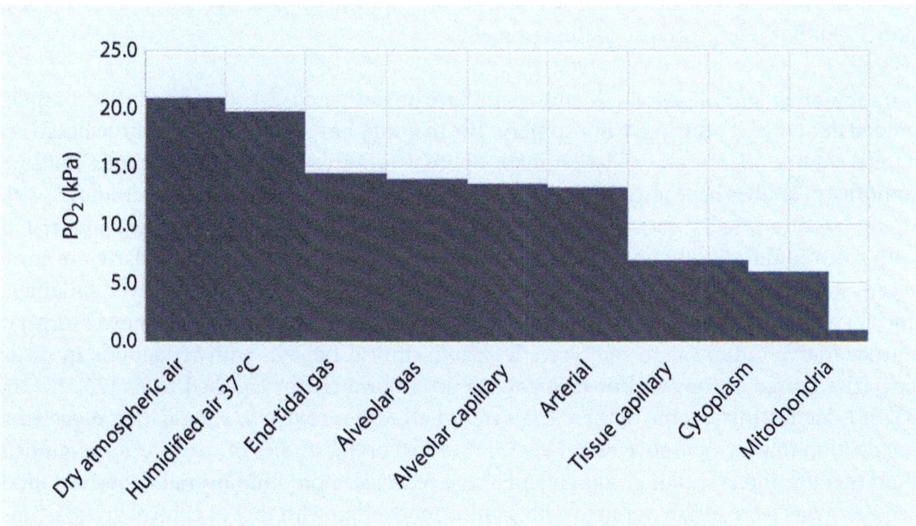

Fig. 36.3 Oxygen cascade. Gradual reduction in oxygen partial pressure from atmospheric air to the mitochondria, at which PO_2 is between 1 and 5 kPa. Note the large step down from arterial to capillary level, showing the critical role of the microcirculation in cellular oxygen delivery

and there is abundant data indicating profound disruption of the microcirculation in shock. These include a decrease in the proportion of perfused vessels smaller than 20 µm, mostly capillaries, whereas the perfusion of larger vessels is preserved. The exact relationship between the global circulation and microvascular flow has not been fully elucidated. Abnormal microvascular flow may be an early trigger in the evolution of sepsis-induced multi-organ failure. Reductions in microvascular blood flow during surgery may also be associated with an increased incidence of post-operative complications [12–14]. Animal studies suggest that the use of cardiac output-related haemodynamic goals for fluid resuscitation may improve both microvascular flow and oxygen tension in gut tissue [15]. These findings are consistent with those of recent clinical studies which suggest that fluid and inotropic therapy may have important effects on microvascular flow in patients with septic shock [16–18] and in high-risk surgical patients [19].

36.5 Haemodynamic Optimisation in Surgical Patients

Preoperative optimisation Most early trials utilised pulmonary artery catheter-derived data to optimise oxygen delivery commencing before major surgery and then continuing into the early post-operative period. The first of these was performed by Shoemaker's group [20]. The intervention was associated with a significant reduction in mortality, but the trial was criticised for several important methodological flaws including poorly defined control and intervention group care and a lack of clear randomisation procedures. Subsequent investigators repeated this work in more robustly designed trials. In these high-mortality groups, haemodynamic optimisation was again associated with mortality reductions, although some trials failed to show any benefit, particularly in the case of vascular surgery [6, 21–25]. The logistical challenges of delivering haemodynamic optimisation before surgery starts have prevented the widespread use of this approach.

Intraoperative optimisation Many trials have investigated the use of cardiac output-guided fluid therapy during major surgery. The majority have utilised an algorithm based on stroke volume measurement to estimate optimal requirements for intravenous fluid. A minority of studies have also employed inotropic agents to increase cardiac output [26–29]. In hip fracture surgery, early studies suggested that this treatment approach was associated with reduced duration of hospital stay but no change in clinical outcomes [30, 31]. A more recent study in patients having spinal anaesthesia for hip fracture repair showed no difference in either hospital stay or clinical outcomes [32]. In patients undergoing bowel surgery, intraoperative optimisation may have a clearer clinical benefit, with reductions in post-operative complications and/or hospital stay in a number of published trials [26, 27, 30, 33–35]. Interestingly, some of these trials report an earlier return to enteral diet, suggesting a reduction in post-operative ileus [33–35]. In most of the studies of stroke volume-guided fluid therapy, intervention group patients have received more fluid overall. However, fluid requirements were highly variable with significant overlap with that of control groups. This approach may provide a more accurate estimate of fluid requirements, avoiding both inadequate and excessive intravenous fluid administration. However, as baseline care has evolved, with more laparoscopic surgery, lower morbidity rates and an emphasis on protocolised fluid management as part of enhanced recovery pathways, more recent intraoperative optimisation trials have not always shown benefit [28, 36–38]. Evidence syntheses have underlined the preponderance of heterogeneous small, single-centre trials in this field [39, 40]. The potential clinical benefit of intraoperative haemodynamic optimisation therefore needs exploring in larger clinical effectiveness trials. Such trials have been recently completed or are in progress and have moved towards haemodynamic optimisation algorithms encompassing the intra- and early post-operative periods.

Post-operative A major obstacle to the implementation of perioperative haemodynamic therapy is the logistical difficulty of arranging ICU admission prior to surgery. The findings of three trials have suggested that optimisation strategies may also be effective when commenced in the immediate post-operative period [41–43]. Two of these trials were undertaken in patients following cardiac surgery [41, 42] and the other following abdominal surgery [43]. The findings of these trials are of particular importance to high-risk surgical patients for whom post-operative resuscitation is an important but often neglected area of care. The optimal approach to perioperative intravenous fluid administration has been further confused by the contradictory findings of trials comparing 'liberal' and 'restrictive' fluid regimes prescribed according to body mass [44–46]. However, whilst maintenance fluid can and should be prescribed according to body mass, this is not a rational method of estimating fluid requirements for optimal resuscitation. The findings of these trials can only guide the more straightforward aspects of perioperative haemodynamic management.

Most recently the multicentre OPTIMISE trial has been completed, the largest such trial ever performed [40]. The intervention algorithm consisted of stroke volume-guided fluid therapy and low-dose inotrope (dopexamine) during and for 6 h after surgery. The primary outcome (moderate or major post-operative complications at 30 days) was met by 37% (134 of 366) of patients in the intervention group and by 43% (158 of 364) of patients in the usual care group (relative risk 0.84 [0.71–1.01]; $p = 0.07$). Infective post-operative complications including wound, organ space, lung, urinary or bloodstream infection occurred in 24% of intervention patients compared with 30% of control patients (RR 0.80 [0.63–1.02]; $p = 0.08$). Health economic analysis suggests the intervention was likely to be cost-effective [32, 47]. The findings of this trial neither confirm nor disprove the possible benefit of this treatment approach, possibly because the trial was underpowered.

The previous Cochrane systematic review has now been updated with the findings of OPTIMISE and other published trials (Fig. 36.4) [40]. Complications were less frequent among patients treated according to a haemodynamic therapy algorithm (Intervention 488/1548 [31.5%] vs Controls 614/1476 [41.6%]; RR 0.77 [0.71–0.83]). The intervention was associated with a reduced incidence of post-operative infection (Intervention 182/836 patients [21.8%] vs Controls 201/790 patients [25.4%]; RR 0.81 [0.69–0.95]) and a reduced duration of hospital stay (mean reduction 0.79 days [0.62–0.96]). There was a nonsignificant reduction in mortality at longest follow-up (Intervention 267/3215 deaths [8.3%] vs Controls 327/3160 deaths [10.3%]; RR 0.86 [0.74–1.00]). However, there remains a risk of bias due to the large number of small trials in the systematic review. More than half the included studies were published more than 10 years ago and may not be representative of current practice. Furthermore, the important patient group undergoing emergency abdominal surgery has not been represented within the current evidence base.

These data highlight the uncertainty surrounding the possible benefits of perioperative haemodynamic therapy algorithms and the need for definitive large multicentre clinical trials in both elective and emergency surgery to resolve this.

Source	Intervention No. of events	Intervention Total no.	Control No. of events	Control Total no.	Risk ratio (95% CI)	Weight %
Shoemaker et al,[20] 1988	8	28	30	60	0.57 (0.30–1.08)	1.7
Berlauk et al,[21] 1991	11	68	9	21	0.38 (0.18–0.79)	1.3
Mythen et al,[22] 1995	0	30	6	30	0.08 (0.00–1.31)	0.1
Sinclair et al,[23] 1997	1	20	1	20	1.00 (0.07–14.90)	0.1
Ueno et al,[24] 1998	4	16	5	18	0.90 (0.29–2.78)	0.5
Wilson et al,[25] 1999	38	92	28	46	0.68 (0.48–0.95)	6.2
Lobo et al,[26] 2000	6	19	12	18	0.47 (0.23–0.99)	1.3
Jerez et al,[27] 2001	53	181	65	209	0.94 (0.70–1.28)	7.6
Conway et al,[28] 2002	5	29	9	28	0.54 (0.20–1.40)	0.8
Pearse et al,[14] 2005	27	62	41	60	0.64 (0.46–0.89)	6.3
Wakeling et al,[29] 2005	24	67	38	67	0.63 (0.43–0.93)	4.8
Noblett et al,[30] 2006	1	51	8	52	0.13 (0.02–0.98)	0.2
Donati et al,[31] 2007	8	68	20	67	0.39 (0.19–0.83)	1.3
Smetkin et al,[32] 2009[a]	1	20	4	20	0.25 (0.03–2.05)	0.2
Jhanji et al,[6] 2010	57	90	30	45	0.95 (0.73–1.23)	10.4
Mayer et al,[33] 2010	6	30	15	30	0.40 (0.18–0.89)	1.1
Cecconi et al,[34] 2011	16	20	20	20	0.80 (0.64–1.02)	12.8
Challand et al,[35] 2012	10	89	13	90	0.78 (0.36–1.68)	1.2
Brandstrup et al,[36] 2012[a]	23	71	24	79	1.07 (0.66–1.71)	3.1
Salzwedel et al,[37] 2013[a]	21	79	36	81	0.60 (0.39–0.93)	3.6
Goepfert et al,[38] 2013[a]	34	50	42	50	0.81 (0.65–1.01)	13.7
OPTIMISE, 2014	134	368	158	365	0.84 (0.70–1.01)	21.8
Total	488	1548	614	1476	0.77 (0.71–0.83)	100.0

Heterogeneity: $\chi^2_{21}=30.44$; $P=.08$; $I^2=31\%$

Test for overall effect: $z = 6.22$; $P<.001$

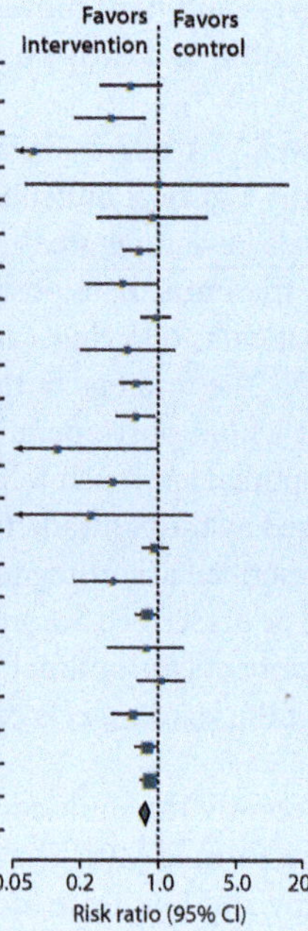

Fig. 36.4 Meta-analysis of number of patients developing complications after surgery. Systematic review of published randomised trials of 'perioperative increase in global blood flow to explicit defined goals and outcomes following surgery'. (From Ref. [40], with permission)

Take-Home Messages

Optimisation of global oxygen delivery is just one approach to haemodynamic resuscitation. Like all resuscitation treatments, benefit is difficult to demonstrate in patients who do not require haemodynamic resuscitation or those in whom the chance of survival is unlikely to change. The inconsistent findings of the many clinical trials of this treatment can be explained by differences in treatments, haemodynamic goals, timing and patient population. However, the current evidence base neither confirms nor refutes the proposed clinical benefits of this treatment. Early theories regarding the mechanisms through which haemodynamic optimisation may lead to improved clinical outcomes now appear unlikely, whilst emerging evidence strongly suggests improved microvascular flow may play a central role. Several multicentre studies of haemodynamic optimisation strategies are now planned. It seems likely that, after 25 years of debate, the definitive evidence for or against the use of haemodynamic optimisation will soon be available.

References

1. Weiser TG, Haynes AB, Molina G, Lipsitz SR, Esquivel MM, Uribe-Leitz T, et al. Estimate of the global volume of surgery in 2012: an assessment supporting improved health outcomes. Lancet Lond Engl. 2015;385(Suppl 2):S11.
2. The International Surgical Outcomes study group. Global patient outcomes after elective surgery: prospective cohort study in 27 low-, middle- and high-income countries. BJA: Br J Anaesth. 2016;117(5):601–9.
3. Clowes GH Jr, Vucinic M, Weidner MG. Circulatory and metabolic alterations associated with survival or death in peritonitis: clinical analysis of 25 cases. Ann Surg. 1966;163(6):866–85.
4. Shoemaker WC, Montgomery ES, Kaplan E, Elwyn DH. Physiologic patterns in surviving and nonsurviving shock patients. Use of sequential cardiorespiratory variables in defining criteria for therapeutic goals and early warning of death. Arch Surg. 1973;106(5):630–6.
5. Harvey S, Harrison DA, Singer M, Ashcroft J, Jones CM, Elbourne D, et al. Assessment of the clinical effectiveness of pulmonary artery catheters in management of patients in intensive care (PAC-Man): a randomised controlled trial. Lancet. 2005;366(9484):472–7.
6. Sandham JD, Hull RD, Brant RF, Knox L, Pineo GF, Doig CJ, et al. A randomized, controlled trial of the use of pulmonary-artery catheters in high-risk surgical patients. N Engl J Med. 2003;348(1):5–14.
7. Richard C, Warszawski J, Anguel N, Deye N, Combes A, Barnoud D, et al. Early use of the pulmonary artery catheter and outcomes in patients with shock and acute respiratory distress syndrome: a randomized controlled trial. JAMA. 2003;290(20):2713–20.
8. Pinsky MR. Hemodynamic evaluation and monitoring in the ICU. Chest. 2007;132(6):2020–9.
9. MacDonald N, Ahmad T, Mohr O, Kirk-Bayley J, Moppett I, Hinds CJ, et al. Dynamic preload markers to predict fluid responsiveness during and after major gastrointestinal surgery: an observational substudy of the OPTIMISE trial. BJA: Br J Anaesth. 2015;114(4):598–604.
10. Shepherd SJ, Pearse RM. Role of central and mixed venous oxygen saturation measurement in perioperative care. Anesthesiology. 2009;111(3):649–56.
11. Hanique G, Dugernier T, Laterre PF, Dougnac A, Roeseler J, Reynaert MS. Significance of pathologic oxygen supply dependency in critically ill patients: comparison between measured and calculated methods. Intensive Care Med. 1994;20(1):12–8.
12. Jhanji S, Lee C, Watson D, Hinds C, Pearse RM. Microvascular flow and tissue oxygenation after major abdominal surgery: association with post-operative complications. Intensive Care Med. 2008;35(4):671–7.
13. Miyazaki T, Kuwano H, Kato H, Yoshikawa M, Ojima H, Tsukada K. Predictive value of blood flow in the gastric tube in anastomotic insufficiency after thoracic esophagectomy. World J Surg. 2002;26(11):1319–23.
14. Vignali A, Gianotti L, Braga M, Radaelli G, Malvezzi L, Di Carlo V. Altered microperfusion at the rectal stump is predictive for rectal anastomotic leak. Dis Colon Rectum. 2000;43(1):76–82.
15. Kimberger O, Arnberger M, Brandt S, Plock J, Sigurdsson GH, Kurz A, et al. Goal-directed colloid administration improves the microcirculation of healthy and perianastomotic colon. Anesthesiology. 2009;110(3):496–504.
16. Trzeciak S, McCoy JV, Phillip Dellinger R, Arnold RC, Rizzuto M, Abate NL, et al. Early increases in microcirculatory perfusion during protocol-directed resuscitation are associated with reduced multi-organ failure at 24 h in patients with sepsis. Intensive Care Med. 2008;34(12):2210–7.
17. De Backer D, Creteur J, Dubois M-J, Sakr Y, Koch M, Verdant C, et al. The effects of dobutamine on microcirculatory alterations in patients with septic shock are independent of its systemic effects. Crit Care Med. 2006;34(2):403–8.
18. Jhanji S, Stirling S, Patel N, Hinds CJ, Pearse RM. The effect of increasing doses of norepinephrine on tissue oxygenation and microvascular flow in patients with septic shock. Crit Care Med. 2009;37(6):1961–6.
19. Jhanji S, Vivian-Smith A, Lucena-Amaro S, Watson D, Hinds CJ, Pearse RM. Haemodynamic optimisation improves tissue microvascular flow and oxygenation after major surgery: a randomised controlled trial. Crit Care. 2010;14(4):R151.
20. Shoemaker WC, Appel PL, Kram HB, Waxman K, Lee TS. Prospective trial of supranormal values of survivors as therapeutic goals in high-risk surgical patients. Chest. 1988;94(6):1176–86.

21. Bender JS, Smith-Meek MA, Jones CE. Routine pulmonary artery catheterization does not reduce morbidity and mortality of elective vascular surgery: results of a prospective, randomized trial. Ann Surg. 1997;226(3):229–36; discussion 236–237.
22. Berlauk JF, Abrams JH, Gilmour IJ, O'Connor SR, Knighton DR, Cerra FB. Preoperative optimization of cardiovascular hemodynamics improves outcome in peripheral vascular surgery. A prospective, randomized clinical trial. Ann Surg. 1991;214(3):289–97; discussion 298–299.
23. Bonazzi M, Gentile F, Biasi GM, Migliavacca S, Esposti D, Cipolla M, et al. Impact of perioperative haemodynamic monitoring on cardiac morbidity after major vascular surgery in low risk patients. A randomised pilot trial. Eur J Vasc Endovasc Surg. 2002;23(5):445–51.
24. Boyd O, Grounds RM, Bennett ED. A randomized clinical trial of the effect of deliberate perioperative increase of oxygen delivery on mortality in high-risk surgical patients. JAMA. 1993;270(22):2699–707.
25. Valentine RJ, Duke ML, Inman MH, Grayburn PA, Hagino RT, Kakish HB, et al. Effectiveness of pulmonary artery catheters in aortic surgery: a randomized trial. J Vasc Surg. 1998;27(2):203–11; discussion 211–212.
26. Donati A, Loggi S, Preiser J-C, Orsetti G, Münch C, Gabbanelli V, et al. Goal-directed intraoperative therapy reduces morbidity and length of hospital stay in high-risk surgical patients. Chest. 2007;132(6):1817–24.
27. Lobo SM, Salgado PF, Castillo VG, Borim AA, Polachini CA, Palchetti JC, et al. Effects of maximizing oxygen delivery on morbidity and mortality in high-risk surgical patients. Crit Care Med. 2000;28(10):3396–404.
28. Cecconi M, Fasano N, Langiano N, Divella M, Costa MG, Rhodes A, et al. Goal-directed haemodynamic therapy during elective total hip arthroplasty under regional anaesthesia. Crit Care. 2011;15(3):R132.
29. Van der Linden PJ, Dierick A, Wilmin S, Bellens B, De Hert SG. A randomized controlled trial comparing an intraoperative goal-directed strategy with routine clinical practice in patients undergoing peripheral arterial surgery. Eur J Anaesthesiol. 2010;27(9):788–93.
30. Sinclair S, James S, Singer M. Intraoperative intravascular volume optimisation and length of hospital stay after repair of proximal femoral fracture: randomised controlled trial. BMJ. 1997;315(7113): 909–12.
31. Venn R, Steele A, Richardson P, Poloniecki J, Grounds M, Newman P. Randomized controlled trial to investigate influence of the fluid challenge on duration of hospital stay and perioperative morbidity in patients with hip fractures. Br J Anaesth. 2002;88(1):65–71.
32. Moppett IK, Rowlands M, Mannings A, Moran CG, Wiles MD, NOTTS Investigators. LiDCO-based fluid management in patients undergoing hip fracture surgery under spinal anaesthesia: a randomized trial and systematic review. Br J Anaesth. 2015;114(3):444–59.
33. Gan TJ, Soppitt A, Maroof M, el-Moalem H, Robertson KM, Moretti E, et al. Goal-directed intraoperative fluid administration reduces length of hospital stay after major surgery. Anesthesiology. 2002;97(4):820–6.
34. Noblett SE, Snowden CP, Shenton BK, Horgan AF. Randomized clinical trial assessing the effect of Doppler-optimized fluid management on outcome after elective colorectal resection. Br J Surg. 2006;93(9):1069–76.
35. Wakeling HG, McFall MR, Jenkins CS, Woods WGA, Miles WFA, Barclay GR, et al. Intraoperative oesophageal Doppler guided fluid management shortens postoperative hospital stay after major bowel surgery. Br J Anaesth. 2005;95(5):634–42.
36. Challand C, Struthers R, Sneyd JR, Erasmus PD, Mellor N, Hosie KB, et al. Randomized controlled trial of intraoperative goal-directed fluid therapy in aerobically fit and unfit patients having major colorectal surgery. Br J Anaesth. 2012;108(1):53–62.
37. Lai CW, Starkie T, Creanor S, Struthers RA, Portch D, Erasmus PD, et al. Randomized controlled trial of stroke volume optimization during elective major abdominal surgery in patients stratified by aerobic fitness. Br J Anaesth. 2015;115(4):578–89.
38. Brandstrup B, Svendsen PE, Rasmussen M, Belhage B, Rodt SÅ, Hansen B, et al. Which goal for fluid therapy during colorectal surgery is followed by the best outcome: near-maximal stroke volume or zero fluid balance? Br J Anaesth. 2012;109(2):191–9.
39. Grocott MPW, Dushianthan A, Hamilton MA, Mythen MG, Harrison D, Rowan K. Perioperative increase in global blood flow to explicit defined goals and outcomes following surgery. Cochrane Database Syst Rev Online. 2012;11:CD004082.

40. Pearse RM, Harrison DA, MacDonald N, Gillies MA, Blunt M, Ackland G, et al. Effect of a perioperative, cardiac output-guided hemodynamic therapy algorithm on outcomes following major gastrointestinal surgery: a randomized clinical trial and systematic review. JAMA: J Am Med Assoc. 2014;311(21):2181–90.
41. Polonen P, Ruokonen E, Hippelainen M, Poyhonen M, Takala J. A prospective, randomized study of goal-oriented hemodynamic therapy in cardiac surgical patients. Anesth Analg. 2000;90(5):1052–9.
42. McKendry M, McGloin H, Saberi D, Caudwell L, Brady AR, Singer M. Randomised controlled trial assessing the impact of a nurse delivered, flow monitored protocol for optimisation of circulatory status after cardiac surgery. BMJ. 2004;329(7460):258.
43. Pearse R, Dawson D, Fawcett J, Rhodes A, Grounds RM, Bennett ED. Early goal-directed therapy after major surgery reduces complications and duration of hospital stay. A randomised, controlled trial [ISRCTN38797445]. Crit Care. 2005;9(6):R687–93.
44. Holte K, Klarskov B, Christensen DS, Lund C, Nielsen KG, Bie P, et al. Liberal versus restrictive fluid administration to improve recovery after laparoscopic cholecystectomy. Ann Surg. 2004;240(5): 892–9.
45. Brandstrup B, Tønnesen H, Beier-Holgersen R, Hjortsø E, Ørding H, Lindorff-Larsen K, et al. Effects of intravenous fluid restriction on postoperative complications: comparison of two perioperative fluid regimens. Ann Surg. 2003;238(5):641–8.
46. Nisanevich V, Felsenstein I, Almogy G, Weissman C, Einav S, Matot I. Effect of intraoperative fluid management on outcome after intraabdominal surgery. Anesthesiology. 2005;103(1):25–32.
47. Sadique Z, Harrison DA, Grieve R, Rowan KM, Pearse RM, OPTIMISE study group. Cost-effectiveness of a cardiac output-guided haemodynamic therapy algorithm in high-risk patients undergoing major gastrointestinal surgery. Perioper Med Lond Engl. 2015;4:13.

In a Patient Under ECMO

Darryl Abrams and Matthieu Schmidt

M. R. Pinsky et al. (eds.), *Hemodynamic Monitoring*, Lessons from the ICU,
https://doi.org/10.1007/978-3-319-69269-2_37

Learning Objectives

- To understand the mechanisms of different ECMO settings and their implication on hemodynamics
- To select appropriate tools to hemodynamically monitor a patient on ECMO
- To learn how to proceed a weaning trial on venoarterial ECMO

37.1 Introduction

Both the assessment of hemodynamic status and the choice of hemodynamic therapy in patients with severe cardiopulmonary failure supported with extracorporeal membrane oxygenation (ECMO) are affected by many factors. Patients with severe respiratory failure, in whom venovenous ECMO is used to support gas exchange, may, generally speaking, be monitored and managed hemodynamically in a way comparable to patients with respiratory failure without extracorporeal support. For patients in whom venoarterial ECMO is employed for management of cardiogenic shock, many of the more conventional methods of hemodynamic monitoring are either affected or unnecessary in the presence of ECMO. Regardless, ECMO, when used for either respiratory or cardiac support, will have an impact on the reliability or applicability of certain hemodynamic monitoring techniques, which in turn will have implications for how patients are managed.

37.2 General Considerations

ECMO consists of an extracorporeal circuit in which deoxygenated blood is drained from a cannula situated in a central vein by way of a centrifugal pump. The blood then passes through a gas exchange device, commonly referred to as a membrane oxygenator, in which gas exchange occurs across a semipermeable membrane that separates blood from fresh gas, referred to as sweep gas. Oxygen diffuses down a gradient from the gas compartment, across the membrane, into the blood compartment, and carbon dioxide diffuses in the opposite direction from the blood compartment into the gas compartment [1, 2]. The well-oxygenated, decarboxylated blood is then reinfused into the patient. The presence of the membrane oxygenator means that gas exchange is always supplied by the ECMO circuit, provided there is sweep gas flowing through the membrane. However, the location of the reinfusion cannula dictates how much, if any, hemodynamic support will be provided by the circuit.

In venovenous ECMO, blood is drained from a central vein and reinfused back into a central vein. Because blood is drained from and reinfused into the venous system, venovenous ECMO does not directly provide any hemodynamic support, but rather provides gas exchange support alone. In contrast, venoarterial ECMO reinfuses blood directly into an artery, thereby providing circulatory support by pumping blood directly into the systemic circulation [3]. Because this distinction has significant ramifications on the appropriate type of hemodynamic monitoring and therapy employed for patients receiving extracorporeal support, going forward we will consider the effects of venovenous and venoarterial ECMO separately.

37.3 Venovenous ECMO

Because venovenous ECMO has no direct impact on the systemic circulation, much of the modalities used to assess hemodynamic status in conventionally managed patients can also be used in patients receiving venovenous ECMO support for severe respiratory failure. Many of these modalities (e.g., systemic blood pressure, heart rate, lactate, markers of end-organ perfusion, echocardiographic data, etc.) have been reviewed in earlier chapters within this text. Likewise, certain principles employed in conventional management of severe acute respiratory failure appear to hold true in the management of venovenous ECMO-support patients, such as a restrictive fluid management strategy [4, 5]. In a study of 172 patients treated with ECMO, 57 of whom had refractory respiratory failure, positive fluid balance on day 3 of ECMO was an independent predictor of mortality.

In the presence of an extracorporeal circuit, certain hemodynamic principles and monitoring modalities may be difficult to employ, inadequate, or otherwise invalidated. Pulmonary artery catheters, used as an invasive method to assess cardiac output, right-sided pressures, and etiology of shock [6], are frequently inserted in the neck, traversing an internal jugular vein, or in the groin through a femoral vein, with the catheter tip positioned in the pulmonary artery. However, the reinfusion cannula of venovenous ECMO is likewise most commonly positioned in the superior vena cava, while the drainage cannula is optimally positioned in the intrahepatic inferior vena cava [7]. In fact, placement of the drainage cannula in the inferior vena cava and reinfusion into the superior vena cava is the preferred configuration to maximize systemic oxygenation when a dual-site venovenous approach is utilized [8]. The presence of an ECMO reinfusion cannula, often on the order of 20 French or larger in the internal jugular vein and superior vena cava, and often 23 French or larger when used for drainage in the femoral vein, may limit the space for the passage of a pulmonary artery catheter. The use of a bicaval, dual-lumen cannula, which is of a larger caliber than either traditional drainage or reinfusion cannulae in order to accommodate both drainage and reinfusion, will make concomitant placement of a pulmonary artery catheter even more problematic. Bifemoral venous cannulation for venovenous ECMO, although potentially suboptimal from an extracorporeal oxygen delivery standpoint, may afford the easier placement of a pulmonary artery catheter, depending on the ultimate position of the ECMO cannulae within the superior vena cava and right atrium [9].

Thermodilution techniques, be it through a pulmonary artery catheter or by way of a device that allows for transpulmonary thermodilution, have been employed to estimate cardiac output [10, 11]. Conceptually, cardiac output is determined by changes in blood temperature over time after infusion of a cooled injectate. Because the extracorporeal circuit, by way of ambient air, may result in cooling of blood below a patient's core temperature, any effort to use changes in blood temperature as a means of estimating cardiac output will be affected by the presence of reinfused extracorporeal blood into the venous system, particularly if part of the thermal signal is lost in the ECMO blood flow when part of the thermal filament is situated in the right atrium [12].

There are additional limitations to pulmonary artery catheter, and central venous catheter, interpretations in the presence of venovenous ECMO. Because ECMO in a venovenous configuration reinfuses well-oxygenated blood into the vicinity of the superior vena caval-right atrial junction, traditional assessments of central venous oxygen saturation

($ScvO_2$) or mixed venous oxygen saturation ($SmvO_2$) as a gauge of oxygen delivery and consumption are no longer applicable during venovenous ECMO support because of the artificially elevated oxygen saturation levels [7]. The saturation of venous blood entering the drainage cannula (SvO_2), which can be measured immediately before passage into the membrane oxygenator, is instead reflective of the amount of recirculation of oxygenated blood reentering the ECMO circuit [7]. The amount of recirculation mainly depends on the ECMO settings used (e.g., greater recirculation with a femoro-femoral configuration) and the amount of ECMO blood flow (i.e., the higher the ECMO blood flow, the greater the recirculation). For a patient actively receiving venovenous ECMO support, there are several ways to determine the amount of recirculation [13]. However, the only direct way of measuring $ScvO_2$ is by temporarily discontinuing the sweep gas flow (and thus the oxygen supply to the circuit) while using the ventilator to achieve an arterial oxygen saturation equivalent to what was achieved with ECMO support [14]. The SvO_2 can then be measured from blood just before it enters the membrane oxygenator and may be a more accurate representation of venous oxygen saturation.

Despite the general principle that venovenous ECMO does not directly impact or support hemodynamics, there are certain circumstances in which venovenous ECMO may have an indirect impact on hemodynamics and systemic circulation. The acute respiratory distress syndrome (ARDS), for which venovenous ECMO is most commonly employed [15], can lead to increases in pulmonary vascular resistance in the setting of hypoxemia, hypercapnia, and increased airway pressures [16–18]. These physiological derangements may, in turn, lead to right ventricular dysfunction as a consequence of increased right ventricular afterload. Correction of hypoxemia and hypercapnia, along with reductions in mean airway pressure, through the use of venovenous ECMO, can reverse this effect on the pulmonary vasculature and right ventricle, as has been demonstrated in a cohort of patients with ARDS receiving venovenous ECMO [12]. The initiation of venovenous ECMO resulted in a rapid reduction in mean pulmonary artery pressure and increase in cardiac index, which most directly correlated with changes in $PaCO_2$ and SvO_2. The association between hypercapnia and elevated pulmonary artery pressures has previously been demonstrated by Schmidt et al. in decremental sweep gas flow studies [2], lending further evidence to support that venovenous ECMO has the potential to reduce right ventricular afterload in the acute setting. These findings, in turn, have implications for the choice of ECMO configuration when patients have severe hypoxemic or hypercapnic respiratory failure complicated by cardiogenic shock due to right ventricular failure. In the absence of evidence of chronic pulmonary hypertension and right ventricular dysfunction, venovenous ECMO may be sufficient at supporting such patients without the need for the hemodynamic support of venoarterial ECMO [12].

A second, rather unique, circumstance in which venovenous ECMO may have an indirect impact on systemic circulation is in patients with decompensated pulmonary arterial hypertension with a concomitant interatrial defect, in whom there is simultaneous right heart failure and hypoxemia. A bicaval dual-lumen cannula may be placed in an internal jugular vein, with the reinfusion jet directed across the interatrial defect, in order to allow for decompression of the right heart while simultaneously providing an oxygenated right-to-left shunt [19–21]. In patients with pulmonary hypertension without a preexisting interatrial defect, a septostomy, combined with a bicaval dual-lumen approach, may be considered [22, 23].

Aside from the exceptions of providing hemodynamic support in venovenous ECMO mentioned above, initial hemodynamic management of patients in shock who are receiving venovenous ECMO should entail the use of vasopressor agents and inotropic support, as appropriate, just as one would do in patients in shock who are managed without extracorporeal support, and as has been discussed in other chapters within this text. In patients receiving venovenous ECMO in whom concomitant severe, refractory cardiogenic shock develops, consideration should be made for the addition of an arterial limb to the circuit through a Y-connector in the venous reinfusion limb. The resulting circuit, so-called venovenous arterial ECMO (or venoarterial venous ECMO when a venous reinfusion limb is added to an existing venoarterial circuit), is a hybrid configuration that provides upper-body gas exchange through venous reinfusion coupled to native cardiac output and circulatory support through arterial reinfusion [24]. This setting is frequently used in the context of ARDS with sepsis-induced cardiomyopathy, when cardiac recovery, which generally occurs quicker than lung recovery, results in the so-called Harlequin syndrome (i.e., inadequate oxygenation of the upper body contrasting with adequate oxygen delivery to the lower body by the arterial cannula) [25]. In less severe forms of cardiogenic shock during venovenous ECMO, consideration could be made for the addition of a percutaneous, coaxial ventricular assist device (i.e., Impella, ABIOMED Inc., Danvers, MA, USA). However, given the preexisting ECMO circuit, the addition of an arterial limb may be the more practical approach when mechanical circulatory support is warranted for concomitant cardiogenic shock, as such an approach can be done at the bedside without the need for advanced imaging [26]. In addition, such a device in the context of ARDS may generate or increase the risk of the Harlequin syndrome.

Weaning from venovenous ECMO support requires correction of the underlying gas exchange impairment to the point where native gas exchange is sufficient to meet the patient's needs for ventilation and oxygenation without excessive reliance on invasive mechanical ventilation. In general, this weaning process does not require particular consideration of the hemodynamic status of the patient. Exceptions to this rule apply when there is concern for underlying right ventricular dysfunction, with or without concomitant pulmonary hypertension. Any excess hypoxemia, hypercapnia, or elevation in airway pressures upon decannulation from ECMO (particularly when there is excess reliance on the ventilator to maintain gas exchange) may worsen underlying right ventricular failure and cause hemodynamic instability. Additionally, weaning and decannulation could lead to right ventricular failure when the decannulation strategy involves reinfusion of extracorporeal circuit blood volume back to the patient during decannulation (in an effort to conserve patient blood volume), where the extra preload could increase right ventricular loading conditions [27]. The administration of diuretics immediately prior to decannulation may help mitigate that risk.

37.4 Venoarterial ECMO

In contrast to venovenous ECMO, the monitoring and management of hemodynamic dysfunction in venoarterial ECMO is inherently more complex given that hemodynamic instability is the primary circumstance during which its use is employed. However, there are some aspects to hemodynamic monitoring that hold true in both venovenous and venoarterial ECMO, such as the potential invalidation of thermodilution techniques in the presence of extracorporeal blood flow (though pulmonary artery catheters remain commonly employed for assessment of right atrial, right ventricular, and pulmonary arterial pressures) [28]. Likewise, assessing whether end-organ perfusion and oxygen delivery are adequate, be it through lactate production or end-organ function, remains as relevant for venoarterial ECMO as it does for venovenous ECMO. Recently, there has been increasing interest in the use of sublingual microcirculation in venoarterial ECMO as a surrogate for adequate tissue perfusion and as a potential predictor of survival. In a small, single-center prospective study of patients receiving venoarterial ECMO for cardiogenic shock for various etiologies ($n = 24$), more favorable microcirculatory parameters at initiation of ECMO were associated with improved ICU survival, despite no significant difference in macrocirculatory parameters (e.g., heart rate, blood pressure, lactate, hemoglobin) [29]. Microcirculatory parameters performed better than left ventricular ejection fraction (LVEF), troponin, and lactate in predicting survival, suggesting a potential role for microcirculatory assessments as a predictor of success of venoarterial ECMO, though such a strategy requires further investigation.

Those assessments aside, there are important potential physiological consequences of venoarterial ECMO support that warrant discussion. Most frequently, and in essentially all emergent cases, venoarterial ECMO is initiated through femoral venous and arterial cannulation. Venous drainage from the intrahepatic inferior vena cava helps to decrease cardiac preload. However, reinfusion flow of oxygenated blood, in a femoral configuration, is directed retrograde in the descending aorta. In the absence of any native cardiac function, e.g., extracorporeal cardiopulmonary resuscitation during cardiac arrest [30], reinfusion flow will not mean any resistance from anterograde flow from the left ventricle, and oxygenated blood can reach the ascending aorta and carotid and coronary circulation. When there is residual native left ventricular function, the ascending aorta and great vessels may instead be supplied by blood from the native cardiac circulation, which may, in turn, be poorly oxygenated if there is impairment in native gas exchange [24]. Addition of a venous reinfusion limb may help mitigate upper-body hypoxemia by supplying well-oxygenated blood through the native cardiac circulation, which will improve the amount of oxygenated blood being ejected by the left ventricle (i.e., venoarterial venous ECMO). Alternative approaches to mitigate the differential hypoxemia associated with femoral venoarterial ECMO include upper-body configurations (e.g., internal jugular venous drainage combined with axillary, subclavian, or innominate arterial reinfusion via a graft) [31, 32], central venoarterial ECMO with drainage from the right atrium and reinfusion into the left atrium [33], and pumpless pulmonary arterial-to-left atrial arteriovenous ECMO [34], though these latter two approaches are reserved for patients with pulmonary hypertension who require venoarterial ECMO support but have preserved left ventricular function.

37

The retrograde reinfusion of blood through the aorta, particularly in femoral venoarterial ECMO but present to some degree in all peripherally cannulated venoarterial ECMO configurations, has additional implications, particularly in patients with underlying left ventricular dysfunction. Retrograde reinfusion flow increases left ventricular afterload, making it difficult for an already compromised left ventricle to eject blood, which in turn may lead to left ventricular overdistention [35]. Overdistention of the ventricle will have several potential consequences: increased wall stress and myocardial oxygen demand, impeding recovery; stagnation of blood in the ventricle, increasing risk of thrombus formation; and increased left ventricular end-diastolic pressure with resultant pulmonary edema [36, 37]. Because of these potential risks, it is important to consider the amount of venoarterial ECMO blood flow provided and what the appropriate physiological goals should be. Simultaneous assessment of both cardiac function and extra-cardiac organ function is essential. End-organ perfusion should be adequate, but not at the expense of excess left ventricular distention. There are several approaches to ensure the minimization of left ventricular overdistention. Aortic valve opening and pulse wave tissue Doppler imaging by transthoracic echocardiogram are noninvasive ways to assess whether the left ventricle is achieving at least a minimal amount of contractility and emptying. If there is inadequate left ventricular contraction, then an attempt should be made to reduce ECMO blood flow, thereby decreasing left ventricular afterload. If reduced ECMO blood flow is inadequate in achieving sufficient end-organ perfusion, necessitating blood flow rates that will lead to left ventricular overdistention, or if there are clinical sequelae of overdistention despite aortic valve opening, then other approaches for left ventricular decompression should be pursued. Such approaches include balloon atrial septostomy and mechanical left ventricular decompression, which includes intra-aortic balloon pump (IABP), Impella device placement across the aortic valve, and direct cannulation of and drainage from the left ventricle [38–43]. In a recent retrospective single-center study ($n = 259$), the addition of an IABP to venoarterial ECMO, compared to venoarterial ECMO alone, was independently associated with reduced risk of pulmonary edema and a trend toward reduced mortality [39]. The concomitant use of inotropic agents, such as dobutamine or milrinone, during venoarterial ECMO support may also aid in left ventricular ejection.

In addition to the effect of ECMO blood flow on afterload, certain clinical situations may increase the likelihood of left ventricular overdistention, further increasing the risk of pulmonary edema necessitating decompression. Early management strategies for cardiac arrest or septic shock often involve aggressive fluid resuscitation, which can be problematic when there is post-resuscitation or sepsis-associated cardiomyopathy. A recent cohort study of 195 patients receiving venoarterial ECMO found that survival was significantly associated with lower fluid balance and those above the 75th percentile of fluid balance within the cohort at 3 h post-cannulation had a sixfold increased risk of death compared to the average survival of the cohort [44].

Weaning from venoarterial ECMO, when the intention is for ECMO as bridge to recovery rather than bridge to ventricular assist device or transplantation, is notably different than with venovenous ECMO. In venoarterial ECMO, there is a need to predict adequate cardiac function post-decannulation without being able to temporarily discontinue support, as opposed to venovenous ECMO, in which one can temporarily interrupt sweep gas flow to assess native gas exchange. Proposed criteria for candidacy for weaning from venoarterial ECMO include pulsatile arterial waveform for at least 24 h, mean arterial pressure greater than 60 mmHg with no more than low-dose catecholamines, absence of major metabolic disturbance, and sufficiently preserved native gas exchange [45]. Weaning venoarterial ECMO predominantly focuses on gradually reducing extracorporeal blood flow down to a minimum of 1–1.5 L/min, with resultant increases in right ventricular preload and decreases in left ventricular afterload. Reported predictors of successful weaning from ECMO have included maintenance of mean arterial pressure greater than 60 mmHg, aortic velocity-time integral (VTI) of at least 10 cm, LVEF greater than 20–25%, and tissue Doppler lateral mitral annulus peak systolic velocity (TDSa) of at least 6 cm/s at the minimum acceptable ECMO blood flow rate (Table 37.1) [45–47]. Of note, sublingual microcirculation has also been studied as a potential predictor of successful venoarterial ECMO weaning, with a recent study showing certain microcirculation parameters to perform comparably to LVEF and VTI in predicting successful weaning [48]. Unrecognized interdependence between the right and left ventricles, which may manifest by right ventricular overdistention during ECMO weaning, may lead to recurrent cardiac failure post-decannulation. Assessment of ventricular interdependence during ECMO support may help select optimal candidates for weaning from ECMO [49]. The use of pulmonary vasodilators, such as inhaled nitric oxide, to reduce right ventricular afterload during or soon after weaning from venoarterial ECMO may help facilitate weaning success.

Table 37.1 Hemodynamic, pulmonary, and Doppler echocardiographic criteria for venoarterial ECMO weaning test

Gradually decreased ECMO flow to a minimum of 1 L/min		
Hemodynamic stability	**Pulmonary stability**	**Doppler echocardiographic criteria**
Pulsatile arterial waveform for >24 h	No desaturation when ECMO flow is decreased to 1 L/min	LVEF ≥ 20–25%
MAP >60 mmHg with no or low dose of catecholamine	No desaturation when FmO_2 is decreased to 30%	Aortic VTI ≥12 cm
No major metabolic disturbance		TDSa ≥ 6 cm/s
If all criteria are satisfied, consider ECMO removal		

Conclusion

ECMO presents unique challenges in hemodynamic monitoring and management but also offers unique opportunities to support patients with severe, refractory cardiac, and respiratory failure. Although certain traditional measures of hemodynamics are rendered inaccurate or irrelevant in patients supported with ECMO, and will vary depending on the type and amount of extracorporeal support provided, the core principle of ensuring adequate tissue perfusion remains a fundamental goal in extracorporeal support.

Take-Home Messages

- Thermodilution techniques are not efficient/suitable on ECMO.
- Hemodynamic management of patients in shock who are receiving venovenous ECMO should be managed as one would do in patients in shock who are managed without extracorporeal support.
- Retrograde reinfusion flow in venoarterial ECMO increases left ventricular afterload, making it difficult for an already compromised left ventricle to eject blood, which in turn may lead to left ventricular overdistention.
- Venoarterial ECMO weaning tests are based on hemodynamic, respiratory, and Doppler echocardiographic criteria.

37

References

1. Brodie D, Bacchetta M. Extracorporeal membrane oxygenation for ARDS in adults. N Engl J Med. 2011;365(20):1905–14.
2. Schmidt M, Tachon G, Devilliers C, Muller G, Hekimian G, Brechot N, et al. Blood oxygenation and decarboxylation determinants during venovenous ECMO for respiratory failure in adults. Intensive Care Med. 2013;39(5):838–46.
3. Abrams D, Combes A, Brodie D. Extracorporeal membrane oxygenation in cardiopulmonary disease in adults. J Am Coll Cardiol. 2014;63(25PA):2769–78.

4. Wiedemann HP, Wheeler AP, Bernard GR, Thompson BT, Hayden D, deBoisblanc B, et al. Comparison of two fluid-management strategies in acute lung injury. N Engl J Med. 2006;354(24):2564–75.
5. Schmidt M, Bailey M, Kelly J, Hodgson C, Cooper DJ, Scheinkestel C, et al. Impact of fluid balance on outcome of adult patients treated with extracorporeal membrane oxygenation. Intensive Care Med. 2014;40(9):1256–66.
6. Swan HJ, Ganz W, Forrester J, Marcus H, Diamond G, Chonette D. Catheterization of the heart in man with use of a flow-directed balloon-tipped catheter. N Engl J Med. 1970;283(9):447–51.
7. Abrams D, Bacchetta M, Brodie D. Recirculation in venovenous extracorporeal membrane oxygenation. ASAIO J. 2015;61(2):115–21.
8. Rich PB, Awad SS, Crotti S, Hirschl RB, Bartlett RH, Schreiner RJ. A prospective comparison of atrio-femoral and femoro-atrial flow in adult venovenous extracorporeal life support. J Thorac Cardiovasc Surg. 1998;116(4):628–32.
9. Burrell AJC, Pilcher DV, Pellegrino VA, Bernard SA. Retrieval of adult patients on extracorporeal membrane oxygenation by an intensive care physician model. Artif Organs. 2018;42(3):254–62.
10. Monnet X, Teboul JL. Transpulmonary thermodilution: advantages and limits. Crit Care. 2017;21(1):147.
11. Saugel B, Vincent JL. Cardiac output monitoring: how to choose the optimal method for the individual patient. Curr Opin Crit Care. 2018;24(3):165–72.
12. Reis Miranda D, van Thiel R, Brodie D, Bakker J. Right ventricular unloading after initiation of venovenous extracorporeal membrane oxygenation. Am J Respir Crit Care Med. 2015;191(3):346–8.
13. Cornish D, Clark R. Principles and practice of venovenous extracorporeal membrane oxygenation. In: Zwischenberger J, Bartlett R, editors. ECMO, extracorporeal cardiopulmonary support in critical care. Ann Arbor: ELSO1995; 1995. p. 87–107.
14. van Heijst AF, van der Staak FH, de Haan AF, Liem KD, Festen C, Geven WB, et al. Recirculation in double lumen catheter veno-venous extracorporeal membrane oxygenation measured by an ultrasound dilution technique. ASAIO J. 2001;47(4):372–6.
15. Thiagarajan RR, Barbaro RP, Rycus PT, McMullan DM, Conrad SA, Fortenberry JD, et al. Extracorporeal life support organization registry international report 2016. ASAIO J. 2017;63(1):60–7.
16. Zapol WM, Snider MT. Pulmonary hypertension in severe acute respiratory failure. N Engl J Med. 1977;296(9):476–80.
17. Vieillard-Baron A, Schmitt JM, Augarde R, Fellahi JL, Prin S, Page B, et al. Acute cor pulmonale in acute respiratory distress syndrome submitted to protective ventilation: incidence, clinical implications, and prognosis. Crit Care Med. 2001;29(8):1551–5.
18. Balanos GM, Talbot NP, Dorrington KL, Robbins PA. Human pulmonary vascular response to 4 h of hypercapnia and hypocapnia measured using Doppler echocardiography. J Appl Physiol. 2003;94(4):1543–51.
19. Javidfar J, Brodie D, Sonett J, Bacchetta M. Venovenous extracorporeal membrane oxygenation using a single cannula in patients with pulmonary hypertension and atrial septal defects. J Thorac Cardiovasc Surg. 2012;143(4):982–4.
20. Abrams DC, Brodie D, Rosenzweig EB, Burkart KM, Agerstrand CL, Bacchetta MD. Upper-body extracorporeal membrane oxygenation as a strategy in decompensated pulmonary arterial hypertension. Pulm Circ. 2013;3(2):432–5.
21. Rosenzweig EB, Brodie D, Abrams DC, Agerstrand CL, Bacchetta M. Extracorporeal membrane oxygenation as a novel bridging strategy for acute right heart failure in group 1 pulmonary arterial hypertension. ASAIO J. 2014;60(1):129–33.
22. Hoopes CW, Gurley JC, Zwischenberger JB, Diaz-Guzman E. Mechanical support for pulmonary veno-occlusive disease: combined atrial septostomy and venovenous extracorporeal membrane oxygenation. Semin Thorac Cardiovasc Surg. 2012;24(3):232–4.
23. Camboni D, Akay B, Sassalos P, Toomasian JM, Haft JW, Bartlett RH, et al. Use of venovenous extracorporeal membrane oxygenation and an atrial septostomy for pulmonary and right ventricular failure. Ann Thorac Surg. 2011;91(1):144–9.
24. Biscotti M, Lee A, Basner RC, Agerstrand C, Abrams D, Brodie D, et al. Hybrid configurations via percutaneous access for extracorporeal membrane oxygenation: a single center experience. ASAIO J. 2014;60(6):635–42.
25. Brechot N, Luyt CE, Schmidt M, Leprince P, Trouillet JL, Leger P, et al. Venoarterial extracorporeal membrane oxygenation support for refractory cardiovascular dysfunction during severe bacterial septic shock. Crit Care Med. 2013;41(7):1616–26.

26. Pieri M, Contri R, Winterton D, Montorfano M, Colombo A, Zangrillo A, et al. The contemporary role of Impella in a comprehensive mechanical circulatory support program: a single institutional experience. BMC Cardiovasc Disord. 2015;15:126.
27. Agerstrand CL, Burkart KM, Abrams DC, Bacchetta MD, Brodie D. Blood conservation in extracorporeal membrane oxygenation for acute respiratory distress syndrome. Ann Thorac Surg. 2015;99(2):590–5.
28. Doufle G, Ferguson ND. Monitoring during extracorporeal membrane oxygenation. Curr Opin Crit Care. 2016;22(3):230–8.
29. Kara A, Akin S, Dos Reis Miranda D, Struijs A, Caliskan K, van Thiel RJ, et al. Microcirculatory assessment of patients under VA-ECMO. Crit Care. 2016;20(1):344.
30. Pineton de Chambrun M, Brechot N, Lebreton G, Schmidt M, Hekimian G, Demondion P, et al. Venoarterial extracorporeal membrane oxygenation for refractory cardiogenic shock post-cardiac arrest. Intensive Care Med. 2016;42(12):1999–2007.
31. Biscotti M, Bacchetta M. The "sport model": extracorporeal membrane oxygenation using the subclavian artery. Ann Thorac Surg. 2014;98(4):1487–9.
32. Chicotka S, Rosenzweig EB, Brodie D, Bacchetta M. The "central sport model" extracorporeal membrane oxygenation using the innominate artery for smaller patients as bridge to lung transplantation. ASAIO J. 2017;63(4):e39–44.
33. Haushofer M, Abusabha Y, Amerini AL, Spillner J, Nix C, Autschbach R, et al. Oxygenated shunting from right to left: a feasibility study of minimized atrio-atrial extracorporeal membrane oxygenation for mid-term lung assistance in an acute ovine model. Interact Cardiovasc Thorac Surg. 2013;17(1):44–8.
34. de Perrot M, Granton JT, McRae K, Cypel M, Pierre A, Waddell TK, et al. Impact of extracorporeal life support on outcome in patients with idiopathic pulmonary arterial hypertension awaiting lung transplantation. J Heart Lung Transplant. 2011;30(9):997–1002.
35. Cheng R, Hachamovitch R, Kittleson M, Patel J, Arabia F, Moriguchi J, et al. Complications of extracorporeal membrane oxygenation for treatment of cardiogenic shock and cardiac arrest: a meta-analysis of 1,866 adult patients. Ann Thorac Surg. 2014;97(2):610–6.
36. Makdisi G, Hashmi ZA, Wozniak TC, Wang IW. Left ventricular thrombus associated with arteriovenous extra corporeal membrane oxygenation. J Thorac Dis. 2015;7(11):E552–4.
37. Soleimani B, Pae WE. Management of left ventricular distension during peripheral extracorporeal membrane oxygenation for cardiogenic shock. Perfusion. 2012;27(4):326–31.
38. Seib PM, Faulkner SC, Erickson CC, Van Devanter SH, Harrell JE, Fasules JW, et al. Blade and balloon atrial septostomy for left heart decompression in patients with severe ventricular dysfunction on extracorporeal membrane oxygenation. Catheter Cardiovasc Interv. 1999;46(2):179–86.
39. Brechot N, Demondion P, Santi F, Lebreton G, Pham T, Dalakidis A, et al. Intra-aortic balloon pump protects against hydrostatic pulmonary oedema during peripheral venoarterial-extracorporeal membrane oxygenation. Eur Heart J Acute Cardiovasc Care. 2018;7(1):62–9.
40. Koeckert MS, Jorde UP, Naka Y, Moses JW, Takayama H. Impella LP 2.5 for left ventricular unloading during venoarterial extracorporeal membrane oxygenation support. J Card Surg. 2011;26(6):666–8.
41. Cheng A, Swartz MF, Massey HT. Impella to unload the left ventricle during peripheral extracorporeal membrane oxygenation. ASAIO J. 2013;59(5):533–6.
42. Takeda K, Garan AR, Ando M, Han J, Topkara VK, Kurlansky P, et al. Minimally invasive CentriMag ventricular assist device support integrated with extracorporeal membrane oxygenation in cardiogenic shock patients: a comparison with conventional CentriMag biventricular support configuration. Eur J Cardiothorac Surg. 2017;52(6):1055–61.
43. Takeda K, Garan AR, Topkara VK, Kirtane AJ, Karmpaliotis D, Kurlansky P, et al. Novel minimally invasive surgical approach using an external ventricular assist device and extracorporeal membrane oxygenation in refractory cardiogenic shock. Eur J Cardiothorac Surg. 2017;51(3):591–6.
44. Staudacher DL, Gold W, Biever PM, Bode C, Wengenmayer T. Early fluid resuscitation and volume therapy in venoarterial extracorporeal membrane oxygenation. J Crit Care. 2017;37:130–5.
45. Aissaoui N, El-Banayosy A, Combes A. How to wean a patient from veno-arterial extracorporeal membrane oxygenation. Intensive Care Med. 2015;41(5):902–5.
46. Aissaoui N, Luyt CE, Leprince P, Trouillet JL, Leger P, Pavie A, et al. Predictors of successful extracorporeal membrane oxygenation (ECMO) weaning after assistance for refractory cardiogenic shock. Intensive Care Med. 2011;37(11):1738–45.

47. Aissaoui N, Guerot E, Combes A, Delouche A, Chastre J, Leprince P, et al. Two-dimensional strain rate and Doppler tissue myocardial velocities: analysis by echocardiography of hemodynamic and functional changes of the failed left ventricle during different degrees of extracorporeal life support. J Am Soc Echocardiogr. 2012;25(6):632–40.
48. Akin S, Dos Reis Miranda D, Caliskan K, Soliman OI, Guven G, Struijs A, et al. Functional evaluation of sublingual microcirculation indicates successful weaning from VA-ECMO in cardiogenic shock. Crit Care. 2017;21(1):265.
49. Aissaoui N, Caudron J, Leprince P, Fagon JY, Lebreton G, Combes A, et al. Right-left ventricular interdependence: a promising predictor of successful extracorporeal membrane oxygenation (ECMO) weaning after assistance for refractory cardiogenic shock. Intensive Care Med. 2017;43(4):592–4.

The manufacturer's authorised representative in the EU is Springer Nature Customer Service Centre GmbH, Europaplatz 3, 69115 Heidelberg, Germany. If you have any concerns regarding our products, please contact ProductSafety@springernature.com

Printed and bound by CPI Group (UK) Ltd, Croydon, CR0 4YY
09/04/2026
02086910-0006